Proceedings in Life Sciences

Lesion-Induced Neuronal Plasticity in Sensorimotor Systems

Edited by
H. Flohr and W. Precht

With 168 Figures

Springer-Verlag
Berlin Heidelberg New York 1981

Professor Dr. HANS FLOHR
Universität Bremen
Bibliothekstraße
2800 Bremen 33, FRG

Professor Dr. WOLFGANG PRECHT
Institut für Hirnforschung der Universität Zürich
August-Forel-Straße 1
8029 Zürich, Switzerland

The cover illustration shows the pattern of regional deoxyglucose uptake in the frog's brain stem following unilateral labyrinthectomy. It was obtained by microdensitometric analysis of the autoradiograph d in Fig. 2 on p. 156.

ISBN 3-540-10747-9 Springer-Verlag Berlin Heidelberg New York
ISBN 0-387-10747-9 Springer-Verlag New York Heidelberg Berlin

Library of Congress Cataloging in Publication Data. Main entry under title: Lesion-induced neuronal plasticity in sensorimotor systems. (Proceedings in life sciences) Bibliography: p. Includes index. 1. Developmental neurology. 2. Neural circuitry – Adaptation. 3. Sensory-motor integration. 4. Nervous system – Regeneration. I. Flohr, H. (Hans), 1936–. II. Precht, W., 1938–. III. Series. QP363.5.L47 599.01'88 81–9074 AACR2.

Offsetprinting and bookbinding: Brühlsche Universitätsdruckerei, Gießen.
2131/3130-543210

Preface

Sensorimotor systems are not rigidly wired predetermined networks but rather highly plastic structures that learn and modify their entire performance in response to changes in external or internal conditions. Lesions or distortions of the system's input, which initially cause a functional disorganization, induce an active reorganization which often leads to a recovery of function.

Examples of lesion-induced neural plasticity have been known for some hundred years; however, an awareness of their value as research tools is relatively new. This current interest is a consequence of rapidly changing ideas concerning the nature of CNS organization. Out of these, concepts are emerging which describe neural nets as modifiable, highly dynamic, self-organizing structures.

This trend is clearly reflected in this volume, which contains the proceedings of a symposium held in Bremen in July 1980 as a satellite meeting of the XXVIIIth International Congress of Physiological Sciences. The first part of this conference was devoted to some general aspects of plasticity, discussing the current theories of functional recovery as well as morphological, neurochemical, physiological, molecular, and ontogenetic aspects. The second part dealt with lesion-induced plasticity in specific sensorimotor systems of the spinal cord, brain stem, and cerebral cortex.

The meeting was organized with the financial assistance of the University of Bremen, for which both the editors and the participants are grateful. We are also indebted to the staff of the Neurobiology Unit of the University of Bremen for its valuable support in organizing the symposium. We particularly want to thank Ms Helga Kortmann for her highly skilled and tireless efforts in organizing the conference and in preparing this volume. The support of the Springer-Verlag in preparing this publication is very much appreciated.

Bremen/Zürich, May 1981

H. Flohr
W. Precht

Contents

I. General Aspects of Lesion-Induced Neuronal Plasticity

II. Sensorimotor Subsystems: Experimental Models and Techniques
a. Recovery from Spinal Lesions

IIb. Recovery from Vestibular Lesions

IId. Plasticity in the Visual and Olfactory System

Contributors

You will find the addresses at the beginning of the respective contribution

I. General Aspects of Lesion-Induced Neuronal Plasticity

The Significance of Neuronal Cell Death During the Development of the Nervous System

G. RAGER[1]

1 Introduction

It would seem to be a paradox that death of neurons should play a significant role during ontogenesis. Therefore it is understandable that it took a long time for this phenomenon to be generally accepted. Cell death was reported at the beginning of this century by Collin (1906) and by Mühlmann (for references see Ernst 1926). In 1926 Ernst, stimulated by Kallius, published an extensive study on cell death in vertebrates during normal development, after he had carefully investigated no less than 1000 serially sectioned specimens from 32 species. He found that cell death was such a common and widespread phenomenon that it needed systematic investigation to be understood. Although Ernst speculated about endogenous and exogenous factors which might cause embryonic cell death, these factors were not generally accepted. Kallius (1931) emphasized another viewpoint. Instead of looking for mechanisms leading to cell death, he analyzed cell death as a mechanism involved in morpho-, histio- and phylogenesis. Twenty years later, Glücksmann (1951), a former student of Kallius, continued with his teacher's ideas and classified cell degenerations according to their developmental functions. He distinguished morphogenetic, histiogenetic and phylogenetic degenerations. Morphogenetic degenerations were thought to precede or accompany changes in the form of organs; histiogenetic degenerations occur during differentiation of tissues; phylogenetic degenerations are related to vestigial organs and to the regression of larval structures. These distinctions are, however, merely descriptive and do not reveal any developmental mechanisms leading to cell death. Our interest is now to further the ideas of Ernst and search for mechanisms leading to neuronal cell death.

2 Degeneration of Neuroepithelial Cells

In the nervous system two types of cell death can be distinguished: death of undifferentiated neuroepithelial cells and death of young neurons. The mechanisms involved

---

1 Max-Planck-Institut für biophysikalische Chemie, Am Faßberg, 3400 Göttingen-Nikolausberg, FRG

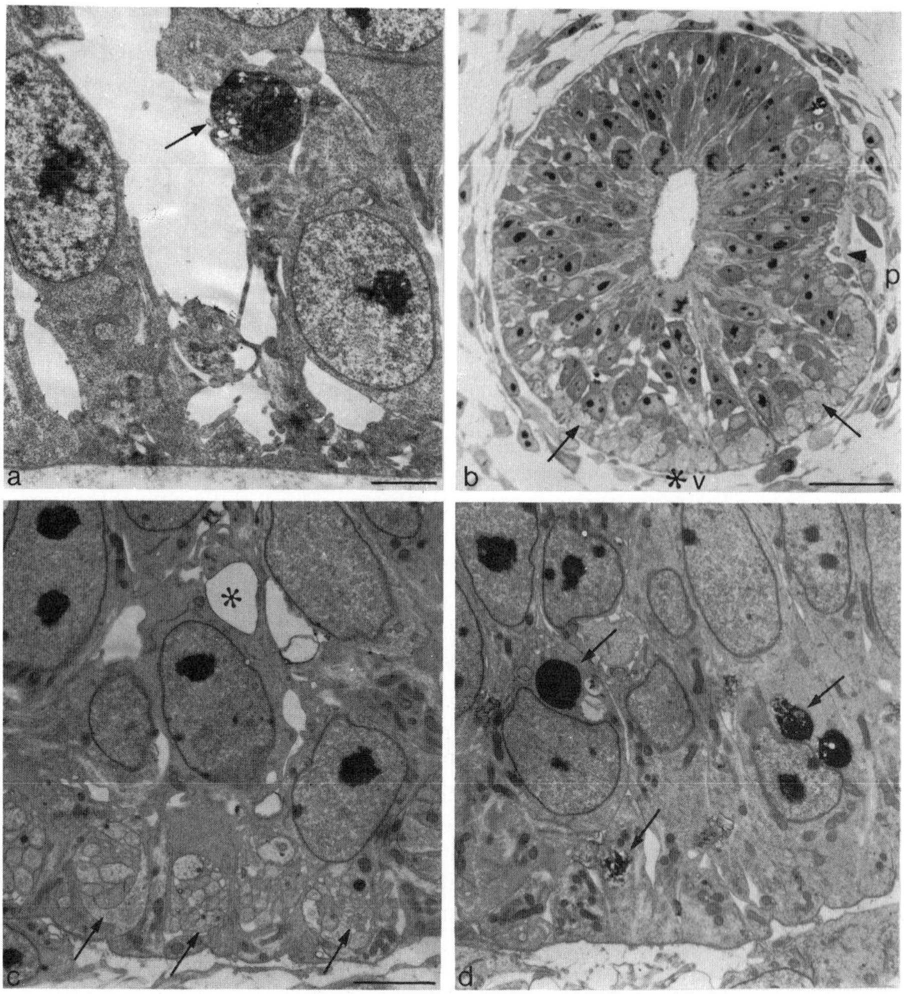

Fig. 1. a Central retina of a chick embryo at embryonic day 3 (E3, HH 20). Large intercellular spaces and intracellular inclusions containing cellular debris (*arrow*) can be seen here. Bar 2 μm. **b** Semithin cross section of the optic stalk at E4 (HH 23). The central (*v*) and ventro-posterior (*p*) rim is occupied by bundles of ganglion cell axons (*arrows*). Wide intercellular spaces lie dorsal to this crescent of fiber bundles. The *asterisk* and the *arrowhead* on the pial border of this section indicate the sites of the electron micrographs shown in **c** and **d**, respectively. Bar 20 μm. **c** Fiber bundles of the ventral crescent (*arrows*) and intercellular spaces (*asterisk*) are shown with the electron microscope. This ultrathin section is cut from the same block as the semithin section shown in **b**. Bar 4 μm. **d** Regions just dorsal to the areas invaded by retinal fibers have normal intercellular spaces but also show a number of degenerating profiles (*arrows*) many of which are already phagocytosed. Same magnification as in **c**

in degeneration of neuroepithelial cells are still far from being understood, but the importance of this type of cell death for the maturation of the nervous system is now beginning to be recognized. The death of these cells could, for example, be related to the formation of topographic projections. We found that debris of degenerating cells appear together with wide intercellular spaces first in the posterior part of the chick retina where first ganglion cells are generated, and begin to settle near the vitreal surface of the retina and to form an axon (Fig. 1a). The retinal periphery, however, does not show any holes or degenerating profiles at this stage. Similarly, we observed holes and degenerating cells in the ventral part of the optic stalk just before the first retinal fibers arrive, whereas in the neighboring regions neuroepithelial cells seem to be closely apposed to each other (Fig. 1b–d). This pattern shifts with time and distance from the retina. The arriving fibers fill the holes in the ventral half of the optic stalk gradually. Degenerating cells can be found more and more dorsally (Rager 1980). Thus degeneration of neuroepithelial cells and the formation of intercellular spaces seem always to precede the ingrowth of fibers. It turned out that these intercellular channels form long tunnels which are oriented in the direction of the stalk (Silver and Sidman 1980). These tunnels may constitute preformed pathways to guide growing axons (Silver 1978; Silver and Robb 1979) and thus contribute to the maintenance of order in the fiber pathway.

3 Degeneration of Competent Neurons

3.1 The Size of the Target

We shall now focus exclusively on the second type of degeneration which occurs in competent young neurons. I define a young neuron as competent when its perikaryon has reached a certain level of maturation of its metabolism reflected in the elaboration of the rough endoplasmic reticulum (RER) and when its axon has arrived at the target area and is able to interact with other neurons.

There is much evidence which implicates the size of the peripheral field as a important influence on the degeneration of young neurons. This was first suggested by Hamburger and Levi-Montalcini (1949) who found large-scale degeneration in cervical and thoracic spinal ganglia, whereas in limb innervating ganglia no such degeneration occurred. Limb extirpation also resulted in massive degeneration of limb ganglia. This observation led to the conclusion that "the periphery provides for conditions necessary for continued growth and maintenance of neurons in stages following the first outgrowth of neurites" (l.c. p. 498). Later on, Hamburger (1958) studied the development of the motor column in the spinal cord and the effects of radical extirpations of leg and wing primordia. Some neuronal degeneration normally takes place also in the brachial and lumbo-sacral segments. After limb bud extirpation, increased cell degeneration nearly eliminates the normal population of the lateral motor column. The process of degeneration reaches its maximum at approximately the same time as in the normally occurring cell death. Hamburger concluded that the size of the motor column which ultimately reflects the number of motor neurons is adjusted to the size of the peripheral field by cell death. Similar evidence was obtained in the Nucleus trochlearis (Cowan and Wenger 1967) and in the Nucleus isthmo-opticus (Cowan and Wenger 1968; Clarke et al. 1976) where 50%–30% of neurons degenerate normally. The relation between the size of the periphery or target area, the onset of innervation, and the cell loss has also been established in several other systems (Piatt 1946; Prestige

1967a, b; Landmesser and Pilar 1974a, b; Hughes and LaVelle 1975; Landmesser 1976; Landmesser and Pilar 1976; Chu-Wang and Oppenheim 1978a, b).

The importance of the size of the innervation area has then been positively demonstrated by experimental enlargement of the periphery. Shieh (1951) was able to prevent the normally occurring degeneration of some neurons in the ventro-lateral column of the cervical spinal cord by transplanting these segments in the place of thoracic segments. Here the cells could find additional postsynaptic targets. Hollyday and Hamburger (1976) transplanted a supernumerary leg into a chick embryo. Subsequently the death of motoneurons was considerably reduced compared with the control side (cf. also Lamb 1979b). These results suggest not only a target size-cell death relationship but also a new interpretation of the morphogenesis of the spinal cord; the cervical and lumbar enlargements do not develop primarily because of a hyperplasia but of a "hypothanasia" of motor neurons which have an enlarged innervation space in the extremities.

3.2 Ultrastructural Changes During Degeneration

It has been asked whether there is any difference between normal and experimentally induced cell death. Therefore, the ultrastructural changes during cell degeneration have been carefully described in the last few years. Pilar and Landmesser (1976) (in the ciliary ganglion) and Chu-Wang and Oppenheim (1978a) (in spinal motoneurons) found essentially two types of degeneration.

Type I degeneration is characterized in its initial phase by the increase in density of the nuclear chromatin. Cytoplasmic changes begin with the dissociation of polyribosomes, detachment of ribosomes from the RER, fragmentation of the Golgi apparatus and swelling of mitochondria. The whole cell becomes progressively darker or electron dense. In the intermediate phase of degeneration the cytoplasm shrinks and increases further in electron density. The nuclear chromatin condenses to homogeneous masses, the fibrillar and the coarse granular components of the nucleolus become separated. In the late phase of degeneration the nuclear membrane breaks down, nucleoplasm and cytoplasm become mixed and finally only amorphous clumps of debris remain.

Type II degeneration begins with the dilatation of the cisternae of RER, Golgi apparatus, and the nuclear envelope, while the polyribosomes remain intact for a while. Nuclear changes appear only in a late phase of degeneration. In both types the cellular debris are finally phagocytosed mainly by glial cells, but also by mononuclear leukocytes which can transform into tissue macrophages.

Pilar and Landmesser (1976) provided some evidence that Type I degeneration occurs in peripherally deprived neurons; the dissociation of polyribosomes and the early nuclear changes would indicate that protein synthesis is stopped in these neurons. Type II degeneration is suggested to be characteristic of normally occurring cell death; all neurons dying without surgical interference developed a well-organized RER at the same time when peripheral synapses are formed; it has, therefore, been suggested that transmission-related proteins will accumulate if peripheral synapses cannot be formed or maintained; this accumulation could lead to cisternal dilatation and eventual cell death. Although this interpretation is not generally accepted (Chu-Wang and Oppenheim 1978a), it could provide a basis to search for mechanisms involved in degeneration of neurons.

4 Competition and Neuronal Cell Death

4.1 The Competition Hypothesis

The time when axons of certain projecting cells arrive at their target area and begin to form synaptic contacts marks a critical period in neuron development. At that time neurons become competent and will either continue to mature in their cytoplasmic structure (Landmesser and Pilar 1974a), or expand their axonal arbor; their axons increase in diameter as a function of this terminal arborization (Rager 1976a, b; Rager and von Oeynhausen 1979).

As we have seen, neuronal cell death seems to be related to the size of the innervation space. Since the essential features of the innervating competent cells are axonal arborization and synapse formation, we may formulate the hypothesis that these cells compete for an adequate termination space which may be equivalent to a minimum number of synaptic contacts. Only those cells which are able to establish a minimum number of synaptic contacts will survive. The concept of competition was already used by Ramón y Cajal (1929) and is discussed more recently by several other authors (e.g., Prestige 1970; Cowan 1973; Hamburger 1975; Prestige and Willshaw 1975; Jacobson 1978).

4.2 Testing the Competition Hypothesis in the Retino-Tectal System of the Chick

Neuronal cell death has been investigated mainly in motor systems. In order to test the generality of the competition hypothesis, we have tested it in a sensory system, namely the retino-tectal system of the chick. One advantage of this system is that here we know precisely when axons originating in certain retinal regions arrive at certain tectal sites and begin to arborize and to form synaptic contacts (Crossland et al. 1975; Rager and von Oeynhausen 1979; McGraw and McLaughlin 1980; Rager 1980). A first step in this analysis would be to determine the number of retinal ganglion cells present at various times during development. Unfortunately, there are a number of problems in obtaining a direct count of neurons. Firstly, much of the apparent disappearance of neurons is due to the fact that at the earliest stages glial cells can be misidentified as neurons (Cowan 1973). Secondly, since cell counts are usually performed by counting nucleoli, whose number per nerve cell changes with developmental age, correction factors have to be introduced which are an additional source of errors. Thirdly, since quite a number of displaced amacrine cells are located in the ganglion cell layer (Ramón y Cajal 1911; Binggeli and Paule 1969; Ehrlich and Morgan 1980), it would be extremely difficult to evaluate the percentage of ganglion cells at the various stages of development. To avoid these problems, we determined the total number of fibers in the optic nerve where these fibers do not form collaterals so that a one-to-one correspondence between ganglion cell perikarya and their axons is given. We counted optic nerve fibers from embryonic day 5 until 100 days after hatching (Rager 1978; Rager and Rager 1978) and found that the total number of fibers increases nearly exponentially until E8 reaching a maximum value of 4 million fibers on E10 and E11. Thereafter the total number decreases rapidly and reaches a final value of about 2.4 million by E18. This is a reduction of about 40% from the maximum.

There is a possibility that the reduction in the number of axons is not congruent with the reduction in the number of ganglion cell perikarya; these ganglion cells could have been transformed into anaxonic or amacrine cells (Hinds and Hinds 1978). Therefore, we examined the ganglion cell layer of the retina with the electron microscope. We found degenerating cells from E8 to E18 (Rager and Rager 1978; Hughes and McLoon 1979). Thus we conclude that at least some of the degenerating axons have their counterpart in degenerating ganglion cell perikarya.

In the next step we localized the degenerating cells with a light microscope. In the early phase (E9) a considerable number of dying cells can be found around the papilla with special emphasis on the centro-temporal retina. This is 1 day after the first retinal axons have begun to invade the central tectal area and to form branches (Rager and von Oeynhausen 1979). At that time axo-dendritic contacts can first be detected (McGraw and McLaughlin 1980; Rager 1980). Three days later (E12), when degeneration has attained its highest rate, dying cells are distributed over the whole retina with a lower density in the central area. On E15, when degeneration begins to wane, they are present mainly in more peripheral zones. A few days later synapse formation is established over the whole tectal surface (Crossland et al. 1975).

These results can be summarized as follows: (1) Degeneration of neurons does not occur before fibers invade the optic tectum, form terminal arbors, and start to make synaptic contacts. (2) The topography of dying ganglion cells closely resembles the topography of tectal innervation. (3) Degeneration of ganglion cells is heaviest in the central and the centro-temporal portions of the retina. The axons of these cells, which arrive first, encounter a more unfavorable situation than the peripheral ones arriving later which corresponds well to the mode of maturation of the optic tectum.

From these results we draw the following conclusions: (1) The degeneration of ganglion cells does not seem to be preprogramed, but to depend on a large extent on the direct interaction with their target neurons in the optic tectum. (2) Axons compete for their subsistence minimum, namely a minimum number of synaptic contacts. Based on this formulation of the competition hypothesis, a mathematical model was developed which fits the measured values with a high coefficient of determination (Rager 1978), indicating that the competition hypothesis is sufficient to interprete the phenomena not only on a qualitative, but also on a quantitative level.

4.3 Additional Factors Contributing to Cell Death

Recently, the hypothesis of competition for peripheral targets was seriously attacked (Lamb 1979a, 1980). Experiments with developing limb motoneurons in Xenopus suggested "that the contact must be made with regions of the limb for which the motoneurons have been specified" (Lamb 1980, p. 349). If motoneurons die because of wrong connections, the errors lie probably in the relation between the choice of the target muscle and the set of central inputs to the motoneuron (Lewis 1980). This assumption may be useful for the spinal motor system and indicate that a number of different factors may contribute to neuronal cell death, but it does not rule out the competition hypothesis. In addition, it does not seem to apply to the retino-tectal system of the chick, because most of the degeneration process is completed before ganglion cell dendrites receive synaptic contacts (Rager 1980), and because no signs of spontaneous activity in ganglion cells could be detected before light signals can be transmitted in the retina which is on E18 (Rager 1979); this indicates that degeneration of retinal ganglion cells may be independent of any special input and activity pattern of these cells. Thus, the competition hypothesis still remains as a reasonable explanation for the events in the retino-tectal system, although it is perhaps not the only possible one for all examples of neuronal cell death occurring during ontogenesis.

5 Molecular Aspects of Competition

The competition hypothesis may have an explanatory value on the cellular level, but our interest now is to understand its molecular basis. Changeux and Danchin (1976) presented a model to explain the phenomenon that certain fibers are able to establish and stabilize synaptic contacts while others fail to do so. This model is called the selective stabilization hypothesis. It is assumed that labile receptor molecules are distributed over the cell membrane at early stages of development. When nerve terminals arrive, an anterograde factor, probably the neurotransmitter, is liberated during activity of the nerve terminal. In cooperation with an internal coupling factor the receptor molecules in the postsynaptic membrane are converted into their stable form, while the synthesis of the labile extrasynaptic receptors is stopped with the onset of electric activity. At the same time a retrograde factor is liberated which might be able to stabilize the nerve terminal. We could imagine that this factor also serves as a molecular signal necessary for the maturation of the metabolism in the projecting cell.

Several experiments have been carried out to investigate the role of receptor molecules for the stabilization of synapses and consequently for neuronal cell death by blocking nicotinic postsynaptic receptors with α-neurotoxins and d-tubucurare (Giacobini et al. 1973; Oppenheim et al. 1978; Pittman and Oppenheim 1978; Creazzo and Sohal 1979; Betz et al. 1980). The results, however, were not unambiguous. In addition, it turned out that the stabilization process is probably more complicated and puzzling than assumed initially. For example, the transformation of receptor molecules from a labile to a stable state occurs much earlier than the transformation of electric gating properties from immature to mature forms (Michler and Sakmann 1980). This indicates that there are perhaps several different properties of receptor molecules which develop at different developmental periods and, therefore, not all of them are directly linked to the stabilization of synapses. Thus, although a promising progress has been made in elucidating the molecular mechanisms of competition or selective stabilization, a completely satisfactory answer has not yet been obtained.

6 The Significance of Neuronal Cell Death

Degeneration of neurons during ontogenesis has been found in so many places that it could be a nearly universal phenomenon in the developing nervous system of vertebrates. This implies that in many places many more cells are produced than needed for constructing the complex neuronal network. A consequence of this overproduction is that the sizes of projecting and receiving systems do not match initially; the matching is subsequently brought about by degeneration. Thus, the complex structure of the nervous system is probably not determined in the genes with respect to the fate of every single cell, but rather is a consequence of the interaction of its elements. The generation, maturation, and degeneration of cells, the mechanism of axonal growth towards their targets (Rager 1980), and the interaction of cells at synaptic sites seem not to be strictly determined, but to follow probabilistic rules. The development as well as the maintenance of the nervous system of vertebrates result more from a balance of forces than from a rigid plan. Thus, plasticity is an intrinsic or essential property of such a system. If one element of the balanced system is impaired or destroyed, the remaining elements rearrange themselves and achieve a new equilibrium. This occurs not only after surgical manipulations but also during the normal course of development (e.g., Knyihar et al. 1978). Thus, death of neurons during ontogenesis is not a paradox; it is instead a significant and necessary part of normal ontogenesis.

References

Betz H, Bourgeois J-P, Changeux J-P (1980) Evolution of cholinergic proteins in developing slow and fast skeletal muscles in chick embryo. J Physiol 302: 197–218

Binggeli RL, Paule WJ (1969) The pigeon retina: quantitative aspects of the optic nerve and ganglion cell layer. J Comp Neurol 137: 1–18

Changeux J-P, Danchin A (1976) Selective stabilisation of developing synapses as a mechanism for the specification of neuronal networks. Nature (London) 264: 705–712

Chu-Wang IW, Oppenheim RW (1978a) Cell death of motoneurones in the chick embryo spinal cord. I. A light and electron microscopic study of naturally occurring and induced cell loss during development. J Comp Neurol 177: 33–58

Chu-Wang IW, Oppenheim RW (1978b) Cell death of motoneurones in the chick spinal cord. II. A quantitative and qualitative analysis of degeneration in the ventral root, including evidence for axon outgrowth and limb innervation prior to cell death. J Comp Neurol 177: 59–86

Clarke PGH, Rogers LA, Cowan WM (1976) The time of origin and the pattern of survival of neurons in the isthmo-optic nucleus of the chick. J Comp Neurol 167: 125–142

Collin R (1906) Recherches cytologiques sur le dévelopment de la cellule nerveuse. Névrae 8: 181–308

Cowan WM (1973) Neuronal death as a regulative mechanism in the control of cell number in the nervous system. In: Rockstein M (ed) Development and aging in the nervous system. Academic Press, London New York, pp 19–41

Cowan WM, Wenger E (1967) Cell loss in the trochlear nucleus of the chick during normal development and after radical extirpation of the optic vesicle. J Exp Zool 164: 267–280

Cowan WM, Wenger E (1968) Degeneration in the nucleus of origin of the preganglionic fibers to the chick ciliary ganglion following early removal of the optic vesicle. J Exp Zool 168: 105–123

Creazzo TL, Sohal GS (1979) Effects of chronic injections of α-bungarotoxin on embryonic cell death. Exp Neurol 66: 135–145
Crossland WJ, Cowan WM, Rogers LA (1975) Studies on the development of the chick optic tectum. IV. An autoradiographic study of the development of retino-tectal connections. Brain Res 91: 1–23
Ehrlich D, Morgan IG (1980) Kainic acid destroys displaced amacrine cells in post-hatch chicken retina. Neurosci Lett 17: 43–48
Ernst M (1926) Über Untergang von Zellen während der normalen Entwicklung bei Wirbeltieren. Z Anat Entwicklungsgesch 79: 228–262
Giacobini G, Filogamo G, Weber M, Boquet P, Changeux JP (1973) Effects of a snake α-neurotoxin on the development of innervated skeletal muscles in chick embryo. Proc Natl Acad Sci USA 70: 1708–1712
Glücksmann A (1951) Cell deaths in normal vertebrate ontogeny. Biol Rev 26: 59–86
Hamburger V (1958) Regression versus peripheral control of differentiation in motor hypoplasia. Am J Anat 102: 365–409
Hamburger V (1975) Cell death in the development of the lateral motor column of the chick embryo. J Comp Neurol 160: 535–546
Hamburger V, Levi-Montalcini R (1949) Proliferation, differentiation and degeneration in the spinal ganglia of the chick embryo under normal and experimental conditions. J Exp Zool 111: 457–501
Hinds JW, Hinds PL (1978) Early development of amacrine cells in the mouse retina: an electron microscopic, serial section analysis. J Comp Neurol 179: 277–300
Hollyday M, Hamburger V (1976) Reduction of the naturally occurring motor neuron loss by enlargement of the periphery. J Comp Neurol 170: 311–320
Hughes WF, LaVelle A (1975) The effects of early tectal lesions on development in the retinal ganglion cell layer of chick embryos. J Comp Neurol 163: 265–284
Hughes WF, McLoon SC (1979) Ganglion cell death during normal retinal development in the chick: Comparisons with cell death induced by early target field destruction. Exp Neurol 66: 587–601
Jacobson M (1978) Developmental neurobiology. Plenum, New York
Kallius E (1931) Der Zelluntergang als Mechanismus bei der Histio- und Morphogenese. Verh Anat Ges Suppl Anat Anz 72: 10–22
Knyihar E, Csillik B, Rakic P (1978) Transient synapses in the embryonic primate spinal cord. Science 202: 1206–1209
Lamb AH (1979a) Evidence that some developing limb motoneurones die for reasons other than peripheral competition. Dev Biol 71: 8–21
Lamb AH (1979b) Ventral horn cell counts in a Xenopus with naturally occurring supernumerary hind limbs. J Embryol Exp Morphol 49: 13–16
Lamb AH (1980) Motoneurone counts in Xenopus frogs reared with one bilaterally-innervated hindlimb. Nature (London) 284: 347–350
Landmesser LT (1976) The role of the periphery in cell death. Neurosci Res Prog Bull 14: 295–301
Landmesser L, Pilar G (1974a) Synapse formation during embryogenesis on ganglion cells lacking a periphery. J Physiol (London) 241: 751–736
Landmesser L, Pilar G (1974b) Synaptic transmission and cell death during normal ganglionic development. J Physiol (London) 241: 737–749
Landmesser L, Pilar G (1976) Fate of ganglionic synapses and ganglion cell axons during normal and induced cell death. J Cell Biol 68: 357–374
Lewis J (1980) Death and the neurone. Nature (London) 284: 305–306
McGraw CF, McLaughlin BJ (1980) Fine structural studies of synaptogenesis in the superficial layers of the chick optic tectum. J Neurocytol 9: 79–93
Michler A, Sakmann B (1980) Receptor stability and channel conversion in the subsynaptic membrane of the developing mammalian neuromuscular junction. Dev Biol in press
Oppenheim RW, Pittman R, Gray M, Maderdrut JL (1978) Embryonic behaviour, hatching and neuromuscular development in the chick following a transient reduction of spontaneous motility and sensory input by neuromuscular blocking agents. J Comp Neurol 179: 619–640

Piatt J (1946) The influence of the peripheral field on the development of the mesencephalic V nucleus in Amblystoma. J Exp Zool 102: 109–141

Pilar G, Landmesser L (1976) Ultrastructural differences during embryonic cell death in normal and peripherally deprived ciliary ganglia. J Cell Biol 68: 339–356

Pittman RH, Oppenheim RW (1978) Neuromuscular blockade increases motoneurone survival during normal cell death in the chick embryo. Nature (London) 271: 364–366

Prestige MC (1967a) The control of cell number in the lumbar spinal ganglia during the development of Xenopus laevis tadpoles. J Embryol Exp Morphol 17: 453–471

Prestige MD (1967b) The control of cell number in the lumbar ventral horns during the development of Xenopus laevis tadpoles. J Embryol Exp Morphol 18: 359–387

Prestige MC (1970) Differentiation, degeneration, and the role of the periphery: Quantitative considerations. In: Schmitt FO (ed) The neurosciences: Second Study Programme. Rockefeller Univ Press, New York, pp 73–82

Prestige MC, Willshaw DJ (1975) On a role for competition in the formation of patterned neural connexions. Proc R Soc London Ser B 190: 77–98

Rager G (1976a) Morphogenesis and physiogenesis of the retino-tectal connection in the chicken. I. The retinal ganglion cells and their axons. Proc R Soc London Ser B 192: 331–352

Rager G (1976b) Morphogenesis and physiogenesis of the retino-tectal connection in the chicken. II. The retino-tectal synapses. Proc R Soc London Ser B 192: 353–370

Rager G (1978) Systems-matching. II. Interpretation of the generation and degeneration of retinal ganglion cells by a mathematical model. Exp Brain Res 33: 79–90

Rager G (1979) The cellular origin of the b-wave in the electroretinogram. A developmental approach. J Comp Neurol 188: 225–244

Rager G (1980) The development of the retinotectal projection in the chicken. Adv Anat Embryol Cell Biol 63: in press

Rager G, Oeynhausen B von (1979) Ingrowth and ramification of retinal fibres in the developing optic tectum of the chick embryo. Exp Brain Res 35: 213–227

Rager G, Rager U (1978) Systems-matching by degeneration. I. A quantitative electronmicroscopic study of the generation and degeneration of retinal ganglion cells in the chicken. Exp Brain Res 33: 65–78

Ramón y Cajal S (1911) Histologie du systéme nerveux de l'homme et des vertébrés, vol II. Maloine, Paris

Ramón y Cajal S (1929) Ètudes sur la neurogenése de quelques vertébrés. Inst Ramón y Cajal, Madrid

Shieh P (1951) The neoformation of cells of preganglionic type in the cervical spinal cord of the chick embryo following its transplantation to the thoracic level. J Exp Zool 117: 359–396

Silver J (1978) Cell death during development of the nervous system. In: Jacobson M (ed) Development of sensory systems, pp 419–436

Silver J, Robb RM (1979) Studies on the development of the eye cup and optic nerve in normal mice and in mutants with congenital optic nerve aplasia. Dev Biol 68: 175–190

Silver J, Sidman RL (1980) A mechanism for the guidance and topographic patterning of retinal ganglion cell axons. J Comp Neurol 189: 101–111

The Critical Afferent Theory: A Mechanism to Account for Septohippocampal Development and Plasticity

C.W. COTMAN, E.R. LEWIS, and D. HAND[1]

1 Introduction

Synaptic connections are established with a high degree of specificity. They are specific with respect to the cell they contact but also often with respect to particular parts of that cell, e.g., a particular zone on a dendritic field. Such laminar specificity is particularly well illustrated in the dentate gyrus of the hippocampal formation where nearly all inputs terminate within defined laminar boundaries (Fig. 1).

The major inputs to the molecular layer are those from entorhinal and CA4 hippocampal neurons. Entorhinal fibers project to the outer 3/4 of the molecular layer while

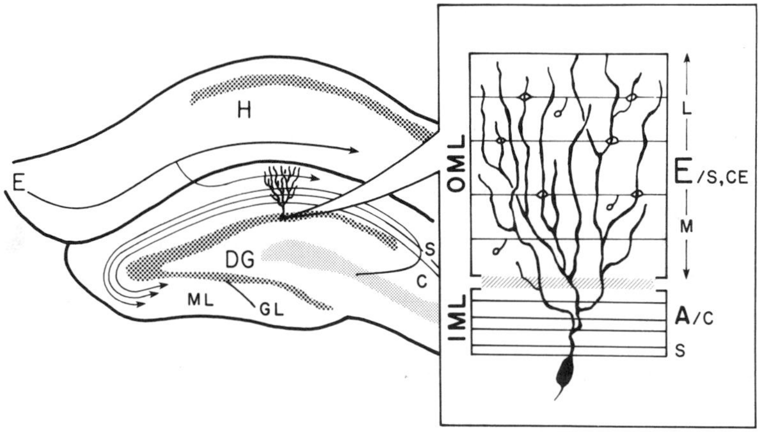

Fig. 1. Organization of afferent inputs to the molecular layer (*ML*) of the dentate gyrus (*DG*). Granule cells, the major cell type of the dentate, are arranged in a layer (*GL*) with their dendrites extending into the molecular layer. Ipsilateral associational fibers (*A*) and contralateral commissural fibers (*c*) from CA4 pyramidal cell innervate the inner 1/4 of the molecular layer. The outer 3/4 of the molecular layer consists primarily of fibers from the entorhinal cortex (*E*). Septohippocampal fibers (*S*) form a relatively dense supragranular innervation immediately above the granular cell layer; a less dense input is intermixed with entorhinal fibers. Septohippocampal fibers are absent from the *A*/*c* zone

1 Department of Psychobiology, University of California, Irvine, CA 92717/USA

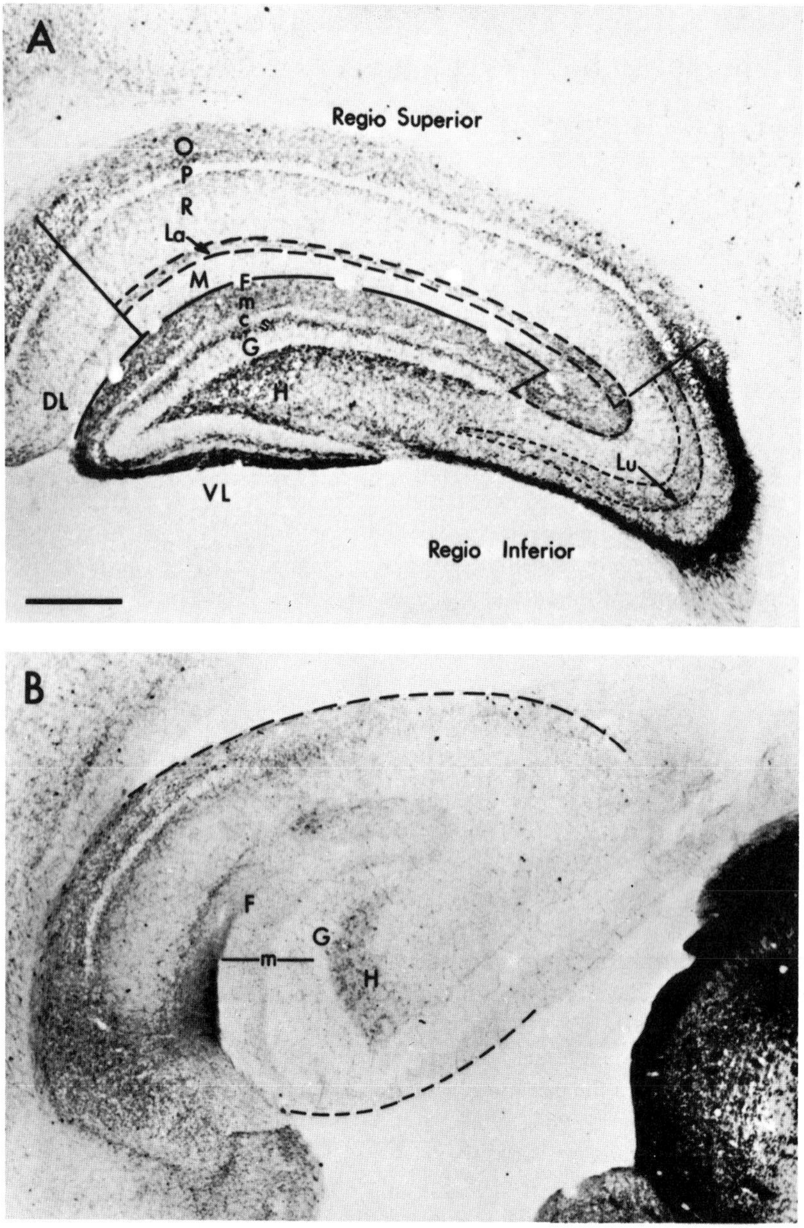

Fig. 2A, B. Acetylcholinesterase staining pattern of the hippocampus in naive rats (**A**) and rats whose fimbria has been transected (**B**), thereby cutting incoming septal fibers. Note the trilaminar staining pattern in the dentate molecular layer in A (see also Fig. 4A). Transection of the fimbria causes the disappearance of AChE activity in the molecular layer in **B**. *G* granule cell layer; CA4 zone; *m* molecular layer; *F* hippocampal fissure (Lewis et al. 1980)

CA4 neurons project to the inner 1/4. Septohippocampal fibers, a prominent cholinergic pathway, coinhabit the molecular layer along with several other minor inputs. A supragranular band of septal fibers is found just beneath CA4 fibers, while a moderately dense outer zone coexists along with entorhinal fibers. The CA4 zone contains very few if any septal fibers.

At present very little is known about the mechanisms which account for the development and plasticity of laminar patterns. Most studies and nearly all theories focus on cell-to-cell specificity. In this chapter we will describe the development and lesion-induced plasticity of septohippocampal fibers, and we will provide a unity theory which appears to account for these facts.

The septal system is a suitable system for analysis because of the large amount of information available on it, and also because it can be readily followed by histochemical methods which stain for acetylcholinesterase activity (AChE) (Fig. 2). AChE histochemistry reveals a trilaminar pattern: a dark supragranular band immediately above the granule cell layer followed by a very lightly stained zone above it. The outer 3/4 of the molecular layer stains at an intermediate intensity. Microchemical analyses of choline acetyltransferase activity also show a trilaminar pattern (Fonnum 1970; Storm-Mathisen 1970). We have used a combination of histochemical and microchemical methods to monitor the development and plasticity of this pathway.

2 Normal Development

At 2–3 days after birth neither AChE activity nor high affinity choline uptake appear to be detectable in the dentate, indicating that septal fibers have not yet arrived (Matthews et al. 1974; Nadler et al. 1974; Shelton et al. 1979). On the other hand, entorhinal and CA4 projections are both present in the dentate at this time (Fricke and Cowan 1977; Loy et al. 1977). Some AChE staining, however, is present in rostral portions of hippocampal area CA3.

By 4 days after birth AChE activity is detectable though it is still very low (Matthews et al. 1974). The areas of staining in the dentate gyrus are continuous with a slightly darker area superficial to the granule cell layer. The molecular layer is rudimentary at 4 days and in the internal leaf is discernible only at the apex of the granule cell arch. In fact, at this age the dentate gyrus consists primarily of undifferentiated granule cells (Altman and Das 1965, 1966).

At 6–11 days the staining pattern is similar to 4 days except that the supragranular band increases in intensity relative to the light diffuse staining of the remainder of the molecular layer. In both leaves this light deposit in the more superficial part of the developing molecular layer is continuous with the supragranular band.

At later ages the intensity of AChE staining increases and the zones of staining become more sharply delineated. At about 16 days of age the unstained commissural associational zone of the molecular layer first becomes detectable although it is not clearly visible until about 25 days.

Development of the CA4 zone separates the intensified supragranular band from the more highly stained superficial 3/4 of the molecular layer. It is the last of the lam-

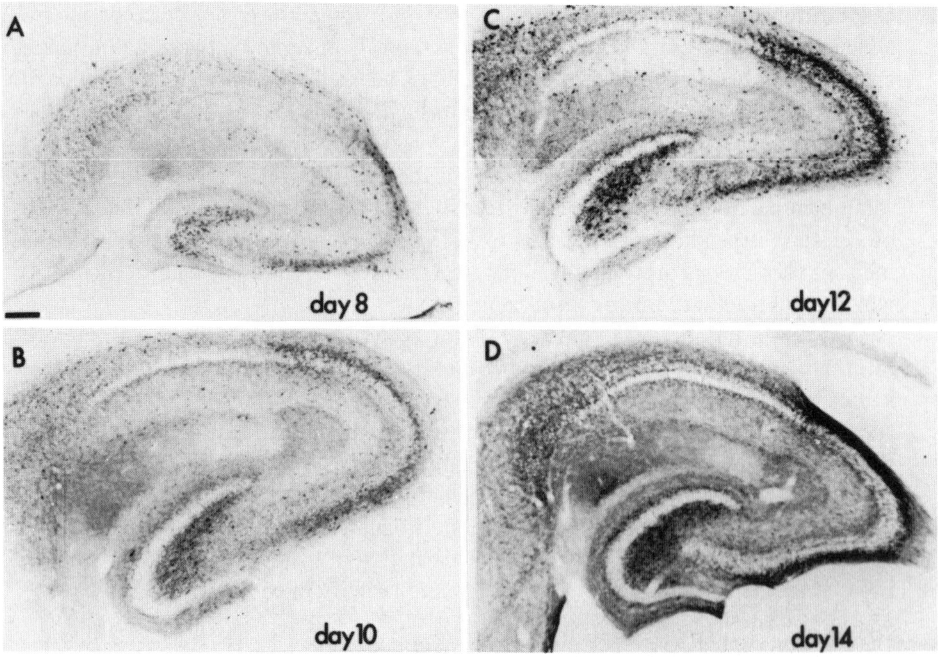

Fig. 3A–D. AChE staining patterns in the developing rat brain. Initially the molecular layer stains uniformly. A supragranular band becomes evident soon thereafter. The clear CA4 zone appears only after day 14

inar zones to differentiate (Matthews et al. 1974). The development of AChE activity is illustrated in Fig. 3.

Thus the pattern of AChE begins as a rather diffuse one and gradually takes on its trilaminar features. This sharpening of innervation pattern is not unlike that which occurs during the development of the neuromuscular junction. Neuromuscular development also begins as a diffuse innervation over most of the muscle surface and over time becomes restricted to the end plate area. Perhaps similar mechanisms such as selective stabilization are responsible for the development of the septohippocampal pattern.

3 Lesion-Induced Plasticity

The removal of the entorhinal cortex either during development or as an adult dramatically changes the pattern of septohippocampal projections. When the entorhinal cortex is removed at 11 days of age AChE staining in the molecular layer shows a transient and general increase throughout which begins almost immediately and lasts for about 24 h (Cotman et al. 1973; Nadler et al. 1977a). Shortly afterwards a strong band of intense staining develops in the outermost zone (approximately the outermost 1/5) which persists for as long as 2 years, the longest time point we have examined. Microchemical analyses show that this outer band contains additional ChAc activity (Nadler et al. 1974), accumulates more choline via high affinity transport and synthesizes more ACh (Nadler et al. 1979). Electron microscopic analysis reveals the presence of more AChE staining synaptic boutons in the outer zone (Cotman et al. 1973).

A detailed analysis was made of the exact requirements of the entorhinal lesion necessary to produce the increase in septal input in the outer zone (Nadler et al. 1977b). A complete entorhinal lesion always causes an outer band of AChE intensification but only certain partial lesions are successful. A lateral entorhinal lesion which denervates the outer 1/3 produces an effect like that of a complete lesion. However, a

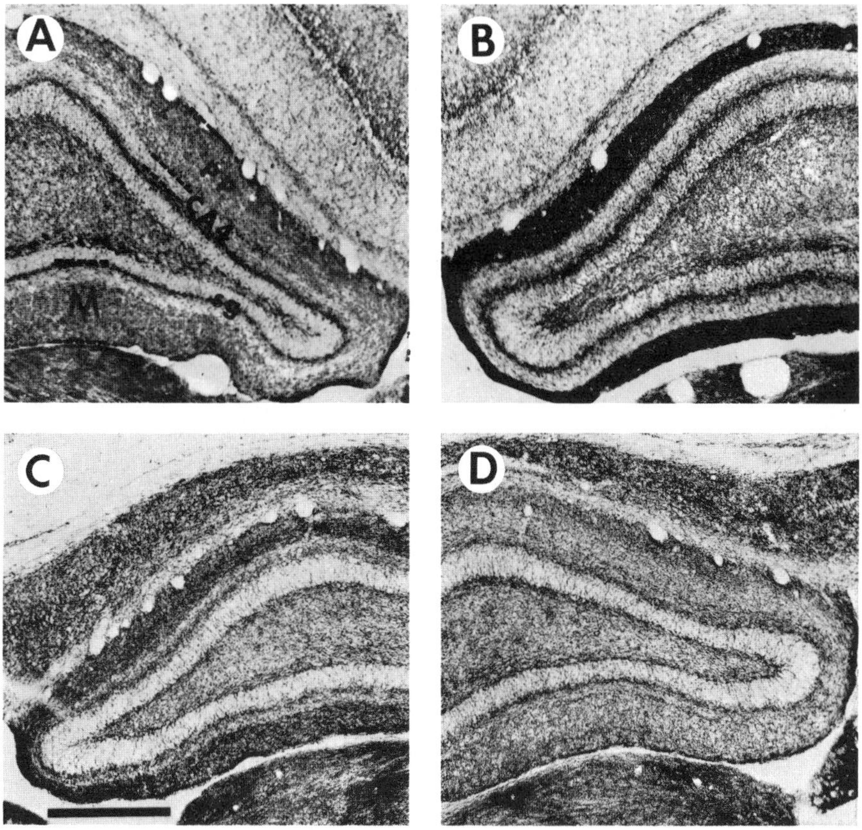

Fig. 4A–D. AChE staining pattern of the dentate gyrus. **A** Normal pattern showing the dark supragranular band (*sg*), the clear CA4 zone and the moderately stained entorhinal area (*pp*). **B** Pattern ipsilateral to an entorhinal lesion. Note the intensified staining in most of the former entorhinal zone and the expansion of the subjacent CA4 terminal zone. **C** Ipisilateral to an entorhinal lesion made 30 days after a bilateral kainic acid (KA) lesion. Note the presence of an AChE intensification in this entorhinal zone but the absence of expansion of the CA4 zone. **D** Contralateral to entorhinal lesion made 30 days after a bilateral KA lesion. Note slight intrusion of dark staining into outer part of CA4 terminal zone and greater staining throughout this zone. Scale bar 0.5 mm (Nadler et al. 1980)

medial lesion which denervates the middle 1/3 of the molecular layer is completely ineffective. This selectivity to a lateral lesion suggests that available septal fibers are somehow prohibited from growing in the middle zone when it is denervated.

An entorhinal lesion performed in adult rats also elicits an AChE intensification in the outer molecular layer, but the pattern is unlike that seen in developing rats (Lynch et al. 1972). As shown in Fig. 4, the reaction product is greatly intensified in the outer 1/2 of the molecular layer. In addition, the lightly stained zone in the inner molecular layer expands its width and perhaps also becomes somewhat lighter (Lynch et al. 1972; Storm-Mathisen 1974). It appears that these septal fibers retract or are displaced from the inner zone in addition to proliferating in the outer zone. Microchemical analyses of ChAc confirm the notion that septal fibers translocate from the middle zone to the outer (Storm-Mathisen 1974). It should be pointed out that this septal translocation is one of the few known instances in the CNS where a lesion produces both growth and regression.

Septal fibers retain their responsiveness to an entorhinal lesion throughout life, though in aged (2-year-old) rats this intensification appears somewhat reduced in intensity (Scheff et al. 1980). This probably corresponds to a general decline in lesion-induced reactive growth with age.

4 Role of Directional Growth and Time of Arrival on Septohippocampal Development

Having described the development and plasticity of septal fibers in the dentate, we will now consider the possible mechanisms underlying the development and plasticity of the laminar patterns. Mechanisms which have been proposed to account for the precision of connections include those which fall into the general categories of positional, temporal, and specificity factors. The evaluation of positional and temporal factors has been studied in nonmammalian species by grafting or rotating organs, thereby changing the position of the afferent relative to the target. Temporal factors have been examined during normal development by placing exogenous structures into host animals of various ages (see Jacobsen 1978).

Accordingly we have used tissue implants in the immature rat brain as a means to elucidate the mechanisms which specify the development of septohippocampal connections. The idea that neural tissues could survive transplants into a host mammalian brain has existed since the turn of the century (Dunn 1916; Le Gros Clark 1940). Only recently, however, have the technical difficulties of the approach been overcome and successfully applied (Stenevi et al. 1976). We have used these techniques to transplant the septal region of an embryonic donor (E16-18) into the occipital or entorhinal cortex of a 3-day-old neonatal host. Simultaneously the fimbria is cut so as to eliminate native septal afferents. Septal fibers are visualized by staining for AChE activity (Lewis and Cotman 1980; Lewis et al. 1980).

When placed in the occipital cortex, septal implants innervate specific laminar zones within the host hippocampus and dentate gyrus; these are the same laminar zones that receive septal efferents in the normal animal (Fig. 5). Septal implants placed

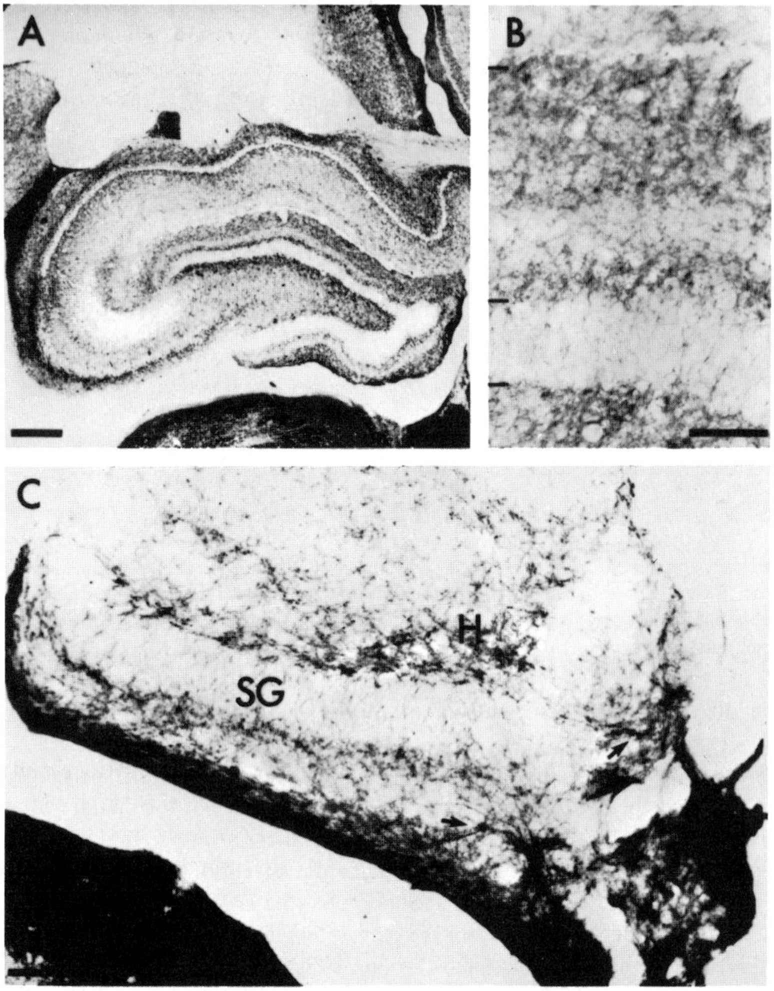

Fig. 5. A Low power micrograph of hippocampus from animal with implant in occipital cortex stained for AChE. Implant cavity can be seen in cortex dorsal to hippocampal formation. **B** High power photomicrograph showing laminar pattern of AChE staining in dentate molecular layer from hippocampal formation shown in **A. C** Dentate gyrus stained for AChE. Despite damage to hippocampus, implanted tissues lying adjacent to dentate neuropil forms a distinct laminar staining pattern. *Arrows* denote darkly stained cell bodies displaced from the implant. Calibration bars: 500 μm (**A**), 100 μm (**B** and **C**) (Lewis and Cotman 1980)

in the entorhinal cortex also produce a pattern of AChE staining in the host hippocampus which is similar to that seen in the normal hippocampus. However, the unstained CA4 zone is expanded similarly to the pattern seen after an entorhinal lesion.

These findings indicate that the location of the presynaptic cell in relation to the target organ is not critical to the mechanism guiding septal axons to their terminal fields. Septal efferents reach the hippocampus regardless of whether their cells of ori-

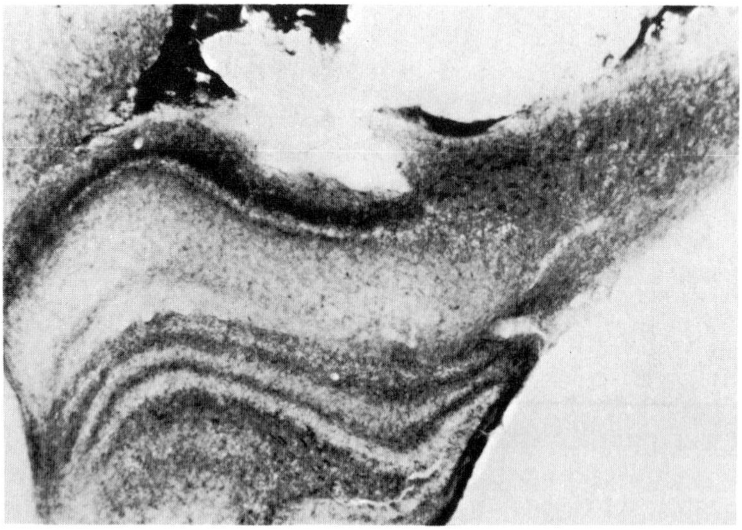

Fig. 6. Photomicrograph from an adult animal with a septal implant placed in the entorhinal cortex 3 days after a cavity was made to receive the implant. This delayed implant paradigm illustrates that the time of implantation is not a critical factor underlying the formation of the AChE pattern

gin are located anterior (as in the normal animal), dorsal, or postero lateral to the hippocampus.

It also seems unlikely that a close temporal correspondence between the arrival of the septal afferents and the maturation of the dendritic membrane of the dentate granule cells is responsible for specifying septohippocampal connections. It appears that septohippocampal fibers normally arrive in the dentate gyrus of the rat between 4 and 7 days postnatal (Matthews et al. 1974; Shelton et al. 1979). Based on the presence of AChE reaction product, fibers from the grafted tissue do not arrive in the dentate gyrus until about day 12 (Lewis and Cotman 1980). Thus implant fibers experience altered temporal events. The lack of critical temporal role can be further demonstrated using a delayed implant paradigm (Lewis et al. 1980). Septal tissues can be implanted into the entorhinal area with a 3–6 day interval between time of surgery and implantation. In this paradigm, septal fibers grow into the dentate and form a pattern indistinguishable from that of an implant paradigm with no delay (Fig. 6). The results using either a 3- or 6-day interval are identical. These data suggest there is considerable flexibility in the timing of afferent growth and pattern formation. It should be mentioned in passing that the delayed implant paradigm also shows that the presence of degenerating axons does not guide the ingrowth of septal axons. Degenerating axons have been removed by the time the implant is placed.

Thus our results argue against temporal competition between several afferent systems as the factor specifying the laminar development of septal fibers. In the case of the occipital placement, fibers from the implant are able to gain access to space along the dendritic membrane despite their delayed arrival. If the laminar pattern of terminal contacts results from a general temporal competition between several major afferent

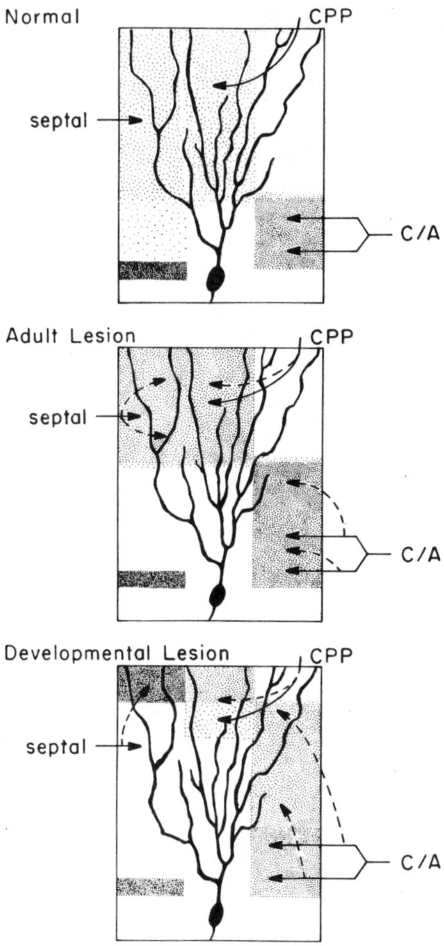

Fig. 7. Schematic showing organization of inputs in the dentate of normal animals and those with entorhinal lesions made during development or adulthood. Note that septohippocampal fibers are absent in the CA4 zone (C/A) (Cotman and Nadler 1978)

systems, it would be expected that the relatively sparse afferents from the implant would be "outcompeted" by the ingrowing entorhinal or CA4 axons. It appears that some specific mechanism exists.

5 The Critical Afferent Theory: A Special Role for CA4 Fibers

Several lines of evidence suggest that the CA4 system plays a pivotal role in establishing the organization of septal fibers in the molecular layer. This hypothesis appears to explain the data on the normal and lesion-induced reorganization of septal afferents. Septohippocampal fibers are always sparse in areas rich in commissural associational fibers (Fig. 7), as if these fibers exclude septohippocampal ones. For example, the expansion of the AChE clear zone following an adult entorhinal lesion corresponds exactly to the widening of the CA4 fibers plexus. It appears that this exclusion is specific to CA4 fibers. Thus, for example, a partial entorhinal lesion causes septal reactivity and a proliferation of contralateral entorhinal and probably other fibers in that zone, but it does not lead to a loss of septal innervation.

It appears that one system can establish that of another: CA4 fibers appear to serve as the critical afferent that establishes the pattern of septal growth and reorganization. A hierarchy of interactions exists probably established during development and retained throughout life. We have called this model the critical afferent theory of lamination; it is where a special type of competition mechanism where the critical afferent enjoys a special advantage (Cotman 1979; Lewis and Cotman 1980).

6 Consequence of Manipulation of CA4 Fibers on Septohippocampal Lamination

A direct test of the critical afferent theory is to remove the CA4 system and examine the response of septal fibers. When CA4 cells are removed in developing animals by kainic acid, septal fibers fill the CA4 zone and the clear zone fails to form. Furthermore, when an adult entorhinal lesion is preceded by a bilateral kainic acid injection to remove CA4 neurons, septal fibers appear to proliferate in the entorhinal area but the clear zone fails to develop (Fig. 4c) (Nadler et al. 1980). Thus it appears that CA4 fibers can somehow exclude septal fibers from their territory. Complete removal of CA4 input with no entorhinal lesion permits septohippocampal fibers to proliferate in that zone (Fig. 4d). Septal fibers can then replace CA4 fibers as expected. If some CA4 neurons survive the kainic acid treatment, however, septal fibers will not proliferate, suggestive again of their powerful suppressive effect on septal growth.

It would be desirable to demonstrate that CA4 fibers interact with septal fibers without having to resort to experimental intervention. Fortunately, the mutant mouse "reeler" has an abnormally positioned CA4 system. In the reeler, CA4 fibers terminate within the hilus of fascia dentata (Stanfield et al. 1979). The major input to the dentate molecular layer appears to be of entorhinal origin. The critical afferent theory predicts that in reeler no lamination of septal fibers should exist. Indeed, this is the case in agreement with the prediction (Fig. 8).

7 Summary

In this chapter we have described the development and plasticity of septohippocampal fibers and shown that their pattern appears to be established by that of CA4 fibers. CA4 fibers appear to be the critical variable which establishes septohippocampal organization in the dentate molecular layer. This conclusion has several implications for molecular theories of specificity. It may be that CA4 fibers directly retard the growth of septal fibers, perhaps through the release of specific growth-retarding substances. Alternatively, CA4 fibers may induce a membrane surface characteristic on their target

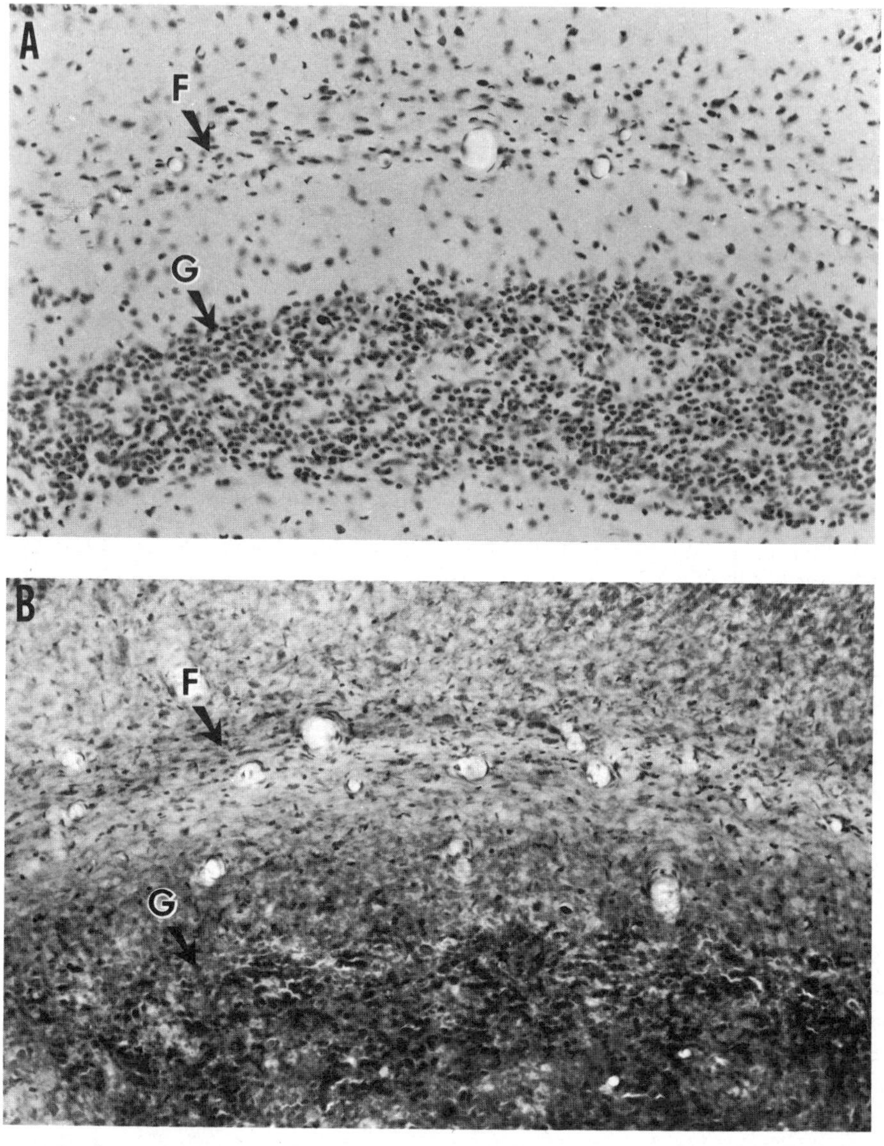

Fig. 8A, B. The dentate gyrus of the "reeler" mouse. **A** Distribution of cell bodies; **B** AChE staining pattern. Note the absence of lamination in the molecular layer. *F* hippocampal fissure, *G* upper edge of granule cell layer

cell that is incompatible with septal input. Thus, it is not necessary to have a specific affinity or other specificity which pre-exists for septal or for that matter other afferents.

The critical afferent theory can be extended to account, at least in principle, for the development of other afferent fields in dentate. It would be predicted, for example,

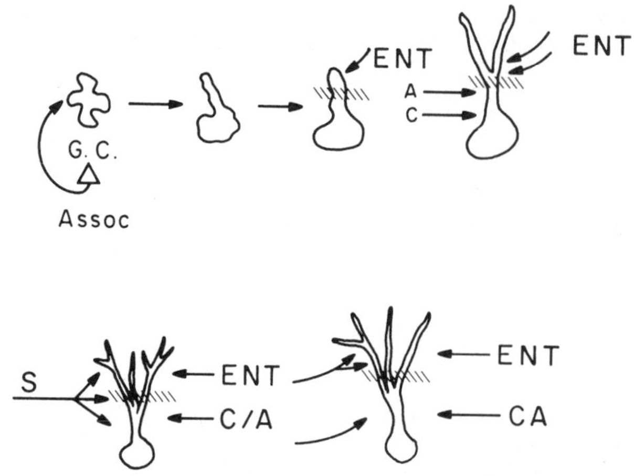

Fig. 9. Hypothetical scheme for the formation of CA4 (C/A) and entorhinal (ENT) lamina. A hierarchy of afferent interactions may exist. Entorhinal fibers may selectively prevent the proliferation of CA4 fibers but not alter the growth of septohippocampal fibers. CA4 fibers, though, retard septohippocampal growth

that associational CA4 fibers are the earliest major afferent to arrive in the molecular layer. Entorhinal fibers could act as a critical afferent to CA4 fibers. Entorhinal fibers growing from the opposite direction establish synapses on the expanding dentrites and perhaps arrest the spread of CA4 fibers over the entire dendritic surface (Fig. 9). It is predicted that other critical afferent combinations exist; however, these have yet to be identified.

In a sense, the critical afferent theory is a special case of the selective stabilization hypothesis previously described for the neuromuscular junction. In a multiinnervated system, a mechanism must exist to select the different inputs individually. A critical afferent such as described for the septohippocampal system could provide the selection mechanism. The critical afferent theory contains postulates for which there is reasonable evidence in other systems where cell-cell recognition is involved. The so-called "interaction modulation" hypothesis was proposed by Curtis and van de Vyver (1971) to explain the specificity of developmental cell psoitioning and patterning. It is also denominated the "morphogen" theory, and its present state has been recently reviewed (Curtis 1978a,b). According to this theory, cells secrete diffusible substances that diminish the adhesion of unlike cells, thus excluding them or allowing them to escape their own environment. Gradients of concentration of these substances (morphogens) would be set up that would determine the position of the different types of cells. The secretion by actively metabolizing cells of soluble factors that diminish the adhesiveness of other cell types, not only to themselves but to other surfaces, has been shown to occur in five widely different groups of organisms, e.g., sponges, chicken neural retina and liver cells, rat and human B and T lymphocytes and mouse liver, echinoderm embryos, and cellular slime molds (see Curtis 1978a). A version of this theory also constitutes the main ingredient in a model proposed by Fraser and Hunt to account for the development of the retinotectal pattern of projection. The fact that similar mechanisms have been suggested for other cases strengthens our contention that the critical afferent theory may have general applicability to the development of laminated terminal fields.

Acknowledgment. This work was supported by grants NS08957 and MH19691. We appreciate the secretarial assistance of Ms. Susanne Bathgate.

References

Altman J, Das GD (1965) Autoradiographic and histological evidence of postnatal hippocampal neurogenesis in rats. J Comp Neurol 124: 319–336

Altman J, Das GD (1966) Autoradiographic and histological studies of postnatal neurogenesis. J Comp Neurol 126: 337–390

Cotman CW (1971) Specificity of synaptic growth in brain: Remodeling induced by kainic acid lesions. In: Akert K, Baumgartner G, Bloom F, Kreutzberg G, Cuenod M (eds) Development and chemical specificity of neurons, progress in brain research, vol 51. Elsevier/North Holland, Amsterdam, pp 203–215

Cotman CW, Nadler JV (1978) Reactive synaptogenesis in the hippocampus. In: Cotman CW (ed) Neuronal plasticity. Raven Press, New York, pp 227–271

Cotman CW, Matthews DA, Taylor D, Lynch G (1973) Synaptic rearrangement in the dentate gyrus: Histochemical evidence of adjustments after lesions in immature and adult rats. Proc Nat Acad Sci USA 70: ~~343–347~~ 3473–3477

Curtis ASG (1978a) Cell-cell recognition: psoitioning and patterning systems. Soc Exp Biol Symposium 32. Cambridge University Press, Cambridge, pp 51–82

Curtis ASG (1978b) Cell Positioning. In: Garrod DR (ed) Receptors and recognition, specificity of embriological interactions, Series B, vol 4. Chapman and Hall, London, pp 157–195

Curtis ASG, van de Vyver (1971) The control of cell adhesion in a morphogenetic system. J Embryol Exp Morphol 26: 295–312

Dunn EG (1916–1917) Primary and secondary findings in a series of attempts to transplant cerebral cortex in the albino rat. J Comp Neurol 27: 565–582

Fonnum F (1970) Topographical and subcellular localization of choline acetyltransferase in rat hippocampal region. J Neurochem 17: 1029–1037

Fraser SE, Hunt RK (1980) Retinotectal specificity: models and experiments in search of a mapping function. Ann Rev Neurosci 3: 319–352

Fricke RA, Cowan WM 91977) An autoradiographic study of the development of the entorhinal and hippocampal afferents to the dentate gyrus of the rat. J Comp Neur 173: 231–250

Jacobsen M (1978) Developmental neurobiology, 2nd ed. Plenum Press, New York

Le Gros Clark WE (1940) Neuronal Differentiation in implanted fetal cortical tissue. J Neur Psychiatr 3: 263–272

Lewis ER, Cotman CW (1980) Mechanisms of septal lamination in the developing hippocampus revealed by outgrowth of fibers from septal implants: I. Positional and temporal factors. Brain Res 196: 307–330

Lewis ER, Kelly P, Cotman CW (1980a) Absence of degenerative debri guidance in the specific growth of septal tissue grafts implanted into neonatal hosts. Abstr Soc Neurosci 6: 161.6

Lewis ER, Mueller JC, Cotman CW (1980b) Neonatal septal implants: Development of afferent lamination in the rat dentate gyrus. Brain Res Bull 5(3): 217–221

Loy R, Cotman CW, Lynch G (1977) The development of afferent lamination in the fascia dentate of the rat. Brain Res 121: 229–243

Lynch G, Matthews D, Mosko S, Parks T, Cotman CW (1977) Induced acetylcholinesterase-rich layer in rat dentate gyrus following entorhinal lesions. Brain Res 42: 311–318

Matthews DA, Nadler JV, Lynch GS, Cotman CW (1974) Development of cholinergic innervation in the hippocampal formation of the rat. I. Histochemical demonstration of acetylcholinesterase activity. Dev Biol 36: 130–141

Nadler JV, Matthews DA, Cotman CW, Lynch GS (1974) Development of cholinergic innervation in the hippocampal formation of the rat. II. Quantitative changes in choline acetyltransferase and acetylcholinesterase activities. Dev Biol 36: 142–154

Nadler JV, Cotman CW, Lynch G (1977a) Histochemical evidence of altered development of cholinergic fibers in the rat dentate gyrus following lesions. I. Time course after complete unilateral entorhinal lesion at various ages. J Comp Neurol 171: 589–604

Nadler JV, Paoletti C, Cotman CW, Lynch G (1977b) Histochemical evidence of altered development of cholinergic fibers in the rat dentate gyrus following lesions. II. Effects of partial entorhinal and simultaneous multiple lesions. J Comp Neurol 171: 589–604

Nadler JV, Shelton DL, Cotman CW (1979) Lesion-induced plasticity of high affinity choline in the developing rat fascia dentata. Brain Res 164: 207–216

Nadler JV, Perry BW, Cotman CW (1980) Interaction with CA4-derived fibers accounts for distribution of septohippocampal fibers in rat fascia dentata after entorhinal lesion. Exp Neurol 68: 185–194

Scheff SW, Bernardo LS, Cotman CW (1980) Decline in reactive fiber growth in the dentate gyrus of aged rats compared to young rats following entorhinal cortex removal. Brain Res 199: 21–38

Shelton DL, Nadler JV, Cotman CW (1979) Development of high affinity choline uptake and associated acetylcholine synthesis in the rat fascia dentata. Brain Res 163: 263–275

Stanfield BB, Caviness VS, Cowan WM (1979) The organization of certain afferents to the hippocampus and dentate gyrus in normal and reeler mice. J Comp Neurol 185: 461–484

Stenevi U, Bjorkland A, Svengaard N-A (1976) Transplantation of central and peripheral monoamine neurons to the adult rat brain: techniques and conditions for survival. Brain Res 114: 1–20

Storm-Mathisen J (1970) Quantitative histochemistry of acetylcholinesterase in rat hippocampal region correlated to histochemical staining. J Neurochem 17: 739–750

Storm-Mathisen J (1974) Choline acetyltransferase in fascia dentata following lesion of the entorhinal afferents. Brain Res 80: 181–197

The Regulation of Sprouting in the Adult Hippocampus: Some Insights from Developmental Studies

C. GALL[1] and G. LYNCH[2]

1 Introduction

Sprouting, the reinnervation of partially denervated targets by residual afferents, has been observed in a number of brain areas in a variety of species (see Gall and Lynch 1980). The existence of this phenomenon has led to general acceptance of the idea that intact axons in the mammalian central nervous system retain some capacity for growth well into adulthood. However, recent studies have emphasized that sprouting in the adult is restricted in its extent and rather sluggish in its time course; these apparent limitations on the sprouting response raise a number of questions as to the nature of the factors which initiate, direct, and shape growth in the adult brain.

Axon sprouting has been intensively studied in the dendritic field (molecular layer) of the granule cell population which forms the dentate gyrus of the rat hippocampus. Within this rather homogeneous cell-free layer the principal afferent systems terminate within adjacent but nonoverlapping lamina; the ipsilateral entorhinal cortex densely innervates the distal 73% of the molecular layer, whereas the hippocampal commissural and ipsilateral associational systems dominate the remaining proximal dendritic zone (see Fig. 1). Deafferentation of the outer molecular layer in the adult rat (by lesions of the ipsilateral entorhinal cortex) initiates a complex but orderly and highly reliable sequence of events, a sequence which leads to sprouting and ultimately reinnervation. Ultrastructural signs of axonal and terminal degeneration are evident by 20–30 h postlesion, and by electron microscopic criteria are most numerous 48–72 h later (Matthews et al. 1976; Lee et al. 1977). The onset and development of degeneration is accompanied by a period of intense glial activity. By 30 h after entorhinal cortex ablation, microglia cells proliferate throughout the hippocampal formation. This mitotic response continues into the third day postlesion and is followed by a gradual migration of the microglial cells into the deafferented zone (Gall et al. 1979c). At about the same time the microglia begin dividing, that is by 30 h postlesion, the astrocytes within the deafferented hippocampus become detectably hypertrophied. This reaction reaches its height by 4 to 5 days postlesion after which a gradual atrophy ensues (Rose et al. 1976).

1 Department of Neurology, State University of New York at Stony Brook, Long Island, NY, USA
2 Department of Psychobiology, University of California, Irvine, CA, USA

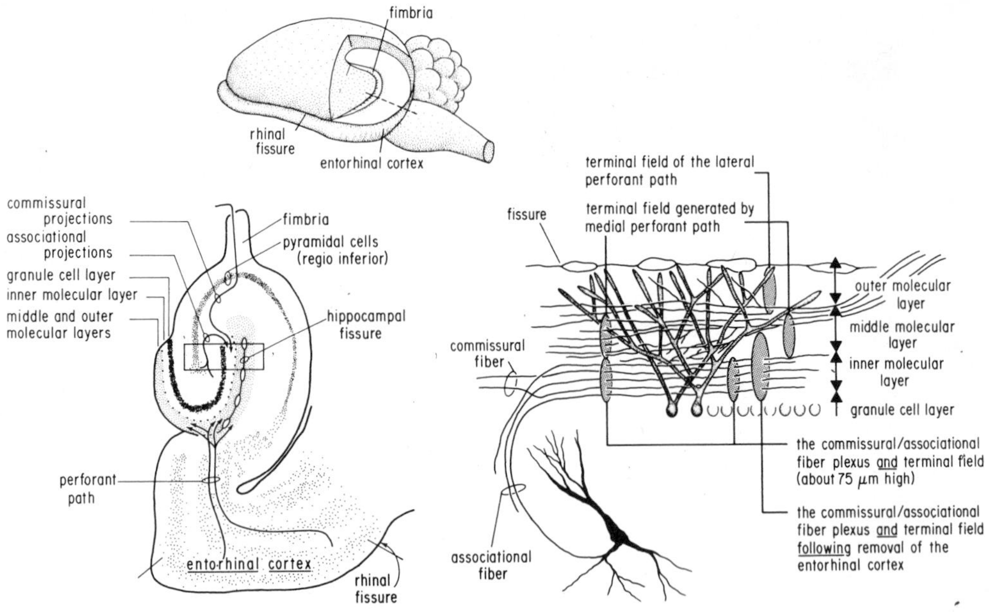

Fig. 1. Schematic illustration of the position and organization of the rat dentate gyrus. The sketch on the ***upper left*** indicates the position of the hippocampal formation as seen from a lateral view of a rat brain in which the caudolateral quadrant of the neocortex has been removed. The ***dashed line*** indicates the plane of the hippocampal cross-section drawn on the ***lower left***. Here one can see the relative position of the dentate gyrus and its major sources of extrinsic afferent input: from the ipsilateral entorhinal cortex via the perforant path and from the contralateral hippocampal formation via the fimbria. The third principal afferent to the dentate gyrus molecular layer, the associational projection, arises within the ipsilateral hippocampal ***regio inferior*** (homotopic to the source of the commissural input). The pattern of afferent termination within both the normal and "reorganized" molecular layer is schematized on the ***lower right***. As indicated, the shared commissural/associational afferent zone normally lies adjacent and proximal to the field of entorhinal innervation. Following deafferentation of the outer zone by ipsilateral entorhinal ablation in the adult rat, the commissural/associational systems sprout distally into the middle molecular layer but fail to penetrate the full depth of the dennervated territory

It is not until 5 days postlesion, after the period of glial activity has largely passed, that an expansion of the commissural and associational afferents into the deafferented zone is observed (Lynch et al. 1977). It should be recalled that the normal entorhinal and commissural-associational terminal fields do not overlap; this clear segregation makes the first inroads of commissural-associational innervation within the distal zone conspicuous and quantifiable. Corroborative autoradiographic (Gall et al. 1979b), electron microscopic (Lee et al. 1977), and axonal staining (Lynch et al. 1977) studies all describe this sprouting response as exhibiting the 5–6 day delay just mentioned and further show that it is limited in its extent. This last point is illustrated in Fig. 1. As shown, the perforant path lesion eliminates the great majority of synapses in the outer 73% of the molecular layer, roughly the region from 75 μm to 300 μm above the granule cells; however, the expanded commissural-associational plexus expands outwards no more than 50 μm and thus fails to gain access to the greater part of the vacated dendritic space (Lynch and Cotman 1975).

While the above described studies have provided a reasonable characterization of sprouting within context of the 'deafferentation syndrome' they raise a number of questions regarding the basis of the specific parameters of the growth response. Why is there a 5 day delay before the onset of sprouting? Does this represent a period in which the deafferented field becomes prepared to receive growth (e.g., degeneration is removed), or it it the time needed for the responsive axons to mobilize for growth? Similarly, does the rate of reinnervation (once sprouting has started) reflect the capacity of the growing axons, or does reinnervation keep pace with extrinsic processes such as degeneration removal? Why is there a sharp limit on the extent of commissural-associational penetration of the deafferented field? Does this reflect a "ceiling" on the capacity of the commissural and associational neurons to effect and sustain a larger-than-normal axonal arborization, or is it due to differences in the growth environment, differences which make the marginal zone more "hospitable" to commissural-associational innervation?

The following fundamental question is involved in each of these issues: *To what extent are the parameters of the sprouting response a function of the properties and capacities of the growing axons themselves, and to what extent are these parameters attributable to events or elements within the neuropil?*

In the following sections we will consider one approach to the investigation of this question, namely an analysis of the development of the parameters of sprouting in the above described dentate gyrus system. Ontogenetic studies have the potential to resolve questions regarding "capacity" or genetically determined absolute limits on growth. Thus if, as suggested by several reports (e.g., Lynch et al. 1973; Zimmer 1973), immature axons are able to generate and sustain into adulthood greatly expanded projection fields, then the failure of adult fibers to do so cannot be due simply to inherent limitations in the metabolic or synthetic capabilities of the neuron. Instead, it would be necessary to postulate that development alters the axon or its targets such that the growth response falls short of that which the cell was once capable of sustaining. If sprouting at different ages produces comparable terminal fields and synaptic numbers, then the hypothesis that absolute limits on capacity are important "regulators" would be strengthened. Ontogenetic analyses also provide opportunities for establishing correlations between the development of specific parameters of adult sprouting and other structural and biochemical events in the maturing hippocampus. This type of information may prove invaluable in identifying candidates for the processes responsible for shaping the mature form of sprouting.

2 The Extent of Sprouting

The original studies on sprouting in the dentate gyrus noted a dramatic difference in the extent to which commissural fibers would invade the outer molecular layer after that zone had been denervated by lesions placed in the neonate and the adult (Lynch et al. 1973; Zimmer 1973). As mentioned above, the commissural axons grow about

50 μm into the deafferented territory following entorhinal cortex removal in the adult rat, but these axons reinnervate the full depth of this field after comparable lesions in rats up to 14 days of age (Gall and Lynch 1978; Gall et al. 1979a,b; Gall et al. 1980). The extent of sprouting is intermediate with lesion placement at 21 days postnatal (dpn); the commissural axons clearly grow further into the deafferented field than seen with adult deafferentation, but the sprouted projection is sparse and seems to fail to reach the hippocampal fissure.

Following lesion placement at 2 weeks of age, sprouting into the deafferented field is sufficiently dense to return the synaptic bouton density of the area to near normal levels (Gall et al. 1979a). The commissural afferents contribute approximately 37% of the new synapses, a value which is essentially equivalent to their contribution to the innervation of the inner molecular layer. Moreover, this expanded innervation is accomplished with no loss of commissural input to their normal target, the inner molecular layer (Gall et al. 1979a). This is a most important finding since it indicates that sprouting after lesions at 14 dpn produces a genuine hypertrophy rather than a redistribution of the commissural projection. Thus, these afferents to the dentate gyrus are capable, during development, of growing and sustaining into adulthood a much larger terminal field than is generated during normal development or following deafferentation in the adult rat.

Studies using anterograde transport methods and, in particular, tritiated amino acid autoradiography, have shown that the sprouted commissural system is evenly distributed throughout the molecular layer following entorhinal lesions at 7 days postnatal; the interface between the normal commissural projection field in the inner molecular layer and the sprouted projection which develops in the middle and outer zones cannot be detected. A very different situation is found after entorhinal cortex ablation in 14-day old rats. In these cases the density of the commissural projection in the middle and outer molecular layer never reaches that found in the inner molecular layer and retains a "shelved" appearance even with extended survival periods (Fig. 2; Gall et al. 1980). This uneven distribution seen with light microscopic autoradiography does not reflect the density of commissural *synapses* since, as discussed above, electron microscopic studies have shown that the number of commissural connections is roughly equivalent in normal and sprouted segments of the projection following lesions at 14 dpn.

A possible explanation for the difference between the distribution of the commissural projection seen with the autoradiographic and electron microscopic techniques is that although commissural synapses are equally dense throughout the molecular layer, the commissural axons are not. The autoradiographic method labels both axons and terminals, and it is possible that commissural *axons* are more prevalent in the proximal zone, thereby generating the unequal distribution of grains across the depth of the molecular layer. This suggestion is substantiated by the distribution of axons within the dentate gyrus molecular layer as seen in tissue processed with the Holme's stain for fibers. In the normal dentate gyrus molecular layer the commissural and associational afferent systems generate a prominent and measurable fiber plexus that conforms to the boundary of their terminal field. Following entorhinal cortex removal in the adult rat, this fiber plexus expands into the adjacent deafferented region again coming into conformation with the now-expanded commissural-associational terminal

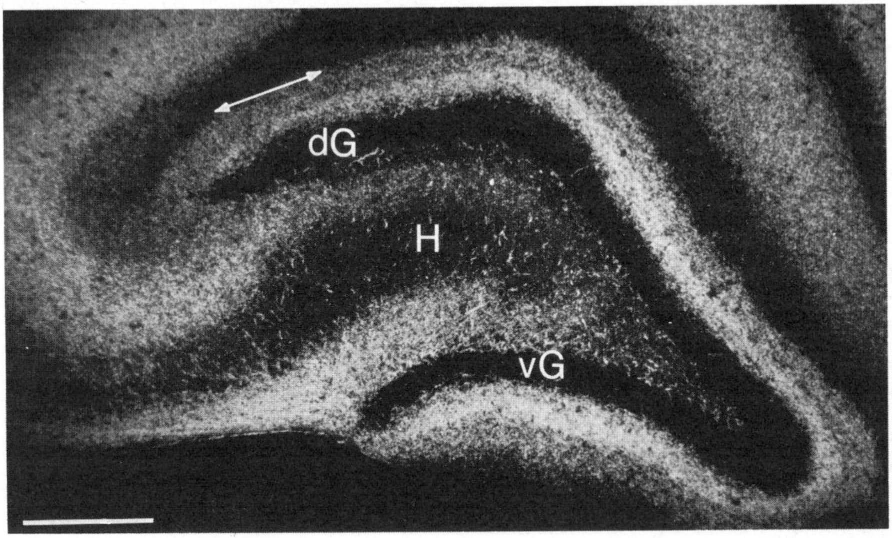

Fig. 2. Dark field autoradiograph of the "sprouted" commissural projection to the dentate gyrus of an adult rat which had been subjected to ipsilateral entorhinal cortex ablation at 14 days of age. The commissural-associated autoradiographic grains can be seen to have a shelved distribution within the dentate gyrus molecular layer. The grains are very dense in the inner molecular layer, adjacent to the outside of the curving layer of granule cells, and are relatively less dense in the more distal outer molecular layer. The densely labeled proximal zone is the normal target for the commissural afferents, whereas the distal zone, here deafferented by the entorhinal ablation, receives no commissural input in the normal rat. *vG* ventral granule cell layer, *dG* dorsal granule cell layer, *H* hilus. The *arrow* indicates the position of the hippocampal fissure. (Calibration: 300 μm)

field (Lynch et al. 1977). The expanded fiber plexus is homogeneous and the sprouted portion cannot be distinguished from the normal projection.

A very different fiber distribution pattern emerges following lesions of the entorhinal cortex placed at 7 dpn. In this case, the commissural-association plexus in the inner molecular layer gives rise to a large population of thick collaterals which invade and travel for great distances (millimeters) in the denervated territory giving off branches that reach the furthest extent of the molecular layer. These collateral sprouts fasciculate and generate a secondary plexus in the middle of the outer molecular layer about 50 μM above the normal plexus in the inner molecular layer. Thus two commissural-associational plexuses form in the dentate gyrus after entorhinal lesions at one week of age: the inner molecular layer plexus which appears more or less normal and a secondary plexus in the middle dendritic zone composed of sprouted collaterals.

Following lesions of the entorhinal cortex at 14 dpn, the commissural-associational fibers assume a pattern which incorporates features found after the lesions placed at 1 week postnatal and in adult rats. Specifically, the inner molecular layer plexus exhibits the uniform 50 μm expansion into the middle molecular layer that is found in the adult but in addition it sends a sparse population of long collaterals which reach throughout the denervated dendritic territory. The number of such collaterals appears to be considerably less than that found after neonatal lesions and the long branches do not fasciculate to form a secondary plexus (Gall and Lynch, in press). In summary, both adult and neonatal forms of sprouting are found after lesions at 14 dpn.

What do these observations on the extent of commissural sprouting following entorhinal ablation at different ages tell us about the factors which restrict the adult sprouting response? Clearly, the commissural projection is capable of sustaining a much more extensive termination within the dentate gyrus molecular layer than that seen in the normal or adult-deafferented rat. Therefore, it seems that a genetic limit on the size of the commissural axon's arborization is not responsible for the limited sprouting response seen in the adult. Secondly, the fact that commissural axons can innervate the distal granule cell dendrites after the destruction of entorhinal innervation in the immature rat suggests that it is not a specificity mismatch that excludes this innervation following adult deafferentation. And finally, since some fibers at 14 dpn appear to engage in the immature form of sprouting while others exhibit the adult type, it seems unlikely that a generalized change in the dentate gyrus (e.g., the invasion of glial cells) is by itself responsible for the restricted growth found in the adult. It is perhaps more probable that maturation alters the developing fibers such that their growth responses are altered and/or made responsive to elements in the neuropil.

3 Delay in the Onset of Sprouting

In addition to the spatial constraints that are placed on axon sprouting with development, the time course of this growth process also reflects the age at which the lesion is delivered. The delay from the time of the lesion to the onset of sprouting has been measured in the adult rat with a variety of anatomical techniques (Lee et al. 1977; Lynch et al. 1977; Gall et al. 1979b). Recently, the time course for commissural sprouting following entorhinal cortex removal in the two-week old rat pup has been studied with results very different from those found in adults. At 14 dpn the normal commissural projection to the dentate gyrus molecular layer is confined to a well-defined lamina beginning immediately above the granule cell layer and extending about 40 μm into the molecular layer. Within 13 h of ipsilateral entorhinal cortex removal it is evident that the commissural axons exceed the distal boundary of this zone and occupy "patches" of the adjacent deafferented field. This incursion proceeds so that commissural-associated autoradiographic grains extend more than 50 μm into the denervated field by 24 h postlesion and reach the hippocampal fissure by the end of postlesion day 2 (Gall and Lynch 1978; Gall et al. 1980).

Electron microscopic work corroborates this light microscopic description of a very rapid sprouting response in the immature rat. The density of intact synapses in the deafferented middle molecular layer falls to 20% of the normal level within 20 h of entorhinal cortex ablation in the 14-day old rat; 10 h later an increase in the number of intact synapses is already in evidence (Gall et al. 1980). Therefore, it seems that with this early lesion placement entorhinal terminal degeneration, commissural collateralization, and finally reinnervation, all proceed without any significant postlesion delay.

These results raise the question as to when the 5 day postlesion delay in the onset of sprouting appears. Using the Holmes stain for normal axons, we have found evidence in the 14-day lesion case that the component of the inner plexus axons that shows the restricted adult-like sprouting also exhibits a postlesion delay to sprouting onset. It will be recalled that with entorhinal cortex removal in the 14-day old rat two forms of axonal adjustment were seen. The first involved the extension of long, thick axon collaterals into the most distal molecular layer, whereas the second consisted of a limited expansion of the inner molecular layer fiber plexus. This plexus expansion is not present at 4 days postlesion but is complete by postlesion day 8 and sustained thereafter (Gall and Lynch, in press). Therefore, at 14 days postnatal, an age where rapid and extensive commissural sprouting has been demonstrated with autoradiographic and electron microscopic techniques, the Holmes fiber stain impregnates a population of inner plexus axons that exhibit the limited and delayed form of growth seen in the adult.

4 Rate of Reinnervation by Sprouting Fibers

The rate of outer molecular layer reinnervation has not been thoroughly examined in the adult rat; however, the available data indicate that reinnervation begins with the onset of sprouting (5 days postlesion), proceeds at a pace of about 1 synapse per 100 μm^2 per day for several days, and then continues at a slower rate for several weeks (Lee et al. 1977). A more detailed time course has been established for the reinnervation of the dentate gyrus inner molecular layer, presumably by the associational fibers, following removal of the commissural projections. As with the entorhinal lesion case, reinnervation does not begin in this system until after 5 days postlesion. Synaptogenesis then follows at a rate of about 1.3 synaptic boutons (SB)/100 μm^2/day for several days but slows until only 0.4 SB/100 μm^2 are added per day (McWilliams and Lynch 1978, 1979). It seems that a negatively accelerating rate of reinnervation, as seen in this case, may be typical. Unfortunately, the extensive data for sprouting in the inner molecular layer may not be an entirely appropriate adult comparison for the neonatal commissural sprouting after entorhinal lesions. In the former instance the lesion removes less than half of the innervation to the area under study, whereas the latter involves the elimination of about 90% of the outer molecular layer innervation. As will be seen below, the residual intact synapse density may have a strong influence on the rate of reinnervation.

In light of the autoradiographic data demonstrating rapid and extensive commissural sprouting with entorhinal cortex removal in the 14-day old rat, it is not surprising that, as mentioned above, reinnervation is also accomplished quite rapidly following lesions at this age. As can be seen in Fig. 3, the density of intact synapses within the dentate gyrus outer molecular layer falls to 16% of the normal level by 20 h postlesion. A return of intact synapses is evident by 30 h postlesion, after which reinnervation proceeds rapidly so that most of the lost synaptic population is recovered by postlesion day 4 (Gall et al. 1980).

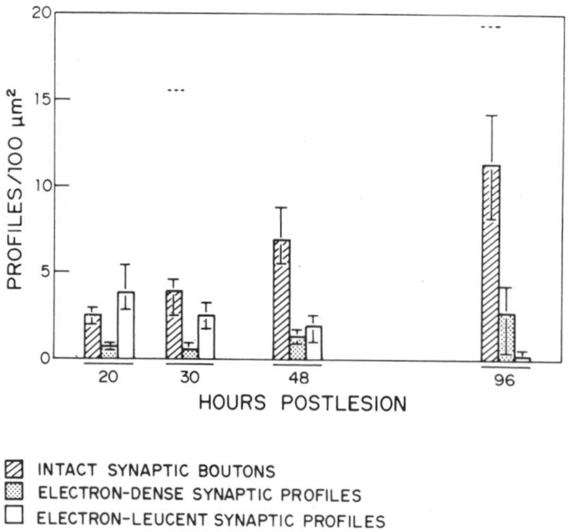

Fig. 3. Bar graphs illustrating the changes seen in the density of intact, electron-lucent, and electron-dense presynaptic profiles in the deafferented dentate gyrus middle molecular layer during the 4 days following removal of the ipsilateral entorhinal cortex in the 14-day old rat. Each *bar* represents the mean value from several cases. The *broken lines* above the bars at 30 and 96 h postlesion indicate the mean intact synapse density observed in control rats at these ages. (From data presented in Gall et al. 1980)

Secondary lesion studies have demonstrated that most of this reinnervation is accomplished by the commissural-associational systems (Gall et al. 1979a). From 15 to 18 days postnatal, these systems normally add 1.3 synaptic boutons/100 μm^2/day to the inner molecular layer (i.e., to their normal targets). In the instance of the 14-day lesion these same afferent systems add synapses to the deafferented field at a rate 2.9 synapses per 100 μm^2 per day over the period 20–96 h postlesion. (The rate is higher still 30–48 h postlesion.) Moreover, the reinnervation is accomplished without any slowing of the normal pace of synaptogenesis within the inner molecular layer (Gall et al. 1980).

Two important conclusions can be drawn from these data. First, the abnormally high rate of synaptogenesis within the deafferented field demonstrates that the commissural-associational afferents are capable of forming new contacts at a rate in excess of that seen in normal development. Secondly, the concurrence of the rapid reinnervation of the outer molecular layer with a normal pace of innervation in the inner molecular layer indicates that the rate of synapse formation by components of the same afferent system, and possibly collaterals of the same axon, can vary depending on the "local conditions" within the target region.

The importance of local conditions in determining the rate of synapse formation can also be argued on the basis of the shape of normal innervation and post-deafferentation reinnervation curves. The normal innervation of the molecular layer has been reported to be much more rapid early in development, when the synaptic density is low, than is the case somewhat later even though during this later interval a large proportion of the total innervation is yet to be realized (Crain et al. 1973; McWilliams et al., in prep.) Similarly, in the case of the inner molecular layer reinnervation following removal of commissural input in the adult, the rate of synaptogenesis slowed as reinnervation progressed (McWilliams and Lynch 1979). In the case of outer molecular layer deafferentation by entorhinal ablation in the 14-day old rat, the initial pace of reinnervation was quite rapid: synapses were added at a rate of 4 SB/100 μm^2/day during the interval 20–48 h postlesion while 48–96 h a gain of 2.1 synapses per 100 μm^2/

day was observed. Again the rate was most rapid when the local synaptic density was lowest and slowed as reinnervation progressed.

The results suggest that a kind of density inhibition may play a major role in dictating the rate of synaptogenesis during normal development as well as during sprouting in the adult and immature brain. The question whether developmental factors also influence the pace with which sprouting adds synapses has not yet been adequately resolved; answers will require a careful analysis of the rate of reinnervation in dendritic zones which have been deafferented to the same extent in animals of different ages.

5 Comment

The above described results indicate that sometime after the first week of postnatal life a fundamental change occurs in the hippocampus such that a rapid, extensive form of sprouting is replaced by a slower restricted version (Fig. 4). Understanding the cellular mechanisms behind these changes should serve to explain much about the nature of growth responses in the adult brain. For purposes of discussion we will group the factors potentially responsible for the shift from the immature to mature forms of sprouting into variables intrinsic and extrinsic to the sprouting axon although, as will be evident, this dichotomy cannot be considered absolute.

Extrinsic Factors. It is at least logically possible that, as far as growth is concerned, axons retain their immature properties into adulthood but that these become increasingly regulated by factors in the neuropil (e.g., by the dendrites or glial cells). However, this hypothesis in its strictest sense appears to be excluded by the experiments showing that the adult and immature variants of the sprouting response are both present at 14 dpn. There is, however, reason to suspect that a modified version of the idea

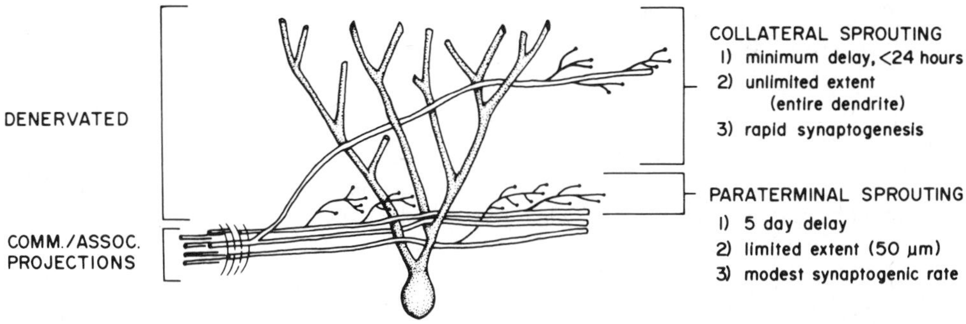

Fig. 4. The two forms of axon sprouting exhibited by the commissural afferents to the dentate gyrus of the rat. The more extensive form, here labeled "Collateral Sprouting", predominates with entorhinal lesion placement during the first week of life, whereas the more limited form, labeled "Paraterminal Sprouting", is the only form of axonal growth seen with similar deafferentation in the adult rat. Both types of adjustment are present following deafferentation in the 14-day old rat, suggesting that the maturational state of the individual axons determines the pattern of their sprouting response

may be correct. It was noted in the introduction that sprouting in the adult hippocampus begins at about the same postlesion time as the astroglial cells undergo a marked change in their morphology (Rose et al. 1976) and phagocytotic activity decreases (McWilliams and Lynch 1979). While our studies on astroglial ontogeny are still incomplete, the data that we have collected thus far indicate that the appearance and maturation of these cells corresponds reasonably well with the development of the mature version of sprouting. Astroglia migrate into hippocampus at the end of the first week of postnatal life and from day 10 on begin the elaboration of their dendritic arbors (Gall, Ishibashi, and Lynch, unpubl.). Possibly then the delay in the onset of the sprouting response recorded for the mature hippocampus reflects an inhibitory effect of the hypertrophied astroglial cells. This, however, would have to occur in conjunction with a change in the sprouting fibers such that they become responsive to the glial reaction since, as described, some axons at 14 dpn appear to ignore any limits on their collateralization. The available data, then, can be gathered into the following "working" hypothesis: *axonal maturation renders the sprouting process sensitive to the activities of the astroglial cells.* Further and more detailed analyses of the time courses for the development of both the astroglia (and their hypertrophic response to denervation) and sprouting should strengthen this hypothesis or eliminate it altogether. It may also prove to be possible to manipulate the development of the astroglial population and, if so, test for predicated effects on sprouting.

Intrinsic Factors. As discussed, the evidence suggests that at least some part of the effects of maturation on sprouting is due to changes in the properties of the growing fibers. But what these changes might be remains totally unexplored; this question, in fact, raises the much broader and poorly understood issue of which mechanisms are used by development to stop growth under normal circumstances (i.e., what is maturity).

It has been suggested that axonal maturation consists of a slowing and cessation of elongation accompanied by an increase in the diameter of the fiber (cf. Lasek and Hoffman 1979). It has also been noted that the neurofilaments make their appearance during this maturational period (Peters and Vaughn 1967). The addition of neurofilaments could serve to "stabilize" the cytoskeleton and its relationship to the membrane; perhaps relevant to this, severed axons in hippocampus (Gall, McWilliams, and Lynch, unpubl.) and elsewhere in the brain (Schoenfeld et al. 1979) disappear extremely quickly in 7-dpn animals but persist for days or weeks in older ones. Possibly then the addition of specific cytoskeletal elements such as neurofilaments renders the axon more stable and hence less able to emit collateral and paraterminal branches. According to this idea, sprouting in the adult requires the removal of the conditions which caused the fiber to stop elongating and collateralizing during the late developmental period. This does not necessarily imply that sprouting in the adult is a simple resurrection of axonal growth as seen in the neonate; the relationship of the mature parent branch to its "sprout" is certain to be different from that which exists between the various aspects of a developing axonal arborization.

References

Crain B, Cotman C, Taylor D, Lynch G (1973) A quantitative electron microscopic study of synaptogenesis in the dentate gyrus of the rat. Brain Res 63: 195–204

Gall C, Lynch G (1978) Rapid axon sprouting in the neonatal rat hippocampus. Brain Res 153: 357–362

Gall C, Lynch G (1980) The regulation of fiber growth and synaptogenesis in the developing hippocampus. In: Hunt RK (ed) Current topics in developmental biology 15: 159–180

Gall C, Lynch G (1981) Fiber architecture of the dentate gyrus following ablation of the entorhinal cortex in rats of different ages: Evidence for two forms of axon sprouting in the immature brain. Neuroscience, in press

Gall C, McWilliams R, Lynch G (1979a) The effect of collateral sprouting on the density of innervation of normal target sites: Implications for theories on the regulation of the size of developing synaptic domains. Brain Res 175: 37–47

Gall C, McWilliams R, Lynch G (1979b) Maturational changes in the dynamics of postlesion axonal growth in the dentate gyrus of the rat. Anat Rec 193: 554

Gall C, Rose G, Lynch G (1979c) Proliferative and migratory activites of glial cells in the partially deafferented hippocampus. J Comp Neurol 183: 539–550

Gall C, McWilliams R, Lynch G (1980) Accelerated rates of synaptogenesis by "sprouting" afferents in the immature hippocampal formation. J Comp Neurol 193: 1047–1062

Lasek R, Hoffman P (1978) The neuronal cytoskeleton, axonal transport, and axonal growth. In: Goldman P, Pollard I, Rosenbaum J (eds) Cell motility. Cold Spring Harbor Laboratories, New York, pp 1021–1049

Lee K, Stanford E, Cotman C, Lynch G (1977) Ultrastructural evidence for bouton proliferation in the partially deafferented dentate gyrus of the adult rat. Exp Brain Res 29: 475–485

Lynch G, Cotman CW (1975) The hippocampus as a model for studying anatomical plasticity in the adult brain. In: Issacson R, Pribram K (eds) The hippocampus, vol I. Plenum Publ Co, New York, pp 123–155

Lynch G, Stanfield B, Cotman C (1973) Developmental differences in postlesion axonal growth in the hippocampus. Brain Res 59: 155–168

Lynch G, Gall C, Cotman C (1977) Temporal parameters of axon sprouting in the brain of the adult rat. Exp Neurol 54: 179–183

Matthews DA, Cotman C, Lynch G (1976) An electron microscopic study of lesion-induced synaptogenesis in the dentate gyrus of the adult rat: I: Magnitude and time course of degeneration. Brain Res 115: 1–21

McWilliams JR, Lynch G (1978) Terminal proliferation and synaptogenesis following partial deafferentation: The reinnervation of the inner molecular layer of the dentate gyrus following removal of its commissural afferents. J Comp Neurol 180: 581–615

McWilliams JR, Lynch G (1979) Terminal proliferation in the partially deafferented dentate gyrus: Time course for the appearance and removal of degeneration and the replacement of lost terminals. J Comp Neurol 187: 191–198

Peters A, Vaughn JE (1967) Microtubules and filaments in the axons and astrocytes of early post natal rat optic nerves. J Cell Biol 32: 113–119

Rose G, Cotman CW, Lynch G (1976) Hypertrophy and redistribution of astrocytes in the deafferented hippocampus. Brain Res Bull 1: 87–92

Schoenfeld T, Street C, Leonard C (1979) Maturation of Wallerian degeneration: An EM study in the developing olfactory tubercle. Neurosci Abstr 5: 177

Zimmer J (1973) Extended commissural and ipsilateral projections in postnatally de-entorhinated hippocampus and fascia dentata demonstrated in rats by silver impregnation. Brain Res 64: 293–311

Formation and Regression of Synaptic Contacts in the Adult Muscle

A. WERNIG, A.P. ANZIL, and A. BIESER[1]

1 Sprouting and Synapse Formation in Adult Muscles Under Abnormal Conditions

1.1 Motoneurone Sprouting

A large amount of information has been accumulating over the last 30 years indicating that the *adult* motoneuron is capable of producing extensive peripheral sprouting under a variety of conditions. Sprouts can reoccupy abandoned synaptic sites, form new ones, or might remain or be withdrawn without forming synaptic contacts. Such abnormal outgrowth of branches, which was first described after partial denervation of a muscle (van Harreveld 1945; Weiss and Edds 1945; Edds 1950; Hoffman 1950), includes collateral sprouts which originate from the nodes of Ranvier, preterminal sprouts and sprouts from the endplate itself ('ultraterminal' sprouts). Consequently, when searching for sprouts most investigators have been looking for nerve branches which appear "abnormal" in the sense that they leave the vicinity of the parent endplate and do not regularly occur under normal conditions (see Sect. 2.1). This is demonstrated in Fig. 1, which shows a typical endplate from a normal mouse muscle (Fig. 1A) and an endplate after local application of tetanus toxin (Fig. 1B); in the latter unusual branches are present (*arrows*) which leave the endplate area, often to reach neighboring muscle fibers (cf. Duchen and Tonge 1973).

Such unusual sprouting has been observed after blockade of transmitter release by presynaptically acting substances [like tetanus toxin and botulinum toxin (Duchen and Strich 1968; Duchen and Tonge 1973) see Fig. 1B] and blockade of propagation of the action potential (by tetrodotoxin applied to the axons) quite remote from the synapse (Brown and Ironton 1977). Partial denervation of a muscle (e.g., Haimann et al. 1976; Brown and Ironton 1978; for a review see Edds 1953), or even denervation of nearby muscles (Rotshenker 1979), also results in extensive sprouting of the remaining motoneurons. Barker and Ip (1966), and Brown et al. (1978) found unusual sprouting after cutting the dorsal roots supplying a muscle. It is not quite clear whether or not interruption of synaptic transmission by blocking acetylcholine receptors causes sprouting (Pestronk and Drachman 1978; Holland and Brown 1980; Wernig et al. 1980a).

A common feature of the above-mentioned investigations appears to be that some or all of the muscle fibers in a muscle (or a nearby muscle) are inactivated over a cer-

1 Max-Planck-Institut für Psychiatrie, Kraepelinstraße 2, 8000 München 40, FRG

tain period of time (owing to anatomical or functional denervation), or are at least reduced in activity (presumably after deafferentation.). From this fact it can be concluded that the muscle fiber's activity "controls" the production of diffusable substances which trigger or inhibit sprouting by the motoneuron. This idea seems rather well supported by findings that direct muscle stimulation in such cases prevents the production of massive sprouting (Brown and Holland 1979). It has been pointed out that some of these conditions could suggest that factors released from the nerve rather than from the muscle control motoneuron sprouting (Guth 1968).

In autonomic ganglia there is evidence for an influence of the *postsynaptic* cell in sprouting of the presynaptic neuron (see Purves and Lichtman 1978).

In addition, it is important to note the evidence for the sprout-inducing capability of locally acting products of nerve degeneration and phagocytosis (Hoffman 1950; Brown et al. 1978; see also Cangiano et al. 1977). These last findings might indicate that abnormal sprouting is a more general reaction of the motoneuron to a *number* of stimuli. This notion could account for the increase in numbers of terminal branches observed after repeated injection of albumine-Ringer solution (Pestronk and Drachman 1978) or lipids (Tweedle and Kabara 1977) into the muscle or, e.g., application of cholinesterase blocking agents (Schwartz et al. 1977).

Also, it is noteworthy that besides their transmitter blocking action tetanus and botulinum toxins like axotomy and application of colchicine (which induces sprouting of untreated cells from contiguous areas in the peripheral sensory system; Diamond et al. 1976; and in the hippocampus, Goldowitz and Cotman 1980) all produce chromatolysis of motoneurons (Watson 1968, 1969; Schubert et al. 1973; Dimpfel and Habermann 1973). Axotomy and botulinum increase protein and RNA synthesis in the motoneurons (Watson 1968, 1969) and there is, as well, retraction of the dendrites and substantial loss of presynaptic boutons (Blinzinger and Kreutzberg 1969; Sumner 1977). Qualitatively similar changes occur after colchicine (Hansson and Norström 1971; Schubert et al. 1972), but the studies of the central effects of tetanus toxin leave this point unresolved.

Partial denervation produces functional changes in the unsevered ipsilateral motoneurons (Huizar et al. 1977); contralateral central glial changes have even been reported after nerve section (Watson 1972), which could be of significance in the contralateral sprouting (Rotshenker 1979).

At this stage it is not clear whether these changes in motoneurons are general responses to diverse stimuli or whether they have a close association with the axon growth and sprouting which accompany these various procedures.

1.2 New Formation of Synaptic Contacts

It has repeatedly been reported that after total or partial muscle denervation, reinnervating axons form contacts at the sites of the former endplates (Hoffman 1950; Letinsky et al. 1976; Sanes et al. 1978; Burden et al. 1979). It is quite clear, however, that there is a number of situations in which synapses form at sites on the muscle fiber which did not bear a contact before: this is the case whenever a foreign or the original nerve is implanted into denervated muscle at some distance from the original endplate region (e.g., Frank et al. 1975; Kuffler et al. 1977; Tonge 1977, 1978; Lömo and

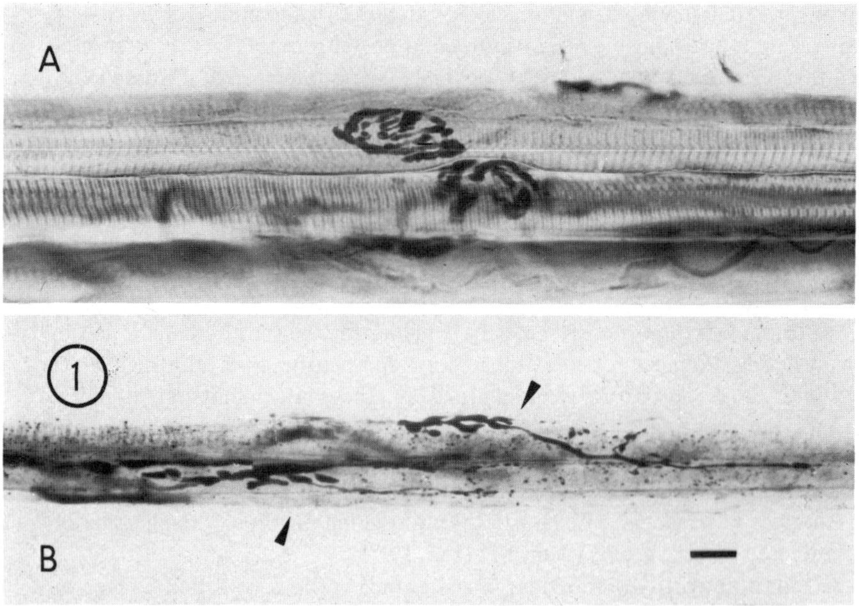

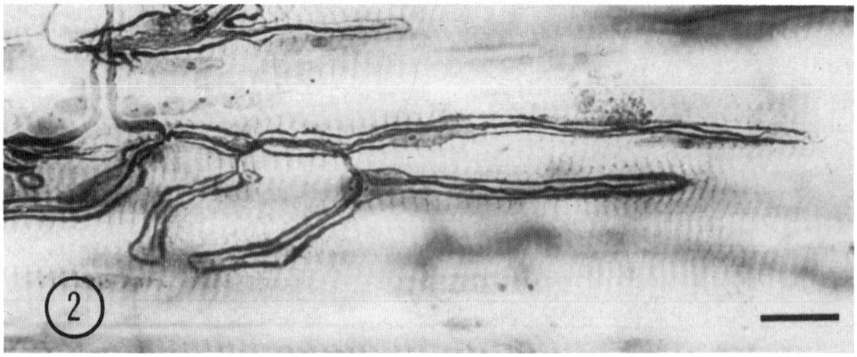

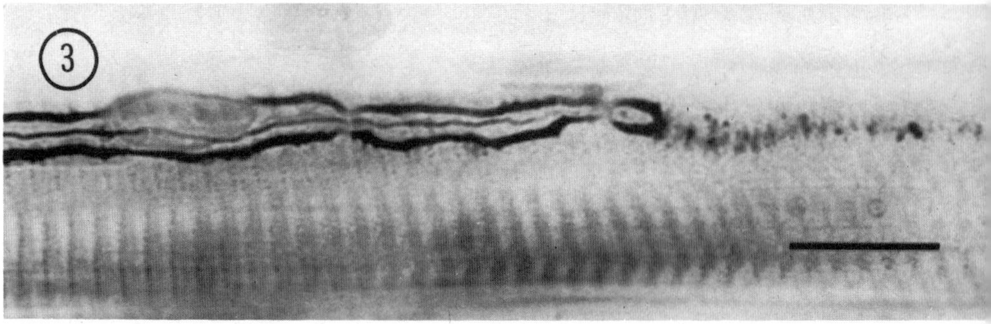

Figs. 1–3

Slater 1978, 1980a,b; Cangiano et al. 1980; Lömo 1980) or after sprouting from the endplate, e.g., after application of botulinum toxin (Duchen 1971, 1973).

Clearly then, the muscle fibers also retain the ability to form typical synaptic contacts during adult life. It is likely that in the adult muscle fiber the formation of secondary clefts occurs considerably later than other features of synaptic contacts (e.g., Duchen 1971, 1973; Koenig 1973); as in embryological development (Teräväinen 1968) secondary clefts probably start as fingerlike membrane indentations which gradually change in size and shape to reach the mature state. In this way morphologists are provided with a "measure" indicating the maturity of a synaptic contact.

2 Signs of Nerve Sprouting and Regression in Muscle of Normal Adult Animals

It is clear from the facts discussed above that the adult mature motoneuron can show extensive sprouting. An attractive idea that follows these observations is that the neuromuscular junction is not at all a static structure but is permanently undergoing some remodeling which could include nerve sprouting, synapse formation and nerve regression with abandoning of synaptic contacts.

2.1 Mammalian Muscle

There is a limited number of reports of sprouting in normal, untreated mammalian muscle in the literature of the last 20 years. Barker and Ip (1966) for example reported the presence of 'abnormal' nerve branches, similar to those described after partial muscle denervation, in normal and deafferented muscles of otherwise untreated mammals (cat, rabbit, rat). Since signs of synapse degeneration were also found in normal muscles, the authors suggested that normally endplates degenerate after a limited lifespan and are replaced by others, which – it is claimed – form at the site of the old endplate or outside it. Counting the number of collaterals contributing to a single

Fig. 1A, B. Teased muscle fibers of mouse soleus (Zn-J-Os staining). **A** Normal endplate, **B** 7 days after local injection into the calf of a high dose of tetanus toxin (~100 × MLD 50) which was 30 min later followed by ~20 I.U. tetanus antitoxin (i.v.). (This is a convenient method to obtain sprouting.) Scale: 10 μm

Fig. 2. 'Normal' synapse on frog cutaneus pectoris muscle after a combined staining of axons (silver) and ChE. The stained argyrophylic elements of the axon delineate the nerve terminal arborizations. With the ChE stain used (Karnovsky and Roots 1964), the reaction product predominantly develops at the lateral edges of the synaptic gutters where these are occupied by presynaptic elements (nerve or Schwann cell). Thus a double line of ChE reaction product accompanies the nerve branches where they presumably are in close contact with the muscle fiber. Bar: 10 μm (Wernig et al. 1980a)

Fig. 3. ChE remnants without axon in distal prolongation of a normal part of the synapse. Bar: 20 μm (Pecot-Dechavassine et al. 1979)

muscle fiber's synapse in cats of different ages, Tuffery (1971) took a more quantitative approach and found their number increasing with age of the animal. Brown and co-workers regularly find apparently similar sprouts in normal muscles (Brown and Ironton 1977, 1978; Brown et al. 1978; Brown and Holland 1979; Holland and Brown 1980). While Duchen (1971, 1973) has provided cogent ultrastructural evidence for formation of new synapses after toxin treatment, apparently no such investigations have been performed on sprouts in normal muscles. Also none of these authors acknowledged the possibility that sprouts might originate and also terminate *within* the complex of a single endplate and would thus not be counted as 'collateral', 'preterminal', or 'ultraterminal' sprouts. Consequently then, no clear information is available about numbers of terminal branches per synapse in animals of different ages, which would be bound to provide a direct measure for sprouting (see below). In fact most investigations on sprouting in *abnormal* situations (see above) ignore the possibility that the number of 'normal'-looking branches constituting an endplate might reflect the degree of sprouting in this synapse (see However Pestronk and Drachman 1978).

2.2 Frog Muscle

In the mammalian neuromuscular synapse a variable number of usually short nerve branches occupy a small area on the muscle fiber (see Fig. 1A), a fact which allows one to talk, strictly, about an 'endplate'. It is quite different in the frog neuromuscular junction where the terminal arborizations may extend over several hundred micrometers and where individual branches are quite separate from each other. One would expect that 'local' processes of nerve sprouting and regression in this synapse would correspondingly be more accessible to observation. In a combined axon and cholinesterase (ChE) staining, which is particularly useful for studying those questions (Wernig et al. 1980a), axon branches in a synapse are usually found to be more or less continuously followed by ChE reaction product (Fig. 2); this indicates that synaptic transmission is continuously present along such branches. When synapses stained with this method are examined in finer detail, striking deviations from the usual picture can be observed.

2.2.1 Signs or Nerve Regression

ChE reaction product is present within the complex of the synapse but not in association with axonal elements (Letinsky et al. 1976; Wernig et al. 1980a,b). The reaction product is either arranged in a single broad band or in a band of palisades (Fig. 3). Such spots are usually located at the distal or proximal end of a synaptic contact of normal appearance or – less frequently – not directly connected to a normal synaptic site. These localizations immediately suggest that ChE is present at sites from which the nerve has retracted or into which the nerve is destined to grow. Serial sections through such a site (Fig. 4) reveal that ChE is located in the depth of a secondary cleft (Fig. 5). Since secondary clefts are only present in mature synapses this site undoubtly is an abandoned synaptic site from which the nerve and the Schwann cell have retracted. Retraction of nerves from synaptic contacts appears to be a local event since other parts in the same synapse retain their normal ultrastructure and retain normal function

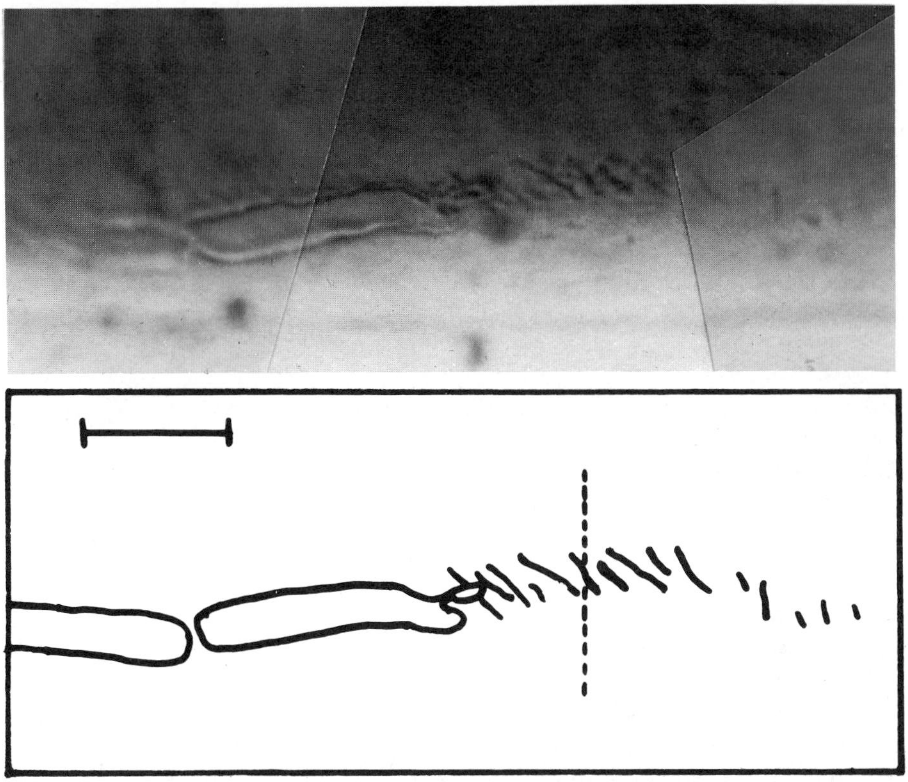

Fig. 4. Light micrograph and camera lucida drawing of the distalmost portion of a synaptic contact followed by ChE remnants (ChE stain only). The *stippled* line indicates the about site where the section shown in Fig. 5 was taken from. Bar = 10 μm (Wernig et al. 1981b)

(Wernig and Bieser, unpubl.). One or several abandoned sites within a synapse are by no means infrequent and were found in as many as 50% of the synapses on muscles in which the extent of ChE remnants ranged from a few to some hundred microns (Wernig et al. 1980a,b)

2.2.2 Signs of Sprouting and New Synapse Formation

The other striking feature observable after combined axon and ChE staining is the arrangement of ChE in one or several small circles rather than continuously along terminal branches (Fig. 6); occasionally the very distal ends of branches are devoid of recognizable amounts of ChE (Wernig et al. 1980a,b). There is good evidence that at least some of those branches are sprouts with newly formed synaptic contacts. In serial sections prepared from such branches, small synaptic sites were observed at which – as a clear sign of immaturity – secondary clefts were either completely absent (Fig. 8C,F), or in a state of early development (Wernig et al. 1981a). This is demonstrated in

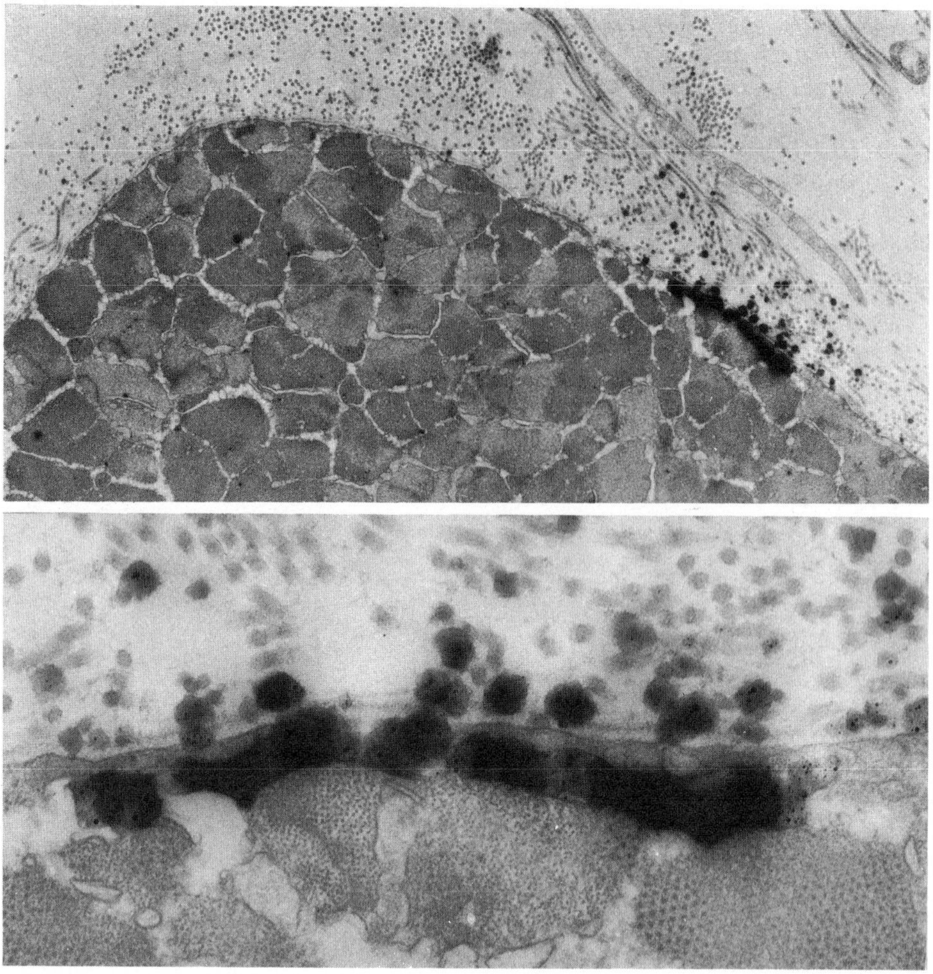

Fig. 5. Electron micrographs showing a secondary cleft filled with ChE reaction product at the abandoned synaptic site visible in Fig. 4. (12250×, 63750×) (Wernig et al. 1981b)

Fig. 8; which shows representative electron micrographs from serial sections performed on the distalmost part (to the left) of a presumed sprout (Fig. 7).

In the frog, growth in length of the animal continues nonlinearly throughout life (Hk. Müller, pers. comm.), and with this growth significant increases in synapse length and in number of nerve branches per synapse take place (unpublished). Since the enlargement of synapses most likely occurs by means of sprouting, it can be regarded as a common event which takes place more or less continuously. Quite apart from any ontogenetic causes, however, sprouting and nerve regression seem to be controlled also by external factors (cf. Wernig et al. 1980a,b). No information is yet available as to the time course of these changes. Nor is it known yet whether and in what way sprouting

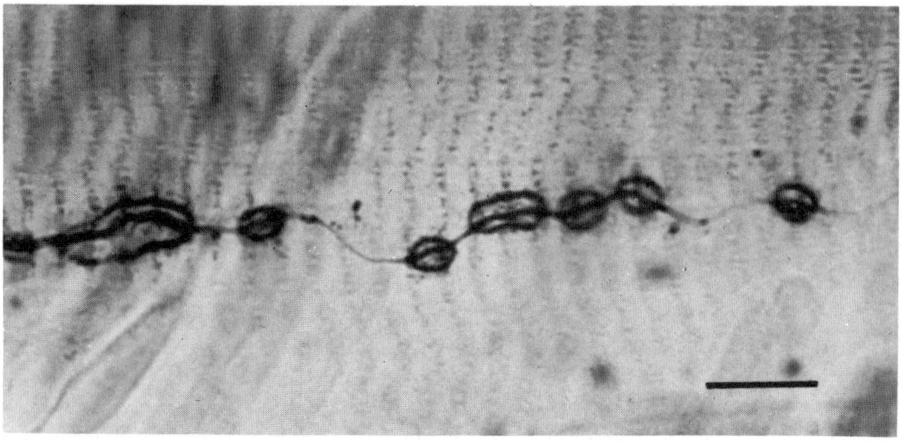

Fig. 6. Presumed nerve sprout. Combined axon and ChE stain. Bar = 10 μm

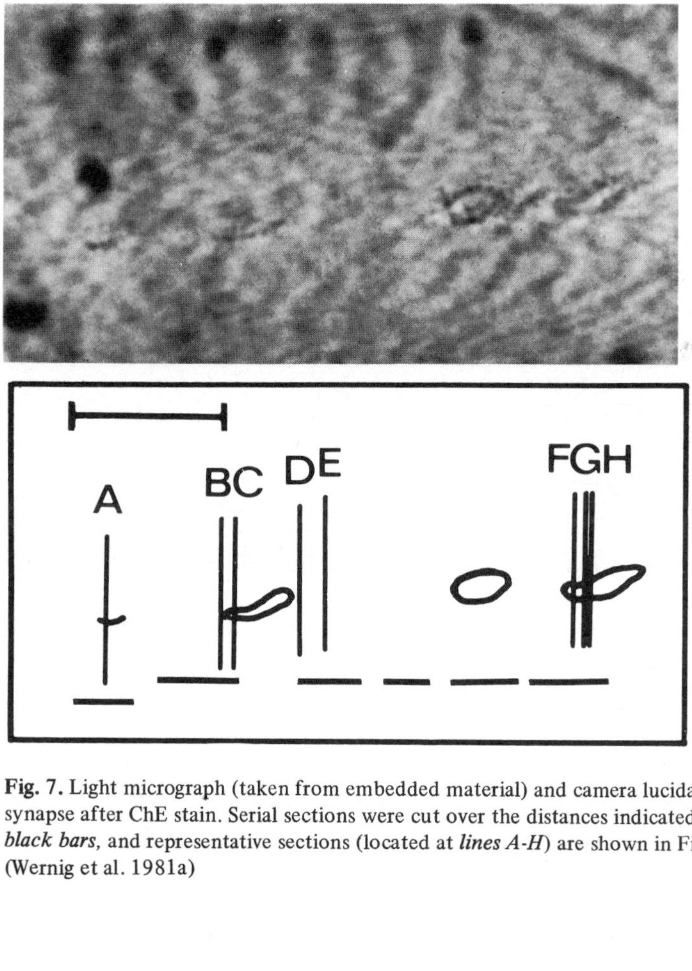

Fig. 7. Light micrograph (taken from embedded material) and camera lucida drawing of part of a synapse after ChE stain. Serial sections were cut over the distances indicated by the *horizontal black bars*, and representative sections (located at *lines A-H*) are shown in Fig. 8. Bar = 10 μm (Wernig et al. 1981a)

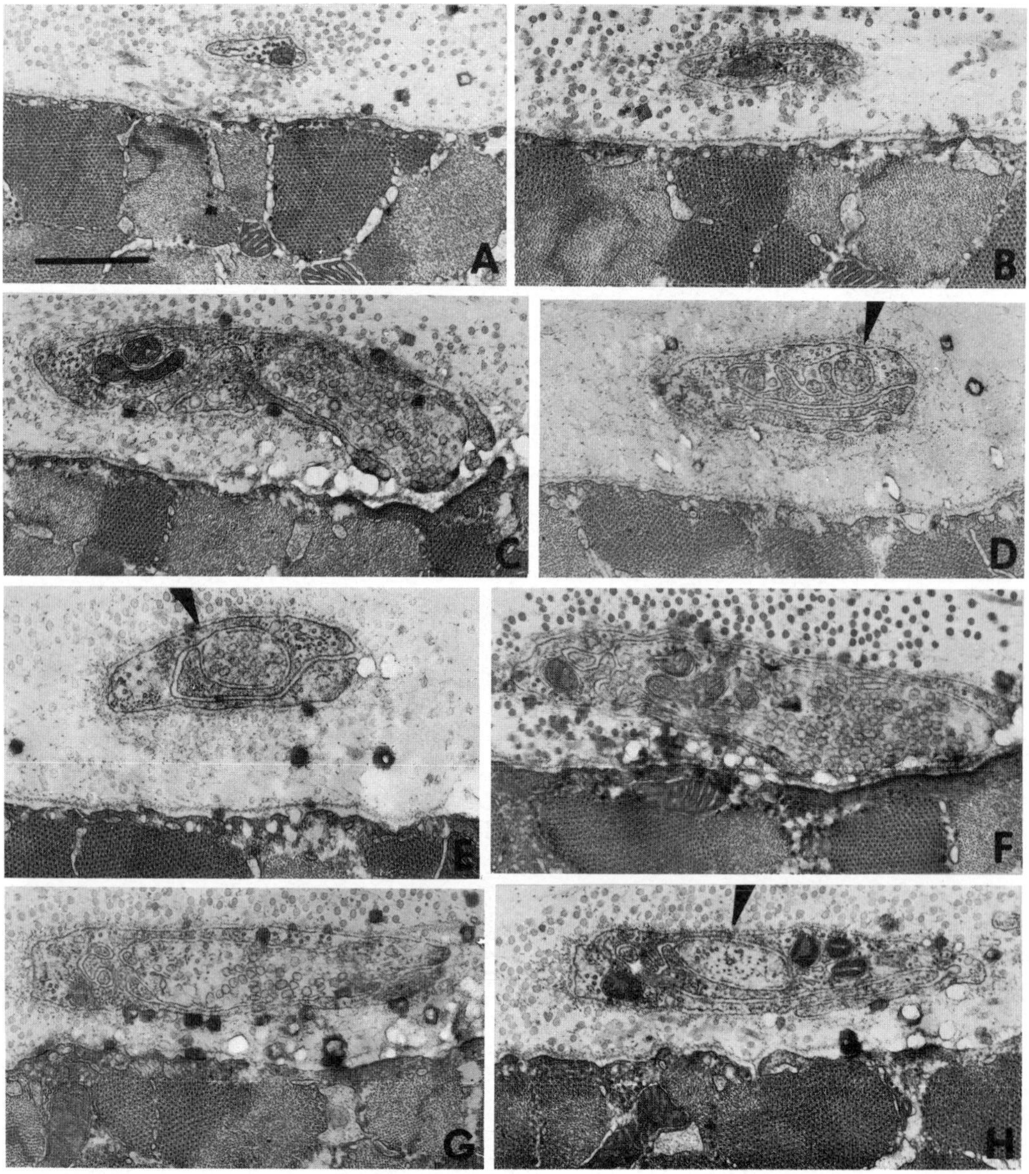

Fig. 8A–H. Selected electron micrographs of serial sections through a presumed nerve sprout (*lines A-H* in Fig. 7). *Arrowheads* point out axon profiles. Bar = 0.5 μm (Wernig et al. 1981a)

is related to nerve regression. The equal presence of ChE remnants in equivalent amounts (proportion of total synapse length) in muscles of differently sized animals (unpublished results) is best explained by assuming that some continuous remodeling of synapses takes place with nerve regression, on the one hand, and sprouting and new synapse formation and possibly reoccupation of abandoned gutters, on the other.

3 Conclusions

The hypothesis is put forward, based on the findings in frog muscles, that in the neuromuscular synapse there is normally continual sprouting of nerve terminals with new formation of synaptic contacts leading to increases in the complexity of individual synapses with time. Synapses are further remodeled in that the nerve retracts from certain contacts within a synapse, forms contacts at new sites and can reoccupy previously abandoned ones. Since this sprouting is confined to the area of the synapse, it will be called "intraterminal" sprouting. It is likely that external factors determine the degree and the rate at which these changes occur. A part of this hypothesis is that "abnormal" sprouting (e.g., after partial muscle denervation) is caused by an excess of physiological conditioning stimuli or still other, imbalancing, factors impinging on the motoneuron.

The marked longitudinal extent of the frog synapse as compared with any mammalian nerve muscle synapse might just make ongoing changes more obvious and thus accessible to simple measurements. Also, these changes might occur to a greater extent in poikilotherm animals because they are more susceptible to environmental influences. No directly comparable observations have been reported from mammalian synapses but the reasons for this might be manifold. Nevertheless, there are a few findings (discussed in Sect. 2.1) which hint at possible similarities. While abandoned synaptic gutters with ChE remnants have not been described, Barker and Ip (1966), Tuffery (1971) and Ip (1974) found features 'resembling degeneration' to be present in normal muscles of cat, rabbit, and rat. Confirmation of these light microscopic findings by corresponding ultrastructural observations is still lacking. From different intensities of ChE stain within a single endplate (and between endplates within a muscle) Ip (1974) suspected that endplates are heterogeneous structures.

Ultrastructural evidence for formation of new synaptic contacts in an endplate of *normal* mammalian muscle is also lacking. Nevertheless, an increase with age of the animal in the average number of collaterals contributing to an endplate has been observed in cat muscle (Tuffery 1971) and also an increase in endplate size (Nyström 1968), and the latter is likely to occur by 'intraterminal' nerve sprouting. The numbers and the length of unmyelinated nerve branches within a synapse should be clear indicators of sprouting; it is not clear from published results whether and in which way these parameters change with age in mammalian muscles. Apart from this, the question could be clarified by electron microscopical observation of serial sections cut through individual endplates.

There is an apparent discrepancy between the present hypothesis and the observations that after implantation into a normally innervated muscle a foreign nerve usually cannot induce synapse formation. Recent findings by Bixby and van Essen (1979) indicate that this might not be true for sites inside the endplate region where foreign nerve synapses *can* form. This, and the restriction of nerve terminal arborizations to circumscribed areas on the muscle fiber, might indicate that formation of new synaptic contacts in the normal muscle fiber is confined to this region. After functional or anatomical denervation this zone spreads to include the whole muscle fiber membrane.

Acknowledgments. The authors thank Theresa Gruber, Susanne Luh, and Brigitte Wernig for their contributions to this work. J.J. Carmody was helpful with preparing this manuscript.

References

Barker D, Ip MC (1966) Sprouting and degeneration of mammalian motor axons in normal and deafferentated skeletal muscle. Proc R Soc London Ser B 163: 538–554

Bixby JL, van Essen DC (1979) Competition between foreign and original nerves in adult mammalian skeletal muscle. Nature (London) 282: 726–728

Blinzinger K, Kreutzberg G (1968) Displacement of synaptic terminals from regenerating motoneurons by microglial cells. Z Zellforsch 85: 145–157

Brown MC, Holland RL (1979) A central role for denervated tissues in causing nerve sprouting. Nature (London) 282: 724–726

Brown MC, Ironton R (1977) Motor neuron sprouting induced by prolonged tetrodotoxin block of nerve action protentials. Nature (London) 265: 549–561

Brown MC, Ironton R (1978) Sprouting and regression of neuromuscular synapses in partially denervated mammalian muscles. J Physiol 278: 325–348

Brown MC, Holland RL, Ironton R (1978) Degnerating nerve products affect innervated muscle fibres. Nature (London) 275: 652–654

Burden SJ, Sargent PB, McMahan UJ (1979) Acetylcholine receptors in regenerating muscle accumulate at original synaptic sites in the absence of the nerve. J Cell Biol 82: 412–425

Cangiano A, Lutzemberger L, Nicotra L (1977) Non-equivalence of impulse blockade and denervation in the production of membrane changes in rat skeletal muscle. J Physiol 273: 325–348

Cangiano A, Lömo T, Lutzemberger L, Sveen O (1980) Effects of chronic nerve conduction block on formation of neuromuscular junctions and junctional AChE in the rat. Acta Physiol Scand in press

Diamond J, Cooper E, Turner C, Macintyre L (1976) Trophic regulation of nerve sprouting. Science 193: 371–377

Dimpfel W, Habermann E (1973) Histoautoradiographic localisation of ^{125}I-labelled tetanus toxin in rat spinal cord. Naunyn-Schmiedeberg's Arch Pharmacol 280: 177–182

Duchen LW (1971) An electron microscopic study of the changes induced by botulinum toxin in the motor end-plates of slow and fast skeletal muscle fibres of the mouse. J Neurol Sci 14: 47–60

Duchen LW (1973) The effects of tetanus toxin on the motor end-plates of the mouse – an electron microscopic study. J Neurol Sci 19: 153–167

Duchen LW, Strich SJ (1968) The ffects of botulinum toxin on the pattern of innervation of skeletal muscle in the mouse. Q J Exp Physiol 53: 84–89

Duchen LW, Tonge DA (1973) The effects of tetanus toxin of neuromuscular transmission and on the morphology of motor endplates in slow and fast skeletal muscle of the mouse. J Physiol 228: 157–172

Edds MV (1950) Collateral regeneration of residual motor axons in partially denervated muscles. J Exp Zool 113: 517–552

Edds MV (1953) Collateral nerve regeneration. Q Rev Biol 28: 260–276

Frank E, Jansen JKS, Lömo T, Westgaard RH (1975) The interaction between foreign and original motor nerves innervating the soleus muscle of rats. J Physiol 247: 725–743

Goldowitz D, Cotman CW (1980) Do neurotrophic interactions control synapse formation in the adult rat brain. Brain Res 181: 325–344

Guth L (1968) "Trophic" influences of nerve on muscle. Physiol Rev 48: 645–687
Haimann C, Mallart A, Zilber-Gachelin NF (1976) Competition between motor nerves in the establishment of neuromuscular junctions in striated muscles of *Xenopus laevis*. Neurosci Lett 2: 15–20
Hansson HA, Norström A (1971) Glial reactions induced by colchicine-treatment of the hypothalamic-neurohypophyseal system. Z Zellforsch 113: 294–310
Hoffman H (1950) Local re-innervation in partially denervated muscle: a histophysiological study. Aust J Exp Biol Med Sci 28: 383–397
Holland RL, Brown MC (1980) Postsynaptic transmission block can cause terminal sprouting of a motor nerve. Science 207: 649–651
Huizar P, Kuno M, Kudo N, Miyata Y (1977) Reaction of intact spinal motoneurones to partial denervation of the muscle. J Physiol 265: 175–191
Ip MC (1974) Some morphological features of the myoneural junction in certain normal muscles of the rat. Anat Rec 180: 605–616
Karnovsky MJ, Roots L (1964) A "direct-coloring" thiocholine method for cholinesterases. J Histochem Cytochem 12: 219–221
Koenig J (1973) Morphogenesis of motor end-plates "in vivo" and "in vitro". Brain Res 62: 361–435
Kuffler D, Thompson W, Jansen JKS (1977) The elimination of synapses in multiply-innervated skeletal muscle fibres of the rat: dependence on distance between end-plates. Brain Res 138: 353–358
Letinsky MS, Fischbeck KH, McMahan UJ (1976) Precision of reinnervation of original postsynaptic sites in frog muscle after a nerve crush. J Neurocytol 5: 691–718
Lömo T (1980) The role of impulse activity in the formation of neuromuscular junctions. In: Taxi J (ed) Ontogenesis and functional mechanisms of peripheral synapses. Elsevier, Amsterdam pp 327–334
Lömo T, Slater CR (1978) Control of acetylcholine sensitivity and synapse formation by muscle activity. J Physiol 275: 391–402
Lömo T, Slater CR (1980a) Control of junctional acetylcholinesterase by neural and muscular influences in the rat. J Physiol 303: 191–202
Lömo T, Slater CR (1980b) Acetylcholine sensitivity of developing ectopic nerve-muscle junctions in adult rat soleus muscles. J Physiol 303: 173–189
Nyström B (1968) Postnatal development of motor nerve terminals in "slow-red" and "fast-white" cat muscles. Acta Neurol Scand 44: 363–383
Pecot-Dechavassine M, Wernig A, Stöver H (1979) A combined silver and cholinesterase method for studying exact relations between the pre- and the postsynaptic elements at the frog neuromuscular junction. Stain Technol 54: 25–28
Pestronk A, Drachman DB (1978) Motor nerve sprouting and acetylcholine receptors. Science 199: 1223–1225
Purves D, Lichtman JW (1978) Formation and maintenance of synaptic connections in autonomic ganglia. Physiol Rev 58: 821–862
Rotshenker S (1979) Synapse formation in intact innervated cutaneous pectoris muscles of the frog following denervation of the opposite muscle. J Physiol 292: 535–547
Sanes JR, Marshall LM, McMahan UJ (1978) Reinnervation of muscle fiber basal lamina after removal of myofibers. J Cell Biol 78: 176–198
Schubert P, Kreutzberg GW, Lux HD (1972) Neuroplasmic transport in dendrites: effect of colchicine on morphology and physiology of motoneurones in the cat. Brain Res 47: 331–343
Schwartz MS, Sargent MK, Swash M (1977) Neostigmin-induced end-plate proliferation in the rat. Neurology 27: 289–293
Sumner BEH (1977) Ultrastructural responses of the hypoglossal nucleus to the presence in the tongue of botulinum toxin, a quantitative study. Exp Brain Res 30: 313–321
Teräväinen H (1968) Development of the myoneural junction in the rat. Z Zellforsch 87: 249–265
Tonge DA (1977) Effect of implantation of an extra nerve on the recovery of neuromuscular transmission from botulinum toxin. J Physiol 265: 809–820
Tonge DA (1978) Prolonged effects of a post-synaptic blocking fraction of "naja siamensis" venom on skeletal muscle of the mouse. Q J Exp Physiol 63: 33–47

Tuffery RA (1971) Growth and degeneration of motor end-plates in normal cat hind limb muscles. J Anat 110: 221–247

Tweedle CD, Kabara JJ (1977) Lipophilic nerve sprouting factor(s) isolated form denervated muscle. Neurosci Lett 6: 41–46

Van Harreveld D (1945) Reinnervation of denervated muscle fibres by adjacent functioning motor units. Am J Physiol 144: 477–493

Watson WE (1968) Observations on the nucleolar and total cell body nucleic acid of injured nerve cells. J Physiol 196: 655–676

Watson WE (1969) The response of motor neurones to intramuscular injection of botulinum toxin. J Physiol 202: 611–630

Watson WE (1972) Some quantitative observations upon the responses of neuroglial cells which follow axotomy of adjacent neurones. J Physiol 225: 415–435

Weiss P, Edds MV (1945) Spontaneous recovery of muscle following partial denervation. Am J Physiol 145: 587–607

Wernig A, Pecot-Dechavassine M, Stöver H (1980a) Sprouting and regression of the nerve at the frog neuromuscular junction in normal conditions and after prolonged paralysis with curare. J Neurocytol 9: 277–303

Wernig A, Pecot-Dechavassine M, Stöver H (1980b) Signs of nerve regression and sprouting in the frog neuromuscular synapse. In: Taxi J (ed) Ontogenesis and functional mechanisms of peripheral synapses. Elsevier, Amsterdam, pp 225–238

Wernig A, Anzil AP, Bieser A (1981a) Light and electron microscopic identification of a nerve sprout in muscle of normal adult frog. Neurosci Lett 21: 261–266

Wernig A, Anzil AP, Bieser A, Schwarz U (1981b) Abandoned synaptic sites in muscles of normal adult frog. Neurosci Lett (in press)

Morphological and Physiological Effects of Axotomy on Cat Abducens Motoneurons

R. BAKER, J. DELGADO-GARCIA, and R. McCREA[1]

1 Introduction

In order to better understand the mechanisms underlying trophic relationships between pre- and postsynaptic elements in respect to neuronal recognition and specificity, the response of mature neurons to axonal section and/or injury is a question of basic importance. There have been many metabolic, anatomic and electrophysiological reviews of injured neurons, which have described specific features of the cellular reaction to axotomy as well as alterations in synaptic transmission (Cragg 1970; Lieberman 1971; Matthews and Nelson 1975; Kuno 1976; Purves and Lichtman 1978; Purves and Noja 1978). The cat abducens nucleus offers an unparalleled substrate in the vertebrate for correlative physiological and ultrastructural studies because its afferent organization is well understood and the functional activity of its constituent neurons during eye movement have been discussed in detail (Baker and McCrea 1979). The morphological and physiological integrity of abducens motoneurons following axotomy and during reinnervation are of interest because these cells are representative cranial motoneurons, and as such they may be compared to prior work on spinal and hypoglossal motoneurons in order to identify general, as opposed to unique, properties of injured cells. The present study has assessed the synaptic and electrophysiological properties of abducens motoneurons including their morphology following axotomy. In addition, physiological excitability and functional synaptic transmission have been examined in the alert behaving cat and correlated with the above observations to further specify the truly "adaptive" features of axotomy.

2 Methods

Experiments were carried out in 16 cats (10 acute, 4 chronic, and 2 for electron microscopy). In all experiments the left VIth nerve was sectioned peripherally in the orbit within 1 mm of lateral rectus muscle innervation. No attempt was made to prevent

1 Department of Physiology and Biophysics, New York University Medical Center, 550 First Avenue, New York, NY 10016, USA

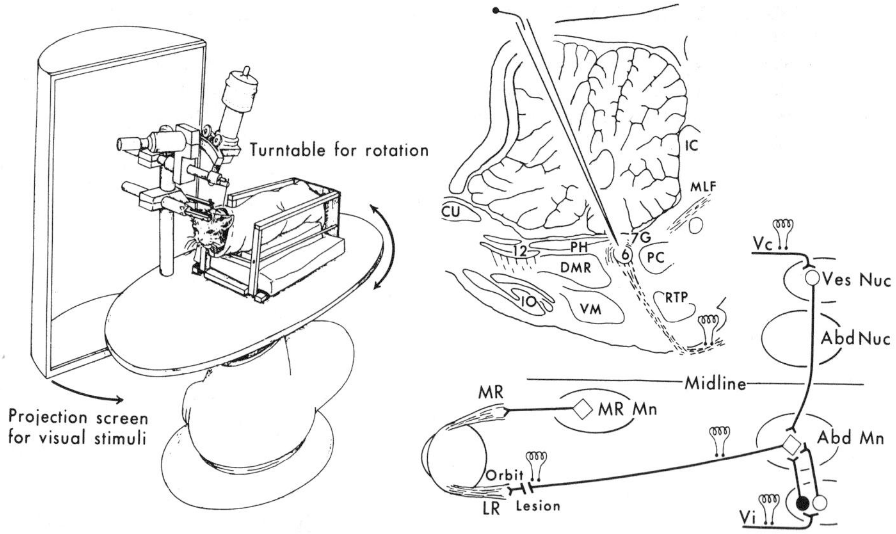

Fig. 1. Experimental paradigm and synaptic connections. On the *left,* head rotation and/or other visual stimuli could be employed as indicated in the alert restrained cat. Access to the VIth nucleus was via a microelectrode angled 30° to the sagittal plane as shown *in the middle.* The inset on the *lower right* illustrates the inhibitory (*filled circle*) and excitatory (*open circles*) vestibular connections to the left abducens nucleus. In all experiments, the VIth nerve was lesioned peripherally near its innervation of the lateral rectus muscle. Stimulation points are indicated

reinnervation, nor was the lateral rectus muscle either injured or removed. In eight experiments the muscle tendon was disinserted from the globe to facilitate clean nerve resection with no apparent differences in the findings. As shown in the schematic diagram in Fig. 1, the bilateral vestibular nerves were electrically stimulated as well as the VIth nerve centrally via an electrode situated about 1 cm from the abducens nucleus. The disynaptic inhibitory and excitatory vestibular pathways to the abducens nucleus have been described (Baker et al. 1969; Schwindt et al. 1973). Access to the abducens nucleus was via the approach shown in the schematic sagittal section. In four chronic experiments a tungsten microelectrode was positioned in the abducens nucleus with the assistance of the antidromic field potential. In the chronic experiments the cats were tested every day for (1) threshold for antidromic activation, (2) maximum amplitude of the field with head rotation in both directions, and (3) excitability changes during saccades and eccentric fixations. Intracellular recordings were obtained from motoneurons with glass microelectodes containing 4 M K acetate and/or a solution containing 10% HRP dissolved in 0.1 M Tris buffer and 0.5 M KCl with electrical impedances of 10–20 MΩ. For visualizing motoneurons injected with HRP, cats were perfused with 1% paraformaldehyde and glutaraldehyde mixture and the reaction product visualized via use of DAB and cobalt chloride.

3 Results and Discussion

The average cat abducens nucleus contains about 1000 motoneurons and 600 internuclear neurons (Spencer and Sterling 1977). The soma-dendritic trees of these neurons are intermingled throughout the nucleus and they share common synaptic input (Baker and McCrea 1979). The major morphological reaction of higher vertebrate neurons to axotomy is that associated with the metabolic event of breaking up of Nissl bodies and the movement of the nucleus of the cells to an eccentric position in the cell body (Watson 1970). These morphological changes were not obvious in adult axotomized abducens motoneurons nor was there any evidence of cell death as has been observed in the superior cervical ganglion and hypoglossal nucleus (see Purves and Lichtman 1978).

3.1 Synaptic Physiology

Undoubtedly, the most significant cellular modification that has been reported following axotomy is the depression of synaptic transmission reported in a variety of vertebrate neurons such as hypoglossal, sympathetic, parasympathetic, and spinal (Eccles et al. 1958; Kuno and Llinas 1970a,b; Sumner 1973, 1975a,b; Mendell et al. 1974, 1976; Purves 1975; Farel 1978; Purves and Thompson 1979). In nearly all the above cases excitatory synaptic transmission was affected. The cat abducens nucleus offers the unique advantage of testing both a potent disynaptic excitatory (EPSP) and an inhibitory synaptic influence (IPSP) on abducens motoneurons. Ten acute experiments ranging 4–20 days following axotomy were carried out before initiating the behavioral work illustrated in Figs. 6 and 7. The extracellular field potential profile of vestibular-evoked excitation (Vc) and inhibition (Vi) is shown in Fig. 2A. In C the intracellular correlates of the field potentials are shown as an EPSP (Vc) and IPSP (Vi). The records in B and D were obtained in the contralateral (left) abducens nucleus 5 days following axotomy of the left VIth nerve. As indicated by the *crossing arrows,* the contralateral vestibular (Vc) extracellular negativity (A and B) and the disynaptic EPSP (C and D) were relatively unchanged. Quite in contrast, comparison of the same set of records for ipsilateral vestibular nerve stimulation (Vi), showed that the inhibition of abducens motoneurons was completely absent. The above was true for 10/10 abducens motoneurons penetrated in that experiment. The complete absence of vestibular inhibition up to 10 days following the axotomy is shown in Fig. 3A, B for another abducens motoneuron in which stimulation of the ipsilateral vestibular nerve produced a disynaptic EPSP of short latency (utricular, see Schwindt et al. 1974) and the typical disynaptic Vc EPSP. Notably, the EPSP's from either ipsi- or contralateral vestibular stimulation were nearly unaltered in (a) rise time, (b) amplitude, and (c) decay from those recorded in normal abducens motoneurons. In addition, membrane polarization produced no visible indication of inhibition; however, in the same experiment the disynaptic Vi EPSP in some motoneurons was followed by membrane hyperpolarization (control in C), which upon the application of a hyperpolarizing current (-15 nA) and depolarizing current (+20 nA) clearly revealed an IPSP. In this experiment (i.e., day 10) 15 abducens motoneurons were penetrated and tested with K acetate electrodes

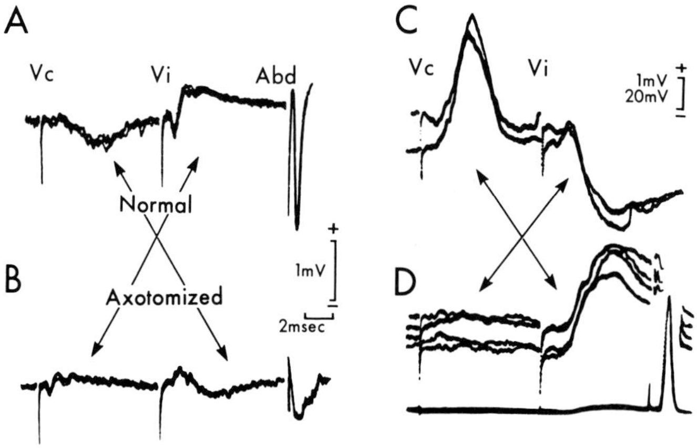

Fig. 2A–D. Extra- and intracellular synaptic potentials in the normal and five day axotomized cat abducens nucleus. **A, C** Records from the normal (right) and **B, D** from the axotomized (left) abducens nucleus. The ***crossing arrows*** facilitate comparison of contralateral (*Vc*) and ipsilateral vestibular (*Vi*) synaptic potentials in the two conditions. Time and voltage calibrations are as indicated for the extracellular (**A, B**) and intracellular (**C, D**) records

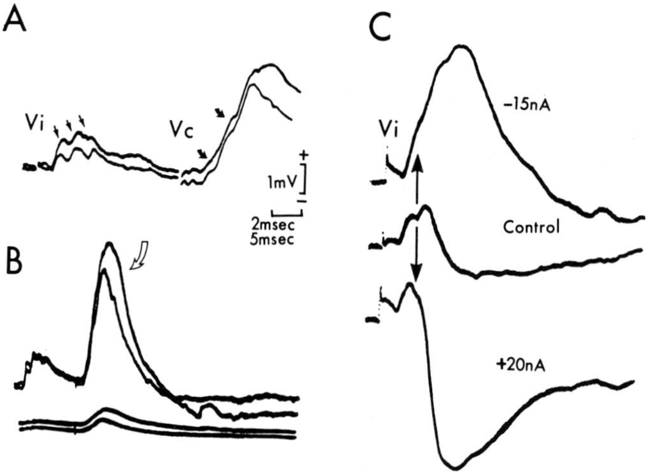

Fig. 3A–C. Intracellular records from abducens motoneurons 10 days after axotomy. **A, B** Disynaptic excitation from utricular nerve (*Vi*) and contralateral (*Vc*) semicircular canal stimulation at fast (**A**) and slow (**B**) sweep speeds to illustrate rise time and course of the synaptic potentials, respectively. **C** An intracellular record from another abducens motoneuron in which the disynaptic EPSP is followed by a membrane hyperpolarization which upon application of depolarizing (+20 nA) and hyperpolarizing (−15 nA) current indicates an IPSP

for the presence of IPSPs. Eight motoneurons were found without IPSP's (like in A) and 7 with IPSPs (like in C).

In conclusion, these results demonstrated that during the entire time course of axotomy there was little modification in excitatory vestibular synaptic transmission to abducens motoneurons (see Fig. 6); however, there was a remarkable alteration in the ipsilateral vestibular inhibitory pathway to the extent that for a brief interval (up to about 8 days) there was complete absence of inhibition. Yet, the inhibition returned gradually (as shown for day 10 in Fig. 3) and essentially was near normal by day 20. These data contrast with all other axotomy studies in that for the first time a selective modification of inhibitory transmission, as opposed to excitatory synaptic transmission, has been found. Secondly, as indicated in Fig. 3B, there was not any evidence for an increase in dendritic excitability, as a matter of fact dendritic and/or partial spike responses were not recorded. Thirdly, since prior electrophysiological studies and more recent intracellular HRP studies have demonstrated that the ipsilateral vestibular inhibitory pathway is largely localized to the soma and proximal dendrites of abducens motoneurons, we can assume that there was relatively selective stripping of these synaptic boutons from abducens motoneurons. This explanation is consistent with the original description by Blinzinger and Kreutzberg (1968) for facial motoneurons and spinal neurons (Hamberger et al. 1970; Chen et al. 1977; Chen 1978). In two experiments HRP was injected into axotomized abducens motoneurons and the soma and proximal dendritic trees were covered with fibrillar astrocytic processes including a reduction in the number of synapses by 50%–60% from normal (Delgado-Garcia et al. 1978). The removal of inhibitory, not excitatory, boutons contrast with those removed from hypoglossal motoneurons in which presynaptic losses were presumably excitatory (Sumner 1975a,b). Although the mechanisms for such synaptic loss and its recovery after axotomy are not well understood (cf. Matthews and Nelson 1975), we believe it does not play a causative role in the excitability changes observed in abducens motoneurons (described below and mentioned in other studies; Farel 1979). However, the synaptic loss and excitability change may result from the same cellular metabolic sequence enlarged on in later discussion.

3.2 Electrophysiology

As illustrated in Fig. 2B (and compared to A), the amplitude of the antidromic field potential, especially the negativity, was remarkably reduced (even absent in two cases) as early as 4 days following axotomy. Figure 4 shows an intracellular record from an abducens motoneuron 6 days after axotomy. Even though the resting potential was in the normal range (50–60 mV) there was failure of antidromic invasion and only a spike in the medullated axon (M-spike) could be recorded (see arrows in A and B). Its amplitude and time course was normal for abducens motoneurons (see Grantyn and Grantyn 1978). As shown in B, membrane depolarization (via DC current) permitted antidromic invasion to occur at a given threshold level. In contrast to spinal motoneurons, the lowest safety factor for antidromic invasion in extraocular motoneurons is between the medullated axon (M) and initial segment (IS; the latter includes both the nonmedullated axon and axon hillock) as opposed to the IS – soma-dendritic (SD) compartment (Baker and Precht 1972; Grantyn and Grantyn 1978). These findings suggested that the excitability of the initial segment had been decreased, and further evidence was found in the records shown in C in which the application of a step depolarizing current initiated IS-SD spikes at nearly the same threshold level as that required for combining the antidromic activation (M-spike) with membrane depolariza-

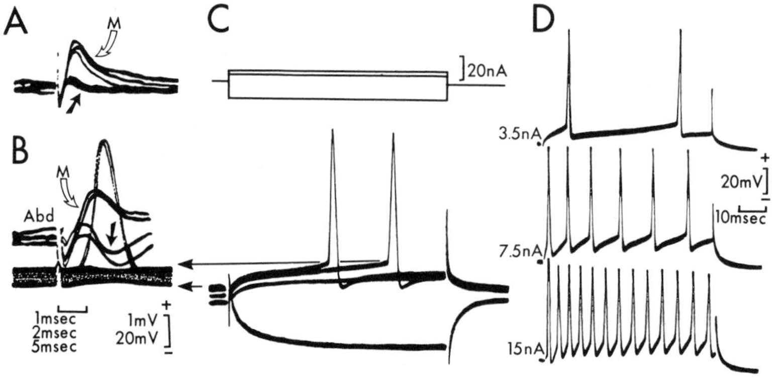

Fig. 4A–D. Antidromic and direct current activation of abducens motoneurons 5 days after axotomy. **A–C** Intracellular records from the same abducens motoneuron. **A** At axon stradling intensity and normal resting potential, the M spike is shown by the *arrow*. **B** At a faster sweep speed, the high gain trace shows the all or none M spike compared to the field potential (*filled arrow*). A step of DC current depolarizes the motoneuron from the level indicated by the *lower arrow* until antidromic initial segment-somadendritic invasion takes place. **C** Two steps of depolarizing and one of hyperpolarizing currrent with intensities indicated in the *upper part* of the figure. The *arrows* comparing **B** and **C** indicate that the threshold for spike initiation is nearly identical. The slope input impedance of this motoneuron was 2 MΩ. **D** Response of a 7-day axotomized abducens motoneuron to 3.5, 7.5, and 15 nA steps of depolarizing current. Discussion in text

tion (compare the arrows connecting B and C). Also, it was not possible to distinguish the IS from the SD component in the directly activated spikes. The range of input impedances in acutely axotomized abducens motoneurons was little different from that reported by Grantyn and Grantyn (1976, 1978; e.g., the motoneuron in Fig. 4 was a 2 MΩ). Not enough neurons were sampled to assess whether the larger input impedances and membrane time constants found by Gustafsson (1979) in axotomized spinal motoneurons are also reflected in abducens motoneurons.

The above decrease in excitability was first noticed in spinal motoneurons by Eccles et al. (1958), described in detail in sympathetic ganglion by Hunt and Riker (1966) and more recently elaborated on in frog spinal motoneurons by Farel (1978). Thus, one may postulate that the excitability change in the initial segment area is common to all classes of neurons studied to date. In spite of this striking change in IS excitability, the axotomized abducens motoneurons responded with repetitive spikes to constant current injections in a nearly normal fashion. Figure 4D shows three current levels, and the interspike voltage trajectories in respect to both scoop and ramp (see Grantyn and Grantyn 1976) were relatively normal. Notably, the first interspike intervals were shorter and the abducens motoneuron reached an adapted state with maintained discharge frequency in 40–50 ms. No obvious changes in after-hyperpolarization (amplitude or time course) and/or frequency-current plots were noted. If anything, the motoneurons tended to be slightly less excitable, as shown by the cell in Fig. 4D (13 spikes per nA at adapted frequency). Given the absence of any large increases in dendritic excitability, the responses of abducens motoneurons are quite comparable to those recently described for spinal motoneurons by Gustafsson (1979) and Mendell et al. (1974, 1976). The important question to be addressed was whether any of the above subtle modifications in electrical properties of motoneurons (as extensively described by Gustafsson 1979) might reflect changes which could be visualized in the alert behaving animal during the normal physiological operation of motoneurons, and whether maintenance of any of the above-mentioned alterations and/or properties were dependent on functional contact with the lateral rectus muscle (Huizar et al. 1975, 1977). Before carrying out the experiments in the alert animal, it was necessary to answer two intriguing questions regarding the morphology of axotomized versus normal motoneurons.

3.3 Morphology

Sumner and Watson (1971) and Sumner (1975a,b) have contended that motoneurons undergo dendritic retraction following axotomy, and re-expansion following re-innervation in the hypoglossal nucleus. In view of normal synaptic potentials and the dendritic location of excitatory synapses as well as electrotonic properties of abducens motoneurons our data suggested that this might not be the case in the abducens nucleus. To examine this possibility we intracellularly injected HRP in pairs of motoneurons in the normal and axotomized nuclei in six experiments to compare soma-dendritic geometry following reconstruction (Fig. 5). Clearly, there did not appear to be any dendritic retraction, nor was there, as indicated by the microphotograph of the axotomized motoneuron, any alteration (or distortion) in cellular size and/or dendritic shape. Although this work needs to be extended in a more quantitative fashion, visual inspection of the material leads to the conclusion that abducens motoneurons do not experience marked retraction and expansion of dendritic trees following axotomy.

Secondly, given the alteration in initial segment electrical properties it would have been nice, but admittedly surprising, to find a morphological correlate at the light microscope level, which in this case might have been expected to be some slight swelling of the initial segment area (especially the nonmyelinated axon). However, comparison of our six pairs of cells indicated, if anything at all, that the axotomized motoneurons exhibited less initial segment-axon hillock area than normal. Clearly, this places the mechanism of excitability modification at a more sophisticated experimental level than that employed in the present studies. Just as the membrane-associated dense material of the postsynaptic site, which is thought to include bouton attachment among its functions, is lost, so also may be the density of Na channel receptor protein and/or undercoating in the initial segment. The likelihood of the above changes in protein occurring at the receptor surface is high because injured neurons have been shown to reduce synthesis of materials related to synaptic transmission (see Reis, this book). Thus, while the neuron is reorganizing itself, the detachment of synapses and decrease in IS excitability (two unrelated physiological events but correlative from the metabolic viewpoint) stress the hierarchial importance of the need to produce other protein than that associated with membrane surface function.

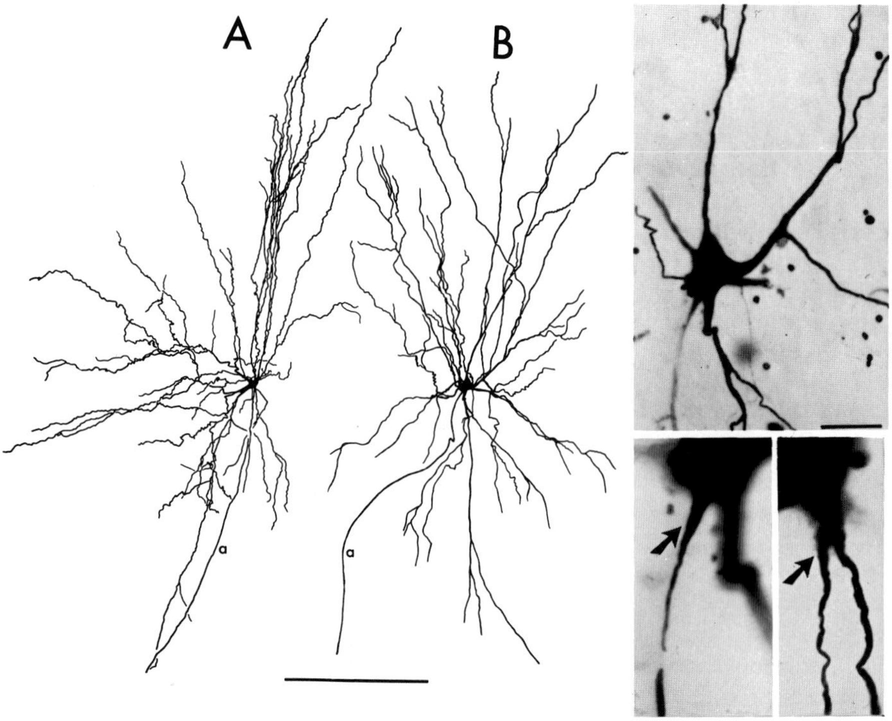

Fig. 5. Microphotograph and reconstruction of a normal (**A**) and axotomized (**B**) abducens motoneuron within the same experiment. The microphotographs *on the right* (from top to bottom) illustrate the normal appearance of the somadendritic tree in the axotomized abducens motoneuron and then compares the initial segment morphology. The calibration bar in **A** and **B** is 0.5 mm, and 50 μ in the inset

3.4 Behavioral Physiology

In four cats a Tungsten microelectrode was positioned superficially (dendritic location) into the abducens nucleus. As shown by the gliosis in the morphological inset in Fig. 7 (arrow), the electrode in the best experiment was located in the posterior dorsomedial aspect of the abducens nucleus. Electrical stimulation of the VIth nerve induced a typical positive-negative field potential (Fig. 6) which at a double shock interval of 0.75 ms selectively blocked the second negative field (IS-SD invasion). Clearly, in the alert cat, the amplitude of this antidromic negativity was reduced to more than 90% within 5 days following axotomy (see inset B at 10 days). Significantly, both the peak of the positive and negative fields had a slightly longer latency, which is consistent with alterations in conduction velocity reported by others (Kuno et al. 1974; Mendell et al. 1976). The above depression in excitability was quite noticeable because in the normal alert cat more than 50%–75% of the abducens motoneurons exhibit a tonic discharge with forward directed gaze, yet the axotomized abducens nucleus was nearly quiescent. The question of whether the absence of spike generation is a desirable (i.e., adaptive)

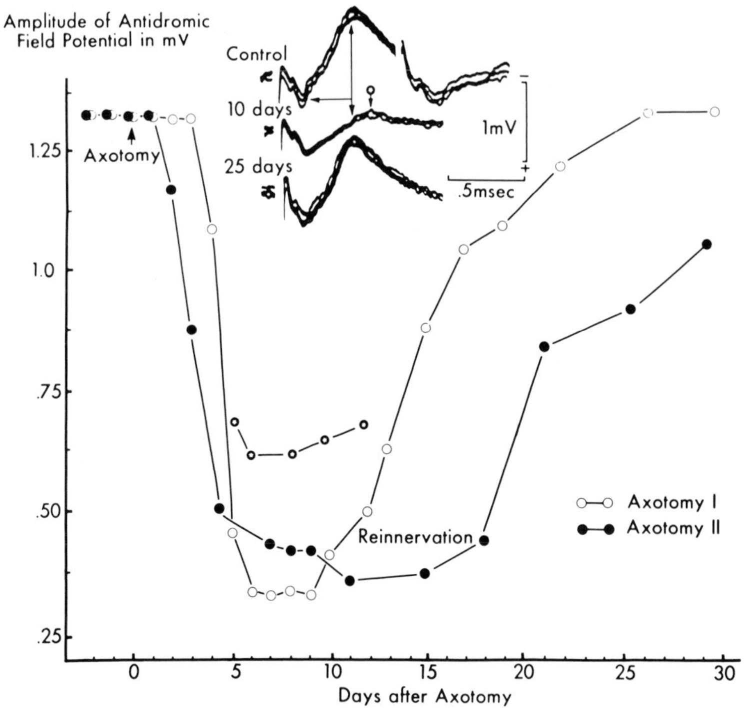

Fig. 6. Amplitude of the antidromic field potential in the abducens nucleus from axotomy to reinnervation. On the ***abscissa*** is days following axotomy and on the ***ordinate*** is the amplitude of the antidromic field potential in mV. The insets in the ***center*** of the figure show the amplitude of the control field potential including blockage of the antidromic negativity following a short interval double shock stimulation (0.75 ms). The amplitude of the field potential at 10 days (peak effect) and at 25 days (recovery) are shown following the first axotomy (*Axotomy 1*). The ***second arrow*** indicates the shift in latency for the antidromic negativity and, as plotted below, a decrease in amplitude

physiological correlate to the absence of muscle innervation, or if it is the consequence of simple metabolic events, cannot yet be answered. However, the above findings reduce the attraction for prior reasoning in which increases in dendritic excitability were suggested as being necessary to maintain normal neuronal excitability in the face of excitatory synaptic bouton loss. Especially in view of the findings that either inhibition and/or excitation may be lost but, in general, motoneuronal excitability (at initial segment only) is reduced. In fact, the above findings disassociate any direct physiological correlation between the synaptic events and the excitability modification. It, therefore, appears that at least in all the cranial motoneurons examined to date (including some with axon collaterals; Evinger et al. 1979) there are significant changes in physiological sensitivity.

Whatever the underlying reason for the excitability change, the remarkable finding demonstrated for the first tim is its complete recovery including return of synaptic connections in such a short time following lesion of the VIth nerve (Fig. 6). The be-

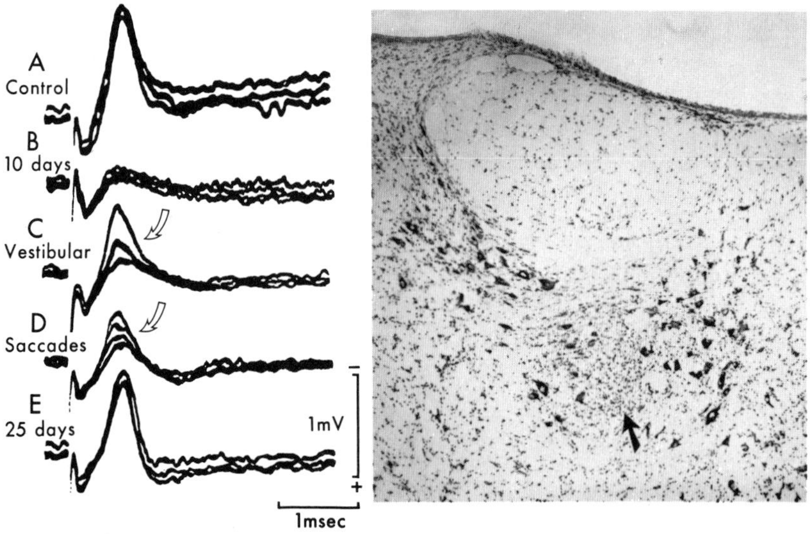

Fig. 7A–E. Modulation of abducens field potential during head rotation and saccadic activity including location of the recording microelectrode in the abducens nucleus. **A** Control, **B** 10 days after axotomy, **C** increase in amplitude of the field potential with head rotation to the right, **D** increase with saccades and fixation to the left, **E** recovery after 25 days. The microphotograph *on the right* illustrates location of the recording electrode near the posterior and central part of the left abducens nucleus. The gliosis is marked by an *arrow*

ginning of recovery within 10 to 15 days following axotomy is much sooner than the 25–50 days reported in the spinal cord by Kuno et al. (1974). Although eye movements have not been quantified yet, it is clear that this recovery in excitability begins long before functional normality has returned to the lateral rectus muscle. As suggested by Kuno et al. (1974), restoration of electrical and synaptic properties begins in motoneurons, and is returned to near normal, long before restoration of normal muscle function. In the above experiment a second axotomy was performed and, as indicated in Fig. 6, the same sequence of events but with somewhat altered time course occurred, suggesting that the rules which govern and underlie the changes in connectivity and excitability are reasonably well specified. We have observed this sequence of events after axotomy in two chronic animals and the depression in excitability for all four. The relative extent to which motoneuronal excitability alters the performance of the abducens motoneurons is much greater than that suggested from the relatively minor change in electrical and discharge properties (firing frequency curves in Fig. 4) and/or synaptic physiology (shown in Figs. 2 and 3) because as illustrated in Fig. 7 even high velocity head rotations to the right or saccades and fixations in eccentric gaze positions (C and D) could not increase excitability enough for more than antidromic invasion of about 50% of the motoneuronal population. As yet, we have not assessed whether the severity of the effect of axotomy is entirely dependent on retrograde trophic signals from the muscles or depends, in part, on peripheral motoneuronal sprouting and reinnervation (Huizar et al. 1975, 1977).

4 Conclusions

Morphological and physiological studies were carried out to evaluate the integrity of abducens motoneurons following axotomy and during reinnervation.

1. From 4 to 20 days following axotomy a marked reduction in antidromic field potential of the VIth nucleus was observed. Intracellular studies indicated a failure of antidromic invasion between the medullated and initial segment, probably due to a decrease in membrane excitability in the non-medullated axon and hillock area.
2. Somatically located vestibular IPSP's were nearly completely removed in axotomized motoneurons from 4 to 7 days; however, they gradually returned coincident with reinnervation over a period of 10–20 days. Proximal and distally located vestibular EPSP's remained with little noticeable alteration in time course and amplitude and without large changes in dendritic excitability.
3. Intracellular HRP injections in normal and axotomized motoneurons showed little change in soma-dendritic morphology at the light microscope level. Retraction and expansion of the dendritic tree as well as any noticeable difference in the initial segment area were absent.
4. Although the cellular electrical properties and firing frequency to constant current injection were not altered very much in the anesthetized cat, abducens motoneurons were relatively quiescent in the alert cat following axotomy. The antidromic field potential remained largely depressed even though normal physiological stimuli such as head rotation and attempted eccentric fixation did produce some increase in excitability.
5. The modification in initial segment excitability and alterations in synaptic input which paralleled the axotomy to re-innervation stage were significant, but it was not possible to conclude whether they were, adaptive, or, epi-phenomenological, in nature (i.e., simply the end effect of alteration in cell surface protein due to metabolic events).
6. Yet it does appear though that the excitability and synaptic input alterations can be disassociated physiologically. Increases in dendritic excitability are apparently not utilized as a mechanism to offset the loss of excitatory synaptic boutons on the soma of the cells in order to maintain normal motoneuronal operation. On the contrary motoneuronal activity is reduced.
7. Plasticity of the above changes was demonstrated by the recovery of both physiological and morphological properties of abducens motoneurons following axotomy. This suggests that the physiological and biochemical sequelae are important cellular processes and may provide a useful model for further studying trophic relationships in the mature mammalian central nervous system.

References

Baker R, McCrea R (1979) The parabducens nucleus. In: Asanuma H, Wilson V (eds) Integration in the nervous system. Igakaku Shoin Ltd, New York, pp 97–122

Baker R, Precht W (1972) Electrophysiological properties of trochlear motoneurons as revealed by IVth nerve stimulation. Exp Brain Res 14: 127–157

Baker RG, Mano N, Shimazu H (1961) Postsynaptic potentials in abducens motoneurons induced by vestibular stimulation. Brain Res 15: 577–580

Blinzinger K, Kreutzberg G (1968) Displacement of synaptic terminals from regenerating motoneurons by microglial cells. Z Zellforsch 85: 145–157

Chen DH (1976) Qualitative and quantitative study of synaptic discplacement in chromatolyzed spinal motoneurons of the cat. J Comp Neurol 177: 635–664

Chen DH, Chambers WW, Liu CN (1977) Synaptic displacement in intracentral neurons of Clarke's nucleus following axotomy in the cat. Exp Neurol 57: 1026–1041

Cragg BG (1970) What is the signal for chromatolysis? Brain Res 23: 1–21

Delgado-Garcia J, Baker R, Alley K, McCrea R (1978) Anatomy and physiology of axotomized cat abducens motoneurons. Neurosci Abstr 4: 602

Eccles JC, Libet B, Young RR (1958) The behaviour of chromatolysed motoneurons studied by intracellular recording. J Physiol 143: 11–40

Evinger C, Baker R, McCrea RA (1979) Axon collaterals of cat medial rectus motoneurons. Brain Res 174: 153–160

Farel PB (1978) Reflex activity of regenerating frog spinal motoneurons. Brain Res 158: 331–341

Grantyn R, Grantyn A (1978) Morphological and electrophysiological properties of cat abducens motoneurons. Exp Brain Res 31: 249–274

Grantyn R, Grantyn A, Schaaf P (1977) Conduction velocity, input resistance and size of cat ocular motoneurons stained with Procion yellow. Brain Res 135: 167–173

Gustafsson B (1979) Changes in motoneurons electrical properties following axotomy. J Physiol 293: 197–215

Hamberger A, Hansson HA, Sjöstrand J (1970) Surface structure of isolated neurons. Detachment of nerve terminals during axon regeneration. J Cell Biol 47: 319–331

Heyer CB, Llinás R (1977) Control of rhythmic firing in normal and axotomized cat spinal motoneurons. J Neurophysiol 40: 480–488

Huizar P, Kuno M, Miyata Y (1975) Differentiation of motoneurons and skeletal muscles in kittens. J Physiol 252: 465–479

Huizar P, Kuno M, Kudo N, Miyata Y (1977) Reaction of intact spinal motoneurones to partial denervation of the muscle. J Physiol 265: 175–191

Hunt CC, Riker WK (1966) Properties of frog sympathetic neurons in normal ganglia and after axon section. J Neurophysiol 29: 1096–1114

Kuno M (1976) Responses of spinal motor neurons to section and restoration of peripheral motor connections. Cold Spring Harbor Symp Quant Biol XL: 457–463

Kuno M, Llinás R (1970a) Enhancement of synaptic transmission by dendritic potentials in chromatolysed motoneurons of the cat. J Physiol 210: 807–821

Kuno M, Llinás R (1970b) Alterations of synaptic action in chromatolysed motoneurones of the cat. J Physiol 210: 823–838

Kuno M, Miyata Y, Munoz-Martinez J (1974) Differential reaction of fast and slow α-motoneurones to axotomy. J Physiol 240: 725–739

Lieberman AR (1971) The axon reaction: A review of the principal features of perikaryal responses to axon injury. Int Rev Neurobiol 14: 50–125

Matthews MR, Nelson VH (1975) Detachment of structurally intact nerve endings from chromatolytic neurones of the rat superior cervical ganglion during the depression of synaptic transmission induced by postganglionic axotomy. J Physiol 245: 91–135

Mendell LM, Munson JB, Scott JG (1974) Connectivity changes of Ia afferents on axotomized motoneurons. Brain Res 73: 338–342

Mendell LM, Munson JB, Scott JG (1976) Alterations of synapses on axotomized motoneurones. J Physiol 255: 67–79
Purves D (1975) Functional and structural changes of mammalian sympathetic neurones following interruption of their axons. J Physiol 252: 429–463
Purves D, Lichtman JW (1978) Formation and maintenance of synaptic connections in autonomic ganglia. Physiol Rev 58: 821–862
Purves D, Noja A (1978) Trophic maintenance of synaptic connections in autonomic ganglia. In: Cotman CW (ed) Neuronal plasticity. Raven Press, New York, pp 27–47
Purves D, Thompson W (1979) The effects of post-ganglionic axotomy on selective synaptic connexions in the superior cervical ganglion of the guinea-pig. J Physiol 297: 95–110
Schadewald M (1940) Number and size of the boutons about the cells of the trochlear and abducens nucleus in the cat after unilateral section of the corresponding nerves. Anat Rec 76: 48–49
Schwindt PC, Richter A, Precht W (1973) Short latency utricular and canal input to ipsilateral abducens motoneurons. Brain Res 60: 259–262
Spencer RF, Sterling P (1977) An electron microscope study of motoneurons and interneurones in the cat abducens nucleus identified by retrograde intraaxonal transport of horseradish peroxidase. J Comp Neurol 176: 65–86
Sumner BEH (1975a) A quantitative analysis of boutons with different types of synapse in normal and injured hypoglossal nuclei. Exp Neurol 49: 406–417
Sumner BEH (1975b) A quantitative analysis of the response of presynaptic boutons to postsynaptic motor neuron axotomy. Exp Neurol 46: 605–615
Sumner BEH (1976) Quantitative ultrastructural observations on the inhibited recovery of the hypoglossal nucleus from the axotomy response when regeneration of the hypoglossal nerve is prevented. Exp Brain Res 26: 141–150
Sumner BEH (1979) Ultrastructural data, with special reference to bouton/glial relationships, from the hypoglossal nucleus after a second axotomy of the hypoglossal nerve. Exp Brain Res 36: 107–118
Sumner BEH, Sutherland FI (1973) Quantitative electron microscopy on the injured hypoglossal nucleus in the cat. J Neurocytol 2: 315–328
Sumner BEH, Watson WE (1971) Retraction and expansion of the dendritic tree of motor neurones of adult rats induced in vivo. Nature (London) 233: 273–275
Watson WE (1970) Some metabolic responses of axotomized neurones to contact between their axons and denervated muscle. J Physiol 210: 321–343

Neuronal Plasticity in the Newborn and Adult Feline Red Nucleus

N. TSUKAHARA[1,2] and Y. FUJITO[1]

1 Introduction

Synaptic plasticity represents one of the possible mechanisms of recovery of functions after brain lesions. Recently we have increased our understanding on the nature of plastic changes in the central synapses. One remarkable phenomenon, axonal sprouting and formation of new synapses, seems to be particularly important for the recovery of functions. Although the phenomenon was first demonstrated in the 1950s (Edds 1953), it has been difficult to demonstrate unequivocally sprouting of central axonal connections. However, recent studies provided convincing evidence that sprouting occurs in central synapses and the newly formed synapses are functionally active (Raisman 1969; Moore et al. 1971; Steward et al. 1973; Tsukahara et al. 1974; Cotman and Lynch 1976; Lund 1978; Tsukahara 1981).

The red nucleus (RN) neurons represent a suitable substrate to determine whether new, functionally effective synaptic connections are formed following lesions. In addition to an advantage for microelectrode studies due to their large size, they have useful features of synaptic organization; they receive two kinds of synaptic inputs, one from the contralateral nucleus interpositus (IP) of the cerebellum on the somatic portion of RN neurons, and the other from the ipsilateral cerebral cortex on the distal dendrites. This synaptic organization characterizes several features of the postsynaptic potentials produced by these synapses (Tsukahara and Kosaka 1968; Tsukahara et al. 1975b).

2 Sprouting and Formation of Functional Synapses in the Kitten Red Nucleus

It is generally agreed that the degree and extent of sprouting is more remarkable after denervation at the neonatal stage than at the adult stage (Cotman and Lynch 1976;

1 Department of Biophysical Engineering, Faculty of Engineering Science, Osaka University, Toyonaka, Osaka, Japan
2 National Institute for Physiological Sciences, Okazaki, Aichi, Japan

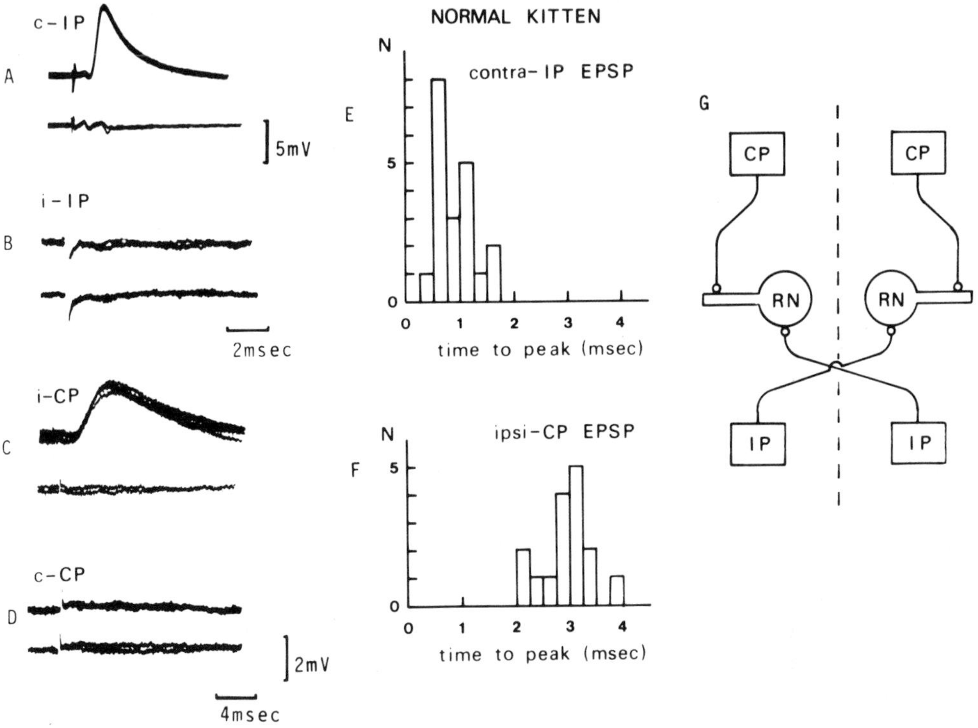

Fig. 1A–G. EPSP's produced in normal kitten red nucleus neurons **A** EPSP's elicited in a RN cell by stimulating the contralateral nucleus interpositus of the cerebellum (*c-IP*) (*upper trace*). Corresponding extracellular traces just outside the cell are illustrated at the lower traces of **A–D. B** Same as **A** but by stimulating the ipsilateral IP (*i-IP*). **C** EPSP's induced by stimulation of the ipsilateral cerebral peduncle (*i-CP*). **D** Same as **C**, but by stimulating the contralateral cerebral peduncle (*c-CP*). **E, F** Frequency distribution of the time-to-peak of the EPSP's elicited in kitten red nucleus 80th day after birth. **E** c-IP, **F** i-CP. **G** Connection of the red nucleus (RN). A *broken line* indicates the midline

Lund 1978; Tsukahara 1981 for the reviews). Recently we investigated the sprouting phenomenon in kitten RN with physiological techniques.

Figure 1 shows synaptic potentials recorded intracellularly in normal kitten RN neurons. Synaptic potentials produced in kitten RN neurons at 2 to 3 months after birth are virtually the same as those recorded in adults. Stimulation of the contralateral IP produces a fast-rising EPSP (Fig. 1A, E). This EPSP was only produced by stimulating the contralateral IP and not from the ipsilateral IP as shown in Fig. 1B. Stimulation of the ipsilateral cerebral sensorimotor cortex (SM) or their fibers at the cerebral peduncle (CP) produces a slow-rising dendritic EPSP as in normal adult cats (Fig. 1C, F). The stimulation of the contralateral CP does not produce any postsynaptic potentials, as shown in Fig. 1D.

After lesions of the contralateral IP by hemicerebellectomy in the early developmental stages within several weeks after birth, new functional connections appeared from the ipsilateral IP. As shown in Fig. 2A, stimulation of the ipsilateral IP produced

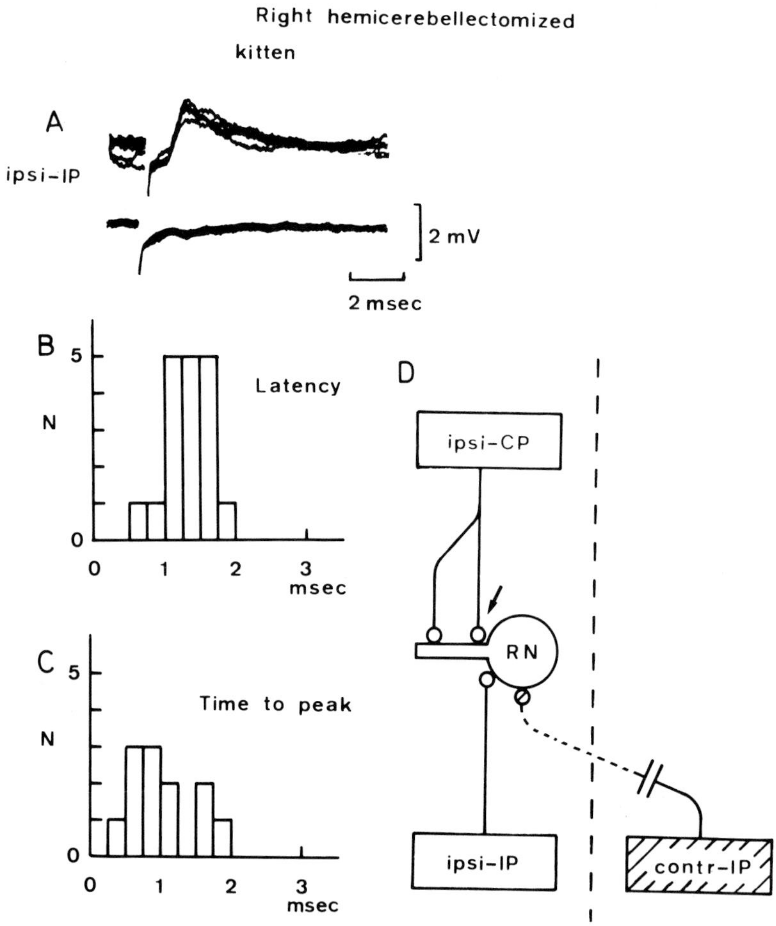

Fig. 2A–D. Sprouting in kitten red nucleus after hemicerebellectomy. **A** Newly appeared EPSP's in a RN cell by stimulation of ipsilateral IP. *Upper trace,* intracellular record. *Lower trace,* corresponding extracellular record. **B, C** Frequency distribution of latency (**B**) and time-to-peak (**C**) of the newly appeared EPSP's. **D** Connections after hemicerebellectomy as illustrated by the *shaded block*. *Arrow* indicates the sprouting of the ipsilateral corticorubral fibers onto the proximal part of the dendrites which can also be seen after IP lesion in adults (cf. Fig. 5)

an EPSP in a RN cell of a cat hemicerebellectomized 27 days after birth with a latency of 1 ms and time to peak of about 0.8 ms. Figure 2B, C illustrates frequency distribution of latency and time to peak of the newly appeared IP-EPSP's. In view of relatively long synaptic delays observed in the central nervous system of the kitten (Purpura et al. 1965), it is likely that these EPSP's were produced monosynaptically.

The most effective site for producing the EPSP's was mapped and determined as the ipsilateral IP. These results were interpreted as due to sprouting and formation of new functional synapses from ipsilateral IP. This conclusion is in agreement with the histological findings in rats (Lim and Leong 1975; Castro 1978) and similar findings on the cerebellothalamic projections in kittens (Kawaguchi et al. 1979).

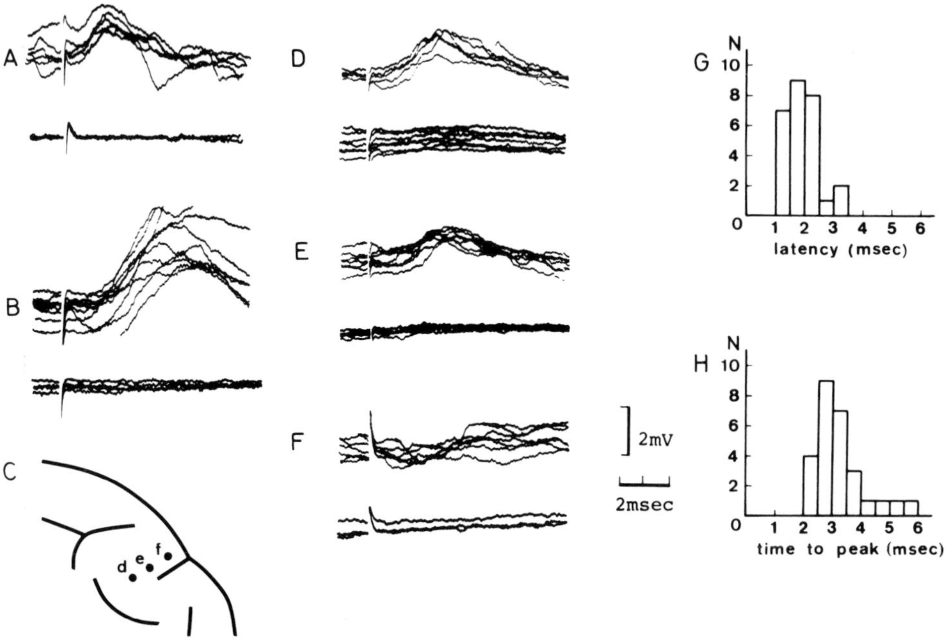

Fig. 3A–H. Sprouting in kitten red nucleus after destruction of the cerebrorubral input. **A** Newly appeared EPSP's induced in a RN cell by stimulating the contralateral cerebral peduncle. **B** Same as in **A** but by stimulating the contralateral sensorimotor cortex. **C–F** Somatotopical organization of the newly appeared corticorubral projection from the contralateral sensorimotor cortex. **C** Sensorimotor cortex in which the stimulating points were labeled as d, e, f, corresponding the intracellular records of d, e, f, respectively. **D–F** Newly appeared EPSP's in a RN cell by stimulating three loci of the contralateral sensorimotor cortex as labeled in **C. G, H** Frequency distribution of latency (**G**) and time-to-peak (**H**) of the newly appeared CP-EPSP's

Cerebral lesions destroying the corticorubral fibers were found to induce sprouting from three sources: (1) most importantly from the contralateral cerebral cortex via the contralateral CP (Nah and Leong 1976a,b), (2) contralateral IP, and (3) ipsilateral IP. As shown in Fig. 3A, stimulation of contralateral CP produces a slow-rising EPSP with latency of 1.4 ms in kittens in which ipsilateral cerebral sensorimotor cortex was ablated at the 17th day after birth. The latency of the contra-CP-EPSP's was 1.8 ± 0.6 ms with time-to-peak of 3.2 ± 0.8 ms (n = 27). Similar slow-rising EPSP's were also produced by stimulating contralateral SM with a longer latency of 2.6 ms, as shown in Fig. 3B. Assuming the conduction distance from SM to CP as 25 mm, the conduction velocities of fibers for the newly appeared EPSP's are about 20 m/s. This value is in the range of that of the normal corticorubral fibers or slow conducting pyramidal tract. EPSP's were followed in some cases, by an IPSP with longer latency (not illustrated), as was found by stimulating the ipsilateral CP in normal cats.

The area producing the slow-rising EPSP's in RN cells is somatotopically organized. Figure 3D, E, F show the corticorubral EPSP's recorded from a RN cell which innervates the upper spinal segment (C-cell) and thus could be antidromically invaded from

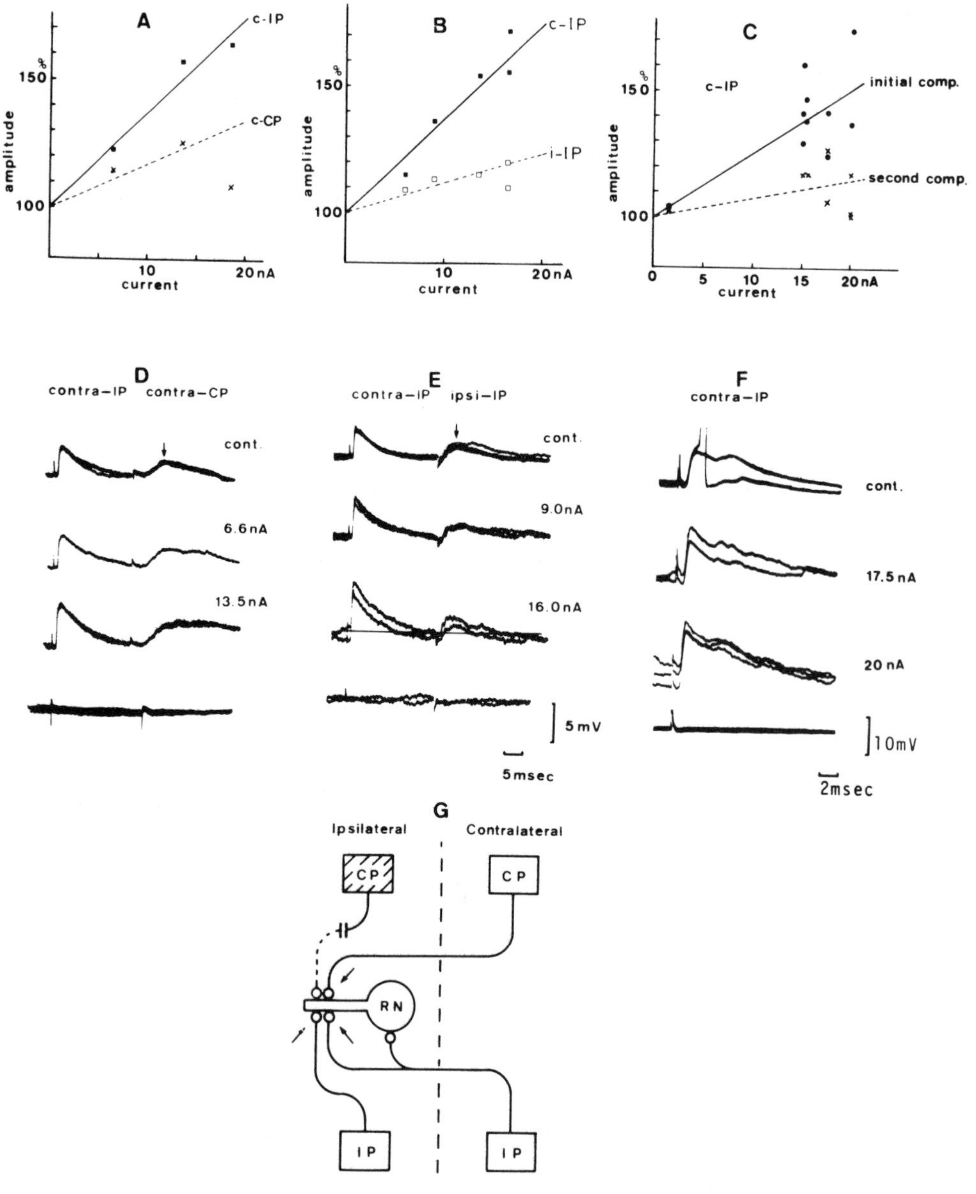

Fig. 4A–G. Sensitivity of amplitude of the newly appeared EPSP's to membrane polarization in kitten with cerebral lesions. **A–C** Relation between amplitude of EPSP's and injected current. **A** Comparison between c-IP-EPSP's (*filled squares*) and c-CP-EPSP's (*crosses*) from experiments partly shown in **D**. Normalized amplitudes as percentage of the control amplitudes (*ordinate*) are plotted against applied polarizing current (*abscissa*). **B** Comparison between c-IP-EPSP's (*filled squares*) and i-IP-EPSP's (*open squares*) from experiments partly shown in **E**. **C** Comparison between initial fast-rising component (*filled circles*) and the second slow-rising component of the c-IP-EPSP's (*crosses*) from experiments partly shown in **F**. **D–F** Specimen records of the EPSP's before (*cont.*) and during membrane hyperpolarization by passing currents labeled in each *trace*. The lowermost *traces* are corresponding extracellular fields. Voltage and time calibration in **E** also apply to **D**. **G** Sprouting in kitten red nucleus after lesion of the ipsilateral corticorubral fibers. *Arrows* indicate three sources of sprouting. Data from a cat with ipsilateral SM lesion at 67th day postnatally

C_1 spinal segment and not from L_1 spinal segment (Tsukahara and Kosaka 1968), receiving EPSP's from the lateral part of the sensorimotor cortex (Fig. 3C). Similarly, in RN cells innervating the lower spinal segment (L-cell) EPSP's were produced predominantly from the medial part of the SM.

The slow-rising EPSP's induced from the contralateral CP are less sensitive to membrane potential displacement than the contralateral IP-EPSP's, as shown in Fig. 4A, D. Therefore, it was concluded that the newly appeared slow-rising EPSP's are produced at sites remote from the soma.

Stimulation of the ipsilateral IP produces in some cases a slow-rising EPSP with mean latency of 1.8 ± 0.4 ms and time-to-peak of 3.1 ± 1.5 ms (n = 7). These EPSP's were also less sensitive to membrane hyperpolarization than contralateral IP-EPSP's (Fig. 4B, E). Therefore, it is likely that ipsilateral IP formed new synaptic contacts on distal dendrites of kitten RN. Furthermore, contralateral IP-EPSP's have additional slow-rising components superimposed on the fast-rising EPSP's. The former had a latency of 1.0 ± 0.3 ms and time-to-peak of 2.9 ± 0.8 ms (n = 13). The slow-rising component is considered to be produced by synapses on distal dendrites, since this component is less sensitive to membrane hyperpolarization than the initial fast-rising component (Fig. 4C, F) Thus sites of sprouting of these three sources after ablation of the ipsilateral SM appear to be dendrites remote from the soma as indicated by arrows in Fig. 4G.

There are interesting features on the possible sources of sprouting following cerebral lesion in kittens. Although three possible sources of sprouting exist as described above, sprouting does not seem to take place from three sources simultaneously in the same cell. Most frequently, only one source gives sprouting in 20 out of 29 RN cells tested. Less frequently, simultaneous sprouting from two independent inputs occurs only in 7 cells out of 29 RN cells. Simultaneous sprouting from three independent sources occurs in 2 out of 29 RN cells. As for frequency of occurrence of these three sprouting sources, the contralateral cerebral cortex represents the most predominant source (18 out of 29 RN cells), and the second is the contralateral IP (15 out of 29 RN cells), and the last possibility is the ipsilateral IP (7 out of 29 RN cells). Although the chance to reach the denervated synaptic sites seems to be equal to these three input fibers, it is likely that one of them would suppress the connection of others on the denervated synaptic sites.

3 Sprouting in the Adult Feline Red Nucleus

In contrast to sprouting after neonatal lesions, which takes place over a considerable physical distance, sprouting after deafferentation in the adult central nervous system is limited in the denervated field of the deafferented neurons. Since sprouting is also less prominent than in young animals, it is more difficult to detect.

One way to demonstrate physiologically sprouting in adult central neurons is to study possible changes in the time course of the EPSP's, which might occur if the synaptic sites of the newly formed synapses differ from the original ones. This method takes advantage of the distortion of the waveform during electrotonic propagation from dendrites to soma.

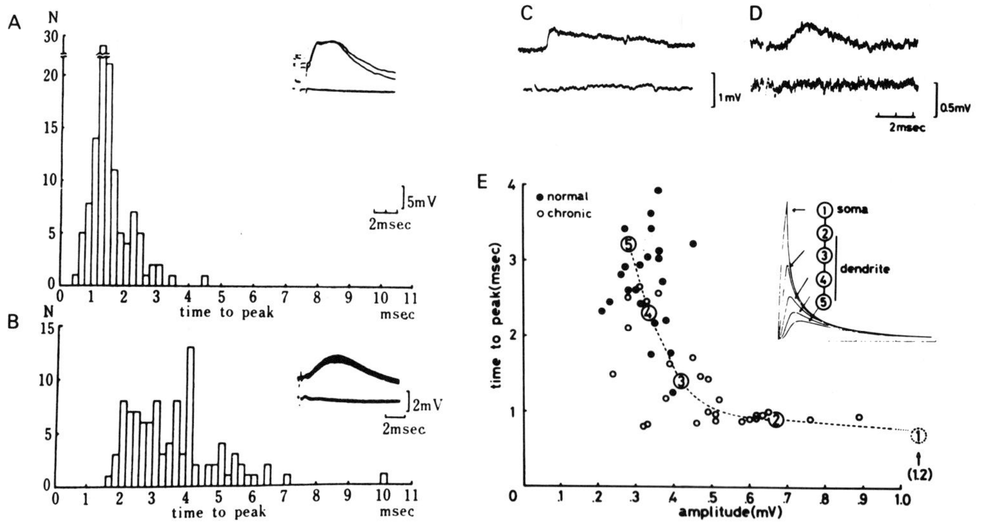

Fig. 5A–E. Sprouting of the adult feline red nucleus. **A** Time-to-peak of the corticorubral EPSP's induced by stimulating the cerebral peduncle (CP) after lesion of the interpositus nucleus (IP). Frequency distribution of the time-to-peak of the CP-EPSP's in operated cats. Specimen records of the intracellular and corresponding extracellular records are shown in the *insert diagram.* **B** Same as in **A** but in normal cats (modified from Tsukahara et al. 1975a). **C–E** Corticorubral unitary EPSP's. **C** Intracellular EPSP evoked by stimulation of sensorimotor cortex at a rate of 1/s in a cat with IP lesion 27 days before acute experiment. **D** Intracellular corticorubral unitary EPSP in a normal cat. *Upper traces* in **C, D**, intracellular potentials. *Lower traces,* extracellular records corresponding to the upper traces. **E** Relation between time-to-peak and amplitude of the unitrary EPSP's. *Open circles* represent unitary EPSP's of operated cats and *filled circles* represent those of normal cats. *Large open circles* represent time-to-peak and amplitudes of theoretical EPSP's derived by Rall's compartment model initiated at each compartment of a five-compartment chain. The time course of the theoretical EPSP's generated in those compartments is shown in the *inset* of the figure. (Modified from Murakami et al. 1977a)

We (Tsukahara et al. 1974; Tsukahara et al. 1975a) have shown that a fast-rising component appeared in the corticorubral EPSP's in RN cells, induced from the sensorimotor cortex or their pathway at the CP two or more weeks after lesion of the IP nucleus, as shown in Fig. 5A. This was taken to indicate that new and effective synapses were formed on the proximal portion of soma-dendritic membrane of RN cells after IP lesion.

In order to characterize the properties of synaptic transmission of the newly formed synapses, unitary EPSP's were analyzed in cats with IP lesion (Murakami et al. 1977a,b). One type seen consisted of corticorubral unitary EPSP's with a shorter time-to-peak and larger amplitude than in normal cats (Fig. 5C), and the other, of unitary EPSP's of normal range.

It should be noted that in normal cats unitary EPSP's showed a longer time-to-peak and smaller amplitude than those of chronic cats. Furthermore, in normal as well as in IP lesioned cats there was a tendency for a larger unitary EPSP to display a shorter time-to-peak. This relation is predicted theoretically by Rall's compartment model

(Rall 1964; Sato and Tsukahara 1976) on calculating the theoretical EPSP's produced at each of five compartments. There was a good numerical agreement between the theoretical curve shown in Fig. 5E (inset) and the experimental points (Fig. 5E). From this curve, new synapses were assumed to be at the proximal portion of the soma-dendritic membrane close to the soma but not on the soma itself. Furthermore, the model predicts that the observed reduction of the electrotonic length accounts for only a minor portion (less than 5%) of the observed decrease of the time-to-peak of the corticorubral EPSP's after IP lesions (Tsukahara et al. 1975a). Therefore, it was concluded that the major portion of the reduced rise time of the corticorubral EPSP's could not be attributable to the reduction of the electrotonic length of neurons, and must be due to sprouting and formation of functional synaptic connections. This conclusion was corroborated by the electron microscopic studies (Nakamura et al. 1974; Hanaway and Smith 1978; see also Nakamura et al. 1978).

Furthermore, the sensitivity of the corticorubral EPSP's with rapidly rising and those with slowly rising time course to the membrane potential displacement was compared. It was found that rapidly rising EPSP's are more sensitive than the slowly rising ones.

The properties of synaptic transmission during and after repetitive stimuli are characteristic of these synapses. Corticorubral synapses show facilitation and post-tetanic potentiation (PTP) in their synaptic transmission. The degree and time course of facilitation of the newly appearing corticorubral EPSP's were not significantly different from those of the old synapses. PTP was also found in newly appearing corticorubral EPSP's and lasted for several minutes, as in normal synapses.

4 Discussion

The degree of plasticity following neonatal lesions of synaptic inputs of RN neurons is in two ways more remarkable than that following adult lesions. First, newly formed corticorubral or interposito-rubral sprouts seem to elongate a considerable distance up to several millimeters after neonatal lesions. This is in sharp contrast to the sprouting in adult IP lesions, in which the remaining corticorubral fibers terminating on distal dendrites give sprouts only a few hundred microns more proximally to the soma-dendritic membrane of RN cells. Secondly, there are three sources of sprouting following lesions of corticorubral fibers after neonatal SM lesions. We found none in the adults after similar lesions.

How specifically the newly formed cerebro-rubral projection is organized? Three kinds of specificity have been investigated in this study as diagramatically illustrated in Fig. 6. First, the "topographic specificity" was found to be preserved since the newly formed corticorubral projections from the contralateral cerebrum were also somatotopically organized as in normal ipsilateral corticorubral projections. Secondly, the "specificity of the synaptic connections" seems to be preserved at least in part. As shown in Fig. 6, ipsilateral fast pyramidal tract neurons project onto the inhibitory interneurons, and slow-conducting pyramidal or corticorubral fibers terminate onto the rubrospinal (RN) neurons (Allen and Tsukahara 1974). In the newly formed corti-

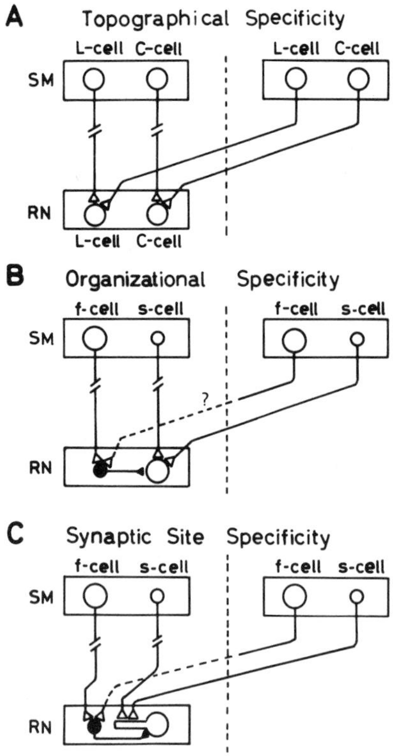

Fig. 6A–C. Specificity of the newly formed cerebrorubral projection. **A** *SM,* Sensorimotor cortex; *RN,* Red nucleus; *L-cell,* Cells innervating lumbosacral spinal cord; *C-cell,* Cells innervating cervicothoracic spinal cord. *Dotted vertical line,* midline. **B** *f-cell,* fast-conducting pyramidal tract cells; *s-cell,* slow-conducting pyramidal tract and corticorubral cells. **C** Same as **B**. *Open circles,* excitatory neurons; *filled circles,* inhibitory neurons

corubral system, the fast-conducting pyramidal tract cells do not project onto the rubrospinal neurons, and slow-conducting pyramidal tract and corticorubral fibers do project onto the rubrospinal cells. Whether the fast-conducting pyramidal tract cells project onto the inhibitory interneurons or not is obscure at present, although it is likely to be so, since we found sometimes IPSP's by stimulation of the contralateral CP. Thirdly, the "specificity of the synaptic location" seems to be preserved for the sprouting after neonatal ipsilateral cerebral lesions. The present studies on the newly formed cerebrorubral map thus seem to have given some insight into hitherto unasked questions in similar experiments.

It is likely that sprouting and formation of functional synapses account at least in some part for the behavioral recovery that cats show after IP lesion (Bromberg and Gilman 1978) and after cross-innervation (Tsukahara 1978) or muscle crossing (Yumiya et al. 1979). Since the phenomena were now recognized to occur widely in the central neurons, sprouting in other synapses, sometimes too small to be detected by the ordinary physiological methods, may also contribute to this recovery.

Sprouting and synaptic reorganization are not limited to cases of removal of the direct synaptic inputs of RN neurons. We attempted to perform cross-innervation experiments and to detect possible synaptic reorganization at the supraspinal level in the red nucleus. After cross-innervation a fast-rising component appeared superimposed on the slow-rising corticorubral EPSP's (Tsukahara and Fujito 1976). There was no appreciable change in the electrotonic length of RN neurons after cross-innervation (Tsukahara et al., unpubl.). These results suggest that sprouting and formation of new synapses occurred on the proximal dendrites after cross-innervation as in the case of IP lesions. Since none of the synaptic inputs of RN neurons are destroyed in the case of cross-innervation experiments, it is likely that sprouting occurs even without lesions of the synaptic inputs and seems to be a more general phenomenon of neurons to the environmental changes.

References

Allen GI, Tsukahara N (1974) Cerebrocerebellar communication systems. Physiol Rev 54: 957–1006

Bromberg MB, Gilman S (1978) Changes in rubral multiunit activity after lesions in the interpositus nucleus of the cat. Brain Res 152: 353–357

Castro A (1978) Projections of superior peduncle and the development of new connections in response to neonatal hemicerebellectomy. J Comp Neurol 78: 611–628

Cotman CW, Lynch GS (1976) Reactive synaptogenesis in the adult nervous system: the effects of partial deafferentation of new synapse formation. In: Barondes S (ed) Neuronal recognition. Plenum Press, New York, pp 69–108

Edds Jr MV (1953) Collateral nerve regeneration. Q Rev Biol 28: 260–276

Goldberger ME, Murray M (1978) Recovery of movement and axonal sprouting may obey some of the same laws. In: Cotman CW (ed) Neuronal plasticity. Raven Press, New York, pp 73–96

Hanaway J, Smith J (1978) Sprouting of corticorubral terminals in the cerebellar deafferented cat red nucleus. Soc Neurosci Abstr 4: 1507

Kawaguchi S, Yamamoto T, Samejima A (1979) Electro-physiological evidence for axonal sprouting of cerebello-thalamic neurons in kittens after neonatal hemicerebellectomy. Exp Brain Res 36: 21–39

Lim KH, Leong SK (1975) Aberrant bilateral projections from dentate and interposed nuclei in albino rats after neonatal lesions. Brain Res 96: 306–309

Lund RD (1978) Development and plasticity of the brain. Oxford Univ Press, New York Oxford

Moore RY, Björklund A, Stenevi U (1971) Plastic changes in the adrenergic innervation of the rat septal area in response to denervation. Brain Res 33: 13–35

Murakami F, Tsukahara N, Fujito Y (1977a) Analysis of unitary EPSPs mediated by the newly-formed cortico-rubral synapses after lesion of the interpositus nucleus. Exp Brain Res 30: 233–243

Murakami F, Tsukahara N, Fujito Y (1977b) Properties of synaptic transmission of the newly formed corticorubral synapses after lesion of the nucleus interpositus of the cerebellum. Exp Brain Res 30: 245–258

Nah SH, Leong SK (1976a) Bilateral corticofugal projection to the red nucleus after neonatal lesions in the albino rat. Brain Res 107: 433–436

Nah SH, Leong SK (1976b) An ultrastructural study of the anomalous corticorubral projection following neonatal lesions in the albino rat. Brain Res 111: 162–166

Nakamura Y, Mizuno N, Konishi A, Sato M (1974) Synaptic reorganization of the red nucleus after chronic deafferentation from cerebellorubral fibers: an electron microscope study in the cat. Brain Res 82: 298–301

Nakamura Y Mizuno N, Konishi A (1978) A quantitative electron microscope study of cerebellar axon terminals on the magnocellular red nucleus neurons in the cat. Brain Res 147: 17–27

Purpura DP, Shofer RJ, Scarff T (1965) Properties of synaptic activities and spike potentials of neurons in immature neocortex. J Neurophysiol 28: 925–941

Raisman G (1969) Neuronal plasticity in the septal nuclei of the adult rat. Brain Res 14: 25–48

Rall W (1964) Theoretical significance of dendritic trees for neuronal input-output relations. In: Reis RF (ed) Neural theory and modeling. Stanford Univ Press, Stanford, pp 73–87

Sato S, Tsukahara N (1976) Some properties of the theoretical membrane transients in Rall's neuron model. J Theoret Biol 63: 151–163

Steward O, Cotman CW, Lynch GS (1973) Re-establishment of electrophysiologically functional entorhinal cortical input to the dentate gyrus deafferented by ipsilateral entorhinal lesions: innervation by the contralateral entorhinal cortex. Exp Brain Res 18: 396–414

Tsukahara N (1978) Synaptic plasticity in the red nucleus. In: Cotman CW (ed) Neuronal plasticity. Raven Press, New York, pp 113–130

Tsukahara N (1981) Synaptic plasticity in the mammalian central nervous system. Annu Rev Neurosci 4: 351–379

Tsukahara N, Fujito Y (1976) Physiological evidence of formation of new synapses from cerebrum in the red nucleus neurons following cross-union of forelimb nerves. Brain Res 106: 184–188

Tsukahara N, Kosaka K (1968) The mode of cerebral excitation of red nucleus neurons. Exp Brain Res 5: 102–117

Tsukahara N, Hultborn H, Murakami F (1974) Sprouting of cortico-rubral synapses in red nucleus neurons after destruction of the nucleus interpositus of the cerebellum. Experientia 30: 57–58

Tsukahara N, Hultborn H, Murakami F, Fujito Y (1975a) Electrophysiological study of formation of new synapses and collateral sprouting in red nucleus neurons after partial denervation. J Neurophysiol 38: 1359–1372

Tsukahara N, Murakami F, Hultborn H (1975b) Electrical constants of neurons of the red nucleus. Exp Brain Res 23: 49–64

Yumiya H, Larsen KD, Asanuma H (1979) Motor readjustment and input-output relationship of motor cortex following cross-connection fo forearm muscles in cats. Brain Res 177: 566–570

Neurochemistry of Synaptic Renewal

J.J. BERNSTEIN[1,2], D. GANCHROW[2], and M.R. WELLS[1]

1 Introduction

The renewal of synapses in the central nervous system (CNS) of mammals, particularly after traumatic deafferentation, has been studied extensively for many decades (reviewed Clemente 1964; Bernstein et al. 1978a,b; Cotman and Nadler 1978). Due to the limited regenerative capacity in the CNS of the adult mammal, it was surprising to find that morphological synaptic renewal could occur and that the new synaptic complexes were physiologically efficacious. While it is clear that the regrowth and subsequent synapse formation demonstrated in such studies is subtended by basic biochemical processes, understanding of these events is very limited. This paper will examine some of the neurochemical data which seem correlated to synaptic renewal in the CNS of adult mammals.

2 Morphological Aspects

2.1 Axonal Regeneration and Sprouting

In the adult mammalian CNS, synaptic renewal must occur as the result of the regeneration of retracted or lesioned fibers or the growth of axon sprouts from intact fibers. The actual regeneration of axon terminals in the CNS of adult mammals is so limited (Windle 1955; Clemente 1964; Puchala and Windle 1977; Bernstein et al. 1978a,b; Cotman 1978) that studies of synaptic renewal due to this process alone have not been possible. Despite the failure of the CNS to regenerate, it is possible to obtain an idea of the potential of the system to grow and re-innervate deafferented structures by the use of tissue grafts. The implantation of peripheral tissues into mammalian brain (LeGros-Clark 1940, 1942; Björklund and Stenevi 1971; Stenevi et al. 1976) has demonstrated that, to some extent, central axons are capable of re-innervating structures

1 Laboratory of Nervous System Injury and Regeneration, VA Medical Center, (151Q) and Department of Neurosurgery and Physiology, George Washington University, College of Medicine, Washington, D.C. 20422, USA

2 Department of Anatomy and Embryology, Hadassah Medical School, Jerusalem, Israel

in a pattern which appears similar to normal. The connections formed may also be functional (Björklund et al. 1975). In other studies (reviewed Björklund and Stenevi 1977; Björklund and Stenevi 1979), the implantation of fetal brain grafts into adult rats has resulted both in the re-innervation of the host tissue by the graft and innervation of the graft by the host. These experiments demonstrate that although regeneration does not normally occur in adult mammals, the central nervous system maintains the potential to grow by recognition of a deafferented target. The specificity of the regrowing nerve fibers into the implant remains to be determined.

Experiments on axonal sprouting also demonstrate a definite, but limited potential for regrowth in the adult mammalian CNS under conditions of traumatic deafferentation (Lynch et al. 1974; Lynch and Cotman 1975; Bernstein et al. 1978a,b; Cotman and Nadler 1978). The potential for a tract to sprout depends on the tract involved and the conditions of deafferentation. Some tracts readily demonstrate the sprouting of intact axons while others do not (Kerr 1972; Lynch and Cotman 1975; Field et al. 1980). In the adult mammal, sprouting of afferents into a deafferented area is often limited to a restricted pattern. Even when adjacent areas are dennervated, intact axons may not extend sprouts beyond defined boundaries (Lynch et al. 1974; Cotman and Lynch 1975; Cotman and Nadler 1978; Field et al. 1980). It is also of interest that tracts which innervate in a strictly defined pattern (e.g., somatotopic) do not seem to sprout as readily as those which innervate in a more diffuse, less organized manner (Goldberger and Murray 1978). These apparent boundaries to sprouting in the adult brain do not pertain if the deafferentation occurs in the neonatal mammal (Lund and Lund 1971; Lynch et al. 1973).

These and similar studies on the sprouting of intact axons in the adult mammalian CNS demonstrate that a limited potential exists for severed or newly growing axons (generates) and axonal sprouts to recognize a deafferented target. In the process of axonal sprouting there is also morphological evidence that the postsynaptic deafferented neuron reacts. Deafferentation of CNS neurons may result in the retraction and/or expansion of the dendritic tree (Parnavelas et al. 1974; Storm-Mathisen 1974; Bernstein and Bernstein 1977; Cotman and Nadler 1978; Bernstein and Standler 1979), and in areas adjacent to a spinal cord injury dendritic varicosities are formed which may act as sites for innervation (Bernstein et al. 1975). These data suggest that the process of synaptic renewal after axon sprouting is best portrayed as an interaction of growth processes in both the axon and its target.

2.2 Cyclic Growth Patterns

Superimposed upon the interaction of the growing axon sprout and its target, there appear to be more complex interactions of the injured nervous system with generalized, perhaps metabolic influences (Wells and Bernstein 1980). In the rat spinal cord after a spinal hemisection, the numbers (Bernstein et al. 1974) and frequency of types (Bernstein and Bernstein 1977) of boutons on chronically deafferented neurons 1.0–1.5 mm rostral to the site of hemisection undergo a cyclic pattern of degeneration and renewal. The numbers of boutons as detected by a silver impregnation for nerve terminals decreased at 10–20 days postoperation on both the operated and unoperated sides of the spinal cord. This was followed by an increase in bouton numbers at 30 days, and a decrease at 45 to 60 days. From time periods of 60 to 90 days postoperation, the alterations in number of boutons varied with the area of spinal cord. This pattern was present on the motoneurons of lamina IX and up to 60 days on lamina IV and VII neuron soma. This coincidence of morphological changes should have some neurochemical coordinating factor(s) (hypothetical at present) which trigger and/or maintain the coordinated pathological events that lead to bouton renewal. It is of interest in the light of the reactions of the deafferented dendrite mentioned earlier that reactions of the deafferented cell may be a confounding factor in the interpretation of the cyclic renewal of boutons in the hemisected spinal cord. After ventral root section in the rat spinal cord, the dendritic trees of axotomized motoneurons undergo a pattern of retraction and growth which is similar to the cyclic renewal of boutons in the hemisected spinal cord (Bernstein and Standler 1979). Since it has been demonstrated that peripherally axotomized neurons alter their presynaptic profile (Blinzinger and Kreutzberg 1968; Sumner 1975), the supposition that the cyclic renewal of boutons in the hemisected spinal cord results from the cyclic sprouting of axons is obscured by the possibility that the cyclic alterations occur as a result of nonspecific direct injury or axotomy of the neurons involved.

In a recent series of experiments on an intrinsic ascending sensory system, the dorsal columns of the rat spinal cord were lesioned bilaterally at T12, and the parameters of bouton numbers on soma and proximal dendrite, cell size and area covered by boutons examined in the nucleus gracilis (Ganchrow et al. 1981) and the lateral ventroposterolateral (VPL) nucleus of the thalamus (Ganchrow and Bernstein 1981) over time periods of 1, 2, 3, 7, 14, 30, 45, 60, 90, and 120 days postoperation. In the nucleus gracilis, a significant fluctuation of bouton numbers occurred in the first week postlesion and over days postoperative (Fig. 1a). In VPL, the alterations in bouton numbers were reflected by similar, apparently transneuronally induced, statistically significant changes in boutons only on the first 5 μm of proximal dendrites (but not soma) after seven postoperative days (Fig. 1b). In the nucleus gracilis, but not VPL, the bouton changes were correlated with significant alterations in soma size (Fig. 1c; Bernstein and Ganchrow 1981). The processes of change in somatic area and bouton numbers in the nucleus gracilis maintains the area of somatic membrane occupied by synapses within narrow limits. These data suggest that in the absence of direct trauma to the deafferented neuron, patterned fluctuations of boutons still occur, and are related to membrane alteration in the postsynaptic cell.

2.3 Summary

Data from tissue grafts into the adult mammalian CNS and from studies of deafferentation-induced axonal sprouting indicate that the adult CNS is capable of limited growth of axons under the proper conditions. The potential for recognition of targets by the growing axon and/or the neuronal specificity of the individual types of neurons are limited but seem to be present in the adult. The process of synaptic renewal in the adult appears to be a complex interaction of pre- and postsynaptic elements. The existence of cyclic patterns of neuronal growth and synaptic renewal in the rat spinal cord suggest that in addition to the local interactions some generalized modulation of synaptic renewal is present.

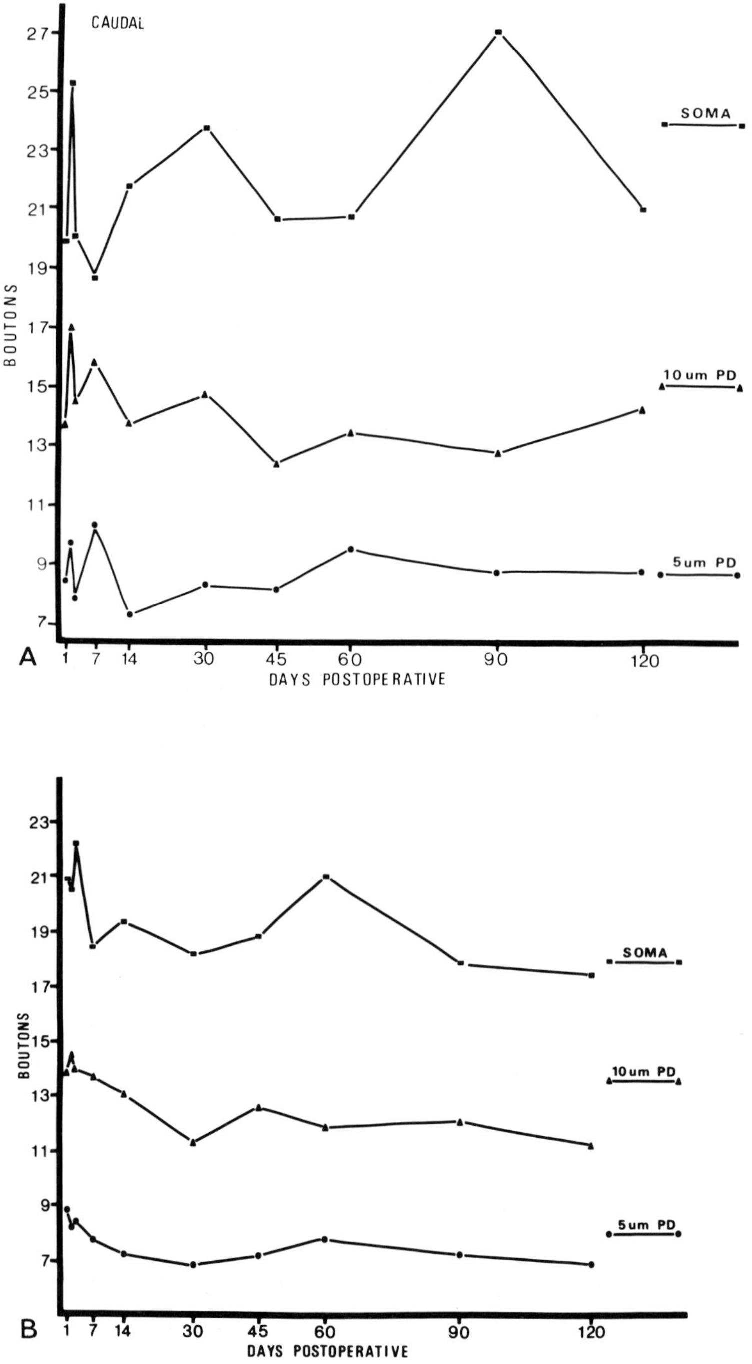
CAUDAL
BOUTONS
SOMA
10 um PD
5 um PD
A
DAYS POSTOPERATIVE
BOUTONS
SOMA
10 um PD
5 um PD
B
DAYS POSTOPERATIVE

Fig. 1A, B

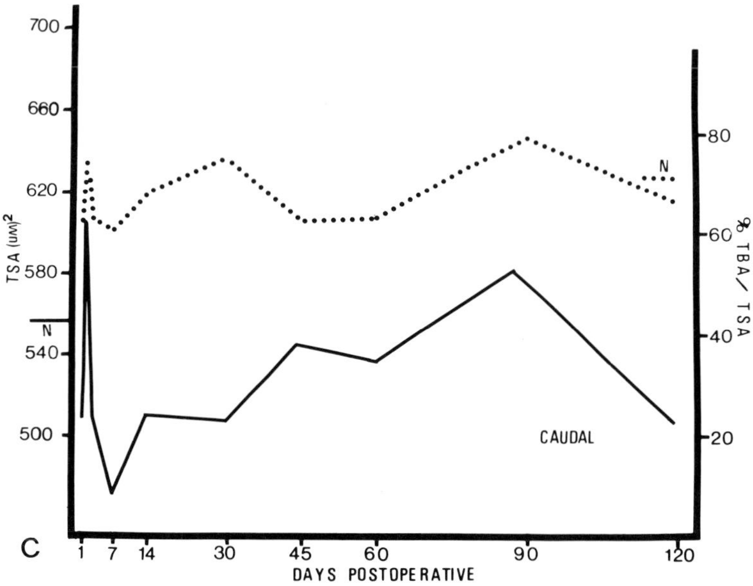

Fig. 1A–C. Average bouton count on neuron soma and proximal dendrite (*PD*) after T12 dorsal column section of rat spinal cord. **A** Neurons in caudal nucleus gracilis (Ganchrow et al. 1981), and **B** lateral ventralis pars lateralis (*VPL*) of the thalamus (from Ganchrow and Bernstein 1981). **C** Total surface area (*TSA, solid line*) of soma of rat caudal nucleus gracilis neurons and percentage of the total somal area occupied by boutons (*TBA/TSA, dotted line;* TBA, total bouton area on soma). N = Normal (Bernstein and Ganchrow 1981)

3 Neurochemical Aspects

3.1 Mechanisms of Growth

The morphological renewal of synapses and nerve terminals offers a static view of a system in a constant state of biochemical flux. Most of the molecular structure of the brain, as in other parts of the body, is in a state of catabolic/anabolic balance. This balance results in a renewal of chemical structure such as that demonstrated for brain protein (Lajtha 1971). In rats, the average half-life of proteins is about 15 days with an enormous range for individual proteins. The same is true for other cellular components. Thus, from a chemical standpoint, the anabolic/catabolic balance of most cellular components provides a constant renewal of synaptic components.

For neuronal processes and terminals, the components for molecular renewal are supplied by cytoplasmic transport in the axon and dendrite (Lasek 1970; Schubert and Kreutzberg 1975). Mechanisms have been best described in the axon. A model for axonal growth and retraction on the basis of axoplasmic transport has been proposed by Lasek and colleagues (Lasek and Hoffman 1976; Lasek and Black 1977). In this model, axonal cytoskeletal elements such as actin and tubulin components of structures such as neurofilaments (Hoffman and Lasek 1975) are transported in the slow components of axoplasmic transport and are essential for axon growth. The continual transport of materials down the axon is balanced by a breakdown of the structural proteins by a calcium dependent protease in the axon terminal. Some evidence has been found for the existence of such a protease in axons (Schlaepfer and Micko 1978, 1979). Alteration of the activity of the protease in the terminal by some means (e.g., calcium concentration) might then produce growth in the axon terminal or retraction through control of the assembly or disassembly of the cytoskeletal elements. It is assumed that other elements of the axon (lipids, glycoproteins, etc.) are modulated in a similar manner.

The supply of cytoskeletal elements in the slow component of axoplasmic transport implies that most of the cytoskeletal elements involved in the regeneration of peripheral nerve is already synthesized at the time of injury (Lasek and Black 1977). The similar rates of slow axoplasmic transport (1–4 mm/day) and peripheral nerve regeneration (1–4 mm/day; Grafstein and McQuarrie 1978) suggest that the supply of cytoskeletal elements may be at least a rate-limiting factor in regeneration if not as intimately involved as proposed by Lasek and colleagues.

The mechanisms of synaptic renewal after axonal sprouting must involve membrane expansion or outgrowth. The extent to which this outgrowth may be controlled by local processes in the synaptic terminal similar to that described above or through the cell body of origin is not known. In the mammalian peripheral nervous system, examination of the outgrowth of axons after lesion and the cell body reaction (Grafstein 1975; Grafstein and McQuarrie 1978) may indicate that more than one response occurs. Outgrowth of some axons may occur as early as 4 to 6 h after axotomy; while substantial vigorous outgrowth does not occur before 24 h. The very early outgrowth, which may be retracted (Grafstein and McQuarrie 1978), may be a local growth process which occurs too rapidly to be under direct biochemical influence of the cell body even by fast axoplasmic transport. The later, maintained outgrowth seems mediated by the neuron soma and its reaction to injury (Lieberman 1971; Grafstein 1975). The early peripheral nerve pattern of outgrowth suggests a limited intrinsic potential for growth to exist in the axon. If a similar potential exists in the CNS, it is possible that paraterminal sprouting and growth over very short distances may be modulated in the axon terminal by intrinsic or extrinsic factors capable of effecting growth.

3.2 Initiation, Guidance, and Recognition

The mediation of synaptic renewal in the central nervous system either as a result of sprouting after trauma or a normal maintenance of synaptic connections should involve processes which are similar to development. Growth must be initiated (or released) and in some manner directed and intercellular recognition and cellular adhesion must occur after growth. Factors which produce the desired effect on the axon could arise from a variety of sources: degeneration products (Ramón y Cajal 1928), reacting neuroglia (Ramón y Cajal 1928), adjacent axons (Diamond et al. 1976; Goldowith and Cotman 1977; Cotman and Nadler 1978), and the postsynaptic cell.

As suggested above, growth in synaptic renewal might be initiated by the presence and action of a stimulating factor(s) directly on the axon terminal or indirectly through the neuron soma. A number of substances have been isolated from the nervous system which may stimulate axonal sprouting (Hoffman and Springel 1951), enhance regeneration (Koechlin 1955), and produce directional growth of neurites in culture (Liu et al. 1979). Many are small diffusable peptides (Koechlin 1955; Liu et al. 1979). Presumably, such substances are released by degenerating tissue, reacting neuroglia, or by the deafferented neuron after injury. Once growth is initiated, the sprout must grow toward its target and initiate a recognition response before synapses can be formed. The mechanism of this process is a subject of study and contention in the areas of development and synaptogenesis. The axon may be guided mechanically (Weiss 1939; Weiss and Hiscoe 1948), by neurotropism (Ramon y Cajal 1928), chemical affinity (Sperry 1963), or by a combination of these factors (Hamburger 1962, 1975; Egar and Singer 1972; Norlander and Singer 1978; Singer et al. 1980). In most, but not all, instances (Liu et al. 1979), there are neurochemical and mechanical interactions between the growing neurite and surface upon which the cell process is growing (either neuronal or neuroglial). This interaction has been implicated as a mechanism of directional growth. Among other surface components, glycoproteins have been implicated as agents involved in directional growth (Singer et al. 1980) and in the intercellular recognition which occurs in synapse formation in nervous system development (Merrel 1976; Marchase 1977). In the adult animal, glycoproteins appear on the external surface of the postsynaptic membrane but are only a minor component of the synaptic junction (Cotman and Nadler 1978). Interestingly, the content of cell surface glycoproteins in the hippocampus is altered during synaptic renewal (Mena and Cotman 1979). These data show a further relationship between the internal structure of the membrane, the surface, components of the membrane, and synaptic renewal.

3.3 General Metabolic Influences

As for any injured tissue, the metabolic state of injured nervous system tissue and the effect of factors capable of influencing it is of great importance in the recovery from injury and in growth. On a cellular level, the importance of the metabolic state of the nerve cell body on axonal regeneration in peripheral nerves (Wells and Bernstein 1977; Grafstein and McQuarrie 1978), and possible sprouting of some central tracts (Scheff et al. 1978), has been demonstrated by the priming lesion phenomenon. In peripheral nerves, outgrowth of lesioned fibers is faster after the second of two lesions spaced two or more weeks apart. In the CNS, sprouting in the rat hippocampus was much faster and to a greater extent if a small priming lesion was made in the entorhinal cortex prior to a complete lesion. The priming lesion effect presumably reflects a metabolic preparation of the cell for outgrowth or reaction to injury (Grafstein 1975; Grafstein and McQuarrie 1978).

The reaction of the neuron to deafferentation or axotomy encompasses wide-ranging alterations of metabolism (Lieberman 1971; Watson 1974; Grafstein 1975; Grafstein and McQuarrie 1978). Included among these alterations are changes in the response to at least one metabolic hormone, triiodothyronine (Cook and Kiernan 1976; Wells et al. 1979). Triiodothyronine altered neuronal metabolism and produced atypical responses to extrinsic factors which are characterized by an attempt of the neuron to increase its metabolism and initiate the growth necessary to mediate recovery. It has been suggested (Grafstein 1975) that these alterations of metabolism create a condi-

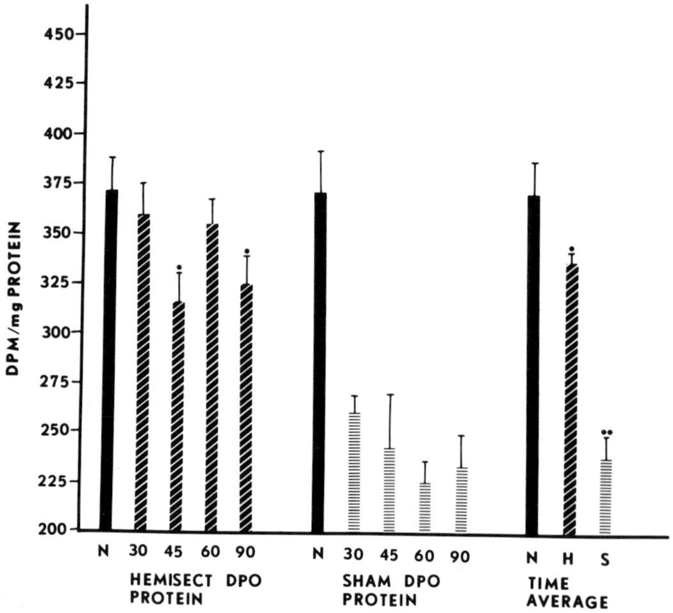

Fig. 2. [^{3}H] lysine uptake of spinal cord T2 hemisected (*H*); normal (*N*) and sham-operated (*S*) rats over days postoperation (*DPO*). Radioactivity is expressed as DPM/mg/protein for trichloroacetic acid (TCA) precipitable protein and soluble fractions. *Bars* represent standard error of means, *asterisks* significant differences ($P<0.05$) (Wells and Bernstein 1980)

tion of metabolic responsiveness in the neuron similar to that in earlier stages of nervous system development.

The presence of a cyclic renewal of synapses in the spinal cord (Bernstein et al. 1978a,b) and dorsal column nuclei of the rat (Ganchrow et al. 1981) after deafferentation and the cyclic dendritic growth after axotomy (Bernstein and Standler 1979) suggests that general metabolic factors may be involved in synaptic renewal which act in addition to the changes in cellular metabolism. Wells and Bernstein (1980) noted that measures of the average incorporation of [^{3}H] lysine into the spinal cord protein of spinal hemisected rats followed a pattern which was very similar to the alterations of bouton numbers at the same time periods (Fig. 2). The patterns in some areas of spinal cord were significantly correlated to changes in lysine uptake. The changes in lysine incorporation occurred both in areas of spinal cord directly affected by the injury and in areas distant to the injury. A similar, but not statistically significant, pattern was also seen in brain. The broad areas over which the metabolic changes occurred again suggest that some general (perhaps hormonal) factors are involved.

3.4 Summary of Neurochemical Aspects

As an extention of the neuronal membrane, the axon and axon terminal are like the rest of the neuron, in a constant anabolic/catabolic balance of its biochemistry. The initiation of growth in the axon and terminal may or may not require a substantial metabolic contribution by the cell body, depending upon the requirements for growth involved. Factors which may initiate axonal or axon terminal growth, particularly in the form of sprouting of intact axons, remain unknown, although preliminary evidence suggests that small diffusable substances released by degeneration of injured tissue or the deafferented postsynaptic neuron may be involved. Once growth of the neurite has been initiated, it is in part directed toward its target by the properties of the substrate upon which is grows and/or by diffusable substances presumably similar to those responsible for growth initiation. Glycoproteins have been suggested as surface agents which may guide the growing axon. They may also be involved in the mutual recognition of the axon for its target in both development and synaptic renewal.

On a broader scale, synaptic renewal may be affected by alterations of nervous system metabolism. Cycles of synaptic renewal have been demonstrated on deafferented neurons in the rat and similar cycles of dendrite growth have been shown on axotomized motoneurons. These patterns of cyclic growth are roughly correlated with alterations of lysine metabolism which occur after spinal cord hemisection. It has been suggested that these cycles of synaptic renewal and growth may be due to a selective stimulation of the injured or deafferented neuron by normally circulating, perhaps hormonal, factors.

4 Conclusion

Observations of synaptic renewal in the adult mammalian central nervous system are largely restricted to the synapses formed by the sprouting of axons after injury. In most instances this growth is limited to relatively strict boundaries defined by the type and area of the injury and the stage of development of the animal. The presence of a defined growth pattern in axonal sprouting and data from peripheral tissue and CNS tissue grafts into the brains of adult animals suggest that a mechanism for mutual recognition of neurite for deafferented target persists in the brain to some extent.

From a biochemical standpoint, the growth necessary for some types of limited axon sprouting may only involve minor alterations in the metabolism of the axon. It is clear, however, that in axonal sprouting requiring substantial growth, the metabolic participation of the cell body is necessary. The similarity of the growth process to the normal metabolism of the axon may account for great difficulty in defining synapses in stages of formation. At present, the mature characteristics of new synaptic complexes are not known either morphologically or chemically.

The processes of growth initiation, guidance, and mutual recognition of cells in the CNS which must be present in synaptic renewal remain vaguely defined. The participation of cell surface proteins and released diffusable substances in these processes have received some experimental support, but are far from conclusive. The existence of cyclic growth patterns in the formation of synapses, the growth of dendrites, and in amino acid metabolism, suggestes that some general, perhaps hormonal, substances may affect long term growth in the injured nervous system.

While the growth involved in axonal sprouting and its mechanisms is not well understood, the fact that it does occur offers hope for the eventual understanding and perhaps manipulation or growth in the central nervous system.

Acknowledgments. Supported in part by funds from the Veterans Administration, National Institutes of Health, NS 16979, the Paralyzed Veterans of America, and the U.S.-Israel Binational Foundation.

References

Bernstein ME, Bernstein JJ (1977) Dendritic growth cone and filopodia formation as a mechanism of spinal cord regeneration. Exp Neurol 57: 419–425

Bernstein JJ, Ganchrow D (1981) The relationship of afferentation and soma size of nucleus gracilis neurons after bilateral dorsal column lesion in the rat. Exp Neurol 71: 452–463

Bernstein JJ, Standler N (1979) Cyclic dendritic degeneration and regeneration of rat motoneurons after ventral root section. Soc Neurosci Abstr 5: 621

Bernstein JJ, Gelderd J, Bernstein ME (1974) Alteration of neuronal synaptic complement during regeneration and axonal sprouting of rat spinal cord. Exp Neurol 44: 470–483

Bernstein JJ, Wells MR, Bernstein ME (1975) Dendrites and neuroglia following hemisection of rat spinal cord: Effects of puromycin. Adv Neurol 12: 439–451

Bernstein JJ, Bernstein ME, Wells MR (1978a) Spinal cord regeneration in mammals: Neuroanatomical and neurochemical correlates of axonal sprouting. In: Waxman SG (ed) Physiology and pathobiology of axons. Raven Press, New York, pp 407–420

Bernstein JJ, Wells MR, Bernstein ME (1978b) Mammalian spinal cord regeneration: Synaptic renewal and neurochemistry. In: Cotman C (ed) Neuronal Plasticity. Raven Press, New York, pp 49–71

Björklund A, Stenevi U (1971) Growth of central catecholamine neurons into smooth muscle grafts in the rat mesencephalon. Brain Res 31: 1–20

Björklund A, Stenevi U (1977) Reformation of the severed septohippocampal cholinergic pathway in the adult rat by transplanted septal neurons. Cell Tissue Res 185: 289–302

Björklund A, Stenevi U (1979) Reconstruction of brain circuitries by neural transplants. In: Trends in neurosciences. Elsevier/North-Holland Biomedical Press, pp 301–306

Björklund A, Johnasson B, Stenevi U, Avendgaard NE (1975) Re-establishment of functional connections by regenerating central adrenergic and cholinergic axons. Nature (London) 253: 446–448

Blinzinger K, Kreutzberg G (1968) Displacement of synaptic terminals from regenerating motoneurons by microglial cells. Z Zellforsch 85: 145–157

Clemente CD (1964) Regeneration in the vertebrate central nervous system. Rev Neurobiol 6: 257–301

Cook RA, Kiernan JA (1976) Effects of triiodothyrorine on protein synthesis in regenerating peripheral neurons. Exp Neurol 52: 514–524

Cotman CW (ed) (1978) Neuronal plasticity. Raven Press, New York, 335 p

Cotman CW, Nadler JV (1978) Reactive synaptogenesis in the hippocampus. In: Cotman CW (ed) Neuronal plasticity. Raven Press, New York, pp 227–271

Diamond J, Cooper E, Turner C, Macintyre L (1976) Trophic regulation of nerve sprouting. Science 193: 371–377

Egar M, Singer M (1972) The role of ependyma in spinal cord regeneration in the urodele, *Triturus*. Exp Neurol 37: 422–430

Field PM, Coldham D, Raisman G (1980) Synapse formation after injury in the adult rat brain: Preferential reinnervation of dennervated fimbrial sites by axons of the contralateral fimbria. Brain Res 189: 103–113

Ganchrow D, Bernstein J (1981) Patterns of reafferentation in rat ventroposterolateral nucleus after thoracic dorsal column lesions. Exp Neurol 71: 464–472

Ganchrow D, Margolin JK, Bernstein JJ (1981) Patterns of reafferentation in rat nucleus gracilis after thoracic dorsal columns lesion. Exp Neurol 71: 437–451

Goldberger ME, Murray M (1978) Recovery of movement and axonal sprouting may obey some of the same laws. In: Cotman CW (ed) Neuronal plasticity. Raven Press, New York, pp 73–96

Goldowitz D, Cotman CW (1977) Does neurotrophic material control synapse formation in the adult rat brain? Neurosci Abstr 3: 534

Grafstein B (1975) The nerve cell body response to axotomy. Exp Neurol 48: 32–51

Grafstein B, McQuarrie IG (1978) Role of the nerve cell body in axonal regeneration. In: Cotman CW (ed) Neuronal plasticity. Raven Press, New York, pp 155–196

Hamburger V (1962) Specificity in neurogenesis. J Cell Comp Physiol Suppl 1 60: 81–92

Hamburger V (1975) Changing concepts in developmental biology. Perspect Biol Med 18: 162–178

Hoffman H, Springell PH (1951) An attempt at the chemical identification of neurocletin (the substance evoking axon-sprouting). Aust J Exp Biol 29: 417–424

Hoffman PN, Lasek RJ (1975) The slow component of axonal transport: Identification of major structural polypeptides of the axon and their generality among mammalian neurons. J Cell Biol 66: 351–366

Kerr FWL (1972) The potential of cervical primary afferents to sprout in the spinal nucleus of V following long term trigeminal dennervation. Brain Res 43: 547–560

Koechlin BA (1955) The neurogenerative factor "NR". In: Windle WF (ed) Regeneration in the central nervous system. CC Thomas, Springfield, Illinois, pp 127–130

Lajtha A (1971) Protein turnover. In: Lajtha A (ed) Handbook of neurochemistry. Plenum Press, New York, pp 551–629

Lasek RJ (1970) Protein transport in neurons. Int Rev Neurobiol 13: 289–324

Lasek RJ, Black MM (1977) How do axons stop growing? Some clues from the metabolism of the proteins in the slow component of axonal transport. In: Roberts et al. (ed) Mechanisms, regulation and special functions of protein synthesis in the brain. Elsevier/North-Holland Biomedical Press, pp 161–169

Lasek RJ, Hoffman PN (1976) The neuronal cytoskeleton, axonal transport and axonal growth. Cold Spring Harbor Conferences on Cell Proliferation, Cell Motil 3: 1021–1049

LeGros-Clark WE (1940) Neuronal differentiation in implanted foetal cortical tissue. J Neurol Psychiatr 3: 263–272

LeGros-Clark WE (1942) The problem of neuronal regeneration in the central nervous system. I. The influence of spinal ganglia and nerve fragments grafted in the brain. J Anat 77: 20–48

Lieberman AR (1971) The axon reaction: A review of the principal features of perikaryal responses to axotomy. Int Rev Neurobiol 14: 49–124

Liu HM, Balkovic ES, Sheff MF, Zacks SI (1979) Production in vitro of a neurotropic substance from proliferative neurolemma-like cells. Exp Neurol 64: 271–283

Lund RD, Lund JS (1971) Synaptic adjustment after deafferentation of the superior colliculus of the rat. Science 171: 804–807

Lynch G, Cotman CW (1975) The hippocampus as a model for studying anatomical plasticity in the adult brain. In: Isaacson RL (ed) The hippocampus: Structure and development, vol I. Plenum Press, New York, pp 123–154

Lynch G, Stanfield B, Cotman CW (1973) Developmental differences in postlesion axonal growth in the hippocampus. Brain Res 59: 155–168

Lynch G, Stanfield B, Parks T, Cotman CW (1974) Evidence for selective post-lesion axonal growth in the dentate gyrus of the rat. Brain Res 69: 1–11

Marchase RB (1977) Biochemical investigations of retinotectal adhesive specificity. J Cell Biol 75: 237–257

Mena EE, Cotman CW (1979) Lesion-induced changes of complex carbohydrates in the rat dentate gyrus. Soc Neurosci Abstr 5: 632

Merrel R (1976) Membranes as a tool for the study of cell surface recognition. In: Barondes S (ed) Neuronal recognition. Plenum Press, New York, pp 249–273

Norlander RH, Singer M (1978) The role of ependyma in regeneration of the spinal cord in the urodele amphibian tail. J Comp Neurol 180: 349–374
Parnavelas JG, Lynch G, Brecha N, Cotman CW, Globus A (1974) Spine loss and regrowth in the hippocampus following deafferentation. Nature (London) 248: 71–73
Puchala E, Windle WF (1977) The possibility of structural and functional restitution after spinal cord injury. A review. Exp Neurol 55: 1–42
Ramón y Cajal S (1928) Degeneration and regeneration of the nervous system. Translated by May RM, vol I. Hafner Publ Co, New York, pp 47–51
Scheff SW, Benado LS, Cotman CW (1978) Effect of serial lesions on sprouting in the dentate gyrus: Onset and decline of the catalytic effect. Brain Res 150: 45–53
Schlaepfer WW, Micko S (1978) Chemical and structural changes of neurofilaments in transected rat sciatic nerve. J Cell Biol 78: 369–378
Schlaepfer WW, Micko S (1979) Calcium-dependent alterations of neurofilament proteins of rat peripheral nerve. J Neurochem 32: 211–219
Schubert P, Kreutzberg GW (1975) [^{3}H] adenosine, a tracer for neuronal connectivity. Brain Res 85: 317–319
Singer M, Norlander RH, Egar M (1980) Axonal guidance during embryogenesis and regeneration in the spinal cord of the newt. The blueprint hypothesis of neuronal pathway patterning. J Comp Neurol 185: 1–22
Sperry R (1963) Chemoaffinity in the orderly growth of nerve fiber patterns and connections. Proc Natl Acad Sci USA 50: 703–710
Stenevi U, Björklund A, Svendgaard NA (1976) Transplantation of central and peripheral monoamine neurons to the adult rat brain: Techniques and conditions for survival. Brain Res 114: 1–20
Storm-Mathisen J (1974) Choline acetyltransferase and acetylcholinesterase in facia dentata following lesion of the entorhinal afferents. Brain Res 80: 181–197
Sumner BEH (1975) A quantitative analysis of the response of presynaptic boutons to postsynaptic motor neuron axotomy. Exp Neurol 46: 605–615
Watson WE (1974) Cellular responses to axotomy and related procedures. Br Med Bull 30: 112–115
Weiss P (1939) Principles of development. Holt Pub. Co, New York, 126 p
Weiss P, Hiscoe HB (1948) Experiments on the mechanism of nerve growth. J Exp Zool 107: 315–395
Wells MR, Bernstein JJ (1977) Amino acid incorporation into rat spinal cord and brain after simultaneous transection and crush or transection followed by crush of sciatic nerve. Brain Res 139: 249–262
Wells MR, Bernstein JJ (1980) Amino acid uptake in the spinal cord and brain of the rat with long-term spinal hemisection. Exp Neurol 68: 122–135
Wells MR, Lofton SA, Bernstein JJ (1979) Effect of triiodothyronine on the amino acid uptake of the brain and spinal cord after spinal hemisection in adult rats. Soc Neurosci Abstr 5: 685
Windle WF (1955) Comments on regeneration in the human central nervous system. In: Windle WF (ed) Regeneration in the central nervous system. CC Thomas, Springfield Illinois, pp 265–272

Changes in Neurotransmitter Synthesizing Enzymes During Regenerative, Compensatory, and Collateral Sprouting of Central Catecholamine Neurons in Adult and Developing Rats

D.J. REIS[1], R.A. ROSS[2], L. IACOVITTI[3], G. GILAD[4], and T.H. JOH[1]

1 Introduction

It is evident that the recovery of function following injury of the central nervous system (CNS) must relate to cellular processes by which synaptic transmission is modified morphologically and also by mechanisms facilitating chemical neurotransmission. While there has been a resurgence of interest in morphological concomitants of recovery of function, less is known about the changes in neurotransmitter biosynthetic enzymes following injury and their possible role in functional recovery.

Over the past several years our laboratory has been studying the reaction of central catecholamine systems to injury either direct (i.e., caused by axonal damage) or indirect (produced by lesions to neurons other than the catecholaminergic), focusing on the effect of such injuries on the activities and amounts of the biosynthetic enzymes TH and DBH (Gilad and Reis 1978, 1980; Iacovitti et al. 1980; Reis et al. 1978a,b; Reis and Ross 1973; Ross and Reis 1974; Ross et al. 1975, 1979). Our studies have provided a number of new and interesting facts about the response of central neurons to injury, challenging a number of previously accepted doctrines and providing new information on the nature of the reorganization of neurons in the brain following neuronal damage.

The reaction to injury of neurons of the CNS, which synthesize, store, and release the catecholamine neurotransmitters dopamine (DA) or norepinephrine (NE), has been examined ever since the discovery of these chemically specific systems in the brain over a decade ago. At first, axonal lesions were utilized only as a tool for mapping the intracerebral distribution of these systems within the brain (Anden et al. 1966; Ungerstedt 1971). More recently, however, central NE and DA systems have been utilized as models for studies of the general processes by which nerve cells, particularly those intrinsic to the brain, respond to injury (see Reis et al. 1978b for review). The advantage of the catecholamine systems as models for such analysis are several: (1) Catecholamine neurons in CNS undergo both regenerative and collateral sprouting (Bjorklund

---

1 Laboratory of Neurobiology, Department of Neurology, Cornell University Medical College, New York, NY 10021, USA
2 Department of Biology, Fordham University, New York, NY, USA
3 Department of Anatomy and Neurobiology, Washington University, St. Louis, MO, USA
4 Department of Isotope Research, Weizmann Institute of Science, Rehovet, Israel

et al. 1971; Bjorklund and Stenevi 1971; Gilad and Reis 1978, 1979, 1980; Iacovitti et al. 1980; Katzman et al. 1971; Moore et al. 1971; Reis et al. 1978a; Reis and Ross 1973; Robinson et al. 1975); (2) the anatomies of these systems are well defined (Ungerstedt 1971; Moore and Bloom 1978); (3) their transmitters can be measured biochemically or visualized by histochemistry; and of particular importance is the fact that (4) the enzymes which specifically subserve the biosynthesis of catecholamines including tyrosine hydroxylase (TH), the enzyme which catalyzes the rate-limiting step in the biosynthesis of all catecholamines, and dopamine-β-hydroxylase (DBH), the enzyme converting DA to NE, have been purified and antibodies produced against them (see Reis et al. 1978b). Such antibodies permit the use of immunochemical techniques for determining the amount of enzyme protein, the relative rates of synthesis, and their localization, by light and electron microscopic immunocytochemistry. The enzymes thus are powerful biochemical probes, representing specific proteins restricted to a particular population of central neurons and easily charted in the cytoplasm.

2 The Reaction of Central Catecholamine Neurons to Axonal Injury

2.1 The Model Systems

The model system which we have utilized for studying the reaction of NE neurons to injury has been that arising from the nucleus of the locus ceruleus (LC). In rat the LC consists of 1400 neurons (Ross et al. 1975) on each side of the brain, which send highly collateralized axons through well-defined trajectories to innervate the upper brainstem, including hypothalamus, telencephalon, cerebellum, and portions of the lower brainstem (Moore and Bloom 1978; Ungerstedt 1971). To study the response of these nerve cells to injury, damage has been produced by electrolytic lesions placed stereotaxically at different sites in the projection path, usually in the lateral hypothalamus. The animals and matched controls are killed at various days after placement of lesions. For biochemical analysis, the brain is removed and dissected. The frontal cortex is removed for analysis of the anterograde reaction; the LC is microdissected for analysis of the retrograde (axon) reaction in parent neurons, while the cerebellum or lower brainstem is isolated for analysis of changes in uninjured collaterals. For histological studies, the animals are killed by perfusion through the heart and regions of terminals, collaterals, or cell bodies examined.

Studies of the DA system have primarily utilized the nigrostriatal (A9) or the mesolimbic (A10) systems (Moore and Bloom 1978; Ungerstedt 1971). In the A9 system the cell bodies are localized in the substantia nigra and project rostrally to innervate, in a topographically organized manner (Moore and Bloom 1978), the striatum. The A10 neurons innervate more widespread regions of the limbic system. In most of our studies we have focused on the innervation of the olfactory bulb provided by a group of A10 cells. The strategy of these studies is similar to that used for studying noradrenergic neurons: lesions are placed and, at various times thereafter, animals are killed and their brains dissected or prepared for histology.

2.2 Anterograde Response

Lesions of cell bodies, axons, or axon terminals of either central NE or of DA neurons result in a characteristic pattern of biochemical and morphological changes in the degenerating axon and nerve terminals. Biochemically, in the terminal field there is a permanent reduction in the content of the neurotransmitter (Erinoff and Heller 1973; Moore and Heller 1967), in the capacities of the terminals to take up and store neurotransmitter via the high affinity uptake system (Zigmond et al. 1971) and in the catalytic activities of the biosynthetic enzymes TH, DBH, and the nonspecific decarboxylating enzyme l-amino acid decarboxylase (Reis et al. 1978a,b). Reduction of the activities of these enzymes is almost, but not entirely complete, and is entirely attributable to loss of enzyme protein.

Qualitatively the changes in the NE and DA systems are comparable. However, quantitatively they differ with respect to time course of degeneration (Fig. 1). While the loss of enzymes in degenerating noradrenergic neurons does not reach a nadir for 14 days (Ross and Reis 1974; Ross et al. 1975), the disappearance of TH enzyme and of transmitter in dopaminergic terminals occurs within 24 to 48 h (Fig. 1) (Reis et al. 1978a), a time course similar to that of the disappearance of transmitter-related molecules in peripheral sympathetic nerves after axonal injury. The molecular basis for the difference in the time for degeneration of transected central NE and DA axons is unknown. Electron microscopic studies have suggested that some of the enzyme in degenerating NE neurons may persist within astroglia (Reis et al. 1978b).

2.3 The Retrograde Reaction in Adults

2.3.1 The Response in NE Neurons

a) Changes in Enzymes. The retrograde response to axonal injury occurring in the cell bodies of central CA neurons has been characterized in both the NE neurons of the LC (Ross et al. 1975, 1979) and DA neurons in the midbrain tegmentum (Gilad and Reis 1978; Reis et al. 1978a). In general, the responses are comparable but have been much more intensively studied in the NE system.

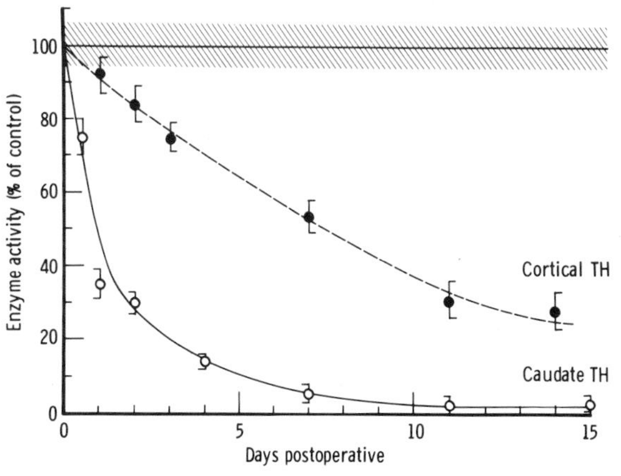

Fig. 1. Time course of fall in TH activity in ipsilateral caudate nucleus and frontal cortex following a unilateral lesion of lateral hypothalamus transecting the DA nigrostriatal and ascending NE pathways. Note the rapid decline of TH in DA projection. Values expressed as mean ± SEM for approximately 6 rats in this and subsequent figures (Reis et al. 1978b)

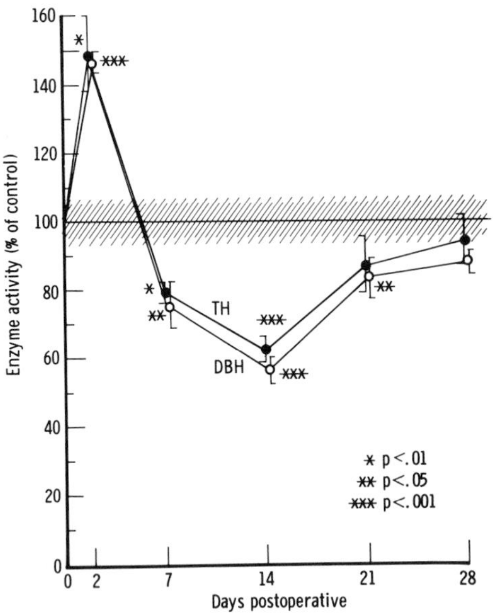

Fig. 2. Time course of changes in TH and DBH activity in LC at various days following axonal transection produced by electrolytic lesions of the lateral hypothalamus in rat (from Reis et al. 1978b). *Asterisks* denote significant differences from control. $^*p < 0.05$; $^{**}p < 0.01$; $^{***}p < 0.001$

Damage of axons of NE neurons of the CNS results in the characteristic pattern of changes in the biochemistry within the parent neurons in the LC (Fig. 2). The changes occur in three distinct phases: (1) a phase of pile-up (days 1–3); (2) a phase of reduced accumulation of neurotransmitter enzymes (days 4–21); and (3) a phase of recovery.

(1) The *phase of pile-up* consists in a marked enhancement in the activities of TH and DBH within the LC, representing most probably an increased accumulation of enzyme protein. Associated is an increase in histofluorescence (Ungerstedt 1971) indicating that the enzyme is catalytically active and producing more transmitter. The increase of enzyme activity in this phase can be almost twofold; it peaks at around 24 h and then rapidly declines, blending into the phase of reduced accumulation of enzyme protein.

The simplest explanation of the pile-up, as the name implies, is mechanical. The interpretation assumes that under steady state conditions the nerve cell is producing sufficient enzyme to maintain relatively constant quantities within the terminal in which to disperse the macromolecules. Hence, they accumulate behind the lesion until the cell readjusts its program of enzyme biosynthesis to accommodate the reduction of cytoplasmic volume. The increased concentration of enzyme per unit of cytoplasm during the pile up phase results in an elevated quantity of neurotransmitter as demonstrated by histofluorescence studies (Ungerstedt 1971).

There may, in fact, be a biologically important concomitant in the phase of pile-up. It is well established by histofluorescence studies that the enhanced amount of neurotransmitter persists long after the time during which enzyme activity is reduced. In view of the fact that the biosynthesis of neurotransmitter enzymes is regulated in part by end product (see, e.g., Burke et al. 1978), i.e., the neurotransmitter itself, pile-up may, in fact, provide the signal to down-regulate the amount of translation of RNA specifically coded for the production of the neurotransmitter biosynthetic enzymes. The reduced biosynthesis of enzyme would lead into the next phase.

(2) The *phase of reduced accumulation* of neurotransmitter enzymes follows immediately after the phase of pile-up. The reduction appears to affect only the specific catecholamine enzymes TH and DBH within the LC neurons, the activities of DDC and the degradative enzyme monoamine oxidase (MAO) not being changed (Ross et al. 1975). The rate for the decline in enzyme activity is much more rapid than the loss of enzymes in the anterograde reaction, falling substantially over only a few days. The time course and magnitude of the retrograde changes of TH and DBH are activities remarkably similar (Fig. 2). The activities of TH fall to about 60% of control where they remain from approximately day 7 to 14, suggesting coordinate regulation.

Reduction in the activities of TH and DBH during the retrograde reaction is entirely a consequence of reduced accumulation of enzyme protein, as can be demonstrated immunochemically (Ross et al. 1975). By pulse labeling DBH and LC neurons in vivo with ^{3}H-amino acids perfused into the IVth ventricle, and then by isolating DBH protein by immunochemical techniques, we have been able to estimate that the reduction of DBH is entirely due to a reduction in the relative rate of biosynthesis of DBH enzyme protein (Ross et al. 1979). Presumably a comparable mechanism accounts for the changes in accumulation of TH.

(3) The *phase of recovery* follows 2 to 3 weeks after axonal lesions. At this time enzyme activity gradually returns to normal. The return to biochemical normalcy is due to recovery of the complement of enzyme within injured nerve cells and not as a consequence of death of some neurons with compensatory exaggeration of content in those that remain (Ross et al. 1975).

b) Changes in Uninjured Collaterals. Biochemical changes also occur in remote uninjured collaterals within the cerebellum in response to damage to LC axons projecting through the hypothalamus (Reis and Ross 1973) (Fig. 3). In parallel with reduced accumulation of TH within LC neurons is a reduction in enzyme activity within the cerebellum comparable in magnitude and in time course to those in the parent cell body. Thus the initiation of reduced accumulation of enzyme in cell bodies by axonal injury results in diminished availability of enzyme molecules for distribution and transport into uninjured collaterals.

c) Morphological Concomitants of the Response. The classical morphological perikaryal response to axotomy comprises the chromotolytic reaction (Cragg 1970; Lieberman 1971, 1974) and consists of neuronal swelling, dissolution of Nissl substance, nuclear eccentricity, and unstacking of the RER. A detailed analysis by light and electron microscopy of LC neurons to injury (Reis et al. 1978b) indicates, however, that there are few and only subtle morphological changes in LC neurons and only detectable by electron microscopy in the face of profound alterations in the accumulation of biosynthetic enzymes. Thus the changes in the amount of neurotransmitter synthesizing enzymes in central NE neurons in response to axonal damage occur without classic signs of chromatolysis, at least by light microscopy.

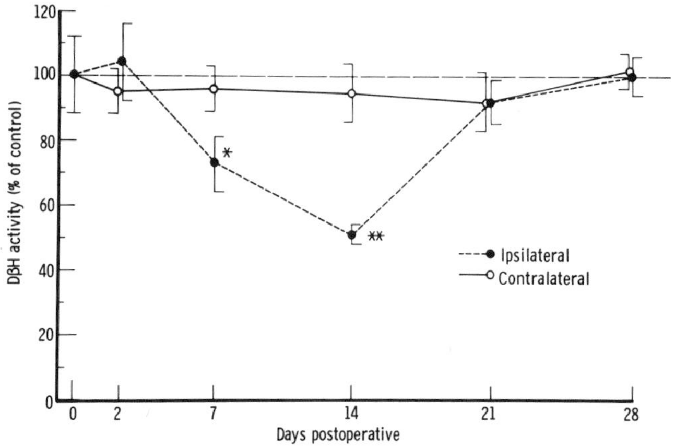

Fig. 3. Time course of changes in DBH activity in cerebellar hemisphere of rat following unilateral lesion of posterolateral hypothalamus. Note that the fall of DBH parallels that in LC (see Fig. 2) (Reis and Ross 1973)

d) Relationship to Regenerative Sprouting. It has often been proposed that in the peripheral nervous system the cellular events of chromatolysis are related to the development of regenerative sprouts from the lesioned axons (Lieberman 1971). One argument for the relationship is based on the temporal association between the appearance of sprouts, usually within 2 to 5 days, and the onset of chromatolysis.

It is well established now that the NE system within the brain, like other monoamine systems, can undergo regenerative sprouting from lesioned axonal tips (Bjorklund and Stenevi 1979). Such regeneration can be elicited by electrolytic lesions or by administration of the neurotoxin 6-OHDA (Bjorklund and Stenevi 1979; Jonsson and Sachs 1976). Fine regenerative sprouts can be seen by 5 to 15 days following the lesion. With mechanical or electrolytic damage the sprouts, which are exuberant, appear to remain indefinitely. The close association of the production of new axoplasm at a time (5–15 days) when the biosynthesis and accumulation of neurotransmitter enzymes are reduced, suggests that one aspect of the retrograde reaction may be a shifting of priorities of protein biosynthesis away from the production of macromolecules required for neurotransmission in favor of those required for the reconstitution of cellular membranes (Reis et al. 1978b).

2.3.2 The Retrograde Reaction in Dopaminergic Neurons

The retrograde reaction in DA neurons is qualitatively similar to that in the central NE neurons (Gilad and Reis 1978; Reis et al. 1978a). The major difference is that lesions which are placed fairly close to the cells of origin will result in neuronal cell death. It is only with remote distal lesions that the recoverable retrograde response can be initiated, a relationship which closely follows the rule of the retrograde response in the periphery, namely that the magnitude and recoverability of the response is indirectly related up to the proximity of the lesion to the cell body (Lieberman 1971, 1974).

Presumably, central DA projections, which are topographically organized (Moore and Bloom 1978) do not have sufficient collaterals emanating from the cell body to permit cellular survival. However, with distal lesions, DA neurons of both the nigrostriatal and the mesolimbic systems exhibit a reversible reduction in accumulation of TH.

2.3.3 The Retrograde Reaction in Young Animals: Compensatory Sprouting and the Role of the Target

The lesions of axons of central NE neurons in developing animals produces effects which are qualitatively different from those observed in the adult (see Iacovitti et al. 1980; Reis and Ross 1973). The earliest observations of this fact were made in a series of studies in which neonatal rats were treated with the systemic administration of the catecholamine neurotoxins 6-hydroxydopamine (6-OHDA) or 6-hydroxydopa (6-OHDOPA) (Jonsson and Sachs 1976). Such treatment resulted in an enduring loss of catecholamine fibers in the forebrain and spinal cord, and the development within the lower brainstem of an increase in the number and distribution of CA-containing fibers as visualized by histofluorescence. The increase of brainstem fluorescence was associated with an increased content of NE, uptake of ^{3}H-norepinephrine into synaptosomes, and with the activities of the CA biosynthetic enzymes TH and DBH. The reactive changes to the neurotoxins were attributed to an outgrowth of sprouts from proximal uninjured branches of NE neurons of the LC after destruction of the distal collaterals. The response was viewed as a special case of a more general principle which governs the reaction of developing neurons to axonal injury: the so-called principle of conservation articulated by Devor and Schneider (1975). According to the principle, neurons are intrinsically programed to elaborate a defined quantity of terminal arborization during development: lesions preventing the growth of one branch of the neuron result in a compensatory overgrowth from other branches, a "pruning effect."

We have recently reinvestigated (Iacovitti et al. 1978, 1980) this question of compensatory sprouting in neonatal rats, asking the question as to whether it is damage to only *one* of the multiple pathways emerging from the LC which is responsible for the reactive sprouting. Our interests were stimulated by the fact that during the growth and development of the projections from LC neurons postnatally [formations of LC neurons occur two-thirds through gestation in the rat (Lauder and Bloom 1974; Nicholson et al. 1973; Specht et al. 1980)], the axons are innervating brain regions in different states of neurogenesis. Thus, one target of the LC, the hippocampus, has entirely completed its neurogenesis prenatally (Altman and Das 1965; Angevine 1965), while another target, the cerebellum, is still undergoing cell division throughout early postnatal life (Altman 1975; Winick 1976). To investigate this question, the effects in developing animals of transection of ascending branches of the LC to hippocampus were compared with those damaging branches to the cerebellum.

Cerebellectomy in 3-day old animals resulted in complete replication of compensatory sprouting in the brainstem and LC comparable in magnitude to that produced by others with the administration of neurotoxins. Thus, there was a persistent elevation within the lower brainstem in the activities of TH and DBH (Fig. 4), in the amounts of TH protein, the Vmax for the high affinity uptake of ^{3}H-NE into homogenates of the lower brainstem, and the intensity in number of catecholamine fluores-

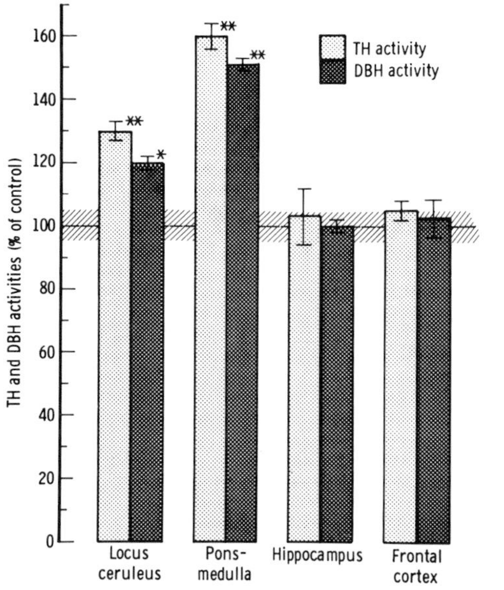

Fig. 4. Changes in the activities of TH and DBH in locus ceruleus, pons medulla, hippocampus, and frontal cortex in rats 30 days after cerebellectomy on day 3 of life. *$p < 0.01$; **$p < 0.001$ (Iacovitti et al. 1980)

cent terminals within the region. This response contrasted with the effects of hemisection of the posterior hypothalamus, which failed to produce any changes in the biochemical and morphological indices of noradrenergic function within the LC, lower brainstem, or cerebellum.

Of greatest interest was the fact that the reactive proliferation of LC neurons only occurred during a critical period of development. The response was gradually attenuated during early postnatal life and disappeared entirely by day 18, interestingly completed (Iacovitti et al. 1978, 1980).

These studies suggest that neonatal lesions of only the cerebellar, but not ascending projections of the LC, result in a proliferative response of processes from cell bodies within the brainstem and that this response only occurs during a critical period of early development. Since the reactive proliferation is lost at a time coincident with cessation of neuronal cytogenesis within the cerebellum, we have suggested that the selective response of LC neurons to injury is a consequence of interruption of projections to a target still in a primitive state of cytodifferentiation. Thus, the proliferative sprouting produced in neonatal animals by axonal injury may be a consequence of interruption of projections to developing target areas rather than an expression of a compulsion of the neuron to express an axonal field of given dimensions.

The nature of the signal from the cytodifferentiating target, which, in fact, appears to hold in check proliferation of the axon terminals, is entirely unknown. One possibility is that replicating cells may indeed produce a factor(s) which may suppress axonal growth. However, whatever the mechanism for the reactive proliferation, it is evident that the amounts of the neurotransmitter biosynthetic enzymes, even in this situation, are carefully calibrated to the size and ramifications of the terminal fields.

It is unknown whether compensatory sprouting also occurs with axonal lesions of central dopaminergic neurons.

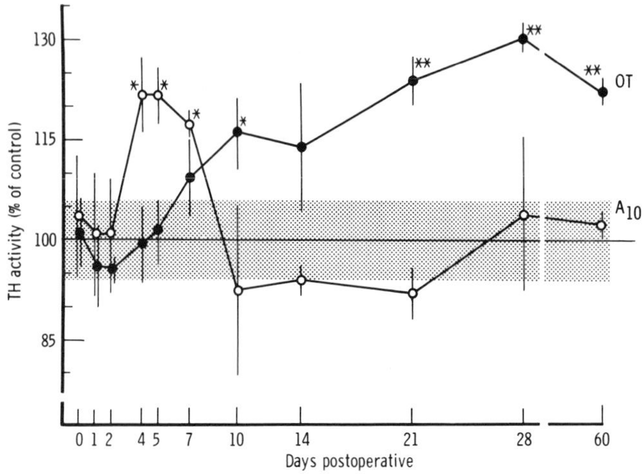

Fig. 5. Time course of changes in TH activity in cell bodies of A10 group and in their terminals in the olfactory tubercle (*OT*) following unilateral bulbectomy. $*p < 0.05$; $**p < 0.005$ (Reis et al. 1978b)

3 Collateral Sprouting in Central Catecholamine Neurons

3.1 Collateral Sprouting Studies in DA Neurons of Adult

It is now well established that catecholamine neurons of both DA and NE systems have the capacity to undergo collateral sprouting (e.g., Bjorklund and Stenevi 1979; Gilad and Reis 1978; Iacovitti et al. 1980; Moore et al. 1971; Reis et al. 1978a,b). The stimulus appears to be degeneration of fibers which are not CA-containing within an area containing CA terminals. As the noncatecholamine fibers disappear, the remaining fibers sprout in an apparent effort to reoccupy abandoned synaptic sites. Thereby they enlarge their terminal fields.

The changes of neurotransmitter enzymes associated with collateral sprouting in the dopaminergic systems have been analyzed by studying the collateral sprouting of mesolimbic DA when initiated by removal of the olfactory bulb whose mitral cells also innervate the tubercle (Gilad and Reis 1978, 1980).

Within one week following olfactory bulb ablation there is substantial evidence of collateral sprouting within the olfactory tubercle. The selective uptake of ^{3}H-DA appears within one week, signaling collateral sprouting, and is followed soon thereafter by a gradual increase in the activity of TH within the terminal field (Fig. 5). The increase of biochemically detectable TH is associated with an increase in the number of TH-containing terminals, as well as an alteration of their normal pattern of distribution as demonstrated by immunocytochemistry.

However, the first event associated with removal of the olfactory bulb occurred in the A10 cell bodies in the midbrain tegmentum. Here there was a surge of TH activity on days 3–7. Although the increase of enzyme activity of the A10 neurons is sufficient (about 30%) to permit analysis by immunochemical titration, an increase of immunocytochemical staining ipsilaterally suggested the presence of more enzyme protein in reacting neurons.

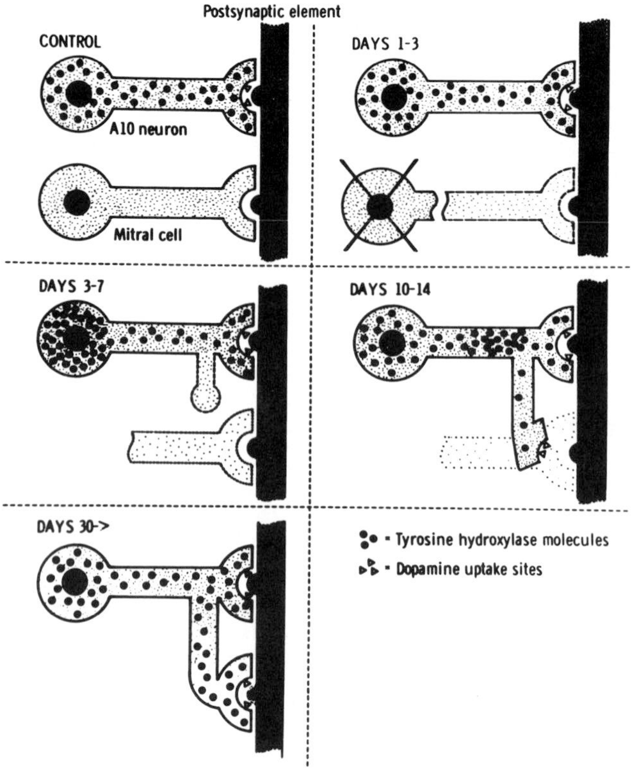

Fig. 6. Proposed mechanism accounting for biochemical changes in TH activity in olfactory tubercle following olfactory bulbectomy. Note lesion of mitral cell results in degeneration of afferents followed by increased accumulation of enzyme in cell body, and transport of surplus enzyme into an enlarging terminal field containing more uptake sites for ^{3}H-DA (Gilad and Reis 1979)

Thus the changes of TH in the cell body during collateral sprouting differ in direction and timing from that seen during regenerative sprouting initiated by axonal damage. The timing of the biochemical events in A10 neurons during collateral sprouting suggests a sequence of events as represented in Fig. 6: namely that along with degeneration of olfactory terminals there is at first sprouting of DA neurons paralleled by a surge of synthesis of TH within the cell bodies. This would be appropriate to tune the neuron to a new level of enzyme biosynthesis in order to accomodate to an enlarged axonal field and to produce enough enzyme protein to fill it.

Thereafter, as axonal sprouts are in place, and with the development of uptake processes, enzyme protein gradually increases to fill up these sprouts. Of particular interest is that this pattern is almost identical to that which is seen during early development of the DA innervation of the neuron, during which time axonal processes are being laid down in an enlarging terminal field (10).

It is of considerable interest that olfactory bulbectomy also results in long-term changes in the activities of the enzymes glutamic acid decarbocylase (GAD) and CAT

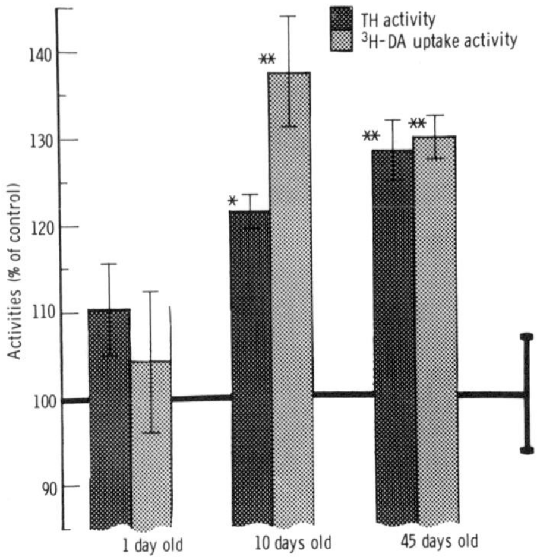

Fig. 7. Changes in TH activity and the uptake of ^{3}H-DA in the ipsilateral olfactory tubercle of adult rats after unilateral ablation of the olfactory bulb at different ages. Note failure of sprouting when lesions are placed in neonate (Gilad and Reis 1980)

within the oflactory bulb (40). GAD activity increases within 2 days and remains elevated for the remainder of the animal's life. CAT activity increases also at the same time; however, it rapidly returns to normal by day 21 at a time when TH activity is fully developed in the olfactory tubercle. An interpretation of these results is that intrinsic GABA neurons in the olfactory tubercle also undergo collateral sprouting in response to removal of mesolimbic structures with the removal of the olfactory bulb, and the sprouts remain in place. Changes of CAT in the cholinergic neurons, also intrinsic in the olfactory tubercle, may reflect formation of temporary synapses replaced by the ingrowing dopaminergic fibers.

3.2 Collateral Sprouting of DA Neurons in Young Animals

The response of young animals to olfactory bulbectomy is qualitatively different from that produced in the adults (Gilad and Reis 1980). Indeed, if the olfactory bulb is removed in animals younger than 7 days of age, the collateral sprouting of DA neurons does not appear as the animal matures (Gilad and Reis 1980). However, when lesions are placed in animals 10 days of age or older, there is abundant sprouting (Fig. 7). The most interesting association of the phenomenon relates to the time of maturation and organization of the olfactory bulb. Full organization of the cellular layering of the olfactory bulb does not occur in young rats until after 7 days of age. Thus the removal of an ingrowing afferent system from the olfactory bulb into an immature target, the olfactory tubercle, fails to initiate the sprouting of the DA innervation. It is only when the OT achieves final cellular organization that such sprouting can occur.

This result is in a sense counter-intuitive for it might be expected that sprouting would be much more abundant in developing neurons in view of their well established plasticity and the fact, from behavioral studies, that recovery of function from brain lesions occurs much more readily when such lesions are inflicted in young rather than old animals. The mechanism which accounts for the failure of collateral sprouting when lesions are produced in developing rats is unknown. Three possible explanations have been proposed. One is that only after the postsynaptic cell has developed a minimal complement of synapses can collateral sprouting occur in response to partial deafferentation. Removal of an input before synapse formation may not lead to differentiation of the postsynaptic cell and thus does not create a stimulus for the sprouting of other inputs.

A second explanation relates to the proximity of the fibers of different classes of neurons to denervated target cells. In early development, as DA fibers are still growing into the olfactory tubercle, it is conceivable that intrinsic neurons have greater access to denervating neurons and can effectively compete for the synaptic sites, thereby occupying them and leaving no further stimulus for growth of dopaminergic fibers. Thus the relative timetable of ingrowth of fibers into the target area may account for competition in the developing animal, with some systems having preeminence over others.

A third possibility is that the state of development of neurons in the region may, in fact, be essential as a stimulus for collateral sprouting, and that target areas still undergoing neuronal organization may not be capable of stimulating collateral sprouts.

4 Summary and Some General Neurobiological Implications of Studies of the Reaction of Central Catecholamine Neurons to Axonal Injury

The reactions of central catecholamine neurons to axonal injury reviewed in this essay not only have enlarged knowledge of the specific behaviors of NE and DA systems, but have provided new facts and provocative hypotheses with respect to the reaction of intrinsic neurons of the CNS to injury. Some of these hypotheses appear to have general implications with respect to the cellular dynamics of neurons during degeneration, regeneration, and development. They must in some manner relate to the cellular mechanisms governing the recovery of function following neuronal injury.

4.1 The Retrograde Reaction in Intrinsic Neurons May Be Reversible

It has long been proposed (Cole 1968; Cragg 1970; Lieberman 1971) that intrinsic neurons of the CNS do not have the capacity to undergo retrograde responses which are reversible. It was generally believed they either underwent retrograde cell death or did not respond at all. Our discovery that reduced and reversible accumulation of neurotransmitter-synthesizing enzymes can occur in the intrinsic NE and DA systems of brain in the absence of chromatolysis demonstrates that the classic view is incorrect. Intrinsic neurons of the CNS in fact do possess the capacity to undergo retrograde changes, and these may be reversible.

4.2 A Reversible Reduction of the Biosynthesis of Neurotransmitter-Synthesizing Enzymes May Be a Specific Biochemical Event Associated with the Retrograde Reaction

Our observation in central NE and DA suggests that a reduction in synthesis, amount, and activity of neurotransmitter-synthesizing enzymes may be a general biochemical feature of the retrograde reaction. In support are observations that comparable reversible reduction in biosynthetic enzymes occur in cholinergic (Wooten et al. 1978) and serotonergic (Reis et al. 1978b) neurons.

4.3 Biochemical Changes of the Retrograde Reaction May Occur Without Evident Morphological Changes of Chromatolysis

Our observation that axonal lesions of NE neurons can lead to a reversible reduction in the amount of TH and DBH in locus ceruleus neurons without chromatolysis demonstrates that the biochemical and morphological changes can be dissociated. Whereas these may represent only matters of the intensity of the reaction (the biochemical events being a more sensitive indicator), they underscore the fact that the absence of chromatolysis does not mean the absence of biochemical components of the axon reaction.

4.4 Changes in Protein Biosynthesis in the Retrograde Reaction May Be Selective

It has generally been believed that during the retrograde reaction there is an increase in net protein and RNA biosynthesis (Lieberman 1971). These findings have suggested therefore that the retrograde reaction was primarily an anabolic event related more to the attempts of the neuron to regenerate by sprouting than to degeneration.

Our finding of a decrease in the synthesis of DBH in central NE neurons during the retrograde reaction, resulting in a reduction in the activity and amount of the enzyme, provides the first direct evidence of selective reordering of protein biosynthesis in neurons undergoing retrograde cell changes. The pattern of biochemical modifications suggests that the response would be characterized by an increase of proteins required for reestablishment of axonal membrane at the expense of those required for the function of the cell in neurotransmission.

4.5 Changes in the Cell Body Initiated by Damage to One Axonal Branch May Be Reflected in Uninjured Collaterals

Hypothalamic lesions damaging ascending branches of a central locus neuron initiate biochemical changes not only in the parent cell body, but in uninjured collaterals in cerebellum. This observation indicates that a whole field of innervation of a neuron is "informed" of damage to a remote collateral. The biological significance of such widespread impairment of neuronal functions is unknown. It could relate to a reduction in the efficacy of the neuron in chemical neurotransmission. Indeed, the widespread reduction in NE neurons following stroke lesions experimentally produced in rats (Robinson et al. 1975) raises the possibility that in pathological states some of the widespread impairment of brain function (diaschesis) may be a consequence of loss of generalized reactivity of the neuron. More intriguing, however, is the possibility that the biochemical changes in remote terminals might be of importance in the recovery of physiological function following brain damage, i.e., may participate in the transfer of recovery of function from one brain area to another, leading thereby to functional compensation.

4.6 Neurotransmitter-Synthesizing Enzymes May Be Regulated by the Size of the Axonal Field

One ancillary finding of our studies is the demonstration that the enzymes responsible for catecholamine neurotransmitter biosynthesis, TH and DBH, are regulated by the integrity of neuronal surface. The surface regulation is an additional mode of long-term regulation of the enzymes. In part, the regulation may relate to cell surface volume, since reduction of the field by axotomy leads to a reduced accumulation of enzyme protein, whereas an enlargement of the field during collateral sprouting or in growth and development will result in a transient elevation of enzyme in cell bodies.

4.7 The Reaction of Neurons to Injury is Qualitatively Different in Young Animals

Thus, in young animals lesions of some neurons may lead to reactive proliferation of collaterals which disappear in aging. Likewise collateral sprouting may not be effective following denervation in some target areas in neonates compared with adults. Thus, variability in the patterning of sprouting may relate, in some as yet uncertain way, to the well-known augmented recovery of neuronal function in young animals. In part, our studies have raised the interesting possibility that targets undergoing neurogenesis may suppress the development of sprouts.

Acknowledgment. Supported by grants from NIH (HL18974 and NS03346).

References

Altman J (1975) Effects of interference with cerebellar maturation on the development of locomotion. An experimental model of neurobehavioral retardation. UCLA Forum Med Sci 18: 41–91

Altman J, Das GD (1965) Autoradiographic and histological evidence of postnatal hippocampal neurogenesis in rat. J Comp Neurol 124: 319–336

Anden N-E, Dahlstrom A, Fuxe K, Larsson K, Olson L, Ungerstedt U (1966) Ascending monoamine neurons to the telencephalon and diencephalon. Acta Physiol Scand 67: 313–326

Angevine JB Jr (1965) Time of neuron origin in the hippocampal region: an autoradiographic study in the mouse. Exp Neurol Suppl 2: 1–70

Bjorklund A, Stenevi U (1971) Growth of central catecholamine neurons into smooth muscle grafts in the rat mesencephalon. Brain Res 31: 1–20

Bjorklund A, Stenevi U (1979) Regeneration of monoaminergic and cholinergic neurons in the mammalian central nervous system. Phys Rev 59: 62–100

Bjorklund A, Katzman R, Stenevi U, West K (1971) Development and growth of axonal sprouts from noradrenalin and 5-hydroxytryptamine neurons in rat spinal cord. Brain Res 31: 21–33

Burke WJ, Davis JW, Joh TH, Reis DJ, Horenstein S, Bhagat BD (1978) The effect of epinephrine on phenylethanolamine-N-methyltransferase in cultured explants of adrenal medulla. Endocrinology 103: 358–367

Cole M (1968) Retrograde degeneration of axon and soma in the nervous system. In: Bourne G (ed) Structure and function of nervous tissue, vol I. Academic Press, London New York, pp 269–298
Cragg BG (1970) What is the signal for chromatolysis? Brain Res 23: 1–21
Devor M, Schneider GE (1975) Neuroanatomical plasticity: the principle of conservation of total axonal arborization. In: Vital-Durand F, Jeannerod M (eds) Aspects of neural plasticity. Inserm, Paris, pp 191–201
Erinoff L, Heller A (1973) Failure of catecholamine development following unilateral diencephalic lesions in the neonatal rat. Brain Res 58: 489–493
Gilad GM, Reis DJ (1978) Reversible reduction of tyrosine hydroxylase enzyme protein during the retrograde reaction in mesolimbic dopaminergic neurons. Brain Res 149: 141–153
Gilad GM, Reis DJ (1979a) Neurochemical plasticity: increased glutamic acid decarboxylase activity in the olfactory tubercle following olfactory bulb removal during postnatal development. Brain Res 177: 200–203
Gilad GM, Reis DJ (1979b) Transneuronal effects of olfactory bulb removal on choline acetyltransferase and glutamic acid decarboxylase activities in the olfactory tubercle. Brain Res 178 (1): 185–190
Gilad GM, Reis DJ (1979c) Collateral sprouting in mesolimbic dopamine neurons: biochemical and immunocytochemical evidence of changes in the activity and distribution of tyrosine hydroxylase in terminal fields and in cell bodies of A10 neurons. Brain Res 160: 17–36
Gilad GM, Reis DJ (1980) Failure to detect collateral sprouting of mesolimbic dompaminergic neurons during early postnatal development. Brain Res 186 (1): 67–81
Iacovitti L, Joh TH, Reis DJ (1978) Prolonged changes in brainstem tyrosine hydroxylase following neonatal cerebellectomy. Neurosci Abstr 4: 474
Iacovitti L, Reis DJ, Joh TH, Reis DJ (1981) Reactive proliferation of brainstem noradrenergic nerves following neonatal cerebellectomy in rats: role of target maturation on neuronal response to injury during development. Brain Res 1: 3–23
Jonsson G, Sachs C (1976) Regional changes in [^{3}H]-noradrenaline uptake, catecholamines, and catecholamine synthetic and catabolic enzymes in rat brain following neonatal 6-hydroxydopamine treatment. Med Biol 54: 286–297
Katzman R, Bjorklund A, Owman C, Stenevi U, West K (1971) Evidence for regenerative axon sprouting of central catecholamine neurons in the rat mesencephalon following electrolytic lesions. Brain Res 25: 579–596
Lauder JM, Bloom FE (1974) Ontogeny of monoamine neurons in the locus coeruleus, raphe nuclei and substantia nigra of the rat. I. Cell differentiation. J Comp Neurol 155: 469–482
Lieberman AR (1971) The axon reaction: a review of the principal features of perikaryal response to axon injury. Int Rev Neurobiol 14: 49–124
Lieberman AR (1974) Some factors affecting retrograde neuronal response to axonal lesions. In: Bellairs R, Gray EG (eds) Essays on the nervous system. Clarendon Press, Oxford, pp 71–105
Moore RY, Bloom FE (1978) Central catecholamine neuron systems: anatomy and physiology of the dopamine system. Annu Rev Neurosci 1: 129–169
Moore RY, Heller A (1967) Monoamine levels and neuronal degeneration in rat brain following lateral hypothalamic lesions. J Pharmacol Exp Ther 156: 12–22
Moore RY, Bjorklund A, Stenevi U (1971) Plastic changes in the adrenergic innervation of the rat septal area in response to denervation. Brain Res 33: 13–35
Nicholson J, Lauder J, Bloom FE (1973) Cell differentiation and synaptogenesis in the locus coeruleus, raphe nuclei, and substantia nigra of the rat. Anat Rec 175: 398–399
Reis DJ, Ross RA (1973) Dynamic changes in brain dopamine-β-hydroxylase activity during anterograde and retrograde reaction to injury of central noradrenergic axons. Brain Res 57: 307–326
Reis DJ, Gilad G, Pickel VM, Joh TH (1978a) Reversible changes in the activities and amounts of tyrosine hydroxylase in dopamine neurons of the substantia nigra in response to axonal injury: As studies by immunochemical and immunocytochemical methods. Brain Res 144: 325–342
Reis DJ, Ross RA, Gilad GM, Joh TH (1978b) Reaction of central catecholaminergic neurons to injury: model systems for studying the neurobiology of central regeneration and sprouting. In: Cotman CW (ed) Neuronal plasticity. Raven Press, New York, pp 197–226

Robinson RG, Shoemaker WJ, Schlumpf M, Valk T, Bloom FE (1975) Experimental cerebral infarction in rat brain: effect on catecholamines and behavior. Nature (London) 255: 332–334

Ross RA, Reis DJ (1974) Effects of Lesions of locus coeruleus on regional distribution of dopamine-β-hydroxylase activity in rat brain. Brain Res 73: 161–166

Ross RA, Joh TH, Reis DJ (1975) Reversible changes in the accumulation and activities of tyrosine hydroxylase and dopamine-β-hydroxylase in neurons of nucleus locus coeruleus during the retrograde reaction. Brain Res 92: 57–72

Ross RA, Joh TH, Reis DJ (1979) Reduced rate of biosynthesis of dopamine-β-hydroxylase in the nucleus locus ceruleus during the retrograde reaction. Brain Res 160: 174–179

Specht L, Pickel V, Joh TH, Reis DJ (1981) Light microscopic immunocytochemical localization of tyrosine hydroxylase in prenatal rat brain. J Comp Neurol in press

Ungerstedt U (1971) Stereotaxic mapping of the monoamine pathways in the rat brain. Acta Physiol Scand 82 (Suppl 367): 1–48

Winick M (1976) Normal cellular growth of the brain. In: Malnutrition and brain development. Oxford Univ Press, New York, pp 35–61

Wooten GF, Park DH, Joh TH, Reis DJ (1978) Immunochemical demonstration of reversible reduction in choline acetyltransferase concentration in rat hypoglossal nucleus after hypoglossal nerve transection. Nature (London) 275: 324–325

Zigmond MJ, Chalmers JP, Simpson JR, Wurtman RJ (1971) Effect of lateral hypothalamic lesions on uptake of norepinephrine by brain homogenates. J Pharmacol Exp Ther 179: 20–28

Effect of a Conditioning Lesion on Axonal Regeneration and Recovery of Function

D.S. FORMAN[1], I.G. McQUARRIE[2,3], B. GRAFSTEIN[3], and D.L. EDWARDS[3]

Axonal regeneration following axotomy may be accelerated in neurons which have undergone a previous axonal injury. When axonal regeneration following an axotomy (the *testing lesion*) is altered as a result of the axon having undergone a previous injury (the *conditioning lesion*), we refer to this change as a *conditioning lesion effect.* The effect of a conditioning lesion is usually (but not always) an acceleration or enhancement of axonal outgrowth. It represents an interesting experimental manipulation which may shed light on the factors which initiate and control axonal regeneration. In this paper, we shall review current knowledge about conditioning lesion effects, present some new data, and discuss possible mechanisms and practical applications of conditioning lesion effects.

1 Types of Neurons Which Display Conditioning Lesion Effects

Effects of conditioning lesions have been demonstrated in several different types of neurons. In the mammalian peripheral nervous system, they have been found in sensory (McQuarrie et al. 1977; Forman et al. 1980), motor (Gutmann 1942; Hall-Craggs and Brand 1977; McQuarrie 1978; Sebille and Bondoux-Jahan 1980), and adrenergic (McQuarrie et al. 1978) neurons. They have also been found in the visual systems of lower vertebrates which are capable of regenerating optic axons, such as the goldfish (Landreth and Agranoff 1977; McQuarrie 1977; Grafstein and McQuarrie 1978; McQuarrie and Grafstein 1978; Edwards et al. 1981; Lanners and Grafstein 1980b) and various amphibia (Agranoff et al. 1976; Brock 1979). Although conditioning lesion effects are seen in many types of neurons, the details of the response are not the same in different types of neurons. For example, the rate of regeneration of the fastest growing axons may increase dramatically, as in the goldfish optic system (Grafstein and McQuarrie 1978; McQuarrie and Grafstein 1978; Table 1), increase slightly or be

1 Naval Medical Research Institute, NNMC, Bethesda, MD 20014, USA
2 Department of Anatomy, School of Medicine, Case Western Reserve University, Cleveland, Ohio 44106, USA
3 Department of Physiology, Cornell University Medical College, New York, NY 10021, USA

Table 1. Effects of a conditioning lesion on regeneration in the goldfish optic system

	Testing lesion alone	Testing lesion preceded by a conditioning lesion 14 days earlier
Rate of axonal elongation (mm/day)[a]	0.34 ± 0.03	0.74 ± 0.13
Initial delay before axonal outgrowth begins (days)[b]	4.3	2.5
Appearance of first axonal sprouts detectable by electron microscopy (days)[c]	2	1
Arrival of axons at optic tectum (days)[d]	16	8

[a] Determined by histological methods. Both conditioning and testing lesions were optic nerve crushes. From McQuarrie (1977)

[b] From extrapolation of histological data in (a)

[c] Electron microscopic data from Lanners and Grafstein (1980a-testing lesion alone and 1980b-testing lesion preceded by a conditioning lesion). Both the testing and conditioning lesions were optic tractotomies

[d] Determined by arrival of radioactively labeled regenerating axons in tectum. Both conditioning and testing lesions were optic nerve crushes. Axons were labeled with radioactive axonally transported proteins by injection of ^{3}H-proline into the eye 3–5 days after the testing lesion. The values given are the day on which the transported radioactivity in the axons which had grown into the tectum reached 10% of the final peak value, and thus represents the time when a substantial population of rapidly growing axons had reached the tectum. From McQuarrie (1977)

unaffected, as in rat sensory axons (McQuarrie et al. 1977; Forman et al. 1980), or even decrease, as in rat adrenergic axons (McQuarrie et al. 1978). Other parameters, such as the delay before initial sprouting, may also be affected to different degrees. Also, the axons which grow most rapidly may be affected differently from the population of axons which grow more slowly (McQuarrie 1978). Our description of the effects of a conditioning lesion is most complete for the regenerating axons of the goldfish retinal ganglion cells. They are especially favorable for studying effects of conditioning lesions because the effects are quite dramatic (described below), and because so much is known about the normal course of regeneration in these neurons (references in Grafstein and McQuarrie 1978).

2 Methods for Studying the Effects of a Conditioning Lesion

Since multiple steps in the process of regeneration may be altered as a result of a prior conditioning lesion, it follows that a variety of methods are needed to analyze its effects on different aspects of regeneration. Light microscopic studies of silver-stained axons (McQuarrie and Grafstein 1973; Wells and Bernstein 1977; McQuarrie 1979) and other histological methods (Mira 1979) have yielded valuable information. It should be realized, however, that in mixed nerves these stains do not distinguish between different populations of axons. Adrenergic axons may be visualized by histochemical methods (McQuarrie et al. 1977). Another technique which can be used to examine the growth of a single type of axon is to label the regenerating axons with axonally transported proteins (Forman and Berenberg 1978; McQuarrie 1978). The pinch test (Young and Medawar 1940; Gutmann et al. 1942; Konorski and Lubinska 1946) is a simple technique for measuring outgrowth of sensory axons that has been useful for analyzing the effects of conditioning lesions (McQuarrie et al. 1977; Forman et al. 1980). In this test, the most distal point on a nerve where a gentle mechanical pinch elicits a withdrawal reflex in a lightly anesthetized animal has been shown to mark the location of the few most rapidly growing sensory axons (Young and Medawar 1940; McQuarrie et al. 1977). Effects of conditioning lesions on regeneration have also been demonstrated with ultrastructural methods (Lanners and Grafstein 1980b), biochemical indices of axonal outgrowth (McQuarrie et al. 1978), and tests for recovery of function (Gutmann 1942; Hall-Craggs and Brand 1977; Edwards et al. 1981; Sebille and Bondoux-Jahan 1980).

In the design of experiments to analyze the effects of a conditioning lesion, an appropriate control is not regeneration in a previously unoperated nerve, but is rather regeneration in a nerve which had received a sham operation at the same time that the experimental group received the conditioning lesion. Nevertheless, no effects of a sham operation on axonal outgrowth have yet been detected; regeneration following a testing lesion appears to be the same in nerves which had received a previous sham operation and in nerves which had received a testing lesion alone. However, effects of a sham operation on some other aspects of neuronal physiology have been found (McQuarrie 1977). The use of contralateral neurons for the controls should be interpreted with caution, since some metabolic effects of experimental axotomies on contralateral neurons have been observed (McQuarrie 1977; Wells and Bernstein 1978).

3 Aspects of Axonal Regeneration Which May Be Affected by a Previous Conditioning Lesion

Effects of a conditioning lesion on the rate of axonal outgrowth have been studied extensively. The largest effect has been found in the goldfish optic system, where the rate doubles (Table 1). However, the rate of regeneration is not increased in all neurons. In the most rapidly growing rat somatosensory neurons there is either a small (McQuarrie et al. 1977) or no (Forman et al. 1980) increase in the rate of growth. Outgrowth of the few most rapidly regenerating motor axons is also not increased after a conditioning lesion, although outgrowth is accelerated for the main population of motor axons which follow behind the leading axons (McQuarrie 1978; Fig. 1). In adrenergic axons in the rat sciatic nerve the rate of growth is actually reduced from 3.9 to 1.8 mm/day (McQuarrie et al. 1978). This is the only situation to date where a conditioning lesion has been found to retard regeneration.

The most consistent effect of a conditioning lesion appears to be a reduction of the initial delay before outgrowth begins. In most experiments, this has not been directly examined microscopically, but instead the initial delay has been estimated by extrapolating the linear axonal growth pattern back to the time of zero growth (e.g., Gut-

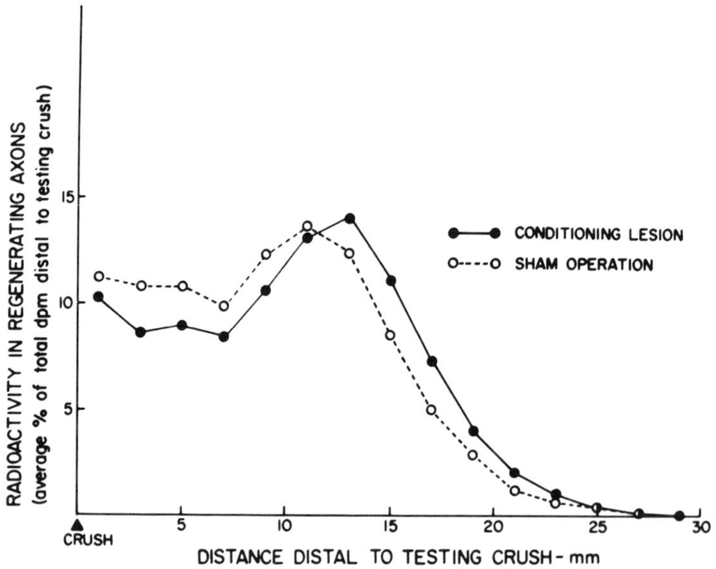

Fig. 1. Effect of a conditioning lesion on regeneration of motor axons in the rat sciatic nerve. The figure shows the distribution of radioactive proteins 8 days after a testing lesion. Fourteen days before the testing lesion the rats received a conditioning lesion (*filled circles*) or sham operation (*open circles*). The conditioning lesion (section of the tibial nerve distally), sham operation, and testing lesion (crush of the sciatic nerve in the upper thigh) were performed as described by McQuarrie et al. (1978) and Forman et al. (1980). Regenerating motor axons were labeled with axonally transported radioactive proteins, as described by Forman and Berenberg (1978). Briefly, ^{3}H-proline was microinjected into the spinal cord ventral horn 7 days after the testing lesion. Twenty-four hours later (i.e., 8 days after the testing lesion) the sciatic nerve was removed and the distribution of radioactive axonally transported protein along the nerve was determined by liquid scintillation counting. In order to normalize for differences in the amount of isotope incorporated by different animals, the radioactivity at each point was expressed as the percent of the total transported radioactivity distal to the testing lesion. These values were then averaged for each group. There were six rats in each group.

The interpretation of the patterns of radioactivity obtained with this technique is discussed in detail in Forman and Berenberg (1978). Current evidence indicates that 24 h after the isotope injection, the regenerating axons are fairly uniformly labeled along their axonal shafts, but are more heavily labeled at their tips. The excess accumulation of label at the endings produces the peak of radioactivity distal to the crush (with maxima at 11 mm in the control group and 13 mm in the group which had received conditioning lesions). The distal shift of this peak of radioactivity in the group with a conditioning lesion shows that most of their motor axons have grown further than in the controls. Note, however, that the locations of the fastest growing axons do not seem to be different in the conditioning lesion and sham-operated groups. The location of the ends of the axons which grew the farthest was determined by regression methods (Forman and Berenberg 1978), and was found to average 26.1 ± 1.0 (SEM) mm distal to the testing lesion in the animals which received a conditioning lesion and 24.7 ± 0.8 mm in the sham-operated controls. This difference is not statistically significant. These results (data of D. Forman) confirm a smaller previous study (McQuarrie 1978) mann et al. 1942). Determined by this approach, the initial delay in the goldfish optic system is reduced, following a testing lesion after a conditioning lesion made 2 weeks previously, from 4.3 to 2.5 days (Table 1). Similarly, with a conditioning interval of 2 weeks, the initial delay for the outgrowth of rat sciatic sensory axons was reduced from 1.6 to 0.9 days (Forman et al. 1980). Even in adrenergic axons, although the growth rate is reduced by a conditioning lesion, the initial delay was shortened from 1.3 to 0.6 days (McQuarrie et al. 1978). The greatly accelerated appearance of neurite outgrowth from explants of retina from goldfish (Landreth and Agranoff 1977) and *Xenopus* (Agranoff et al. 1976) is another manifestation of the earlier onset of axonal sprouting following a conditioning lesion.

In addition to reducing the delay before sprouting begins, a conditioning lesion may accelerate the time course of later sprout formation. For instance, examining silver-stained axons in mouse sciatic nerve, McQuarrie (1979) found that 6 days after a testing lesion which followed a conditioning lesion significantly more sprouts had grown 250 μm beyond the end of the nerve, although by 16 days the number of sprouts was nearly the same in the conditioning lesion and control groups. Lanners and Grafstein (1980a,b) have examined the early sprouts of regenerating goldfish optic axons by electron microscopy. Not only do axonal sprouts appear earlier in axons which had previously received a conditioning lesion, but the sprouts appear more mature morphologically. For example, by two days after the testing lesion, the sprouts in the conditioning lesion group were arranged in bundles and contained numerous microtubules, features not seen in control nerves until 6 days after the testing lesion. An interesting characteristic of the sprouts of nerves which had received a conditioning lesion was a marked increase in the number of coated vesicles.

The fragmentary available evidence suggests that in some systems a conditioning lesion may accelerate sprout formation without increasing the final number of sprouts (McQuarrie et al. 1978; McQuarrie 1979). However, a conditioning lesion can increase the number of regenerating axons which remyelinate in the rat sciatic nerve (Mira 1979). One month after the testing lesion, the number of regenerated myelinated axons was significantly elevated in nerves which had received a conditioning lesion (compared to nerves which had received a testing lesion alone). With two successive conditioning lesions at 21 day intervals, the number of myelinated axons was even greater; however, more than two conditioning lesions did not further increase this number. Most of the excess myelinated axons survived at least 18 months, but reached only 70% of the control fiber diameter.

A conditioning lesion can lead to accelerated recovery of function. In addition to accelerating recovery of motor function (Gutmann 1942), a conditioning lesion has been reported to improve the reinnervation of a muscle transplant (Hall-Craggs and Brand 1977). In one study accelerated recovery of motor function was seen, but only when the denervated muscle was treated by daily electrical stimulation (Sebille and Bondoux-Jahan 1980). The electrical stimulation apparently prevented the muscle atrophy (resulting from the conditioning lesion) which would otherwise have obscured the benefits of accelerated axonal regeneration. A conditioning lesion markedly reduces the time for the return of a visually mediated startle reaction in the regenerating goldfish optic system (Edwards et al. 1981; Table 2), although recovery of more complex visual functions is not markedly improved. It is unclear whether accelerated re-

Table 2. Determination of optimum conditioning interval for recovery of function in the goldfish optic system

Interval between conditioning and testing lesions (days)	Time of recovery of startle reaction following testing lesion (mean days ± SEM) Conditioning lesion = optic nerve crush	Conditioning lesion = optic tract cut
Testing lesion alone	18.5 ± 1.8 (13)	13.0 ± 0.9 (4)
0	19.8 ± 1.5 (17)	15.3 ± 0.5 (12)
7	11.8 ± 1.5[a] (13)	10.3 ± 0.9[a] (16)
14	8.9 ± 2.1[a] (7)	6.5 ± 0.6[a] (16)
21	21.1 ± 1.8 (13)	9.4 ± 0.4[a] (16)

Two types of conditioning lesions were used, crushing the optic nerve and cutting the optic tract. In both cases, the testing lesion was an optic nerve crush. The distance between the nerve crush site and the site where the tracts were cut was about 3 mm. The 0-day group received the conditioning lesion at the same time as the testing lesion. Recovery of function was determined by the presence of a startle reaction to bright light following 20 min of dark adaptation (Edwards et al. 1981). The nonoperated eye was inactivated by injection of 5% lidocaine.

[a] Values where difference from the 0-day group is significant at a level of at least $p < 0.05$. Note that the optimal conditioning interval, 14 days, is the same for both types of conditioning lesions

covery of function after a conditioning lesion is solely a consequence of faster axonal growth, or is also due to greater maturity or other qualitative changes in the regenerating sprouts or end organs.

4 Effects of the Conditioning Interval

Most studies of conditioning lesion effects have used a *conditioning interval* (the time between the conditioning and testing lesions) of 2 weeks. However, Forman et al. (1980) found that outgrowth of rat sensory axons was accelerated (although not maximally) if the conditioning interval was as short as 2 days. A conditioning interval of 1 day was ineffective. The effect of varying the conditioning interval has been explored most thoroughly in the goldfish optic system, using return of the startle reaction to measure recovery of function. In this system, the minimum effective conditioning interval was also 2 days (Edwards et al. 1981). However, the effect was not maximal until 14 days (Table 2), and began to decline by 21 days. Note that the optimal conditioning interval was the same regardless of whether the conditioning lesion was an optic nerve crush or an optic tract cut.

5 Possible Mechanisms Underlying the Conditioning Lesion Effect

Gutmann (1942) originally speculated that the effect of a conditioning lesion might be related to the increased number of Schwann cells induced by multiple injuries. Current evidence suggests instead that the effect is due to responses of the nerve cell body. Continued influence from Schwann cells at the site of the conditioning lesion seems unlikely, since an effect is seen when axons grow into connective tissue following excision of the segment of nerve which sustained the conditioning lesion (McQuarrie and Grafstein 1973; McQuarrie 1979) and when explants are grown in vitro (Agranoff et al. 1976; Landreth and Agranoff 1977). Furthermore, in many studies the testing lesion was made far proximal to the conditioning lesion, so that after the testing lesion any local effects emanating from the conditioning lesion site should be minimal (McQuarrie et al. 1977, 1978; McQuarrie 1978; Forman et al. 1980). Nonspecific metabolic effects between conditioned and uninjured neurons are ruled out by the finding that in a mixed nerve only the motor or sensory axons which receive the conditioning lesion show accelerated growth, while nearby nonconditioned axons are unaffected (McQuarrie 1978; Forman et al. 1980). By elimination, the cell body seems to be the likely locus of the conditioning lesion effect, although some change distributed throughout the entire neuron (e.g., increased membrane fluidity) cannot be ruled out.

That the conditioning lesion effect is mediated through the cell body is consistent with the old observation that chromatolytic changes in the cell body are enhanced by repeated injury (Howe and Bodian 1941). After reviewing clinical and some experimental data, Ducker et al. (1969) concluded that it is desirable to delay reparative peripheral nerve anastomoses until several weeks after the injury. In this situation, the original injury becomes a "conditioning lesion" to the second "testing" axotomy made by the surgeon, who trims the nerve before suturing the ends together. They suggested that the benefits of delay may be related to the development of metabolic responses in the cell body, which "prime" the neuron for regeneration. However, the exact relation between the events in the cell body and axonal outgrowth are not well understood (reviewed by Grafstein and McQuarrie 1978), and we can only speculate as to which components of the cell body response to axotomy produce the conditioning lesion effect.

Some evidence bearing on the mechanism comes from the observation that conditioning lesion effects may be detected after a conditioning interval as short as 2 days. The shortness of the minimal interval would seem to rule out many of the prominent morphological and metabolic changes in the cell body (reviewed by Grafstein and McQuarrie 1978), which take more than a week to develop (although these might play a role in the development of the maximum conditioning lesion effect), and points instead to the earlier responses of the cell body. It also focuses attention on fast axonal transport as a means of communication between the cell body and the injured axon that is rapid enough to be able to mediate the effects of short conditioning intervals. Indeed, one possibility is that the conditioning lesion effect is due to a change in either the amount or composition of the material carried by fast axonal transport. Changes in the amount (Bisby 1978) of the newly synthesized proteins carried by fast transport have been seen in rat sensory axons within 2 days of axotomy. Fast axonal transport in a conditioning lesion paradigm has been studied only in the goldfish optic system

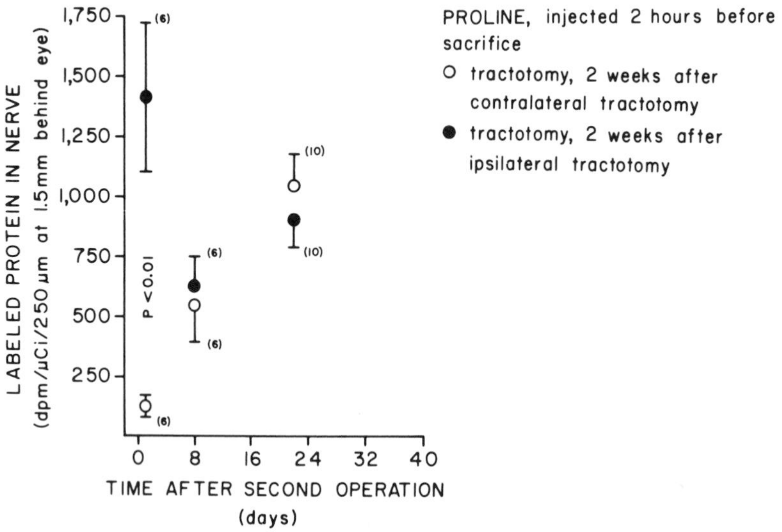

Fig. 2. Effect of a conditioning lesion on the amount of radioactive protein transported into the goldfish optic nerve following a testing lesion. The conditioning lesion was a unilateral section of the optic tract 2 weeks before the testing lesion. The contralateral optic tract served as a sham-operated control since it also incurred the effects of a craniotomy. For testing lesions, both optic tracts were cut at the optic chiasm. Two hours before sacrifice ^{3}H-proline was injected into both eyes. The graph shows the radioactivity in protein in the nerve 1.5 mm behind the eye (dpm per μCi of ^{3}H-proline injected). This was found to be a good index of the amount of radioactive protein carried from the eye by fast axonal transport. For details, see McQuarrie (1977). It can be seen that the amount of protein carried by fast transport 1 day after the testing lesion is greater in the nerve which had received the conditioning lesion than in the contralateral sham-operated nerve (where the values were unchanged from normal). The amount is also 70% greater than that which is transported 15 days after a single tractotomy (data not shown – the average would be about 800 dpm/μCi/250 μm segment). The excess of transported protein might play a role in the earlier sprouting seen in nerves after a conditioning lesion. By 8 days after the testing lesion, the amount of protein transported in the nerves with the conditioning lesion falls to the level seen after a testing lesion preceded by a sham conditioning lesion (*open circles*) or following a testing lesion alone (McQuarrie 1977)

(McQuarrie 1977; McQuarrie and Grafstein 1978). Following a 14-day conditioning interval, the amount of protein carried by fast transport was markedly elevated 1 day after the testing lesion (Fig. 2), but fell to the level found in control nerves by 8 days. The reduction in the initial delay appeared to be correlated with this transient early increase in the amount of newly synthesized protein transported into the axon, occurring prior to any additional increase in protein synthesis triggered by the testing lesion.

In addition to changes in the total amount of protein carried by fast transport, the effect of a conditioning lesion might be due to changes in the transport of specific proteins. Although the pattern of proteins carried by fast transport, as determined by SDS polyacrylamide gel electrophoresis, is remarkably unchanged after axotomy (Bisby 1980; Skene and Willard 1981; reviewed in Forman 1981), a few of the proteins do show significant relative increases within a few days of axotomy (Bisby 1980; Skene and Willard 1980). If these specific proteins are important for axonal sprouting or growth, their earlier or greater supply could enhance regeneration following a testing lesion preceded by a conditioning lesion.

Another response of the cell body which occurs early after axotomy, and therefore might contribute to the effect of a conditioning lesion, is the increase in the pentose phosphate "shunt" metabolic pathway (Härkönen and Kauffman 1974). This pathway produces NADPH that is required for lipid synthesis, and it is conceivable that the synthesis of lipids required for new axolemma during regeneration is suboptimal until the pathway adjusts. A conditioning lesion might accelerate outgrowth from a subsequent testing lesion by increasing the supply of rate-limiting membrane lipids.

6 The Conditioning Lesion Effect and Recovery of Function

Since an appropriately timed conditioning lesion can lead to accelerated axonal outgrowth, it is not surprising that this should lead to accelerated recovery of function provided reinnervation is successful. The possibilities of using this effect to improve surgical repair of severed nerves have not been fully explored; it may have value in special situations, such as muscle (Hall-Craggs and Brand 1977) and limb transplantation. Conditioning lesion effects may also be relevant to axonal growth and recovery of function in the central nervous system. For example, the growth of axons into delayed peripheral nerve grafts in transected spinal cord (Kao et al. 1977) may be facilitated by a conditioning lesion effect due to the delay before the second operation. A phenomenon closely analogous to the conditioning lesion effect is seen in sprouting in the central nervous system (Scheff et al. 1978), where a small lesion that does not lead to much sprouting of undamaged afferents may induce a greatly accelerated and enhanced sprouting response following a second, larger lesion. The time course of this effect on sprouting of central axons (Scheff et al. 1978) is similar to that of the conditioning lesion effect on axonal regeneration, although it is not clear whether these two phenomena share the same underlying mechanisms.

A conditioning lesion is one of the few experimental manipulations which can stimulate axonal regeneration. Analysis of the mechanisms for the effects of a conditioning lesion should shed light on the mechanisms which initiate and control axonal regeneration, and may lead to clinical applications for enhancing recovery of function following lesions in the nervous system.

Acknowledgments. Naval Medical Research and Development Command Research Task No. ZF58.524.013.1023. The opinions and assertions contained herein are the private ones of the writers and are not to be construed as official or reflecting the view of the Navy Department or the Naval Service at large. The experiments conducted herein were conducted according to the principles set forth in the current edition of the "Guide for the Care and Use of Laboratory Animals," Institute of Laboratory Animal Resources, National Research Council.

Supported by USPHS grants NS – 09015 from NINCDS and EY – 02696 from NEI to Dr. Grafstein, NS – 14967 from NINCDS to Drs. Grafstein and McQuarrie, and a grant from the Paralyzed Veterans of America to Dr. McQuarrie.

We are indebted to Ms. Roberta Alpert, Mr. Peter Mandelson, and Mr. David K. Wood for technical assistance, and to Dr. Rochelle Small for help in setting up the tests for recovery of vision. We are grateful to Astra Pharmaceuticals, Inc., for the gift of the lidocaine HCl (Xylocaine).

References

Agranoff BW, Field P, Gaze RM (1976) Neurite outgrowth from explanted *Xenopus* retina: an effect of prior optic nerve section. Brain Res 113: 225–234

Bisby MA (1978) Fast axonal transport of labeled protein in sensory axons during regeneration. Exp Neurol 61: 281–300

Bisby MA (1980) Changes in the composition of labeled protein transported in motor axons during their regeneration. J Neurobiol 11: 435–445

Brock TO III (1979) The effect of a repeated optic nerve lesion on the retinal ganglion cell body response and axon outgrowth in the newt, *Triturus viridescens.* Anat Rec 193: 491

Ducker TB, Kempe LG, Hayes GJ (1969) The metabolic background for peripheral nerve surgery. J Neurosurg 30: 270–280

Edwards DL, Alpert RM, Grafstein B (1981) Recovery of vision in regeneration of goldfish optic axons: enhancement of axonal outgrowth by a conditioning lesion. Exper Neurol, in press

Forman DS (1981) Axonal transport and nerve regeneration: a review. In: Kao CC, Bunge RP, Reier PJ, Grillner S (eds) Fundamentals of spinal cord reconstruction. Raven Press, New York, in press

Forman DS, Berenberg RA (1978) Regeneration of motor axons in the rat sciatic nerve studied by labeling with axonally transported radioactive proteins. Brain Res 156: 213–225

Forman DS, McQuarrie IG, Labore FW, Wood DK, Stone LS, Braddock CH, Fuchs DA (1980) Time course of the conditioning lesion effect on axonal regeneration. Brain Res 182: 180–185

Grafstein B, McQuarrie IG (1978) The role of the nerve cell body in axonal regeneration. In: Cotman C (ed) Neuronal plasticity. Raven Press, New York, pp 155–195

Gutmann E (1942) Factors affecting recovery of motor function after nerve lesions. J Neurol Psychiatr 5: 81–95

Gutmann E, Guttmann L, Medawar PB, Young JZ (1942) The rate of regeneration of nerve. J Exp Biol 19: 14–44

Hall-Craggs ECB, Brand P (1977) Effect of previous nerve injury on the regeneration of free autogenous muscle grafts. Exp Neurol 57: 275–281

Härkönen MHA, Kauffman FC (1974) Metabolic alterations in the axotomized superior cervical ganglion of the rat. II. The pentose phosphate pathway. Brain Res 65: 141–157

Howe HA, Bodian D (1941) Refractoriness of nerve cells to poliomyelitis virus after interruption of their axones. Johns Hopkins Hosp Bull 69: 92–109

Kao CC, Chang LW, Bloodworth JMB Jr (1977) Axonal regeneration across transected mammalian spinal cords: an electron microscopic study of delayed microsurgical nerve grafting. Exp Neurol 54: 591–615

Konorski J, Lubinska L (1946) Mechanical excitability of regenerating nerve fibers. Lancet 1: 609–610

Landreth GE, Agranoff BW (1977) Explant culture of adult goldfish retina: Effect of prior optic nerve crush. Brain Res 118: 299–303

Lanners HN, Grafstein B (1980a) Early stages of axonal regeneration in the goldfish optic tract: an electron microscopic study. J Neurocytol 9: 733–751

Lanners HN, Grafstein B (1980b) Effect of a conditioning lesion on regeneration of goldfish optic axons: ultrastructural evidence of enhanced outgrowth and pinocytosis. Brain Res in press

McQuarrie IG (1977) Axonal regeneration in the goldfish optic system: the role of the nerve cell body. Ph D Thesis, Cornell Univ Graduate School of Medical Sciences, New York

McQuarrie IG (1978) The effect of a conditioning lesion on the regeneration of motor axons. Brain Res 152: 597–602

McQuarrie IG (1979) Accelerated axonal sprouting after nerve transection. Brain Res 167: 185–188

McQuarrie IG, Grafstein B (1973) Axonal outgrowth enhanced by a previous nerve injury. Arch Neurol (Chicago) 29: 53–55

McQuarrie IG, Grafstein B (1978) Protein synthesis and fast axonal transport in regenerating goldfish retinal ganglion cells: effect of a conditioning lesion. Soc Neurosci Abstr 4: 533

McQuarrie IG, Grafstein B, Gershon MD (1977) Axonal regeneration in the rat sciatic nerve: effect of a conditioning lesion and of dbcAMP. Brain Res 132: 443–453

McQuarrie IG, Grafstein B, Dreyfus CF, Gershon MD (1978) Regeneration of adrenergic axons in rat sciatic nerve: effect of a conditioning lesion. Brain Res 141: 21–34

Mira J-C (1979) Quantitative studies of the regeneration of rat myelinated nerve fibres: variations in the number and size of regenerating fibres after repeated localized freezings. J Anat 129: 77–93

Scheff SW, Benardo LS, Cotman CW (1978) Effect of serial lesions on sprouting in the dentate gyrus: onset and decline of the catalytic effect. Brain Res 150: 45–53

Sebille A, Bondoux-Jahan M (1980) Effects of electric stimulation and previous nerve injury on motor function recovery in rats. Brain Res 193: 562–565

Skene JHP, Willard M (1981) Changes in axonally transported proteins during axon regeneration in toad retinal ganglion cells. J Cell Biol 89: 86–95

Wells MR, Bernstein JJ (1978) Amino acid incorporation into rat spinal cord and brain after simultaneous and interval sciatic nerve lesions. Brain Res 139: 249–262

Young JZ, Medawar PB (1940) Fibrin suture of peripheral nerves. Measurement of rate of regeneration. Lancet 2: 126–128

II. Sensorimotor Subsystems: Experimental Models and Techniques

a. Recovery from Spinal Lesions

Primary Afferent Synaptic Modulation as a Mechanism of Behavioral Compensation Following Spinal Cord Lesion in the Frog

A.R. BLIGHT and W. PRECHT[1]

1 Introduction

Direct investigation of neuronal mechanisms responsible for recovery of function following lesions of the central nervous system (CNS) or its peripheral inputs is limited by the need for detailed knowledge of normal functional organization in the system under study. Without this knowledge it is generally impossible to say whether a neuronal change consequent to lesion is a symptom of deficit or an aspect of compensatory self-regulation. Various studies have shown that when a neuron is partly deafferented other inputs to the cell or its region can take over vacant synaptic sites (see, e.g., Cotman, Gall, Tsukahara, this vol.) in a manner analogous to the "sprouting" of motor axon terminals onto denervated muscle fibers. However, it is not easy to demonstrate that such substitution of synaptic input is functionally useful.

We chose to examine the effects of spinal lesions on the input to frog motoneurons (MN's) because this system seemed to offer the possibility of directly correlating changes at the synaptic level with behavior, where such a correlation might be functionally interpretable. Fadiga and Brookhart (1960) established the idea that monosynaptic input from dorsal roots (DR's) to MN's in the frog spinal cord is situated almost exclusively on distal dendrites in the dorsal horn and that it gives rise therefore only to small excitatory postsynaptic potentials (EPSP's), which are relatively slow rising. They contrasted this with the large and faster-rising EPSP's, which could be elicited in the same cells by stimulating the lateral column (LC) of the thoracic cord. The shape, amplitude, and associated negative field potentials of these LC EPSP's suggested synapses restricted to the ventral horn, the somatic and proximal dendritic region of the cell.

It was therefore proposed to deafferent lumbar MN's proximally by cutting the ipsilateral LC and to determine any changes which occurred in the distribution of DR primary afferent projections on the same cells by electrophysiological recording. These might then be related to observed changes in behavior. This investigation showed first that the original interpretation of a segregated input from LC and DR was incorrect (Blight and Precht 1981) but that it was still possible to detect a modulation of primary afferent response, specifically in those MN's involved in the motor deficit follow-

---

1 Max-Planck Institut für Hirnforschung, Deutschordenstraße 46, 6000 Frankfurt/M 71, FRG

ing lesion. This modulation appeared to some extent to be responsible for the process of behavioral recovery.

2 Experimental Approach and Initial Findings

2.1 Lateral Column Lesions

All experiments were performed on grass frogs (*Rana temporaria*) of 30 ± 5 g body weight, acclimatized to laboratory temperatures of 18°–23°C. Animals were anesthetized for surgery by immersion in a solution of tricaine methanesulfonate (MS222–0.5 g/l). LC lesions were made from a dorsal approach, opening a space between thoracic vertebrae IV and V, without laminectomy, making a small opening in dura and pia mater with watchmaker's forceps, and using a fine suction pipette to remove a piece of spinal cord a half-to-one segment in length, close to a full hemisection but leaving the most medial ventral and dorsal tracts intact. Figure 1A shows the extent of a typical lesion from an animal killed 3 months after lesion, with a complete loss of LC fibers at the lesion site. In agreement with the results of other authors (Rensch and Franzisket 1954; Jankowski and Afelt 1964) we saw no evidence of regeneration of long tracts in the frog spinal cord after complete or partial thoracic section. Care was taken to prevent damage to large blood vessels, and capillary bleeding was suppressed with oxycel (Park Davis). Muscle (m. latissimus dorsi) and skin were sutured over the lesion site.

2.2 Behavioral Effects of Lesions

Large lesions of the lateral spinal cord had little effect on the behavior of the frog as long as there was little damage to circulation. Early attempts at lesion-making gave a wide variety of responses, including total paralysis of the hindlimbs and bi- or unilateral loss of postural tone. These effects could be attributed to disruption of circulation and were avoided by more careful techniques. Figure 1B shows that symmetry of posture was not noticeably impaired in operated animals. Locomotion was also little affected and no deficits were seen when the animal swam or walked on a smooth surface. There was little deficit even in the jump, which is the most powerful locomotory activity. The only clear effect was that the hind limb ipsilateral to the lesion frequently showed a delay in being brought under the body at the end of the jump (Fig. 1D), in contrast to the extension phase (Fig. 1C) which was symmetrical, as in the normal animal. This flexion weakness was also seen when the animal walked on surfaces which impeded movement, such as a wire grid. The animal could clearly make the required movements or postural adjustments, usually only a few hundred milliseconds later than the normal animal, but the initial movement was too weak to overcome external resistance, suggesting perhaps a loss of tonic excitation upon flexor MN's.

Detailed motion analysis from video tape records is shown in Fig. 2 for a single frog over the course of 90 days from LC lesion. The frog was placed on a rectangular board (70 × 50 cm) within the field of the video camera and was filmed jumping spontaneously or in response to handclapping. The first ten jumps of a given session were

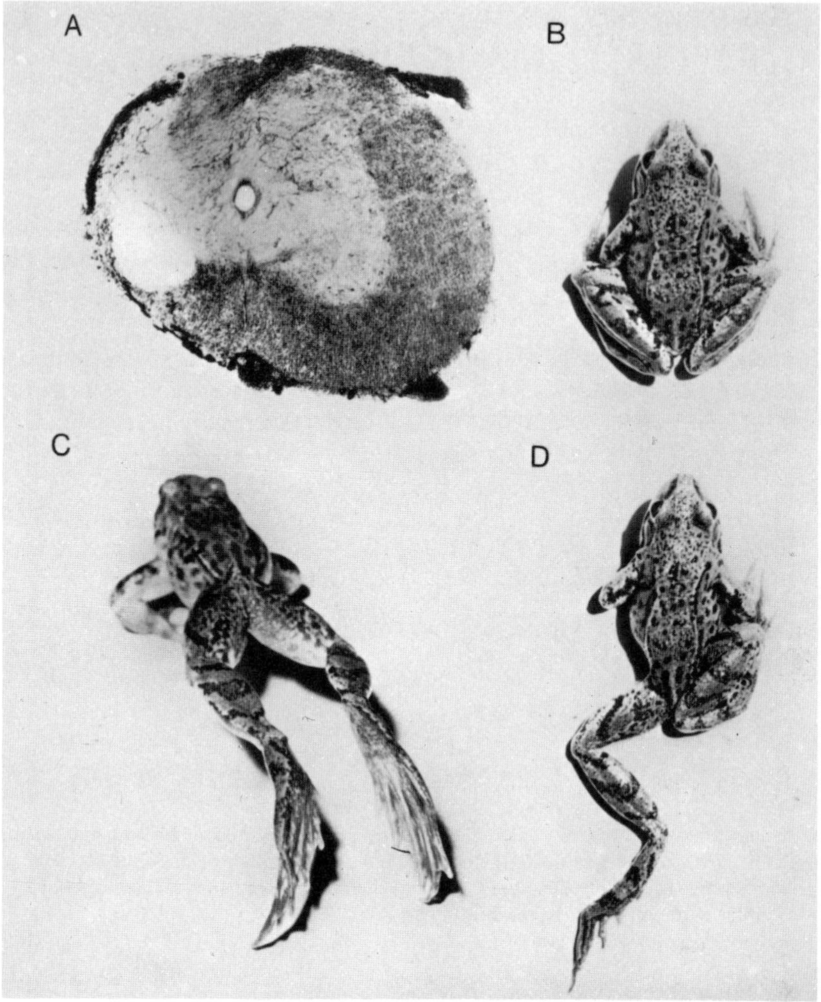

Fig. 1A–D. The lesion and its behavioral effects. **A** Unstained transverse section through lesion site, showing a complete destruction of lateral tract fibers on the left. Dorsal root 4/5 is visible in the upper right. **B** Symmetry of posture is not affected. **C** Extension of hind limbs in the jump seems symmetrical. **D** On landing at the end of a jump the left hind limb may be left extended for a fraction of a second

analyzed for various parameters of the "extension" and "flexion" phases. A second group of ten jumps was sometimes analyzed separately. Extension phases were measured from the frame showing the first displacement of the head from resting position to the frame where the hind limbs left the ground (at 50 frames per second). Flexion phases were measured from forelimbs contacting the ground to the animal reaching a "normal" symmetrical sitting posture.

There was no assymetry of extension except for that normally associated with jumps directed strongly to one side or the other. The extension was often longer in

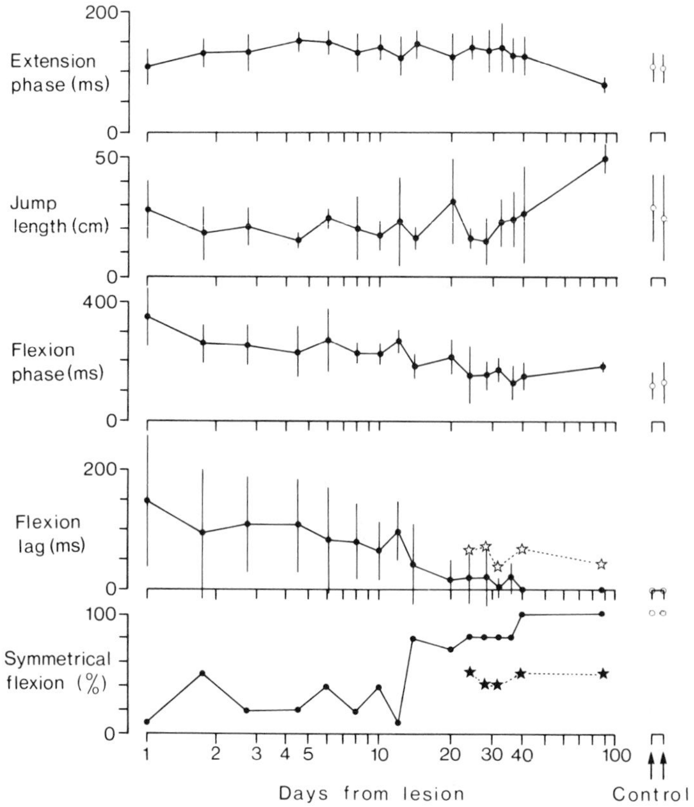

Fig. 2. Graphs indicating the recovery of function in jumping behavior following lesion. Movements were measured from video tape analysis to the nearest 20 ms. "Flexion lag" is the time between right and left hind limbs being fully flexed at the end of the jump. "Symmetrical flexion" shows percentage of jumps with no flexion lag. Details in text (Sect. 2.2)

duration than in control recordings, but this was the result of a tendency for shorter jumps and the normal inverse relation between jump length and extension duration. This tendency was not consistently significant and the first trial was comparable to the control. By contrast, the flexion phase of the jump was consistently slower and heavily asymmetrical, though it improved over the first few weeks and by 1 month post lesion the first ten jumps were close to normal. The mean values for the second ten jumps (asterisks in Fig. 2) show that this behavioral compensation was at least partly reversible, presumably by 'central fatigue'. Again, the fact that the deficit was one of movement power rather than patterning is clear in that a number of jumps were symmetrical less than a day after the lesion.

2.3 Differentiating 'Extensors' and 'Flexors'

For correlation of electrophysiology with behavioral effects it was necessary to differentiate MNs involved in the flexion phase of the jump. The ischiadic nerve divides just above the knee of the frog to form the tibialis nerve which innervates muscles mostly used in the extension of the lower limb and the peroneal nerve which innervates muscles used to flex the toes and ankle (in the jump) and also to extend the knee. The role of some of these muscles is controversial. The largest muscles – peroneus and tibialis anticus longus (TAL) – both extend the knee and flex the ankle. Gaupp (1899) and Cruce (1974) suggested on the basis of anatomy and stimulation experiments that the primary effect of these muscles is to extend the knee during the jump. To clarify the role of the peroneus we made simultaneous electromyographic recordings from peroneus and plantaris longus muscles in frogs free to jump. It was found that though plantaris and peroneus are coactive in the extension phase, the level of activation of the peroneus during extension is only slightly greater than that during the flexion phase, and it is much more strongly activated during a strong flexion movement of the hind limb produced by gentle pinching of the toes. Plantaris activity during jump extension is comparable to that produced by cross extension reflexes (on pinching the toes of the contralateral hind limb). This tibialis-innervated muscle is apparently silent during flexion. The peroneus therefore has an ambiguous function, but the peroneal nerve can be said to innervate predominantly muscles which are used to produce flexion of the limb, whereas the tibialis has an almost purely extensor role (the plantaris acting alone *could* tend to flex the knee, but this tendency is recognized to be slight compared with the primary effect of extending the ankle (Gaupp 1899; Cruce 1974).

We therefore chose to examine the primary afferent input to the two populations of MN's projecting to peroneal and tibial nerves at the knee.

2.4 Primary Afferent Input to Motoneurons

The interpretation of our physiological data was modified by the discovery that the primary afferent EPSP in frog MN's is a mixed chemical and electrotonic potential (Shapovalov and Shiriaev 1978, 1979; Shapovalov et al. 1978; Taugner et al. 1978; Alvarez-Leefmans et al. 1979). Analysis of synaptic potentials in the light of this more recent data, together with the anatomical studies of Székely (1976) led us to conclude that the original description of primary afferent input as primarily distally situated on the MN was no longer acceptable (Blight and Precht 1981). This conclusion seems to be in agreement with the study reported by Shapavalov (1981) on the intracellular staining of single primary afferent fibers with horseradish peroxidase. Primary afferents are probably predominantly proximal on the long MN dendrites of the frog.

It was therefore no longer reasonable to expect changes in DR afferent synapses to be reflected in decreased rise time of EPSP's, associated with the formation of more proximal junctions (analogous to the findings of Tsukahara et al. 1975; Dieringer and Precht 1977, in other systems). For this reason we chose to concentrate on the analysis of maximal amplitudes of DR EPSP's and their distribution in the two MN pools. Fortunately, the primary afferent EPSP amplitude tends to be quite stable with the variations in resting potential we encountered, whilst the rise and fall times are known to be more sensitive to membrane polarization for the mammalian Ia EPSP (see Redman 1979).

Intracellular recordings were made from MN's in the in situ spinal cord of frogs paralyzed with d-tubocurarine (25 mg/kg), 12–24 h after decerebration. The animal's skin was kept moist for cutaneous respiration, which was sufficient to maintain strong circulation and good reflex responses in the spinal cord. MN's were identified by antidromic stimulation of peroneal and tibial nerves at the knee. Glass microelectrodes were filled with 2 mol/l potassium methyl sulphate (to prevent reversal of inhibitory potentials, IPSP's, which occurs when chloride or citrate electrodes are used – Katz and Miledi 1963). DR's 8/9 and 9/10 (i.e., DR's 9 and 10 in the nomenclature of Gaupp 1899) were raised onto bipolar stainless steel hook electrodes under mineral oil which covered the spinal cord.

DR's and spinal nerves were stimulated with 0.1 ms electrical pulses at 1 Hz, with stimulus intensities restricted to 1–2.5 × theshold (T) for the minimal field potential (usually < 1.5 V). MN responses to a given stimulus were recorded intracellularly and averaged over 16 cycles using a signal-averaging computer. A range of stimulus amplitudes was tested, then the electrode was withdrawn just outside the cell and the extracellular fields were averaged at the same stimulus intensities. Fields were subtracted by computer from the intracellular recordings to give the transmembrane potential changes. The "maximal monosynaptic response amplitude" dealt with in this study was calculated by adding linearly the maximal response to stimulation of the two DR's, determined separately. The monosynaptic response was usually maximal at 2 × T.

MN's were sampled at the level of entry of DR 8/9 and one half segment on either side. At this level they showed no response of monosynaptic latency to stimulation of DR 7/8. The very small DR 10/11 was ignored in this study. All recordings, lesions and stimulation sites were restricted to the left side of the body. In a control group of 14 frogs 42 peroneal MN's (PMN's) and 38 tibial MN's (TMN's) were sampled. In 7 frogs with acute LC lesions 23 PMN's and 45 TMN's were sampled (recording 1–12 h postlesion). In 10 frogs with chronic LC lesions 48 PMN's and 42 TMN's were recorded (18 days to 3 months postlesion).

2.5 Defining Monosynaptic Potentials

The identification of monosynaptic potentials from stimulation of a whole DR is difficult and always requires assumptions, though, as we were concerned with comparison of normal and lesioned animals, these assumptions should not greatly influence our comparative conclusions.

Figure 3 shows intracellular recordings from a MN in which it was possible to record large amplitude spontaneous primary afferent EPSP's. The spontaneous potential in Fig. 3A is superimposed in 3C on the just-suprathreshold response to DR stimulation. The range of responses to increasing DR stimulation is shown in Fig. 3B. Transmembrane potentials are superimposed on one another below the corresponding extracellular fields. This allows us to distinguish the two phases of the monosynaptic potentials – electrotonic and chemical – from the disynaptic and polysynaptic potentials which add to their falling phases. Careful analysis with a large number of recordings led us to conclude (Blight and Precht 1981) that the monosynaptic components can be identified fairly reliably on the basis of latency and comparison with the phases of the field potential. This assumes that the primary afferent axons have a reasonably consistent conduction velocity which is greater than about 3 ms^{-1} as a mean between the stimulus site (halfway between cord entry and DR ganglion) and the synapse on the MN.

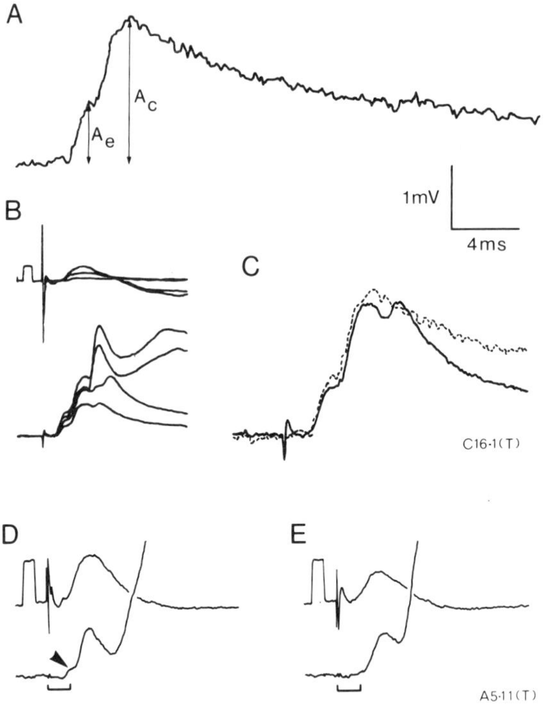

Fig. 3A–E. Characteristics of primary afferent EPSP's in motoneurons. **A** A spontaneous EPSP showing the inflected rising phase, distinguishing the electrotonic and chemical components. A_e and A_c indicate the measurements used for electrotonic and chemical EPSP amplitudes. (Though all the measurements given are for maximal evoked responses.) **B** Superimposed extracellular fields (*above*) and transmembrane potential responses (*below*) to root stimulation of increasing intensity. **C** Superimposition of spontaneous EPSP (*dashed*) and lowest threshold evoked response. **D, E** Field (*above*) and transmembrane (*below*) responses to stimulation of DR's 8/9 and 9/10 respectively in another cell, showing the presence of an electrotonic component in **D** (*arrow*) and a purely chemical monosynaptic EPSP in E. (Both followed by polysynaptic events)

Given this assumption, the electrotonic potential has a latency usually no longer than 2 ms from the stimulus and its initial deflection is closely correlated with the negative dip of the presynaptic field. The chemical monosynaptic component is usually marked by a deflection on the rising phase of the transmembrane potential near the middle of the depolarizing phase of the postsynaptic field (Fig. 3D). Occasionally there is no clear inflection and the latency of the first deflection seems to be that of a purely chemical monosynaptic potential (Fig. 3E). The peak of the monosynaptic potential appears almost invariably to be close to the positive peak of the postsynaptic field. In this study, the monosynaptic chemical EPSP amplitude was measured at the peak of the field if the EPSP peak itself was obscured by a disynaptic potential.

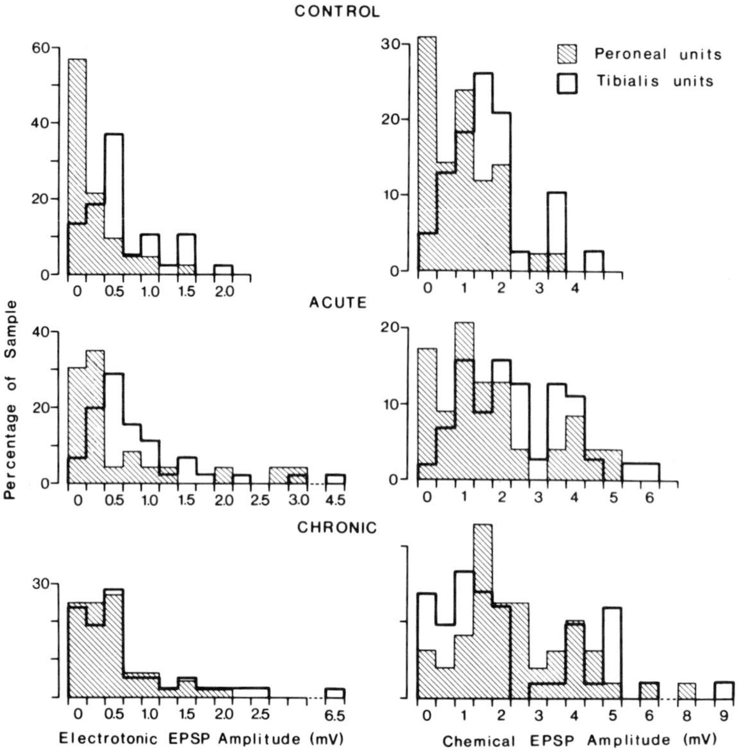

Fig. 4. Histograms showing the distribution of 'maximal monosynaptic DR EPSP amplitudes' in the sampled populations of peroneal and tibialis motoneurons, and the effect of lateral column lesions. Percentages of sample are given to facilitate comparison. Calculation of maximal response is explained in the text (Sects. 2.4, 2.5)

2.6 Primary Afferent Distribution and the Effect of LC Lesion

Figure 4 summarizes the findings from control, acute, and chronic experiments. The histograms show the distribution of maximal monosynaptic DR EPSP amplitudes for the two MN pools and the two components, electrotonic and chemical. In the control records there is a clear difference between the input to PMN and TMN pools ($p < 0.0003$, U-test). The modal value for both electrotonic and chemical components in PMN's in zero (less than background noise) compared to 0.5 and 1.5 mV respectively in TMN's. The amplitude distributions are not simple in either pool, both showing a skew. As they contain motor units from a number of different muscle types, this lack of homogeneity is not surprising though it makes analysis of selective changes more difficult.

The effect of acute LC lesion on these distributions was a general increase in EPSP amplitude, most significant for the chemical component ($p < 0.003$) and least for the electrotonic ($p < 0.3$) in TMN's, whereas the increase was equally significant for the two components in PMNs ($p < 0.03$). The difference between 'extensor' and 'flexor' populations was maintained ($p < 0.02$). A few very large EPSP's were found in both MN types.

Among the units recorded in chronically lesioned animals there were also a few with unusually large EPSP's, but the striking difference from control and acute recordings was the relative change of distributions between PMN's and TMN's. The electrotonic EPSP amplitudes were much more similarly distributed in the two cell groups ($p > 0.2$), and the chemical components showed a relative reversal of primary mode distribution between PMN's and TMN's. Overall, the chronic peroneal distribution was highly significantly changed ($p < 0.002$, electrotonic; $p < 0.00003$, chemical), whereas the tibialis distribution change did not appear significant ($p > 0.3$ for both components) because the population split, a large mode increasing in amplitude and frequency, while the smaller, principle mode decreased. (In this situation the Mann-Whitney U-test registers little change.)

One of the clearest features of the control and acute populations of peroneal units was that the majority had very small primary afferent EPSP's, that is with amplitudes less than the modal values for tibial units. The reason for this is not clear, but we have speculated (Blight and Precht 1981) that it might be related to the ambiguous function of peroneus and TAL muscles in the jump. Given the absence of a separate gamma innervation of muscle spindles in the frog (Gray 1957), the functionally ambiguous feedback from spindles in peroneus and TAL could be modified only centrally. This interpretation must be tested by recording from identified peroneus and TAL MN's.

Table 1 considers only this population of cells with small EPSP amplitudes, comparing the proportion of TMN's and PMN's with EPSP's smaller than the control TMN's modal values. The ratio between peroneal and tibial units is unchanged with acute lesions but is reduced to less than a half for electrotonic, and less then a quarter for chemical components in animals with chronic LC lesions. The primary afferent input to flexor MN's selectively increases and that to extensors possibly decreases at the population level.

Table 1. Distribution of small primary afferent EPSP's between peroneal (flexor) and tibialis (extensor) motoneurons

	Electrotonic EPSP $\leqslant 250\ \mu V$			Chemical EPSP $\leqslant 1$ mV		
	Control	Acute	Chronic	Control	Acute	Chronic
Peroneal MN's	78.4%	65.4%	50.0%	69.2%	47.8%	18.8%
Tibialis MN's	31.6%	26.7%	43.0%	36.7%	24.5%	40.4%
Ratio (P/T)	2.48	2.45	1.16	1.89	1.95	0.47

3 Discussion

3.1 Acute Effects of Lesion

The recordings analyzed in Fig. 4 indicate that there is an effect even within the first few hours of thoracic spinal cord hemisection on the amplitude of DR EPSP's in the two MN populations. The mechanism of the apparent rapid increase in EPSP amplitude is unlikely to be structural (i.e., growth of new synaptic contacts) and cannot be purely pharmacological as both electrotonic and chemical EPSP components are affected. The change may be equivalent to that seen following thoracic section of the cat spinal cord (Mendell, this vol.) where unusually large single fiber Ia EPSP's occur in lumbar MN's. The acute effect in the frog might be explained, however, if under normal circumstances there is incomplete invasion of primary afferent terminals by the action potential (failure at branch points), and if the lesion produces a more complete invasion, for example by elevation of extracellular potassium through cell damage. Such a mechanism would be comparable to that suggested for post-tetanic potentiation at the Ia-MN synapse by Lüscher et al. (1979).

The acute changes affect both extensor and flexor MN populations, so the relation between the two amplitude distributions is not significantly altered (Table 1). Behavioral symptoms of the lesion at this acute stage did not seem to be qualitatively different from those found later in recovery and the functional significance of acute changes is not clear. If the above interpretation of the amplitude increase is correct, it may even have little bearing on function as spike failure at branch points might well be reduced or absent at normal presynaptic firing frequencies.

3.2 Chronic Effects of Lesion

The conditions giving rise to acute changes in DR EPSP's are probably transitory, and the potentials recorded weeks after the lesion is made should be compared with control rather than acute data. There are then at least two striking differences in the amplitude distributions shown in Fig. 4A, C: (1) the presence of more large- and a few very large-amplitude EPSP's in both MN types; (2) a reversal of the differential distribution of smaller amplitudes between peroneal and tibial populations. A large proportion of PMN's have EPSP's of greater amplitude, whereas TMN's show a tendency for reduced monosynaptic input from DR's.

There is therefore an increase in feedback onto MN's involved in hind limb flexion, contrasting with a diminution of spindle feedback to extensors. The former change is directly correlated with the behavioral observation that flexion movements of the hind limb, acutely weakened by the lesion, gradually become stronger over the first few weeks. One of the effects of the stretch reflex mediated by primary afferent feedback is to increase the power of a given movement, especially when this is opposed by some unpredicted force. The increased primary afferent EPSP amplitude *must* therefore contribute to the increased strength of flexion which constitutes behavioral recovery.

The mechanism of the observed increase in response probably involves a structural modification, given the parallel changes in electrotonic and chemical components, possibly a limited 'sprouting' of afferent fibers similar to that seen anatomically in other species (see below). Such sprouting might result from direct deafferentation of MNs activating growth in neighboring input fibers, but the apparent reduction of DR input to extensors is more difficult to interpret. An interesting possibility is that it is triggered by a loss of *inhibitory* input to extensor MN's from the thoracic LC. (A small increase of extensor activity would have been harder to detect behaviorally than the small reduction in the normally much weaker flexor acitivity.) We have seen monosynaptic IPSP's in a few extensor MN's in response to LC stimulation, but the LC input to MN's is not well defined, and we have found it widely variable depending on stimulus site and MN type. These observations may be related to the 'regression of some central synaptic connections' of Ia fibers which had become 'functionally inappropriate' after nerve cross-union in kittens, seen by Eccles et al. (1962).

3.3 Spinal Lesions and Synaptic Plasticity

Behavioral compensation for the effects of spinal lesions has been described for a number of vertebrate species, and parallel anatomical studies have shown that some reorganization of neural connections occurs distal to the spinal section or hemisection (e.g., Murray and Goldberger 1974; Stelzner et al. 1975, 1979; Bernstein et al. 1978). In the terrestrial vertebrates, which show little or no regeneration of long tracts, there seems to be a sprouting of DR afferent fibers (first described in the cat by Liu and Chambers 1958), though such sprouting may be differently organized in different species (Stelzner et al. 1979). The functional significance of these anatomical changes is not clear, though they may parallel behavioral recovery of function.

Electrophysiological studies of the effects of spinal lesions have been made in cats under various conditions. Teasdall et al. (1958) were able to show, from recording action potentials in nerve and muscle, that there is an increase in polysynaptic hind limb reflexes, which occurs within a few days after ipsilateral spinal cord hemisection. They were unable to detect any monosynaptic changes. Pacheco and Guzmán-Flores (1969) appear to have seen a similar effect with intracellular recording from MN's following sensory-motor cortex lesions. Nelson and Mendell (1979) and Nelson et al. (1979) have demonstrated by recording single fiber EPSP's that there are also acute and chronic effects of spinal transection on the *monosynaptic* responses of MN's (see Mendell, this vol.). Again, the functional significance of these neural changes is difficult to assess, but it seems clear that the response to lesion is complex both in its distribution through the nervous system and in its time course.

Our data from the frog demonstrate a change in primary afferent central projection which is directly related to the functional compensation following LC lesion. This examination of functional synaptic plasticity has therefore given us a clearer understanding of the capacity for compensation in the CNS. The relation between the observed neuronal and behavioral changes is unlikely to be simple, however. That we find a change in the afferent system most convenient for study is probably a result of a widespread reaction of the nervous system to damage rather than of unique good fortune. The timing of these changes is also a problem which needs to be faced by repeating the experiments with a range of survival times. It would be interesting to know, for instance, whether DR input changes are only temporary, as they seem to be in the cat after total transection (Mendell, this vol.), and if a return to normal might be correlated with functional modification of other inputs (e.g., does the contralateral LC input eventually increase in effectiveness, thereby obviating the "need" for the functionally less specific DR modulation)?

One of the central questions remaining, even if more detailed mechanistic questions can be answered, is to what degree the behavioral compensation which follows lesions of the CNS is the result of a specific strategy for compensating the loss of input channels due to cell death (perhaps an aspect of the more widespread plasticity present in development) or whether it is an unspecific case of motor learning. We expect the "gain" of reflex responses to be continually modulated during the life of an animal in order that the behavior remain adapted to the changing mechanical requirements of the environment and the body. This requires there be a means by which the overall behavioral performance acts back upon the individual neural components to modify their activity. The kind of change we have seen in the primary afferent input after spinal lesion may be a facet of such "normal" gain modulation in the stretch reflex, brought about by the repeated failure of the overall performance of the limb. In this regard, it would be interesting to attempt the same kind of study replacing CNS lesions with peripheral modifications producing similar behavioral deficits (such as artificial loading of the limb) to see if similar alterations of reflex gain occur by modulation of primary afferent synaptic efficacy.

4 Summary

Following a lesion of the left, mid-thoracic lateral column of the spinal cord in the frog, there is a weakness of flexion movements of the left hind limb. The strength of these movements largely recovers over several weeks, and this recovery is associated with increased monosynaptic input to flexor motoneurons from dorsal roots in the left lumbar cord. It appears that loss of an excitatory input to flexor motoneurons from the destroyed lateral column is functionally replaced, at least partly, by increased synaptic efficacy of segmental feedback. Parallel changes at electrotonic and chemical junctions suggest that this synaptic plasticity represents sprouting of primary afferent terminals.

References

Alvarez-Leefmans FJ, De Santis A, Miledi R (1979) Effects of some divalent cations on synaptic transmission in frog spinal neurones. J Physiol (London) 294: 387–406

Bernstein JJ, Wells MR, Bernstein ME (1978) Spinal cord regeneration: Synaptic renewal and neurochemistry. In: Cotman CW (ed) Neuronal plasticity. Raven Press, New York, pp 49–71

Blight AR, Precht W (1981) Electrical transmission between primary afferents and motoneurons related to function. In: Szentágothai J, Palkovits M, Hámori J (eds) Advances in physiological sciences, vol 1. Regulatory functions of the CNS. Akadémiai Kiadó and Pergamon Press, in press

Cruce WLR (1974) The anatomical organisation of hindlimb motoneurons in the lumbar spinal cord of the frog *Rana catesbiana*. J comp Neurol 153: 59–76

Dieringer N, Precht W (1977) Modification of synaptic input following unilateral labyrinthectomy. Nature (London) 269: 431–433

Eccles JC, Eccles RM, Sheally CN, Willis WD (1962) Experiments utilizing monosynaptic excitatory action on motoneurons for testing hypotheses relating to specificity of neuronal connections. J Neurophysiol 25: 559–580

Fadiga E, Brookhart JM (1960) Monosynaptic activation of different portions of the motor neuron membrane. Am J Physiol 198: 693–703

Gaupp E (1899) A. Ecker's and R. Wiedersheim's Anatomie des Frosches, vol II. 2nd edn. Lehre vom Nerven- und Gefässystem. F. Vieweg, Braunschweig

Gray EG (1957) The spindle and extrafusal innervation of a frog muscle. Proc R Soc London Ser B 146: 416–430
Jankowski K, Afelt Z (1964) Degeneration and regeneration in the chronic spinal preparation of *Rana esculenta*. Acta Biol Exp (Warsaw) 24: 3–11
Katz B, Miledi R (1963) A study of spontaneous miniature potentials in spinal motoneurones. J Physiol (London) 168: 389–422
Liu CN, Chambers WW (1958) Intraspinal sprouting of dorsal root axons. Arch Neurol Psychiatr (Chicago) 79: 46–61
Lüscher H-R, Ruenzel P, Henneman E (1980) How the size of motoneurones determines their susceptibility to discharge. Nature (London) 282: 859–861
Murray M, Goldberger ME (1974) Restitution of function and collateral sprouting in the cat spinal cord: the partially hemisected animal. J comp Neurol 158: 19–36
Nelson SG, Mendell LM (1979) Enhancement in Ia-motoneuron synaptic transmission caudal to chronic spinal cord transection. J Neurophysiol 42: 642–654
Nelson SG, Collatos TC, Niechaj JA, Mendell LM (1979) Immediate increase in Ia-motoneuron synaptic transmission caudal to spinal cord transection. J Neurophysiol 42: 655–664
Pacheco P, Guzmán-Flores C (1969) Intracellular recording in extensor motoneurons of spastic cats. Exp Neurol 25: 472–481
Redman S (1979) Junctional mechanisms at group Ia synaptses. Prog Neurobiol 12: 33–83
Rensch B, Franszisket L (1954) Lang andauernde bedingte Reflexe bei Rückenmarksfröschen. Z Vergl Physiol 36: S318–326
Shapovalov AI (1981) Junctional mechanisms at synapses between primary afferents and vertebrate motoneurones. In: Szentágothai J, Palkovits M, Hámori J (eds) Advances in physiological sciences, vol 1. Regulatory functions of the CNS. Akadémiai Kiadó and Pergamon Press, in press
Shapovalov AI, Shiriaev BI (1978) Electrical coupling between primary afferents and amphibian motoneurons. Exp Brain Res 33: 299–312
Shapovalov AI, Shiriaev BI (1979) Single fibre epsps in amphibian motoneurons. Brain Res 160: 519–523
Shapovalov AI, Shiriaev BI, Velumian AA (1978) Mechanisms of post-synaptic excitation in amphibian motoneurons. J Physiol (London) 279: 437–455
Stelzner DJ, Ershler WB, Weber EB (1975) Effects of spinal transection in neonatal and weanling rats: survival of function. Exp Neurol 46: 156–177
Stelzner DJ, Weber ED, Prendergast J (1979) A comparison of the effect of mid-thoracic spinal hemisection in the neonatal or weanling rat on the distribution and density of dorsal root axons in the lumbosacral spinal cord of the adult. Brain Res 103: 275–290
Taugner R, Sonnhof U, Richter DW, Schiller A (1978) Mixed chemical and electrical synapses on frog spinal motoneurons. Cell Tissue Res 193: 41–59
Teasdall RD, Magladery JW, Ramey EH (1958) Changes in reflex patterns following spinal cord hemisection in cats. Johns Hopkins Hosp Bull 103: 223–241
Tsukahara N, Hultborn H, Murakami F, Fuji Y (1975) Electrophysiological study of formation of new synapses and collateral sprouting in red nucleus neurons after partial denervation. J Neurophysiol 38: 1359–1372

The Role Sprouting Might Play During the Recovery of Motor Function

M.E. GOLDBERGER[1]

A number of mechanisms have been proposed as explanations for the recovery of motor function which follows CNS lesions in adult mammals (for reviews see Goldberger 1974; Lawrence and Stein 1978). One of these is axonal (collateral) sprouting from intact fibers in response to loss of projections to a terminal field in which the damaged and the sprouting axons overlap. Sprouting in the spinal cord of new or additional terminals in a particular system might strengthen the reflex control exerted by that system (cf. Pubols and Goldberger 1980). The resulting enhancement of particular reflexes could mediate recovery of motor function if the enhanced reflexes were substituted for the reflexes lost due to the lesion. According to this scheme the movements which recover might differ in some respects from the movements lost, although their overall adaptive value might be similar to the normal movements. Furthermore, one might anticipate that, after a particular lesion, not all of the remaining reflex systems contribute equally to recovery and that not all systems will respond by sprouting to an equal extent. The system most proximate anatomically to the one damaged and whose function most nearly approximates the function initially lost might be expected to predominate.

Sprouting has been demonstrated repeatedly in the CNS of adult mammals (Liu and Chambers 1958; Raisman 1969; Cotman and Nadler 1978; Goldberger and Murray 1978). It is as yet unclear whether sprouting in the adult CNS is a nonspecific phenomenon elicited from all nearby axons, as in the developing CNS (Gall et al. 1979), or whether the rules governing sprouting in the adult have become stricter during the course of development. The nature of the stimulus for axonal sprouting also remains unclear. Two hypotheses have been advanced: (1) that axonal sprouting is stimulated by products of degeneration (Edds 1954) and may therefore be relatively nonspecific, or (2) that axonal sprouting is stimulated by the presence of post-synaptic sites which have become vacated when the axons degenerate (Raisman 1969; Murray et al. 1979), in which case, some degree of specificity may operate. If sprouting, or at least the final pattern of persistent sprouts is not a random phenomenon, then it should be possible to predict which of several converging systems will respond to a central lesion by increasing their projections. If these new projections are functional, then it should also be possible to predict the extent and nature of the recovery of function following CNS damage, and then perhaps to promote such recovery.

---

1 Department of Anatomy, The Medical College of Pennsylvania, 3300 Henry Avenue, Philadelphia, PA 19129, USA

Four spinal systems contribute to movement of a single hindlimb: ipsilateral dorsal roots, ipsilateral descending systems, contralateral (to the limb) dorsal roots, contralateral descending systems. Following a lesion which interrupts one of these systems, the pattern of recovery seen is similar regardless of which of the systems was destroyed. This pattern can be seen as a three-stage process: (1) a brief period in which a generalized reflex depression is seen (in addition to permanent loss of the reflexes mediated by the system abolished) and locomotion is severely depressed or absent or is executed without the participation of the impaired limb; (2) emergence of surviving reflexes from the generalized depression and recovery of locomotion; (3) enhancement of the reflexes mediated by one (only) of the remaining systems and recovery of accurate limb placement during locomotion. Axonal sprouting of one of the remaining systems may mediate the observed enhancement of specific reflexes and may therefore contribute to the third phase of recovery, i.e., recovery of accurate limb placement.

The classical study of axonal sprouting in the spinal cord described the increased projections of a single dorsal root when all adjacent roots were cut (Liu and Chambers 1958). We have also examined the projection of the L_6 root in chronic spared root preparations (Goldberger and Murray 1978). In these experiments, the unilateral deafferentation, sparing L_6, is performed and then 1 year later the L_6 roots are cut on both sides and their projections mapped and compared. On the control side, this root projects densely into the L_6 segment and, less densely, to all other lumbar segments. The major projection, however, is to the medial 2/3 of laminae III–IV of the dorsal horn at L_6. The lateral 1/3 of the L_6 dorsal horn normally shares a rather sparse projection from the L_6 root with projections from the adjacent roots. In the absence of these adjacent roots, however, the projections of the spared root increase in density in the dorsal horn and intermediate zone. The increased density is most clearly seen in the lateral dorsal horn in the region of maximum overlap among adjacent roots. Unit recordings in the dorsal horn of chronic spared root animals corroborate the anatomical findings and suggest that the sprouts are functional (Pubols and Goldberger 1980). This then represents an example of the specificity of sprouting. There is an increase in the existing projection by the spared root and it is to a region of convergence of the spared root with adjacent roots which were destroyed.

When L_6 spared root preparations are examined by behavioral methods, the importance of the spared root for residual function and recovery of function becomes evident. Initially all reflex function is depressed and the affected limb's participation in locomotion is absent or very poor. By the second day, reflexes mediated by the spared root (e.g., tendon reflexes, cutaneous flexor reflexes) begin to become stronger, and crossed reflexes and reflexes mediated by ipsilateral descending systems (vestibular placing, scratch reflex) emerge from the generalized reflex depression. The affected limb now participates in locomotion and although locomotion becomes faster and more efficient, accurate limb placement (of the spared root limb) is not executed. At this time, proprioceptive placing and monopedal hopping can be elicited by stimulation of the territory of the spared root's peripheral distribution. Tactile placing is absent. On the seventh postoperative day, tactile placing returns (elicited from the spared dermatome only); proprioceptive placing and hopping recover in all directions and accurate limb placement during locomotion is first seen. Thus, the cats can now cross narrow runways (one-inch parallel bars, obstacle courses, etc.) with few "mistakes."

The return of tactile placing and accurate movement is associated with an increase in strength and lowered threshold of reflexes (tendon reflexes, withdrawal responses) elicited by stimulation in the territory of the spared dermatome and with an increase in spinal representation of that dermatome with no change in its peripheral distribution (Pubols and Goldberger 1980). There is, on the other hand, no similar increase in strength of descending reflexes (scratch reflex, vestibular placing) or crossed reflexes other than their early recovery from the initial generalized reflex depression. The role of descending systems in recovery from spared root deafferentation was assessed by performing hemisections (dorsal columns spared) in recovered spared root animals ipsilateral to the initial deafferentation. The results of the combined lesions were first compared with those of hemisection in otherwise intact animals.

The results of hemisection in cats have been described previously by a number of workers (e.g., Teasdall et al. 1958; Stavraki 1961; Jane et al. 1964; Denny-Brown 1966). Only a few additional observations are relevant here. Hemisection sparing the dorsal column results in a severe deficit in all phases of motor behavior, i.e., centrally patterned movement, triggered movement, and reflexes. This is temporary, however. Beginning at about the second day, locomotion, using the impaired limb, reappears. At the same time, all residual reflexes increase somewhat in strength (Murray and Goldberger 1974). Placing and hopping responses are absent and accurate limb placement is not seen. For example, on obstacle courses the affected hindlimb is dragged over the obstacle; on boards with holes the limb often falls through and then cannot be extricated easily. The animals cannot traverse the narrow runways. At about the seventh postoperative day, the first signs of accurate limb placement appear and this is associated with the return of hopping and proprioceptive placing (Goldberger 1979). This is also associated with the onset of enhanced activity of ipsilateral cutaneous and tendon reflexes and sprouting of dorsal roots (Murray and Goldberger 1974). Within two weeks, as fewer and fewer misplacements of the limb occur, the increased accuracy permits the traverse of narrow (2") runways, obstacle courses, etc., at almost preoperative speed. Hopping and proprioceptive placing improve over the same time period. Unlike spared root preparations, tactile placing never recovers after hemisection unless the lesion is made in very young animals (Bregman and Goldberger 1979, 1980). The role of ipsilateral pathways in recovery after spared-root deafferentation can now be assessed.

Hemisection in spared root animals had effects which are similar in most respects to those of hemisection alone. When hemisection was added 6 months to 1 year after spared root deafferentation, an initial profound impairment (no hopping, placing or locomotion using the affected limb) was seen. This was followed in one or two days by recovery of locomotion without recovery of accuracy. On the seventh or eighth postoperative day, as tendon reflexes increased in strength, proprioceptive placing and hopping responses returned. At the same time, accurate limb placement during locomotion on the difficult tasks reappeared (Fig. 1). The ultimate motor status was also similar in hemisected and in spared-root-hemisected animals. The major difference between the two groups was determined by the peripheral distribution of the spared root, revealed by reflex responses of the limb. For example, in animals in which the patellar and tibialis anterior reflexes were preserved, placing and hopping in the forward and lateral directions showed the most recovery and, during locomotion, corrective move-

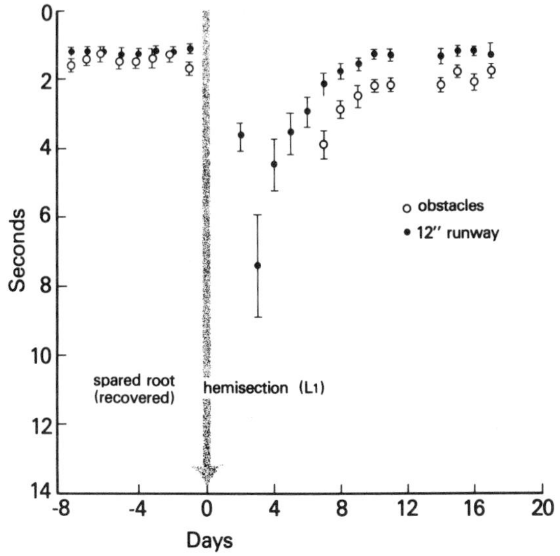

Fig. 1. Recovery of conditioned runway locomotion on simple, 12" runway (•) and an obstacle course (○). Recovery from partial rhizotomy had taken place and the status of locomotion at the time of hemisection is shown on the *left of the arrow*. Hemisection superimposed on spared root rhizotomy caused an initial severe deficit. This is followed in the first post-operative week by a recovery of locomotion and in the second week, by a recovery of accurate locomotion. The recovery reaches a level almost equivalent to preoperative scores. This indicates that recovery in spared root animals is not dependent on ipislateral descending systems

ments in these directions were performed the best. In animals displaying hamstrings, achilles and toe flexor tendon reflexes, backward and medial hopping and placing recovered to the greatest extent. The fact that hemisected and spared-root-hemisected cats recover to a similar extent (with the differences already described) suggests that recovery after spared root deafferentation is not dependent upon a contribution made by ipsilateral descending systems. This is quite different from the situation in completely deafferented hindlimbs.

Following complete unilateral deafferentation and/or ganglionectomy (all lumbar, sacral, and caudal dorsal roots cut and their ganglia removed) the limb is inactive for one or two days. No reflex movements can be elicited and the limb is not used for locomotion. Since this temporary paralysis is also seen following the other lesions studied, it presumably reflects nonspecific effects of the lesion, e.g., spinal shock. Two or three days postoperative, when four-legged locomotion begins, the deafferented limb's movements are unpredictable as to direction and excursion, so that the location of foot placement is unrelated to that required by the center of gravity. At this time, the animals have the motor capacity to cross a wide (12") runway but not a narrow one. The decending reflexes and crossed reflexes are still somewhat depressed. At the end of the first week, the situation is unchanged except that speed of crossing the 12" wide runway has increased to near preoperative levels. By the beginning of the second week (8th–10th day), accurate limb placement begins to appear and the 2" runway can be negotiated. At this early time, the animals make many "mistakes" in limb placement. Each "mistake" costs them a certain amount of time, e.g., for replacement of the limb, regaining balance, etc. As the number of mistakes decreases during recovery, speed increases. The return of accurate movement is accompanied by enhancement of the scratch and the vestibular placing reflexes, i.e., ipsilateral descending reflexes, of the deafferented limb. The crossed segmental (e.g., Phillipson's) or crossed suprasegmental (e.g., crossed placing) reflexes do not increase in strength.

It is not surprising that locomotion should recover since the spinal systems generating locomotion are known to be capable of independent function (Grillner 1976; Grillner and Zangger 1979). The recovery of accurate limb movement without specific training is not self-evident, since topographic feedback (information about the movement itself) from the moving limb is eliminated. Several sources of nontopographic feedback (information about the *results* of the movement) are available for guidance of the limb, however, and this is then an example of recovery by substitution – in this case, cue substitution.

One kind of information which seemed important for the recovery of accurate locomotion is that relating to posture and the center of gravity and this information arises in part from the trunk. Although it is difficult to interfere with posture selectively, a unilateral deafferentation of the trunk could be expected to have effects which are primarily related to the trunk itself. In fact, the disruption of posture and postural reflexes by T_5-T_{13} rhizotomy has profound effects on limb movements, as well as on those of the trunk (Goldberger and Murray 1980). The point to be made here, however, is that if the T_5-T_{13} rhizotomy is made in animals already having recovered from hindlimb deafferentation, the acute effects of hindlimb deafferentation are restored (Goldberger 1977). There is then a second recovery which follows a pattern similar to the first: locomotion begins at about the second day, accurate limb placement during locomotion begins at about the ninth day.

Thus, although postural information, mediated in part by trunk afferents, does indeed contribute to recovery of accurate placement of deafferented hindlimbs, the recovery (from hindlimb deafferentation) does not *depend* upon these trunk afferents. Recovery again takes place after the thoracic rhizotomy.

If, however, the same secondary lesion which was made in spared root cats (hemisection with dorsal columns spared) is made in completely deafferented cats after recovery is completed, not only is the recovery abolished, but the affected hindlimb is never again used for locomotion (Goldberger 1977). The failure of accurate movement to recover from this combination of lesions is, perhaps, not surprising. The failure of any locomotion to recover is. Using treadmill locomotion, it has been shown that neither the descending nor dorsal root systems are essential for locomotion (Grillner and Zangger 1975, 1979). Thus, the failure of the intact systems of the contralateral side to provide any compensation to the deafferented-hemisected partner for overground locomotion is both surprising and at present unexplained. Differences between treadmill and overground locomotion (Wetzel et al. 1976) do not seem great enough to account for this result. We are left with the hypothesis that this complete loss of motor function is the result not only of the loss of excitatory ipsilateral systems, but also of inhibition stemming from the contralateral side of the cord. In fact, if the contralateral white matter is transected in addition to the already existing lesions (deafferentation plus ipsilateral hemisection), crossed reflexes from the afferented to the deafferented limb increase dramatically (Goldberger and Murray 1974), indicating that the crossed reflexes were probably inhibited by contralateral systems. Thus, the effects of hemisection differ markedly in the two groups of animals – spared-root and completely deafferented. Recovery in deafferented hindlimbs is completely dependent on ipsilateral descending systems but in spared-root animals recovery occurs independently of them.

Further differences between spared root and completely deafferented animals can be seen when the anatomical distribution of descending systems is examined. Normally, descending projections of the two sides, demonstrated by degeneration methods after acute transection, are symmetrical. Following chronic unilateral rhizotomy, however, descending projections are denser on the experimental side. This observation is therefore consistent with the interpretation that descending systems sprout in response to the loss of dorsal root input.

When we compare the pattern of sprouting by descending systems elicited by total lumbosacral deafferentation and by the spared root after partial deafferentation, we find that there are regions in the spinal gray in which sprouting can be demonstrated from either descending systems or from the spared root. These regions include the base of the dorsal horn, Clarke's nucleus, and the intermediate zone. In the spared root preparation, the conditions appropriate for sprouting by either dorsal root axons or descending axons, or both are present. We can therefore ask in this preparation whether sprouting from both sources occurs or whether sprouting by one system can block the potential sprouting by a second system. In these experiments, the spinal cords of spared root animals were transected one year post-operatively. The patterns of descending projections in the presence of a single spared root were then compared to the normal pattern of descending projections and also to the descending projections following complete deafferentation. The results show that descending projections are symmetrical throughout the spinal gray matter in the presence of a spared root. Sprouting by the descending systems had therefore been blocked, presumably by the sprouting of the spared root. The results suggest that potential sources of sprouting may compete and this determines which system is successful in forming persistent sprouts.

Although the time course of recovery can be plotted, the time course of sprouting cannot be examined by degeneration methods. The advent of immunocytochemical staining methods for neuropeptides provided us with a way of examining the response of substance P containing systems to deafferentation. Substance P is synthesized in dorsal root ganglion cells and transported in the axon to the terminal region (Mroz and Laman 1979). Within the spinal cord substance P is found in all laminae but it is most densely distributed in laminae I-II and V. It is present as coarse clumps and finely granular material which has been localized to axons and terminals (Cuello et al. 1977; Pickel et al. 1977). Substance P containing cell bodies can also be seen in the gray matter (Tessler et al. 1980a). The dorsal root ganglion cells however are the source of most of the substance P in the dorsal horn (Hockfelt et al. 1976). If the dorsal roots are cut, the amount of substance P staining in the dorsal horn progressively decreases, although it does not disappear entirely. The presence at all times of residual substance P staining even after complete lumbosacral rhizotomy implies the presence of another source of substance P. When we allowed animals to survive after 10 days following

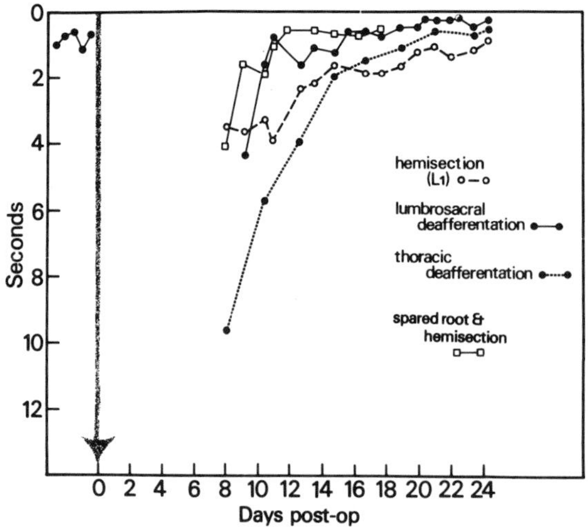

Fig. 2. Recovery of accurate locomotion after four different lesions. Note that the time-course and extent of recovery is similar regardless of the differences in type of lesion or initial severity of the deficit

rhizotomy, we found an increase of substance P in the dorsal horn and lamina V. These observations suggested that other substance P-containing neurons which normally project to this region are stimulated to sprout or to increase their production of substance P as a result of the deafferentation. We have not yet identified the neurons responsible for the return of substance P to the dorsal horn, but interneurons are the most likely candidate (Tessler et al. 1980b). The return of substance P staining appears to be confined to the regions which normally contain dense quantities of substance P, despite the fact that the other laminae are also severely denervated by the deafferentation. The time course with which this occurs appears to be comparable to sprouting by other CNS neurons (Cotman and Nadler 1978). The time-course of substance P increase is also roughly comparable to the time-course of recovery – specifically the recovery of accurate limb placement.

The time-course of recovery is shared by the several lesions described: lumbosacral deafferentation, thoracic deafferentation, spared root deafferentation and partial hemisection (Fig. 2). The initial impairment is severe, temporary (1-2d) and general, affecting all responses of the limb. Since it is similar following diverse lesions it must represent a nonspecific effect. The notion of diaschesis (in the spinal cord, "spinal shock") is frequently introduced in order to explain losses of function which are not permanent. In the spinal cord, shock refers to the temporary loss or depression of spinal reflex activity when the descending systems are damaged but the reflex pathways are not. Although loss of tonic facilitation is usually cited as a cause, the hyperpolarization of motoneurons which is found in spinal shock (Barnes et al. 1962) might be due also to the presence of inhibition (Jankowska et al. 1976a,b). This would suggest that the loss of function is due not only to loss of neural pathways, but to active processes, e.g., inhibition as well. Furthermore, the role of lesion-induced factors of nonneural origin (Cope et al. 1980) remains to be assessed. The early improvement of motor status is also presumed to be due to active processes rather than simply to the "wearing off" of shock. Which cellular mechanisms contribute to recovery in this early phase are uncertain, but included are such diverse phenomena as unmasking of silent synapses

(Merrill and Wall 1978); denervation supersensitivity (Glick 1973; Zigmond and Striker 1977), return of terminals displaced by desynapses (Chen et al. 1977; Chen 1978).

During the second week accurate movements begin to recover and this recovery is associated with the return and increasing strength of one of the placing responses. The nature of the placing response which recovers is selective, depending on the type of lesion made: lumbosacral deafferentation – vestibular placing, spared root or thoracic deafferentation – tactile placing, hemisection (alone or with spared root) – proprioceptive placing. No recovery of placing responses or locomotor function is seen when lumbosacral deafferentation is combined with ipsilateral hemisection regardless of the order of those lesions. The similarities in recovery after each of these lesions suggest that some underlying mechanisms may be common to all of them. Furthermore, the pattern of recovery of placing suggests that its recovery is mediated by mechanisms which permit a degree of selectivity. The selectivity is seen in that the specific reflex responses which recover, e.g., vestibular placing vs. tactile placing, are determined in part by what system was destroyed but also by which systems remain intact. Vestibular placing is *not* enhanced when a spared root is present but tactile placing recovers. Vestibular placing, on the other hand, is enhanced only when the spared root which mediates tactile placing has been cut along with the others. Mechanisms which mediate recovery and which also permit this degree of selectivity are, at present, conjectural.

In order to test the applicability of particular neuronal mechanisms of plasticity to the observed behavioral changes, it will be helpful first to consider the requirements of the recovering behavior, i.e., does the recovery of a particular motor skill depend on recovery of specific mechanisms mediated normally by the damaged pathway or can other mechanisms be used? The recovery of guidance for accurate movement after a lesion does not necessitate restitution of mechanisms identical to those which normally mediate guidance for accurate movement. This is clearest in the case of deafferentation in which topographic somatosensory feedback is substituted for by nontopographic feedback which is mediated by pathways in the ipsilateral lateral and/or ventral funiculi. In the case of partial deafferentation, it seemed clear that the spared root provided information for movements of deafferented parts of the limb, in addition to those parts which already received the spared peripheral innervation. The mechanism(s) by which one system substitutes for another over a specific time-course is not yet known. Our anatomical results (see also Goldberger and Murray 1978) show that in the case of each lesion the system which displays lesion-induced axonal sprouting is the same as the system which is primarily responsible for the recovery of accurate movement. The exception to this is the sprouting of substance P containing processes, which is seen after deafferentation (Tessler et al. 1980a) combined with ipsilateral hemisection (Tessler et al. 1980b) for which no functional expression can be observed unless that function be an inhibitory one (Fig. 3).

Whereas recovery from hindlimb deafferentation was dependent on ipsilateral descending systems, recovery in spared root animals occurred independently of these systems. Furthermore, the reflex responses (scratch, vestibular) which became so active in the deafferented animal failed to do so when one root was spared. In contrast, in the spared root animals, the responses mediated by the spared root (tendon reflexes, tactile placing, hopping) increased in strength without any change in their peripheral distribution (cf. Pubols and Goldberger 1980). Thus, there appears to be some com-

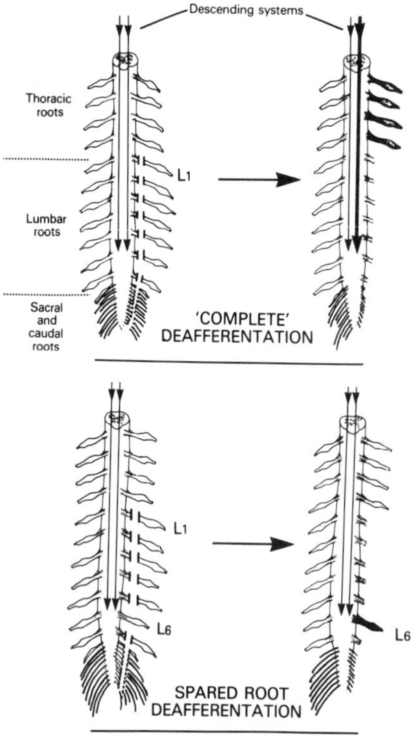

Fig. 3. Diagram summarizing behavioral and anatomical results. After complete lumbosacral deafferentation reflexes mediated by thoracic roots and ipsilateral descending pathways are important for recovery, and sprouting from those pathways can be demonstrated. In spared root animals, the spared root sprouts and appears to be responsible for the mediation of recovery

petitive interaction between the spared root and descending systems in mediating recovery and reflex changes after partial deafferentation. The competition was also observed in the anatomical experiments; the presence of a spared root suppressed the sprouting of descending pathways. The contribution to recovery made by ipsilateral descending systems is far less important in the presence of the spared root and the reflexes mediated by these systems do not increase so long as that root remains intact. This suggests that residual systems capable of mediating recovery are under a control which can be called hierarchical. This model provides an alternative to the idea of mass action (amount of undamaged tissue being the decisive factor) or to the concept that a single system "takes over" for the one that is lost by changing the functions it customarily mediates. The hierarchy may be determined by the factors which control the success or failure of a system to generate enduring terminals by axonal sprouting. Finally, hierarchical control would permit the "choice" of a system to mediate recovery which can do it most efficiently.

References

Barnes CD, Joynt RJ, Schottelius BA (1962) Montoneuron resting potentials in spinal shock. Am J Physiol 203: 1113–1116

Basbaum AI, Clanton CH, Fields HL (1978) Three bulbospinal pathways from the rostral medulla of the cat. J Comp Neur 178: 209–224

Bregman BS, Goldberger ME (1979) Effect of hemisection on motor development in kitten hindlimb. Soc Neurosci Abstracts Vol 5, Abstract #1212, p 364

Chen DH (1978) Qualitative and quantitative study of synaptic displacement in chromatolyzed spinal motoneurons of the cat. J Comp Neurol 177: 635–664

Chen DH, Chambers WW, Liu CN (1977) Synaptic displacement in intracentral neurons of Clarke's Nucleus following axotomy in the cat. Exp Neurol 57: 1026–1041

Cope TC, Nelson SG, Mendell LM (1980) Factors outside the neuraxis mediate "acute" increase in EPSP amplitude caudal to spinal cord transection. J Neurophysiol 44: 174–183

Cotman CW, Nadler JV (1978) Reactive synaptogenesis in the hippocampus. In: Cotman CW (ed) Neuronal plasticity. Raven Press, New York, pp 227: 272

Cuello AC, Jessell TM, Kanazawa I, Iverson LL (1977) Substance P: Localization in synaptic vesicles in rat central nervous system. J Neurochem 29: 747–757

Cuello AC, Galfre G, Milstein C (1979) Detection of substance P in the central nervous system by a monoclonal antibody. Proc Natl Acad Sci USA 76: 3532–3536

Dahlstrom A, Fuxe K (1965) Evidence of the existence of monoaminergic neurons in the central nervous system. Acta Physiol Scand 64: (Suppl 247) 37–84

Denny-Brown DB (1966) Cerebral control of movement University of Liverpool Press, Liverpool

Edds MV (1953) Collateral nerve regeneration. Quart Rev Biol 28: 260–276

Gall CD, McWilliams R, Lyndh G (1979) The effects of collateral sprouting on the density of innervation of normal target sites: implications for theories on the regulation of the size of developing synaptic domaons. Brain Res 175: 37–47

Glick SD (1974) Changes in drug sensitivity during recovery of function after brain damage in functional recovery after lesions of the nervous system. NRP12(2): 252–253

Goldberger M (1977) Locomotor recovery after unilateral hindlimb deafferentation in cats. Brain Res 123: 59–74

Goldberger ME (1979) Hierarchial control of locomotor recovery from the effects of dorsal root lesions. Soc for Neurosci

Goldberger ME, Murray M (1974) Restitution of function and collateral sprouting in the cat spinal cord: the deafferented animal. J Comp Neur 158: 37–54

Goldberger ME, Murray M (1978) Recovery of movement and axonal sprouting may obey some of the same laws. In: Cotman CW (ed) Neuronal plasticity. Raven Press, New York, pp 73–96

Goldberger ME, Murray M (1980) Locomotor recovery after deafferentation of one side of the cat's trunk. Exp Neur 67: 103–117

Grillner S (1976) Some aspects on the descending control of the spinal circuits generating locomotor movements. In: Herman RM, Gillner S, Stein PSG, Stuart DG (eds) Neural control of locomotion. Plenum, New York, pp 351–375

Grillner S, Zangger P (1975) How detailed is the central pattern generation for locomotion. Brain Res 88: 367–371

Grillner S, Zangger P (1979) On the central generation of locomotion in the low spinal cat. Exp Brain Res 34: 241–261

Hokfelt T, Kellerth JO, Nilsson G, Pernow B (1976) Experimental immunohistichemical studies on the localization and distribution of Substance P in cat primary sensory neurons. Brain Res 100: 235–252

Hokfelt T, Terenius L, Kuypers HJM, Dann O (1979) Evidence for encephalin immunoreactive neurons in the medulla oblongate projectory to the spinal cord. Neurosci Lett 14: 55–60

Jane JA, Evans JP, Fisher LE (1964) An investigation concerning the restitution of motor function following injury to the spinal cord. J Neurosurgery 21: 167–171

Jankowska E, Jukes MGM, Lund S, Lundberg A (1976a) The effect of DOPA on the spinal cord. 5. Reciprocal organization of pathways transmitting exitatory action to alpha motoneurons of flexors and extensors. Acta Physiol Scand 70: 369–388

Jankowska E, Jukes MGM, Lund S, Lundberg A (1976b) The effect of DOPA on the spinal cord. 6. Half centre organizations of interneurons transmitting effects from the flexor reflex afferents. Acta Physiol Scand 70: 389–402

Krnjevic K (1977) Effects of substance P on central neurons in cats. In: Von Euler US, Pernow B (eds) Substance P. Raven Press, New York, pp 217–230

Liu CN, Chambers WW (1958) Intraspinal sprouting of dorsal root axons. Arch Neurol Psychiatr 79: 46–61

Loesche J, Steward O (1977) Behavioral correlates of denervation and reinnervation of the hippocampal formation of the rat: recovery of alternation performance following unilateral entorhinal cortex lesions. Brain Res Bull 2: 31–39

Martin RF, Jordan LM, Willis WD (1978) Differential distribution of cat medullary neurons demonstrated by retrograde labeling following spinal cord lesion. J Comp Neur 182: 77–88

Mroz EA, Leeman SE (1979) Methods of Horseradish Radioimmunoassay. In: Jaffee BM, Behramn HR (eds) Substance P. Academic Press, New York, pp 121–137

Murray M, Goldberger ME (1974) Restitution of function and collateral sprouting in the cat spinal cord: The partially hemisected animal. J Comp Neurol 155: 19–36

Ogata N (1979) Substance P causes direct depolarization of neurons of guinea pig interpeduncular nucleus in vitro. Nature 211: 277

Otsuka M, Konishi S (1976) Substance P, an excitatory transmitter of primary sensory neurons. Cold Spring Harbor Symposium Quant Biol 15: 135–146

Pickel VM, Reis DT, Leeman SE (1977) Ulstractural localization of substance P in neurons of rat spinal cord. Brain Res 122: 534–540

Pubols LM, Goldberger ME (1980) Recovery of function in the dorsal horn following partial deafferentation. J Neurophysiology 43: 102–117

Raisman G (1969) Neuronal plasticity in the septal nuclei of the adult rat. Brain Res 14: 25–48

Stavraki GW (1961) Supersensitivity following lesions of the nervous system. University of Toronto Press, Toronto, Canada, pp 205

Teasdall RD, Magladery JW, Ramey EH (1958) Changes in the reflex patterns following spinal cord hemisection in cats. Bull Johns Hopkins Hosp 103: 223–235

Tessler A, Glazer E, Artymyshyn R, Murray M, Goldberger ME (1980a) Recovery of substance P in the cat spinal cord after unilateral lumbosacral deafferentation. Brain Res in press

Tessler A, Artymyshyn R, Murray M, Goldberger ME (1980b) Interneurons as a possible source for the return of substance P after lumbosacral deafferentation. Neurosci in press

Wetzel MC, Atwater AE, Wait JV, Stuart DG (1976) Single hindlimb deafferentation and locomotor programming in cats: a kinematic analysis. J Neurophysiol 39: 667–678

Zigmond MD, Stricker EM (1977) Behavioral and neurochemical effects of central catecholamine depletion: A possible model for "subclinical" brain damage. In: Hanin I, Usdin E (eds) Animal models in psychiatry and neurology. Pergamon, New York

Functional Synaptic Changes Caudal to Spinal Cord Transection

L.M. MENDELL, S.G. NELSON, and T.C. COPE[1]

1 Introduction

Studies on the response of the central nervous system to injury generally require the use of two populations of animals – control and experimental. This places a premium on the choice of an experimental system which is sufficiently well defined to permit unequivocal conclusions that any changes are the result of the experimental manipulation rather than the natural variability of the system.

The present paper centers on a description of the changes which occur in individual monosynaptic EPSP's produced by the action of single medial gastrocnemius (MG) Ia fibers (supplying primary spindle receptors) in homonymous motoneurons caudal to spinal cord transection. This choice was based upon the highly consistent pattern of functional connectivity observed at single synapses in this system in the intact anesthetized cat (Mendell and Henneman 1971; Scott and Mendell 1976; Munson and Sypert 1979). It was hoped that the resolution provided by the ability to study individual EPSP's would provide some insight into the processes which take place after injury to the CNS. Furthermore, physiological studies permit analysis of the time course of the change free from complications introduced by the degeneration and transport anatomical methods (Murray and Goldberger 1974) in systems where histochemical methods (see review by Cotman and Nadler 1978) cannot be used due to lack of knowledge of the transmitter.

These experiments were undertaken with two general aims. First, we were interested in studying the effects of CNS injury on an identified synapse. The effect of spinal cord injury on a synapse known to be important in the mechanism of the stretch reflex (Matthews 1972) was thought to be of particular significance (but see Sect. 10). In addition, we were anxious to examine the consequences of partial denervation of the motoneuron on the action of surviving input. In order to achieve appreciable partial denervation of lumbar motoneurons in the cat, it is necessary to transect the spinal

1 Departments of Physiology (LMM, TCC) and Physical Therapy (SGN), Duke University Medical Center, Durham, N.C. 27710, USA
Present Address (LMM): Department of Neurobiology and Behaviour, SUNY Stony Brook, Stony Brook, NY 11794, USA
Present Address (TCC): Department of Physiology and Biophysics, University of Washington, Seattle, WA 98195, USA

cord relatively close to them, within two to three segments (McLaughlin 1972; Strick et al. 1976). Therefore, cats used in this study underwent cord transection either at T13 or at L5, with the motoneurons under examination located at L7.

2 Experimental Methods

The experimental method which permits examination of EPSP's evoked by the action of single afferent fibers is the spike-triggered averaging technique (Mendell and Henneman 1971). Impulses recorded from a single identified Ia fiber in a dissected but uncut dorsal rootlet are used to trigger a computer which averages the potential recorded simultaneously from a motoneuron identified by antidromic invasion. The spindle is activated by steady stretch on the muscle; impulses in other Ia fibers from that muscle are asynchronous with respect to the trigger impulse and do not contribute to the EPSP which is averaged if the triggering Ia fiber projects to the impaled motoneuron.

The spike-triggered averaging method provides access to three kinds of information which can be used to evaluate changes following experimental manipulation. If an EPSP is recorded from the postsynaptic cell, one can conclude that the afferent fiber makes a functional synapse upon it. A negative result is more difficult to interpret because of the possibility of an EPSP below the noise level. However, current evidence suggests that improvement in the ability to resolve very small EPSP's does not significantly increase the measured connectivity (or projection frequency) (compare Munson and Sypert 1979 to Scott and Mendell 1976). The second piece of information which can be obtained is the amplitude of the averaged EPSP whose mean over a number of synapses can vary independently of the connectivity (Mendell et al. 1976; Nelson and Mendell 1979; see below). Finally, the shape of the EPSP as characterized by the shape indices [time-to-peak (rise time) and duration at half amplitude (half width – Rall 1967)] provides some information concerning the location of the active synaptic terminals of the Ia fiber on the motoneuron soma-dendritic tree. It is difficult to be certain of the absolute location unless a number of additional measurements are made (see Redman 1976); however, it is useful to compare these shape indices in different types of preparations to see if any changes can be detected.

3 Changes in EPSP Properties

3.1 Chronic Changes

Transection of the spinal cord sets off a series of time-dependent changes at MG Ia fiber-motoneuron synapses located caudal to the level of the injury (Nelson and Mendell 1979; Fig. 1). Focusing first on the chronic changes (i.e., $>$ 12 days after transection), we have observed (Fig. 2) that the mean amplitude of averaged EPSP's undergoes a significant increase following transection of the spinal cord at L5 compared to similar values obtained in cats with transection at T13. The mean EPSP in cats with chronic transection at T13 is $114 \pm 8\ \mu V$ with no trend to increase or decrease as a func-

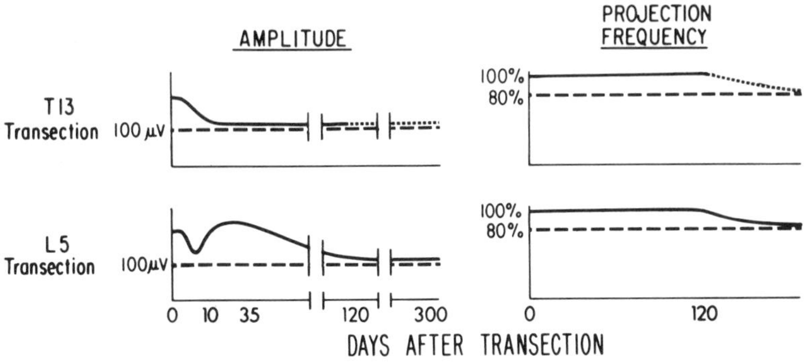

Fig. 1. EPSP amplitude *(left)* and projection frequency *(right)* changes following spinal cord transection at T13 *(top)* and L5 *(bottom)*. Note that EPSP amplitude changes provide evidence for two mechanisms, acute and chronic. Note also the independence of amplitude and projection frequency changes, particularly after chronic transection at T13. Amplitude of 10 μV and projection frequency of 80% represent values in preparations with intact spinal cord against which values in transected preparations can be evaluated. Dotted lines represent postulated results of experiments not yet carried out

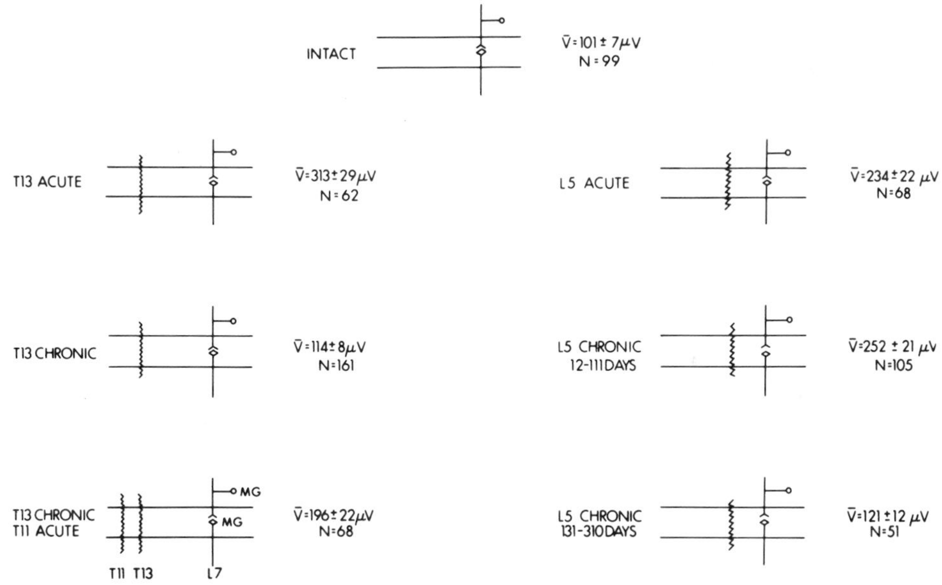

Fig. 2. Mean individual EPSP amplitudes (± SEM) under different experimental conditions. MG Ia fibers and motoneurons throughout. Note increase over intact values following acute transection at T13 and L5 and after chronic transection at L5 (12–111 days) but not T13. Note the recovery in mean amplitude long after transection at L5 (131–310 days). Note also the increase following acute transection at T11 despite presence of chronic transection at T13

tion of time. This is only slightly larger than the mean amplitude in preparations with intact spinal cord studied under the same experimental conditions (101 ± 7 μV; Nelson and Mendell 1979). On the other hand transection at L5 causes a consistent increase in the amplitude of EPSP's which begins 1–2 weeks after injury and reaches a peak in about 30 days. This time course is similar to that for reactive synaptogenesis in the hippocampus following partial deafferentation (see review by Cotman and Nadler 1978). A most unexpected finding is the decrease in EPSP amplitude beginning 7–10 weeks after transection. Normal values are achieved by 120 days.

This clearcut difference between the effects of transection at L5 and T13 on EPSP amplitude is consistent with the hypothesis that the degree of denervation of the motoneuron may contribute to the increase in EPSP amplitudes. However, whatever the mechanism responsible for this increase, it is transient or, alternatively, its action is overcome by the onset of some compensatory mechanism. These issues are discussed more fully in Sect. 7.

3.1.1 Large EPSP's

The considerable enlargement in mean EPSP amplitude occurring 12–111 days following chronic transection of the spinal cord at L5 features the appearance of a population of very large EPSP's never seen in intact preparations studied under these conditions. EPSP's as large as 1 mV have been recorded in contrast to a maximum of 400–500 μV in intact preparations (Scott and Mendell 1976; Munson and Sypert 1979). Another finding consistent with this potentiation is the marked reduction in the proportion of EPSP's smaller than 100 μV. It appears then that there has been a shift in the entire EPSP amplitude distribution under these conditions (Nelson and Mendell 1979). Measurements of motoneuron input resistance and time constant indicate that these increases in EPSP amplitudes cannot be explained by changes in the electrical properties of the motoneurons. This places the locus of the change at the synapse itself, but at present we cannot distinguish between presynaptic and highly localized postsynaptic alterations.

3.1.2 Selectivity of Increase

The increase in EPSP amplitude after chronic L5 transection does not appear to depend on the conduction velocity of the afferent fiber. On the other hand, we find that the potentiation is greatest in small motoneurons, although motoneurons over the entire conduction velocity range participate in the increase. Consistent with this is the finding that the small increase in EPSP amplitude seen after chronic spinal cord transection at T13 is restricted entirely to the smallest motoneurons (Cope et al. 1980). We conclude that increases in EPSP amplitude following chronic transection of the spinal cord occur preferentially, and to the greatest extent, in small motoneurons.

A further example of the selectivity in the increase of EPSP amplitude caudal to chronic L5 transection is provided by the finding that EPSP's with brief rise times are potentiated to a greater extent than those with long rise times (Nelson and Mendell 1979). This is independent of the selective increase in small motoneurons, i.e., small motoneurons do not generate EPSP's with the fastest rise times (see Scott and Mendell 1976). One interpretation is that the EPSP's produced by proximally located Ia terminals are increased to a greater extent than those produced by distal ones, perhaps because these regions are subject to the greatest amount of denervation by the transection. However, it is also possible that synapses with the briefest transmitter release undergo a greater enhancement than those where transmitter release is slower.

3.1.3 Location on Soma-Dendritic Tree

Since the enlargement of EPSP's pursuant to chronic transection may be the result of partial denervation of the motoneurons, it was of interest to explore whether any evidence could be found for a more widespread distribution of the terminals from a single afferent fiber on the motoneuron as has been previously found in the partially deafferented red nucleus (Tsukahara 1978). According to Rall (1967) an increased spread of terminals would be expected to cause an increased half-width for a given rise time, i.e., shift the shape index curve upward. We have seen no evidence for such a shift (Nelson and Mendell 1979), and so we conclude that if the potentiation of the EPSP is associated with the action of new terminals, they must be very close electrically to the ones functioning in the intact preparation.

3.2 Acute Changes in EPSP's

In order to interpret the results seen after chronic transection of the spinal cord, it was important to ascertain the earliest time at which changes in EPSP's could be observed. We found unexpectedly that many acutely transected preparations exhibited mean EPSP amplitudes above normal values (Figs. 1 and 2) with many EPSP's in the range of 500 μV to more than 1 mV (Nelson et al. 1979). This occurred regardless of the level of transection (T13 or L5) indicating a mechanism different from the one responsible for the chronic changes. Experiments, in which the spinal cord was transected while recording an EPSP in a motoneuron, revealed that the increase in amplitude is not an immediate consequence of the injury (Nelson et al. 1979; Cope et al. 1980). Complementary experiments, in which the action of a single fiber was studied in many successively impaled motoneurons over a period of time after transection, indicated that the increase in EPSP amplitude begins only several hours after injury (Nelson et al. 1979).

The delay in the EPSP amplitude increase suggests that release from the action of a tonically active descending system cannot be responsible. We have therefore tested directly whether this phenomenon requires injury to axons which are in synaptic contact with the test segment by making an acute transection at T11 in animals previously (8–12 weeks) transected at T13 (Cope et al. 1980). Surprisingly, substantial elevation in the amplitude of EPSP's in MG motoneurons (located in L7) was caused by transection at T11 despite chronic transection at a level between T11 and L7 (Fig. 2). Together these results are taken to suggest that the effects of acute transection include an important component which does not involve loss of connections from the rostral spinal cord on the brain. We have speculated that "non-neural" or humoral factors may play an important role in this EPSP amplitude increase via liberation of substances from such structures as the pituitary gland or perhaps via the action of the autonomic nervous system (Cope et al. 1980).

4 Increases in Projection Frequency of Afferent Fibers

We have found that projection frequency (pooled from many experiments) increases from a value of about 80% in intact preparations (Scott and Mendell 1976; Munson and Sypert 1979) to 96%–100% within hours after transection (Nelson et al. 1979). This rapid change suggests activation of previously nonfunctional synapses rather than growth of new connections. These high projection frequencies persist into the chronic period (> 12 days after transection) regardless of the level of transection (L5 or T13). It should be recalled that EPSP amplitudes are essentially normal after chronic transection at T13. Therefore the increase in projection frequency in this case cannot be attributed to better resolution of EPSP's, and for this reason we consider increases in projection frequency to be independent of changes in EPSP amplitude. We have hypothesized (Nelson and Mendell 1979) that projection frequency increases may reflect increased access of presynaptic impulses to terminal boutons, whereas the increase in EPSP amplitude may be explained by alterations in synaptic transmission per se.

5 Two Mechanisms – Acute and Chronic (Fig. 1)

Our findings from EPSP amplitude measurements support the view that the acute and chronic changes result from the action of different mechanisms. Increases in EPSP amplitude in the acute period (within several hours of transection) occur regardless of the level of transection and persist for only a few days at most. These might involve the action of humoral mechanisms. After transection at T13, EPSP amplitudes decline to normal values by 12 days. The situation after transection at L5 is more complicated. By 5 days EPSP amplitudes have begun to return towards normal values, but by 12–18 days they become enlarged again. This secondary increase, which may be related to partial denervation of the motoneurons (see above), is not observed in preparations transected at T13.

6 Mechanisms for Increase in EPSP Amplitude in Chronically Transected Preparations

Two processes, which have been suggested to increase the action of surviving input on deafferented spinal neurons, are denervation supersensitivity (Sharpless 1975) and sprouting (Goldberger and Murray 1978). It is difficult to prove the existence of denervation supersensitivity at the Ia fiber-motoneuron synapse, in large part because of our present ignorance of the transmitter at this junction. Another difficulty is that the terminals are not necessarily located on the soma nor in close proximity to one another (Burke et al. 1979). Collateral sprouting from afferent fibers has been shown to occur in the spinal cord of the cat following thoracic spinal cord hemisection (Goldberger and Murray 1978), but mainly onto dorsal horn interneurons rather than motoneurons. This pattern probably resulted from the relative paucity of long descending connections onto motoneurons in the cat.

7 Recovery Processes

One of the most unexpected findings in this series of experiments was the recovery which occurred 3–4 months after transection at L5 (Nelson and Mendell 1979). The failure for the increased EPSP amplitudes or projection frequency to persist is of great significance for the general question of how the CNS reacts to injury. An important issue is whether transection at L5 sets off a transient change beginning by 2 weeks, or whether the change might have been permanent but for the action of some later event which can also influence Ia fiber EPSP's in motoneurons. The persistence of additional dorsal root collaterals for as long as 1 year after hemisection (Murray and Goldberger 1974) suggests that any inactivation occurs in the synaptic region itself.

Previous experiments on denervation supersensitivity in the septate ganglion of the frog (Roper 1976) suggest that it fails to persist even in the absence of reinnervation of the denervated region. Alternatively, in the spinal cord isolated by two transections there is some recent evidence that synapses characteristic of those made by local interneurons first undergo a decrease in number with a later recovery (Pullen and Sears 1978; see also Bernstein and Bernstein 1973). The time course of this change mirrors the change in EPSP amplitudes which we have reported. The recovery in the population of synapses made by local interneurons might influence the potentiated Ia fiber-motoneuron synapse either by diminishing the amount of denervation supersensitivity, or by displacing some of the Ia fiber synapses formed as a result of partial denervation. The latter idea implies a competitive interaction between different synaptic types, with the intrinsic fibers having a greater affinity for some synaptic sites accupied by Ia fibers. Similar processes have been reported following innervation of amphibian muscles by foreign nerve fibers (Bennett and Raftos 1977; Dennis and Yip 1978). The question still remains as to why the presumptive proliferation of these terminals derived from local interneurons should occur much later than those by Ia fiber terminals. Spinal cord interneurons close to transection might suffer more trauma than dorsal root ganglion cells and thus be unable to supply new terminals until much later.

8 The Effect of Disuse

In a recent experiment Kuno and his colleagues (Gallego et al. 1979) reported that disuse of the Ia afferent fiber pathway produced by application of TTX to the peripheral nerve results in a substantial elevation of EPSP's which they evoke in motoneurons. It seems unlikely that this can account for the EPSP enlargement observed after transection. To begin with, the elevation in amplitudes was never seen after transection at T13 although the animals' limbs were as severely incapacitated as after transection at L5 where EPSP enlargement was observed. Furthermore the subsequent decrease in amplitudes back towards normal values was not accompanied by any obvious change in the use of the limb. Finally, in many such preparations we found that Ia fibers possessed tonic activity arguing directly against disuse.

9 Comparison to Effects of Axotomy of Motoneurons

The change in EPSP amplitude and projection frequency is exactly opposite to that observed following motoneuron axotomy. Following transection of a portion of the peripheral nerve supplying the gastrocnemius muscle, Ia fibers which have not been cut are found to generate smaller EPSP's in axotomized motoneurons (Kuno and Llinas 1970; Mendell et al. 1976), and at a later time to become totally disconnected from them (Mendell et al. 1976). The changes following transection are thus opposite from those which follow injury of the motoneuron itself.

10 General Comment

It should be kept in mind that this detailed study of plasticity is limited to a single synaptic type. The emphasis has been on uncovering the mechanisms which operate. Another important issue is the behavioral consequences of such injuries and the way in which the synaptic changes seen here can explain such alterations. However, even the simplest reflex act, such as the tendon jerk, requires knowledge not only of the efficacy of the Ia fiber-motoneuron synapse but also how motoneuron properties (e.g., membrane potential) are affected by the barrage of impulses converging on it. The behavior of the spindle itself will be affected by α-motoneuron outflow. Therefore, to translate the changes studied here into behavioral terms it is required that such information be available for a larger number of synaptic types. This represents an important challenge in further studies of how the function of the CNS is affected by injury.

11 Summary

Synapses which mediate the monosynaptic stretch reflex undergo changes in efficacy caudal to spinal cord transection. Both acute and chronic changes are observed and the latter require the transection to be relatively close to the test segment. The chronic changes seem to require denervation of the motoneuron, and are not permanent. The acute changes may involve the action of a humoral factor.

Acknowledgment. This work was supported by research grant NS-08411 and program grant NS 14899 from the National Institutes of Health (USA). T.C. Cope was supported by the Biological Systems Training Grant awarded to Duke University.

References

Bennett MR, Raftos J (1977) The formation and regression of synapses during reinnervation of axolotl-striated muscles. J Physiol (London) 265: 261–295

Bernstein JJ, Bernstein ME (1973) Neuronal alteration and reinnervation following axonal regeneration and sprouting in mammalian spinal cord. Brain Behav Evol 8: 135–161

Burke RE, Walmsley B, Hodgson JA (1979) Structural-functional relation in monosynaptic action on spinal motoneurons. In: Brooks V, Asanuma H (eds) Integration in the nervous system. Igaku: Shoin, Tokyo, pp 27–45

Cope TC, Nelson SG, Mendell LM (1980) Factors outside the nauraxis mediate the "acute" increase in EPSP amplitude caudal to spinal cord transection. J Neurophysiol 44: 174–183

Cotman C, Nadler JV (1978) Reactive synaptogenesis in the hippocampus. In: Cotman C (ed) Neuronal plasticity. Raven Press, New York, pp 227–271

Dennis MJ, Yip JW (1978) Formation and elimination of foreign synapses on adult salamander muscle. J Physiol (London) 274: 299–310

Gallego R, Kuno M, Nunez R, Snider WD (1979) Disuse enhances synaptic efficacy in spinal motoneurones. J Physiol (London) 291: 191–205

Goldberger ME, Murray M (1978) Recovery of movement and axonal sprouting may obey some of the same laws. In: Cotman C (ed) Neuronal plasticity. Raven Press, New York, pp 73–96

Kuno M, Llinas R (1970) Alterations of synaptic action in chromatolysed motoneurones of the cat. J Physiol (London) 210: 823–838

Matthews PBC (1972) Mammalian muscle receptors and their central actions. Williams and Wilkins, Baltimore

McLaughlin B (1972) Propriospinal and supraspinal projections to motor nuclei of the cat spinal cord. J Comp Neurol 144: 475–500

Mendell LM, Henneman E (1971) Terminals of single Ia fibers: location, density and distribution within a pool of 300 homonymous motoneurons. J Neurophysiol 34: 171–187

Mendell LM, Munson JB, Scott JG (1976) Alterations of synapses on axotomized motoneurons. J Physiol (London) 255: 67–79

Munson JB, Sypert GW (1979) Properties of single fibre excitatory postsynaptic potentials in triceps surae motoneurons. J Physiol (London) 296: 329–342

Murray M, Goldberger ME (1974) Redistribution of function and collateral sprouting in the cat spinal cord: the partially hemisected animal. J Comp Neurol 158: 19–36

Nelson SG, Mendell LM (1979) Enhancement in Ia-motoneuron synaptic transmission caudal to chronic spinal cord transection. J Neurophysiol 42: 642–654

Nelson SG, Collatos TC, Niechaj A, Mendell LM (1979) Immediate increase in Ia-motoneuron synaptic transmission caudal to spinal cord transection. J Neurophysiol 42: 665–664

Pullen AH, Sears TA (1978) Modification of "C" synapses following partial central deafferentation of thoracic motoneurons. Brain Res 145: 141–146

Rall W (1967) Distinguishing theoretical synaptic potentials for different soma-dendritic distributions of synaptic input. J Neurophysiol 30: 1168–1193

Redman SJ (1976) A quantitative approach to the integrative function of dendrites. In: Porter R (ed) International review of physiology: Neurophysiology, vol 10. University Park Press, Baltimore, pp 1–36

Roper S (1976) The acetylcholine sensitivity of the surface membrane of multiply-innervated parasympathetic ganglion cells in the mudpuppy before and after partial denervation. J Physiol (London) 254: 455–473

Scott JG, Mendell LM (1976) Individual EPSPs produced by single triceps surae Ia afferent fibers in homonymous and heteronymous motoneurons. J Neurophysiol 39: 679–692

Sharpless SK (1975) Supersensitivity-like phenomena in the central nervous system. Fed Proc 34: 1990–1997

Strick PL, Burke RE, Kanda K, Kim CC (1976) Tracing spinal neurons projecting to the ventral horn using retrograde transport: possible last order interneurons to medial gastrocnemius motoneurones. Neurosci Abstr 1: 170

Tsukahara N (1978) Synaptic plasticity in the red nucleus. In: Cotman C (ed) Neuronal plasticity. Raven Press, New York, pp 113–130

IIb. Recovery from Vestibular Lesions

Concepts of Vestibular Compensation

H. FLOHR, H. BIENHOLD, W. ABELN, and I. MACSKOVICS[1]

1 Introduction

Peripheral vestibular lesions such as unilateral labyrinthectomy or unilateral vestibular nerve transection result in characteristic gross disturbances of posture and movement. These symptoms disappear spontaneously with time and normal behavior is restored. This compensation process encompasses *all* observed deficits. The pattern of disturbances following the lesion and the time course of the compensation processes are basically similar but not identical in different vertebrates. A detailed description of the similarities and differences in the symptomatology and recovery processes in different species is given by Schaefer and Meyer (1974). The basic phenomena of the compensation process have been well known since the classical investigations of Bechterew (1883) and Ewald (1892). Magnus (1924) realized that compensation must involve an extensive reorganization of the remaining structures of the vestibular system.

More recently it has become evident that these processes reveal an immense capacity for plastic adaptive changes and might well have the potential to become a basic paradigm in the study of lesion-induced neuronal plasticity and, possibly, for the study of plastic processes in general.

The discussion of possible mechanisms underlying vestibular compensation reflects to some extent the present situation of the search for an understanding of neuronal mechanisms in memory and learning. This situation seems to be characterized by a substantial number of possibly relevant experimental data and observations and the complete lack of a hypothesis which orders them coherently.

Some of the difficulties in finding a common thread which connects early and recent observations on vestibular compensation are outlined in this paper.

2 Localization of Changes Underlying Vestibular Compensation

A considerable part of the endeavor to understand the nature of plastic changes consists in attempts to localize them within the nervous system. This has also been the

1 Universität Bremen, 2800 Bremen 33, FRG

purpose of numerous early and more recent investigations on vestibular compensation. The results of this approach are conflicting. They do not lead to simple conclusions and have sometimes caused doubts, similar to those put forward by Lashley (1950), as to whether the underlying hypothesis of a localizable trace is at all tenable (Schaefer and Meyer 1973; Llinás and Walton 1979).

2.1 Role of Vestibular Nuclei

The vestibular nuclei seem to play an important role in the compensation process. They are the first integrative station into which information from both receptors, from other sensory systems (such as visual, somatosensory, and proprioceptive systems), and from various supranuclear motor centers converge. Their output influences many structures related to locomotion and space perception. Following hemilabyrinthectomy an initial bilateral decrease of spontaneous activity in both vestibular nuclei has been observed. The decrease in activity on the intact side has been attributed to cerebellar inhibition (McCabe and Ryu 1969) or to crossed vestibular inhibition (Precht et al. 1966). This initial phase is followed by a period of asymmetrical activity. The activity on the deafferented side is reduced, whereas it is still present or even enhanced on the intact side (Gernandt and Thulin 1952; Trincker 1965; Shimazu and Precht 1966). During compensation the activity on the deafferented side regenerates (Precht et al. 1966; McCabe and Ruy 1969).

2.1.1 Studies with [^{14}C]-2-Deoxyglucose

We have studied the regeneration of resting activity in *Rana temporaria* by means of the [^{14}C]-2-Deoxy-D-Glucose technique (Sokoloff et al. 1977). This technique is based on the use of [^{14}C]-Deoxyglucose as an indicator of glucose consumption. Deoxyglucose is transported from blood to brain by the same carrier which transports glucose and, like glucose, it is phosphorylated by hexokinase. Unlike glucose-6-phosphate, however, it cannot be metabolized further to fructose-6-phosphate and is not a substrate for alternative pathways of glucose metabolism. Once formed, it accumulates in the tissue in a mathematically definable relationship to the rate of glucose uptake. The glucose concentration in the CNS can be determined by means of quantitative autoradiography.

In the present study a modification of Sokoloff's technique was applied. 1-[^{14}C]-2-D-Glucose (53 mCi/mmol, New England Nuclear) was used. 16.7 μCi/100 g body weight suspended in 0.05 ml sterile saline were injected into the dorsal lymph sac. 45 min after injection the animals were sacrificed. The brain was quickly removed and frozen in isopentane, cooled by liquid nitrogen to -160°C. Frozen sections 12 μm thick were cut on a WKF cryotome WK 1150 and picked up with slides. The sections were freeze-dried at -84°C in a vacuum (10^{-6} mbar) for 12 h using a Leybold Heraeus GT 1. Following that, they were brought into contact with emulsion-coated slides and exposed for 20–25 days at -20°C in sealed black boxes containing Drierite. The films were developed (Kodak D-19 developer) and fixed in the usual way after separating them from the sections. The autoradiographs were quantitatively evaluated using a

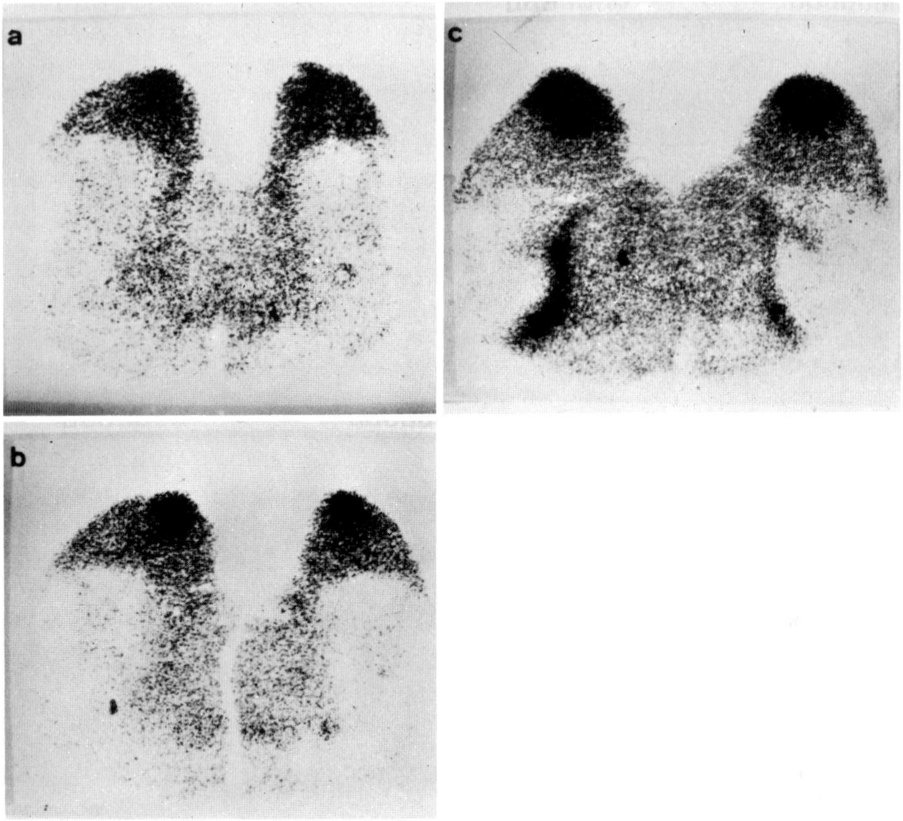

Fig. 1a–c. Autoradiographs showing normal spatial distribution of [^{14}C]-2-Deoxyglucose uptake in the vestibular complex. Transverse sections through caudal (**a**), middle (**b**) and rostral (**c**) thirds of the brain stem of Rana temporaria

television image analyzer (Quantimet 720, Cambridge Instrument) equipped with a densitometer module.

An analysis of the compensation process with this technique leads to the following results:

1. The area of the vestibular nuclei can be seen as a well-defined zone of high activity. Normally the activity is symmetrically distributed (Fig. 1).
2. Immediately after unilateral labyrinthectomy, i.e., in the state of massive postural deficits, there is a considerable asymmetry of metabolic activity. Activity is decreased on the side of the lesion (Fig. 2c,d). This is in line with electrophysiological findings.
3. During compensation recovery of the symmetrical activity is observed. Activity on the side of the lesion increases (Fig. 2e,f).

It is generally accepted that the reappearance of resting activity in the deafferented nucleus is responsible for functional recovery though an exact correspondance with

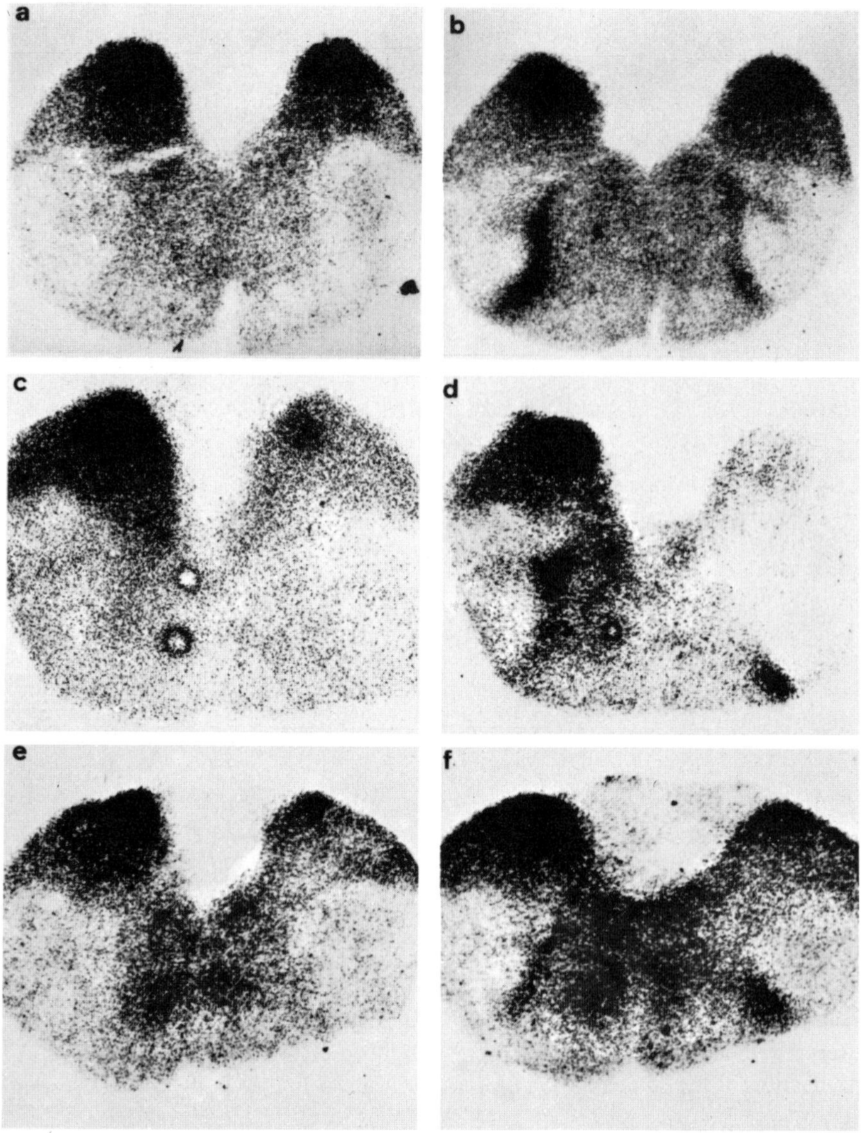

Fig. 2a–f. Spatial distribution of [^{14}C]-2-Deoxyglucose uptake in the vestibular complex of the frog. **a,b** Normal distribution in two different frontal planes (both labyrinths intact). **c,d** Distribution pattern following acute unilateral, right labyrinthectomy. Labyrinthectomy was performed 24 h before DG application. Note the decrease of activity shown in the deafferented N. vestibularis (and in the N. dorsalis). **e,f** Distribution pattern in the compensated state. DG was given 145 days after right side labyrinthectomy and after complete compensation of the head deviation. Note the recovery of the metabolic activity in the deafferented vestibular nucleus (but not in the N. dorsalis)

the disappearance of functional deficits has not been proved beyond doubt. According to our findings, the increase in metabolic activity on the deafferented side and the decrease in the side differences parallel the compensation process, as defined by head deviation, changes with time. The findings of Jensen (1977) and Azzena et al. (1977) support this view that adjustment in bilateral activity is causative in compensation. In decompensation induced by spinal cord transection in fully compensated guinea pigs, it was shown that the activity of the deafferented side again decreases. This recovery of activity, however, does not necessarily prove that the underlying plastic changes are localized in the deafferented nucleus. The source of the regained activity is not known. Compensation can be influenced by interventions into various remote systems preceding labyrinthectomy. Ablation studies indicate that afferents from the cortex (Menzio 1949; Giretti 1971; Schaefer and Meyer 1973), the cerebellum (cf. Schaefer and Meyer 1974), the spinal cord (Kolb 1955; Dal Ri and Schaefer 1957) and the visual system (Kolb 1955; Putkonen et al. 1977; Courjon et al. 1977) are involved. Interventions into these structures can either accelerate or decrease the compensation process.

Following compensation a decompensation, with the reappearance of symptoms, can be produced by destruction of various remote CNS structures. Decompensation, for example, was observed following hemispherectomy (Di Giorgio 1939; Menzio 1949), spinal cord transection (Azzena 1969), bilateral destruction of the fastigial nuclei (Carpenter et al. 1959), chemically induced lesions of the inferior olive (Llinás et al. 1975; Llinás and Walton 1979) and destruction of the intervestibular commissures (Bienhold and Flohr 1978).

It has been concluded from these observations that compensation is not an isolated function of the vestibular system and that the cellular changes basic to vestibular compensation are not unilocular (Schaefer and Meyer 1973; Llinás and Walton 1979), but that more probably widely distributed changes at different locations are responsible for the rearrangement of spatially extended circuits. This would mean that no critical structure exists, and no single trace can be localized. This conclusion, however, is possible but not necessary. Interventions preceding labyrinthectomy affect the velocity of the compensation process positively or negatively, but do not prevent recovery. Ultimately, this only shows that compensatory reorganization can be brought about under different conditions and by means of different strategies, but does *not* necessarily involve structural changes in remote systems. The decompensatory effect of such interventions after compensation cannot be taken as proof of multilocular structural changes involving the organization of spatially extended circuits. It is possible as well that these effects merely indicate that a newly attained functionally sufficient integration of afferents from different systems has been brought about by a reorganization of the vestibular complex into which these afferents converge. Of interest in this connection are the findings of Spiegel and Démétriades (1925) who found that Bechterew compensation due to a second labyrinthectomy after recovery from the first is present if only the deafferented vestibular nucleus is intact. Bechterew nystagmus in cats and rabbits could not be abolished by total ablation of the cerebellum, extirpation of the pros- and diencephalon, injury of the corpora quadrigemina, or destruction of the vestibular nucleus on the side of the second labyrinthectomy. It was, however, abolished by destruction of the vestibular nucleus ipsilateral to the first labyrinthectomy. They concluded from these results that the changes necessary for the development of

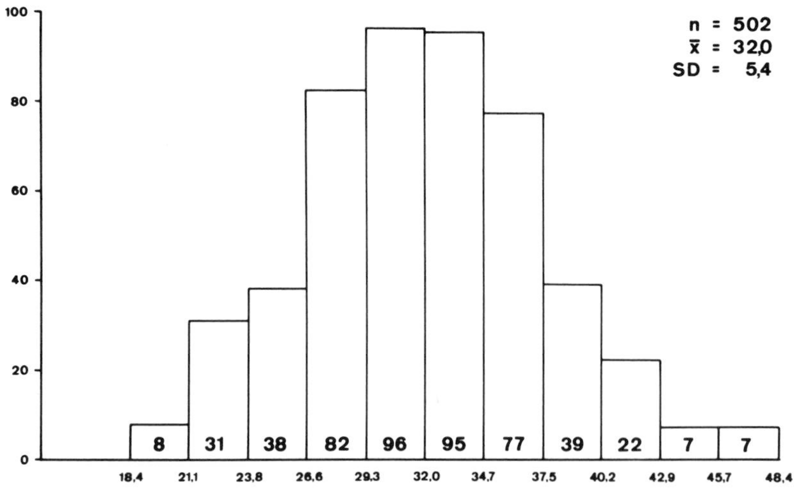

Fig. 3. Distribution of head deviation following unilateral labyrinthectomy in the frog. Measurements of head tilt were performed 24 h after labyrinthectomy. $n = 502$

the Bechterew phenomenon reside exclusively within the ipsilateral nucleus. However, it is questionable whether the persisting predominant activity in the nuclei which were first deafferented, as indicated by the Bechterew phenomenon, is alone responsible for the balanced activity observed in the compensated state (see below).

2.2 Role of Intervestibular Commissures

The restitution of activity in the deafferented vestibular nucleus seems to be necessary for attaining equilibrium between the two sides. However, compensation is more than the restitution of simple symmetry of activity between vestibular nuclei. This may explain some of the recovery phenomena, e.g., the disappearance of the head tilt, but not all of them. To attain a recovery of all vestibular reflexes and locomotor behavior, different circuits must be so organized that the activity of the deafferented nucleus is controlled in a way dynamically equivalent to that previously executed by the ipsilateral labyrinth. Ultimately, this means that the remaining labyrinth must take over control.

It is reasonable to assume that this control is exerted by the intact side via preexisting commissural connections. Physiologically, a close cooperation between the neurons on both sides is required to produce the motor output. It is possible that this cooperation involves inherent plastic properties necessary, for example, in the acquisition of new motor skills or in adjusting asymmetrical inputs from both end-organs. Figure 3 shows that the observed head deviation following unilateral labyrinthectomy in the frog varies considerably, indicating different tonic influences of both labyrinths on the vestibular complex. Obviously, these asymmetries are "compensated for" under normal circumstances. The compensation process after unilateral labyrinthectomy could be an extension of a physiological mechanism.

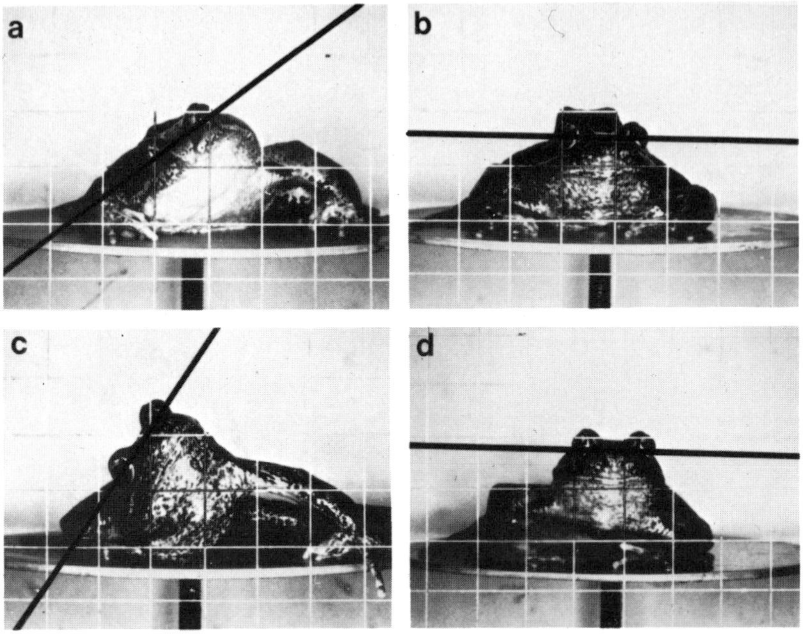

Fig. 4a–d. Decompensation following destruction of the intervestibular commissural connections in the compensated state in the frog. **a** Head deviation immediately after destruction of the right labyrinth; **b** compensated state 100 days after labyrinthectomy; **c** effect of commissurotomy; **d** if the remaining labyrinth is destroyed (5 days later) the decompensatory effect disappears

Bienhold and Flohr (1978) have recently demonstrated the importance of the commissural system. In *Rana temporaria* they have shown that

1. destruction of the commissural fibers after partial or complete compensation was followed by an immediate reappearance of all postural and locomotor symptoms (Fig. 4);
2. this decompensatory effect was independent of the time interval between hemilabyrinthectomy and commissurotomy; it could be observed up to 5 months after complete recovery; it was abolished by a subsequent destruction of the remaining labyrinth (Fig. 4d);
3. no re-compensation could be observed after commissurotomy (Fig. 5).

Dieringer and Precht (1977, 1979) have recently presented convincing evidence that during compensation a profound reorganization of crossed intervestibular connections takes place. In hemilabyrinthectomized frogs the efficacy of excitatory commissural fibers ending on the deafferented neurons increased considerably, and an effective crossed inhibition (which is not present in normal animals) develops via a vestibulo-cerebello-vestibular loop and via the brain stem. For reasons discussed below, these authors assumed that this increased inhibitory and excitatory efficacy of intervestibular commissural connections was due to a reactive synaptogenesis in the deafferented nucleus.

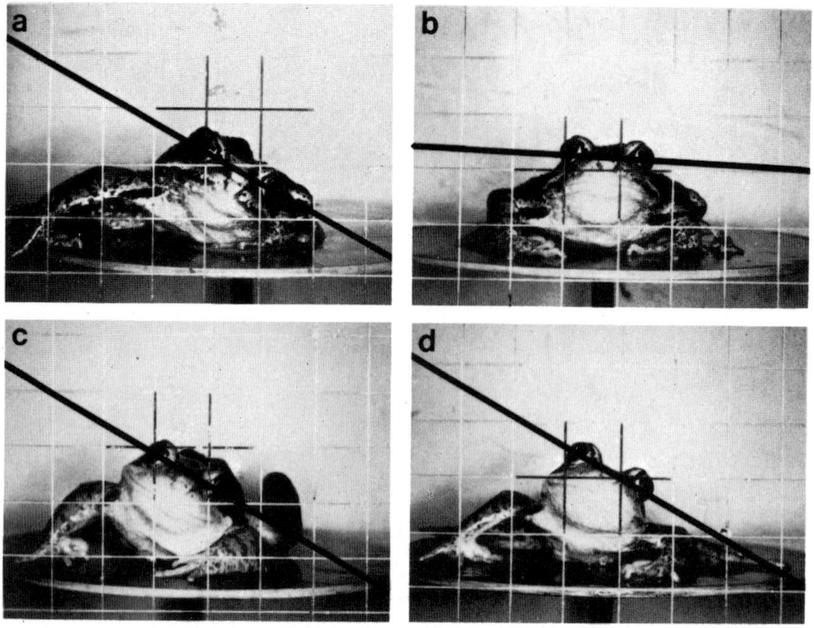

Fig. 5a–d. Decompensation following commissurotomy. **a** Head deviation after acute labyrinthectomy; **b** compensated state; **c** decompensation following commissurotomy; **d** state 80 days after commissurotomy; no second compensation has occurred

In summary, it remains unclear where the changes underlying vestibular compensation occur. The process necessarily involves the reorganization of complex, spatially extended circuits. It does not, however, necessarily demand widely spread multiple structural changes which are probably less well identifiable. At present there is no direct evidence against the assumption that the basic changes are confined to the deafferented nucleus.

3 Nature of Basic Cellular Mechanisms in Vestibular Compensation

Despite Lashley's extensive criticism, connectivistic hypotheses prevail in the present day concepts of long-term storage of information. Moreover, some recent investigations into vestibular compensation have clearly shown that synaptic changes are involved.

3.1 Synaptic Changes

Evidence that synaptic changes are involved comes from electrophysiological and pharmacological studies. Dieringer and Precht (1977, 1979) found that the increased efficacy of excitatory commissural terminals ending at the deafferented neurons was associated with characteristic changes in the spike thresholds and shape indices of the evoked EPSP's (such as amplitude and time-to-peak interval). These changes were best explained by the assumption that after partial denervation the remaining undamaged commissural inputs had sprouted and formed new functional synapses replacing the lost axosomatic labyrinthine synapses. Similarly, they assumed that in increased crossed inhibition Purkinje cell terminals ending at vestibular neurons had formed additional inhibitory synapses on the vacated soma of the deafferented cells.

Observations of Korte and Friedrich (1979) support this view. In the deafferented superior vestibular nucleus of the cat they found that 5–6 days after the lesion a new type of synaptic boutons appeared. These boutons were characterized by vesicles different in size and shape from those found in the intact nucleus and might represent newly formed synaptic endings.

Bienhold and Flohr (1980) presented evidence that cholinergic synapses are involved in the compensation process in *Rana temporaria.* Details are presented by Abeln et al. (this vol.). In brief, it was shown that

1. systemic or intracranial application of cholinesterase inhibitors, such as physostigmine, paraoxon (E 600), parathion (E 605), and diisopropyl fluorophosphate, in fully compensated animals induces an immediate and complete return to the precompensated state;
2. this effect can be obtained in all phases of the compensation process and is dose-dependent;
3. cholinomimetics, such as nicotine, muscarine, and oxotremorine, have the same decompensatory effect;
4. cholinolytics, such as atropine and scopolamine, exert an antagonistic effect, i.e., they diminish the deficit if given during compensation; after full compensation they induce a head deviation to the intact side.

Both observations, electrophysiological and pharmacological, indicate that synaptic changes occur during vestibular compensation and are necessary to maintain the state of compensation. However, several questions remain open. The pharmacological findings indicate that the compensated state results in an asymmetrical distribution of the number and/or efficacy of cholinergic synapses. This does not follow from the assumptions of Dieringer and Precht. The Bechterew phenomenon remains a serious obstacle in attempts to explain compensation as a reorganization of the vestibular complex, which must be postulated for other reasons. This phenomenon cannot be accounted for sufficiently by the assumption that the deafferented neurons come under the control of the intact labyrinth, for it indicates that the activity persisting on the first deafferented side after the second labyrinthectomy is not mediated by the intact side.

3.2 Supersensitivity

It has therefore been proposed that two or perhaps more possible mechanisms exist and that certain nonsynaptic processes, e.g., deafferentation supersensitivity, must be additionally taken into account.

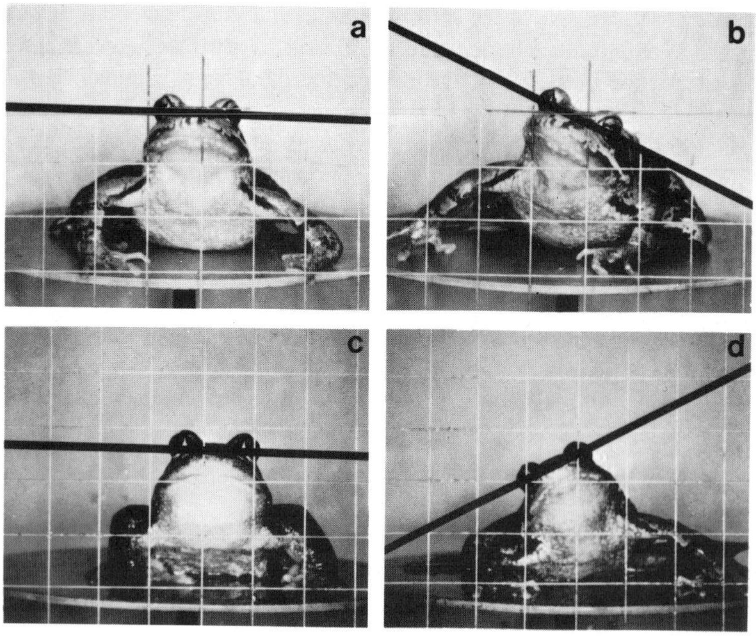

Fig. 6a–d. Bechterew phenomenon in the frog. **a** Normal head position; **b** head deviation after the first labyrinthectomy (left side); **c** compensated state (100 days after first labyrinthectomy); **d** effect of the second labyrinthectomy; head deviation to the second side

3.2.1 The Bechterew Phenomenon

Bechterew phenomena follow the removal of the remaining labyrinth after partial or complete compensation for the deficits of the first lesion. The second lesion causes symptoms that are a mirror image of those observed after the first labyrinthectomy. Figure 6 shows this effect for head deviation in the frog. Quantitatively, the effect develops slowly and depends on the time interval between the first and second labyrinthectomy (Fig. 7). This shows that the resting activity generated during the compensation process in the deafferented nucleus is, at least, in part, independent of the remaining labyrinth. The source of this activity has not been identified. As mentioned above, it develops even if the ipsilateral vestibular nucleus is separated from a number of CNS structures (such as the cerebellum and the cerebral cortex) and, once existing, cannot be abolished by the destruction of various structures, including the contralateral nucleus. However, this activity disappears with time, which is sometimes interpreted as a second compensatory process. Figure 8 shows the time course of this development for the head tilt in *Rana temporaria*, observed for different time intervals between the first and the second labyrinthectomy (Fig. 8, 1–4). As can be seen from the range of variation of the head deviation measured during the second compensation, the gain of the second compensation process depends on the degree of the first compensation (Fig. 8, 2–4). Following simultaneous bilateral labyrinthectomy no compensation takes place. The second compensation is insofar another example for the so-

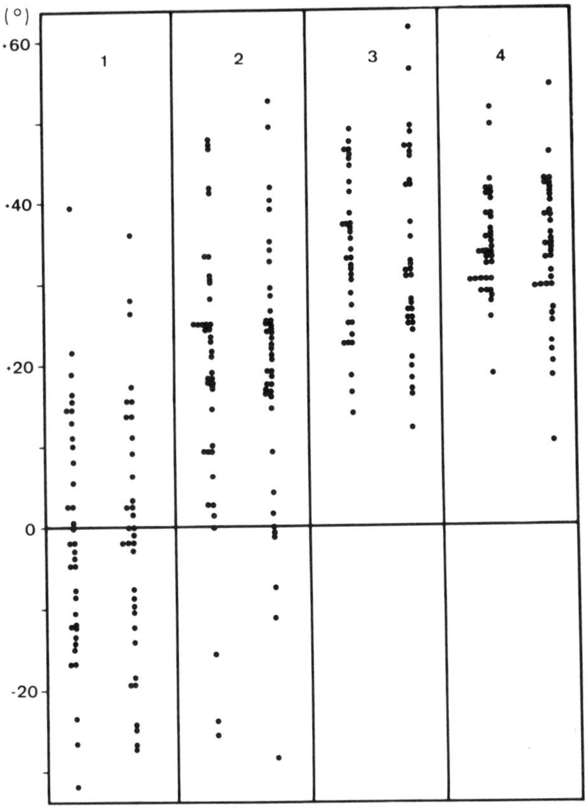

Fig. 7. Dependence of the Bechterew phenomenon on the degree of compensation for the first labyrinthectomy in the frog. The second labyrinthectomy was performed immediately after the first (*box 1*), after 50% (*box 2*), 75% (*box 3*), and 100% (*box 4*) compensation of head tilt. Measurements of the head deviation were performed 1 h (*left vertical row in each box*) and 24 h (*right vertical row*) after the second labyrinthectomy. Positive values indicate a deviation towards the side of the second labyrinthectomy

called serial lesion phenomenon, which means that sequential lesions can be more easily and thoroughly compensated for than one-stage lesions of the same extent.

Usually the Bechterew phenomenon is explained as a persistence of that resting activity which has been built up in the deafferented nucleus to counterbalance the contralateral activity. With this assumption as background, many observations remain enigmatic. For instance, it then remains to be explained why de-compensation can occur after various operative or pharmacological interventions.

However, the above mentioned interpretation is neither necessary nor proven. The Bechterew phenomenon shows that a dominance of the first deafferented side remains following deafferentation of the second nucleus, which is sufficient to elicit the symptoms. But this does not mean that the activity so shown is quantitatively the same as that which is responsible for the balance in the compensated state.

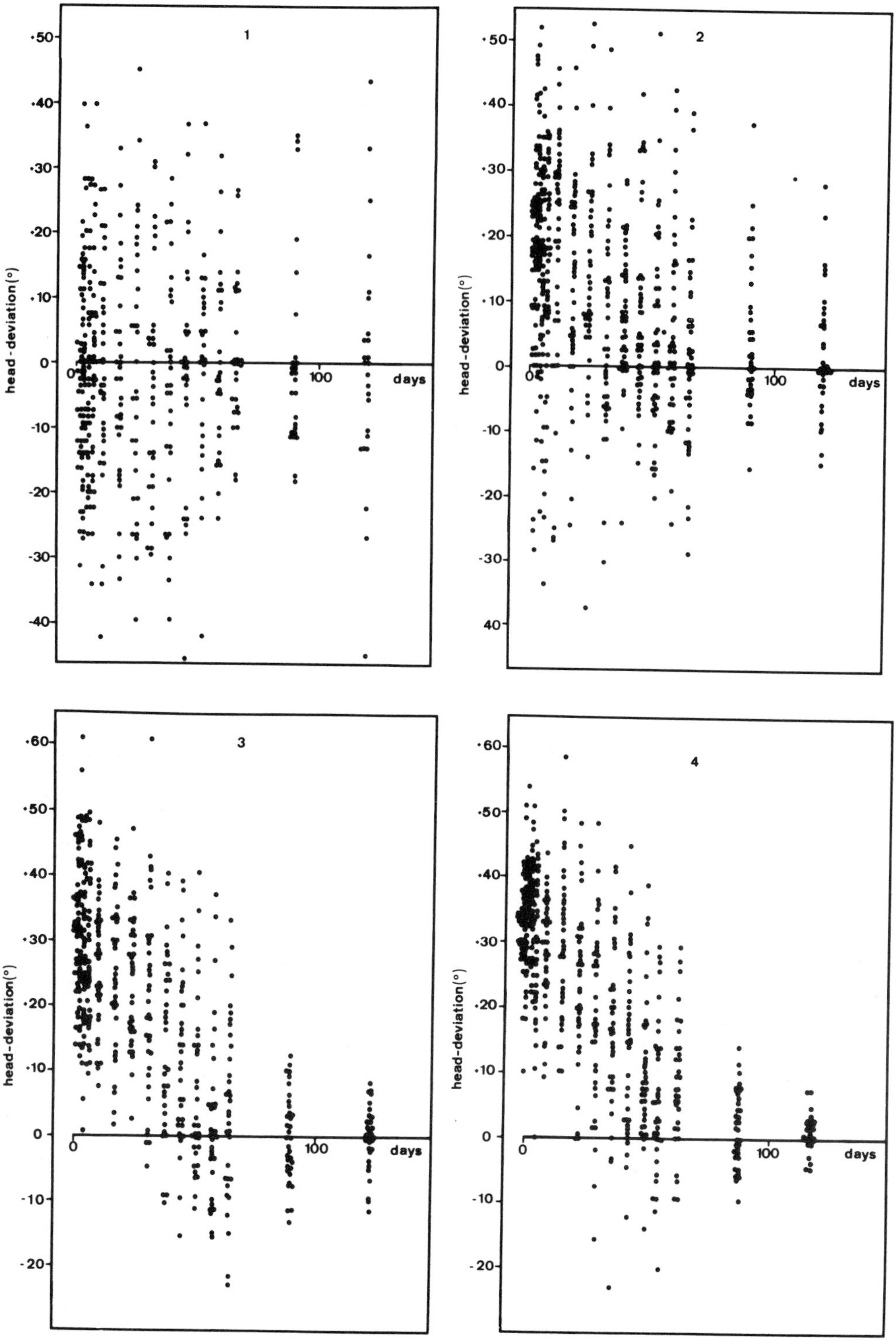

Fig. 8

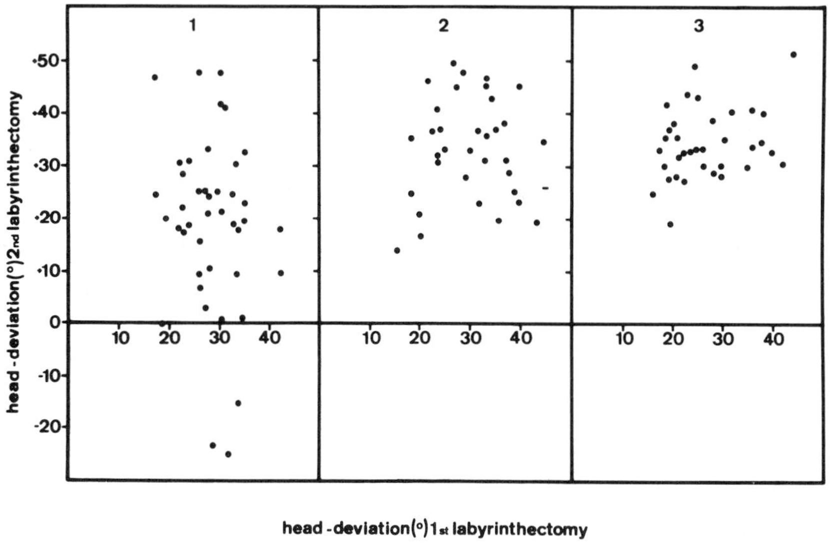

Fig. 9. Head deviation measured immediately after first (*abscissa*) and second (*ordinate*) labyrinthectomy in frogs. The second labyrinthectomy was performed after 50% (*box 1*), 75% (*box 2*), and 100% (*box 3*) compensation for the symptoms following the first ectomy

In fact, it can be shown that the amount of activity indicated by the Bechterew phenomenon cannot quantitatively account for the degree of recovery in different compensation stages. Figure 9, 1–3 shows the degree of head deviation observed in frogs following the first (*abscissa*) and the second (*ordinate*) labyrinthectomy. Labyrinthectomy was perfomed after 50, 75, and 100% of compensation for the first lesion. There is no correlation between the degrees of head tilt in either condition. The equilibrium attained in these compensation stages is therefore not a result of the persisting activity that underlies the Bechterew effect.

An attempt to analyze this situation by means of the deoxyglucose technique is shown in Fig. 10. The tracer was given after full compensation for the first labyrinthectomy and a fully developed Bechterew effect was present following the destruction of the second end organ. In both nuclei there is a severe reduction in activity with only a slightly higher activity on the side of the first labyrinthectomy. The activity on the side of the first lesion is considerably lower than that observed in compensated states with the contralateral labyrinth intact. With chronic animals, in which the Bechterew effect has disappeared, the activity of both sides, as shown by deoxyglucose, remains low (Fig. 11).

Fig. 8. "Compensation" for the Bechterew effect following bilateral labyrinthectomy in the frog. The second labyrinthectomy was performed at different time intervals following the first labyrinthectomy. *Panel 1:* simultaneous bilateral labyrinthectomy, *panels 2, 3, 4:* second labyrinthectomy performed after 50%, 75%, and 100% compensation for head deviation following the first labyrinthectomy

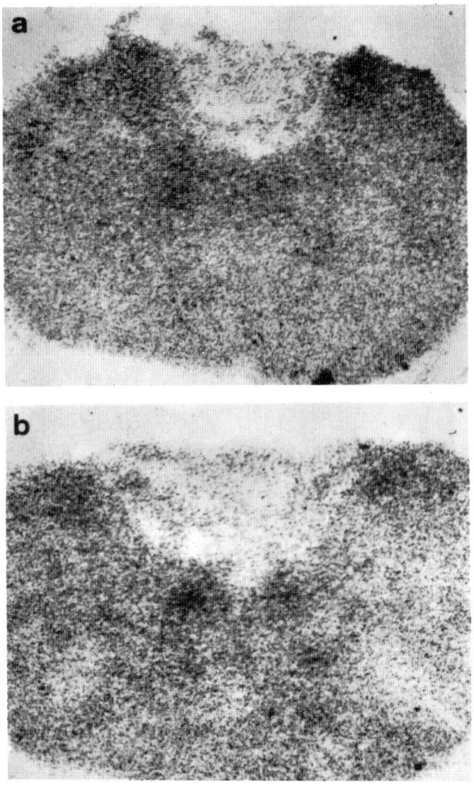

Fig. 10

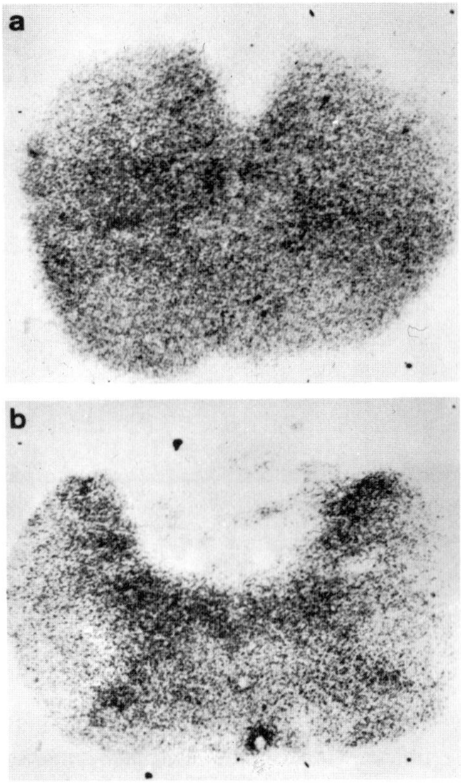

Fig. 11

Fig. 10a, b. Deoxyglucose uptake in the frog brain stem after bilateral labyrinthectomy. The autoradiographs show the DG uptake 24 h after the second labyrinthectomy. First labyrinthectomy was performed on the right side, the second on the left side after full compensation had been achieved. A pronounced Bechterew effect was present. Note the decrease of activity in both vestibular nuclei

Fig. 11a, b. Deoxyglucose uptake of the frog brain stem after bilateral labyrinthectomy. The autoradiographs show the DG uptake 120 days after the second labyrinthectomy. First labyrinthectomy right side, second labyrinthectomy left side in a fully compensated state. At the time of DG administration no consistent head deviation to any side was present

A possible explanation is that the Bechterew phenomenon is elicited by *some sort* of supersensitivity in the deafferented nucleus, which brings about asymmetrical effects of any afferents remaining after bilateral labyrinthectomy. This interpretation of the Bechterew phenomenon would settle many of the difficulties in finding a common denominator for all known observations, it would, e.g., provide an understanding of the decompensatory effects following a reduction of various afferents to the vestibular nucleus. It might also provide an explanation for all observed drug effects.

3.2.2 Denervation Supersensitivity

It has been suggested that denervation supersensitivity in many ways seems to be an ideal candidate for the cellular changes involved in lesion-induced recovery (Lynch et al. 1976). It was first observed by Cannon and Rosenblueth (1949) in the denervated muscle, and has subsequently been observed in various peripheral neurons (Kuffler et al. 1971). Its existence in the central nervous system is still a matter of controversy.

The pharmacological findings, mentioned above are, however, not in line with the assumption that a true denervation supersensitivity to ACh, i.e., an increase in transmitter-receptor sensitivity, develops on the deafferented side. This would lead to greater effects of agonists on the deafferented side and to a decreased response to antagonists on this side. The pharmacological results observed indicate the contrary.

In the "cortical slab" preparation, with which most of the experiments in this field have been carried out, it has been shown that an abnormal sensitivity towards acetylcholine develops, which is not a true supersensitivity but is only due to a reduced acetylcholinesterase activity. Surprisingly, the simple analog assumption, namely that cholinesterase activity is reduced on the deafferented side, leads to a hypothesis which is consistent with most known experimental data. It might explain the decompensatory effects of cholinesterase inhibitors and cholinomimetics. Offered in the same concentration to both sides, they would be more effective on the intact side, where, due to normal acetylcholinesterase activity, relatively low synaptic acetylcholine concentrations exist. Cholinolytics would also be more effective on this side, so that the activity on the deafferented side could then prevail. Moreover, this hypothesis also provides an explanation for the importance of optic, somatosensory, cortical, and spinal afferents to maintain the compensated state and the Bechterew phenomenon, which would simply be an expression of that "supersensitivity". It could also explain an increased efficacy of crossed excitatory afferents. There is a certain discrepancy in the interpretation given by Dieringer and Precht (1977, 1979a,b) of the changes in EPSP parameters observed in chronically deafferented neurons. However, it remains to be proven that these findings exclude the above assumptions.

4 Induction and Control of Plastic Changes

The currently discussed concepts about possible mechanisms for vestibular compensation and for behavioral plasticity in general are unsatisfactory for several reasons. There is no element in them that could explain the adaptive, teleonomic character of these processes. Compensation implies a reorganization of neuronal nets which aims at the elimination of functional deficits and the restitution of normal functions. Obviously, this goal can be reached under different conditions and by different strategies. The description of cellular changes and their localization does not explain how new meaningful neural circuits are established. It is highly improbable that the restitution of complex functional circuits underlying vestibular compensation is a direct consequence of the lesion, as is somehow suggested in discussing supersensitivity or collateral sprouting for instance. Compensation would then be an accidental event. The

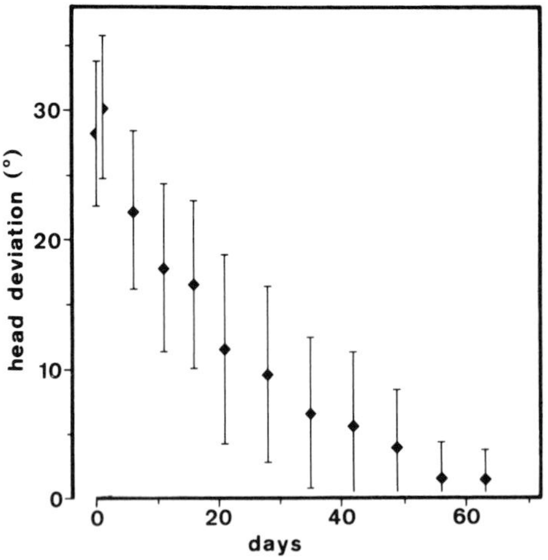

Fig. 12. Time course of compensation for head deviation in *Rana temporaria* following unilateral labyrinthectomy: head deviation was measured by a photographic technique. $n = 131$

changes so induced need not generally benefit the functioning of the organism. Rather their effect would be insignificant or even detrimental. In contrast to the above, it is reasonable to postulate that the elementary plastic modifications are selective and controlled changes. This means that neural nets, capable of recovery or learning, in addition to having components with intrinsic plastic properties also have mechanisms for regulating the initiation and maintenance of such changes. Such mechanisms would include a feedback of the system's output to the structure of the system. This would also include an apparatus for classifying error and producing factors which control the modifiable elements within neural nets.

Such considerations seem to play a minor role in the present day discussion of plasticity. However, many phenomena in vestibular compensation clearly suggest that these aspects are relevant:

1. The characteristic time course of the compensation process could be understood to be the result of an error-controlled process. Figure 12 shows the characteristic course for the symptom head deviation in the frog. Similar curves with other quantifiable criteria of compensation have been reported (e.g., Igarashi et al. 1970).

2. Drugs that induce reversible decompensation in a single injection accelerate the compensation process, if given chronically. Figure 13 shows the results of an experiment with frogs, in which E 600 was given intralymphatically in a dose of 1 mg/kg every fourth day. Each injection induces a brief, separate decompensation, i.e., it increases the system's error. The overall compensation velocity is considerably increased.

3. A chronic activation of the deficient system through an intensified error signal accelerates compensation. Figure 14 shows the result of an experiment in which the experimental animals were placed on an inclined plane, the angle of which was continuously varied during the compensation period. As can be seen, the velocity of the compensation process is significantly increased in comparison with that of a control group which underwent compensation on a fixed horizontal plane.

4. An experimentally manipulated, deceptive feedback signal on the system's error can influence the compensation velocity.

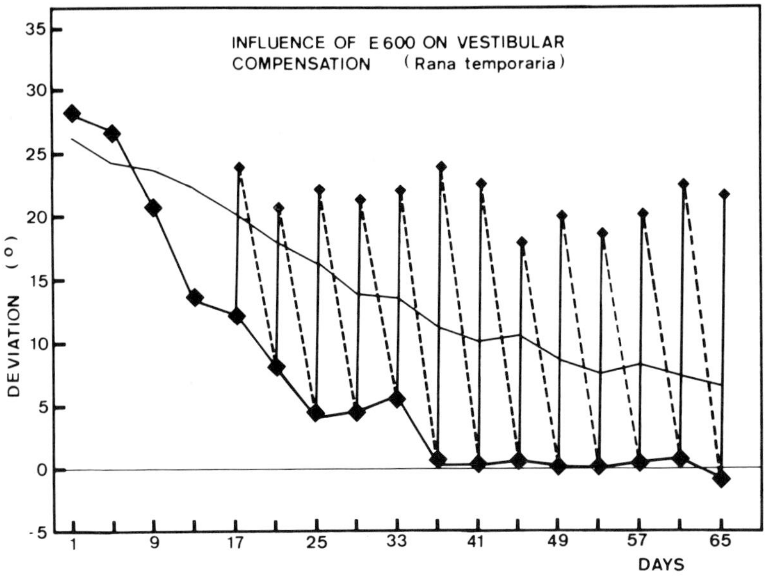

Fig. 13. Effect of chronic E 600 application on compensation velocity in *Rana temporaria.* E 600 (1 mg/kg) was given every fourth day intralymphatically. *Big squares:* head deviation before E 600 injection; *small squares:* head deviation immediately after E 600 injection (n = 20). *Solid line:* control group (n = 28)

The adequate stimulus for the macular hair cells is the tangential shearing force; upon displacement of the head the ciliary tufts are bent as a result of their attachment to the otolithic membrane. This induces positive or negative shifts in the receptor potentials. The shearing force resulting from head deviation is a function of two

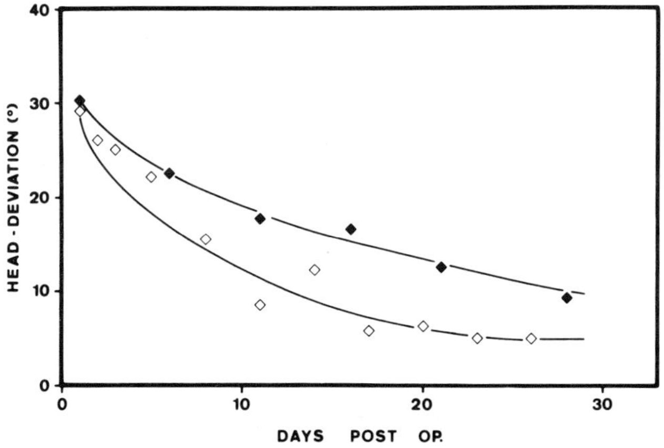

Fig. 14. Effect of chronic vestibular stimulation on compensation velocity (head deviation) in *Rana temporaria.* Following unilateral labyrinthectomy the animals were placed on an inclined plane, the angle of which was continously varied (*open squares; n* = 20). *Solid squares:* control group, compensation under normal conditions (n = 20)

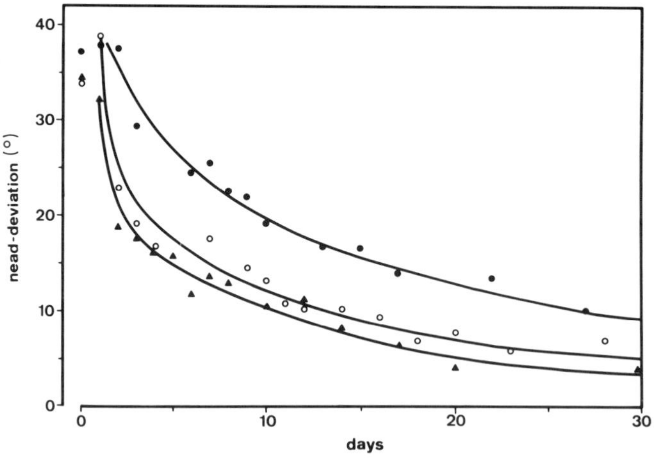

Fig. 15. Effect of increased *g* forces on the compensation velocity (head deviation). Group 1 (*dots*) was kept under normal conditions. ($n = 20$); group 2 (*open circles*) was exposed to 2 *g* for 8 h a day from the 1st to the 11th postoperative day; group 3 (*triangels*) was exposed to 4 *g* for 8 h a day from the 1st to the 8th postoperative day

parameters: the tilting angle and gravitational force. Increase or decrease of the gravitational forces at a given head deviation by centrifugation or zero-g-simulation falsifies the information on the system's error. Figure 15 shows the effects of increased *g* forces on head compensation in the frog. Centrifugation at 2 and 4 *g* was performed for 8 and 11 days, 8 h a day in the first phase of compensation. As can be seen, this causes a considerable acceleration of the compensation process. Similar results were reported by Schön (1950) with fish. Figure 16 shows the result of an attempt to simulate the effects of a zero-*g* situation. Immobilized frogs in dorsal position were exposed to 2 g for 23 h a day. This treatment diminishes or abolishes the actual shear force acting on the hair cells by pulling the otoliths away. As can be seen, this treatment, if started immediately after labyrinthectomy, prevents the onset of the compensation process as long as the treatment is continued. It stops the process and reverses the already attained compensation if started later.

It follows from these observations that the reorganization of the vestibular system is not determined by chance, but is the result of specific changes. The initiation, maintenance, and formation rate of the neuronal modifications responsible for compensation are error-dependent. The structure of the system is governed by the behavioral consequences it produces.

Doubtlessly, this is a key question in understanding plastic processes. At this point, however, the present concepts have significant deficits.

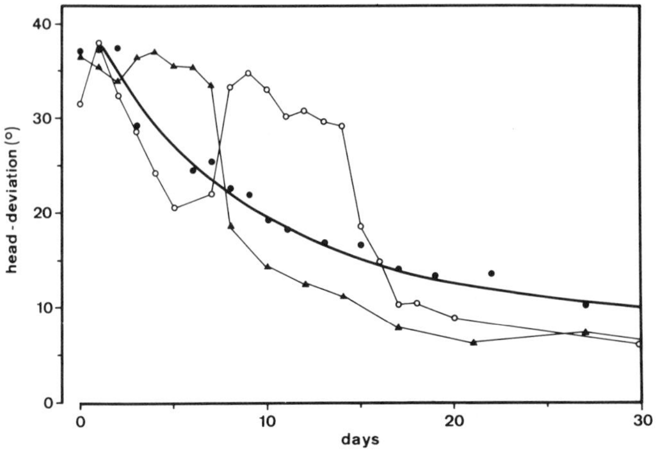

Fig. 16. Effect of 0-*g* simulation on the compensation velocity (head deviation) in *Rana temporaria*. Two groups of animals were exposed to 2 *g* in dorsal position for 23 h a day. Treatment was started immediately following labyrinthectomy and continued for 7 days (*triangles; n* = 20), and after partial compensation for the labyrinthectomy had been achieved (8th–14th day; *open circles; n* = 20). Following treatment the animals were kept under normal conditions. *Dots:* untreated control group (*n* = 20)

References

Azzena GB (1969) Role of the spinal cord in compensating the effects of hemilabyrinthectomy. Arch Ital Biol 107: 43–53

Azzena GB, Mameli O, Tolu E (1977) Vestibular units during decompensation. Experientia 33: 234–235

Bechterew W von (1883) Ergebnisse der Durchschneidung des N. acusticus, nebst Erörterung der Bedeutung der semicirculären Canäle für das Körpergleichgewicht. Pflügers Arch Ges Physiol 30: 312–347

Bienhold H, Flohr H (1978) Role of commissural connexions between vestibular nuclei in compensation following unilateral labyrinthectomy. J Physiol (London) 284: 178P

Bienhold H, Flohr H (1980) Role of cholinergic synapses in vestibular compensation. Brain Res 195: 476–478

Cannon WB, Rosenblueth A (1949) The supersensitivity of denervated structures. McMillan, New York

Carpenter MB, Fabrega H, Glinsman W (1959) Physiological deficits occurring with lesions of labyrinth and fastigial nuclei. J Neurophysiol 22: 222–234

Courjon JH, Jeannerod M, Ossuzio I, Schmidt R (1977) Role of vision in compensation of vestibulo-ocular reflex after hemilabyrinthectomy in the cat. Exp Brain Res 28: 235–248

Dal Ri H, Schaefer K-P (1957) Beeinflussung des Nystagmus durch Stell- und Haltereflexe am nichtfixierten Meerschweinchen. Pflügers Arch Ges Physiol 265: 125–137

Dieringer N, Precht W (1977) Modification of synaptic input following unilateral labyrinthectomy. Nature (London) 269: 431–433

Dieringer N, Precht W (1979a) Mechanism of compensation for vestibular deficits in the frog. I. Modification of the excitatory commissural system. Exp Brain Res 36: 311–328

Dieringer N, Precht W (1979b) Mechanism of compensation for vestibular deficits in the frog. II. Modification of the inhibitory pathways. Exp Brain Res 36: 329–341

Di Giorgio AM (1939) Effetti di lesioni unilaterali della corteccia cerebrale sui fenomeni di compenso da hemislabirintazione. Atti Accad Fisiol Fac Med Siena Ser XI 2: 382–384
Ewald JR (1892) Physiologische Untersuchungen über das Endorgan des N. octavus. Bergmann, Wiesbaden
Gernandt BE, Thulin CA (1952) Vestibular connections of the brain stem. Am J Physiol 171: 121–127
Giretti ML (1971) Spinal compensation of the cerebral release phenomena. Exp Neurol 30: 459–466
Igarashi M, Watanabe T, Maxian PM (1970) Dynamic equilibrium in squirrel monkeys after unilateral and bilateral labyrinthectomy. Acta Oto-Laryngol 69: 247–253
Jensen DW (1977) Vestibular compensation: Influence of spinal cord on spontaneous activity of vestibular nuclei. Soc Neurosci Abstr 3: 543
Kolb E (1955) Untersuchungen über zentrale Kompensation und Kompensationsbewegungen einseitig entstateter Frösche. Z Vergl Physiol 37: 136–160
Korte GE, Friedrich VL (1979) The fine structure of the feline superior vestibular nucleus: identification and synaptology of the primary vestibular afferents. Brain Res 176: 3–32
Kuffler SW, Dennis MJ, Harris AS (1971) The development of chemosensitivity in extrasynaptic areas of the neuronal surface after denervation of parasympathetic ganglion cells in the heart of the frog. Proc R Soc London Ser B 177: 555–563
Lashley K (1950) In search of the engram. Symp Soc Biol 4: 454–482
Llinás R, Walton K (1979) Place of the cerebellum in motor learning. In: Brazier MAB (ed) Brain mechanisms in memory and learning: from the single neuron to man. Raven Press, New York, p 17
Llinás R, Walton K, Hillmann DE (1975) Inferior olive: its role in motor learning. Science 190: 1230–1231
Lynch GS, Smith RL, Cotman CW (1976) Recovery of function following brain damage: a consideration of some neural mechanisms. In: Buerger AA, Tobis JS (eds) Neurophysiologic aspects of rehabiliation medicine. Thomas, Springfield Illinois, p 280
Magnus R (1924) Körperstellung. Springer, Berlin
McCabe BF, Ryu JH (1969) Experiments on vestibular compensation. Laryngoscope 79: 1728–1736
Menzio P (1949) Rapporti fra la corteccia cerebrale ed i fenomeni di hemislabirintazione. Arch Fisiol 49: 97–104
Precht W, Shimazu H, Markham CH (1966) A mechanism of central compensation of vestibular function following hemilabyrinthectomy. J Neurophysiol 29: 996–1010
Putkonen PTS, Courjon JH, Jeannerod M (1977) Compensation of postural effects of hemilabyrinthectomy in the cat. A sensory substitution process? Exp Brain Res 28: 249–257
Reiffenstein RJ, Triggle C (1972) Sensitivity of denervated cerebral cortex to cholinomimetics. Electroencephalogr. Clin Neurophysiol 33: 215–220
Schaefer K-P, Meyer DL (1973) Compensatory mechanisms following labyrinth lesions in guinea-pigs. A simple model of learning. In: Zippel HP (ed) Memory and transfer of information. Plenum Press, New York London, p 203
Schaefer K-P, Meyer DL (1974) Compensation of vestibular lesions. In: Kornhuber HH (ed) Handbook of sensory physiology, vol VI/2. Springer, Berlin Heidelberg New York, p 463
Schön L (1950) Quantitative Untersuchungen über die zentrale Kompensation nach einseitiger Utriculusausschaltung bei Fischen. Z Vergl Physiol 39: 399–417
Shimazu H, Precht W (1966) Inhibition of central vestibular neurons from the contralateral labyrinth and its mediating pathway. J Neurophysiol 29: 467–492
Sokoloff L, Reivich M, Kennedy C, des Rosiers MH, Patlak CS, Pettigrew KD, Sakurada O, Shinohara M (1977) The ^{14}C-Deoxyglucose method for the measurement of local cerebral glucose utilization: Theory, procedure and normal values in the conscious and anesthetized albino rat. J Neurochem 28: 897–916
Spiegel EA, Démétriades TD (1925) Die zentrale Kompensation des Labyrinthverlustes. Pflügers Arch Ges Physiol 210: 215–222
Trincker D (1965) Physiologie des Gleichgewichtsorgans. In: Berendes J, Link R, Zöllner F (eds) Hals-Nasen-Ohren-Heilkunde, vol III/1. Thieme, Stuttgart, p 311

An Ontogenetic Approach to Vestibular Compensation Mechanisms

E. HORN[1]

Unilateral labyrinthectomy has often been performed to analyze the structure and function of the vestibular system by neuroanatomical and physiological methods. Anatomical investigations by means of axon degeneration techniques indicate the location of synapses in the vestibular-spinal and vestibular-ocular reflex arcs. Behavioral methods may be used to determine the formation and maturation of bilateral interactions.

During ontogeny the neural network undergoes many differentiation processes. Recently, Hughes (1976) has reviewed the structural changes of the frog's CNS during metamorphosis. Structural changes during the development of the CNS indicate very high plasticity properties of the network in young animals, which may cause different time courses in the differentiation and maturation of various sensory pathways or reflex arcs. The technique of hemilabyrinthectomy and observation of the subsequent compensation for the defects induced by this operation throw some light on the amount of plasticity and stability of the developing neural structures which are part of the vestibular influenced reflex arcs.

Anurans are suitable animal species to investigate these problems using behavioral methods. Because their larvae are free-swimming, behavioral reactions such as body posture, leg and eye reflexes, or even swimming can be quantitatively measured at developmental stages in which their labyrinths are less differentiated. We[2] use *Xenopus laevis,* the South-African clawed toad, for our experiments, because its development is described in detail by means of morphological characteristics (Nieuwkoop and Faber 1975). There are 66 developmental stages distinguishable. The first free-swimming larvae are called stage 36; 46 is characterized by the initial growth of the hind limbs, stage 48 by that of the fore limbs, which appear at these stages as very small buds. At stage 54 all five toes and all four fingers are discernible; stage 58 is characterized by the fact that the fore limbs break through the body wall and the tip of the tail begins to shrink. At stage 61 the head becomes narrower and the tail shorter; at stage 63 it is only a small triangle, no longer visible from the ventral side (Fig. 1).

Unilateral labyrinthectomy causes the same defects as it does in other vertebrates. When swimming, clawed toads and their tadpoles rotate around their longitudinal axis

---

1 Zoologisches Institut II der Universität, Kaiserstraße 12, 7500 Karlsruhe, FRG

2 The investigations were performed in cooperation with B. Rayer and E. Cagol

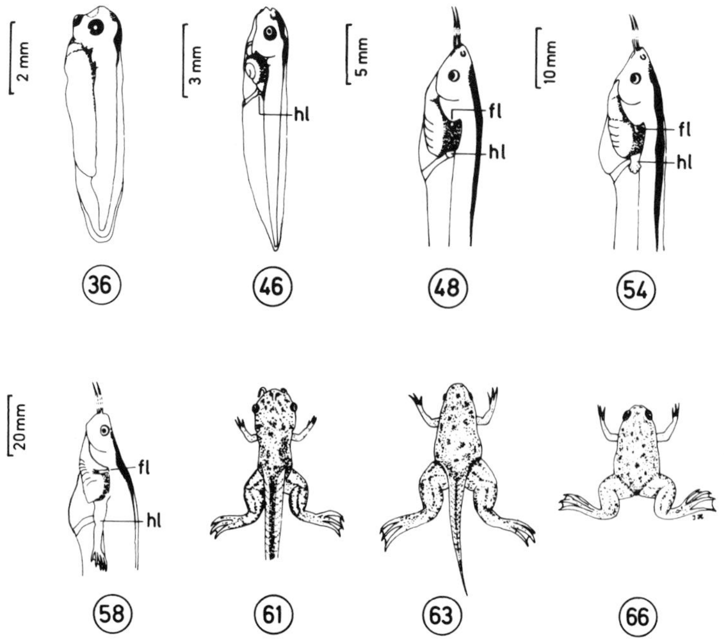

Fig. 1. Some characteristic developmental stages of *Xenopus laevis* which show the typical development of the hind limbs (*hl*), forelimbs (*fl*) and the tail. (After Nieuwkoop and Faber 1975)

after this operation. The eye on the operated side of the body is tilted downwards, whereas the contralateral one is tilted upwards. The leg and the arm on the operated side are bent, whereas the limbs on the intact side of the body are stretched. Often the body is twisted around its longitudinal axis, especially in the hip area. In tadpoles, the tail is curved (Fig. 2).

1 Compensation or Rotatory Movements in Relation to Development

Horn and Rayer (1978) demonstrated that the compensation time t_c, defined by the number of days when 50% of the unilateral labyrinthectomized animals swim normally, depends on the developmental stage at which the operation was performed. The older the tadpoles are on the day of operation, the longer the compensation time is. Tadpoles operated at stage 38 to 46 swim normally 4 to 7 days later, whereas tadpoles operated at stages 60 to 66, and juvenile clawed toads, never swim normally; they even rotate around their longitudinal axis 1–2 years later (Fig. 3). Even light does not improve compensation in *Xenopus*. The visual input seems to influence only the general activity level of the brain, especially of the neural nuclei important in the control of body posture, on which different sensory pathways may converge (Horn 1980). Jahn (1960), for example, pointed out that cutting the optic nerves in unilateral labyrinth-

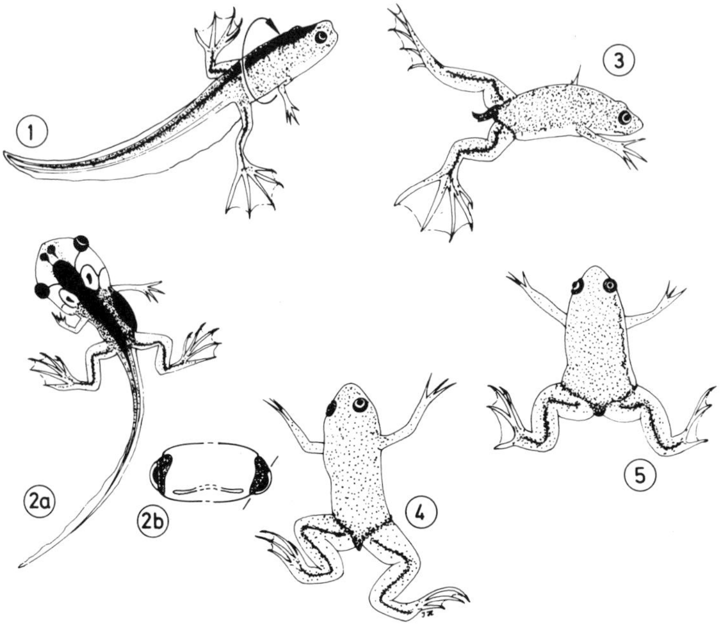

Fig. 2. Defects caused by unilateral (left-side) labyrinthectomy. Five types are distinguishable: rotations during swimming, mostly around the animal's longitudinal axis (*1*); a curved tail (*2a*); a torsion of the body, especially in the hip area (*3*); a flexion and extension of the limbs on the operated and intact body side, respectively; a downward tilt and an upward tilt of the eye on the operated and intact body side, respectively (*2a, 2b, 4, 5*). *Animals 1 to 4:* two weeks after the operation; *animal 5:* 6 months after the operation

ectomized amphibians causes an increase of compensation time, whereas covering the eyes has no significant effect.

The short compensation times up to stages 48/50 point to very great plasticity properties of their CNS. It has to be taken into consideration that the development from stage 38 to stage 46 lasts only 2 days and from 46 to 48 only 3 days. Therefore, the majority of these tadpoles compensate their movement defects before important structural changes in the CNS take place, such as the seperation and internal differentiation of the vestibular nuclei, the migration of Schwann cells into the brain, the myelinization, etc. These differentiation processes are characteristic of the vestibular nuclei of stage-48 tadpoles and older ones (Rayer, pers. comm.). These processes determine the capacities of neurons, but they also limit their plasticity properties. For example, a neuron builds up a dense net of dendrites during its development, but as its maturation proceeds many of these dendrites degenerate (Jacobson 1978). Therefore, the probability of contacting other neurons through dendro-dendritic synapses or axonal sprouting decreases.

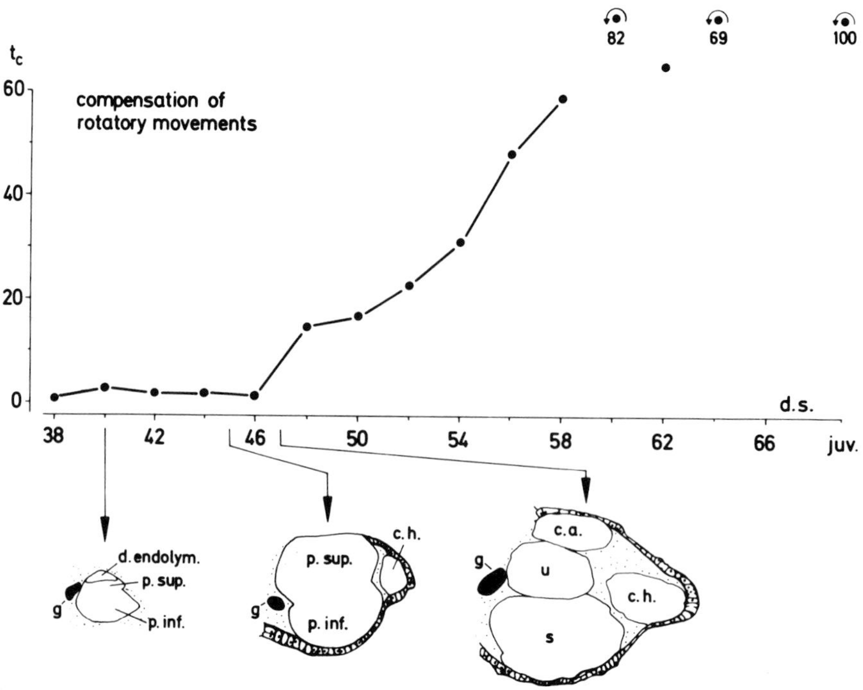

Fig. 3. The relationship between the compensation time (t_c), and the developmental stage (*d.s.*) at which the operation was performed. t_c is defined by the number of days when 50% of the unilateral labyrinthectomized animals swim normally. ↻ the *numbers* indicate the percentage of still rotating animals, 70 days after the operation. *Below the graph:* characteristic stages in the development of the labyrinth in *Xenopus laevis. c.a.*, canalis anterior; *c.h.*, canalis horzontalis; *d. endolymph.*, ductus endolymphaticus; *g* ganglion VIII; *p. inf.*, pars inferior; *p. sup.*, pars superior; *s*, sacculus; *u* utriculus

2 The Relationship Between the Compensation Time of Movement and Eye Position Defects

Systems with different neural networks may be characterized by different developmental times and plasticity properties. Magnus (1924) noticed very early that different defects induced by unilateral labyrinthectomy need different durations of time to be compensated. During the development of the clawed toad there is a short period during which the compensation of the asymmetrical eye positions is considerably retarded compared with that of the rotatory swimming movements. Tadpoles unilaterally labyrinthectomized at stages 48, 52, 56, and 60 were checked daily for movement compensation. Immediately after normal swimming behavior was restored, the angular position of both eyes was determined. The angular position of both eyes was symmetrical ($\Delta\mu = 0°$) in the groups operated at stages 48 and 60. In the other groups, however, there is still a significant asymmetry in the position of the eyes. This difference is independent of the stage at which the tadpoles show complete movement compensation (Fig. 4).

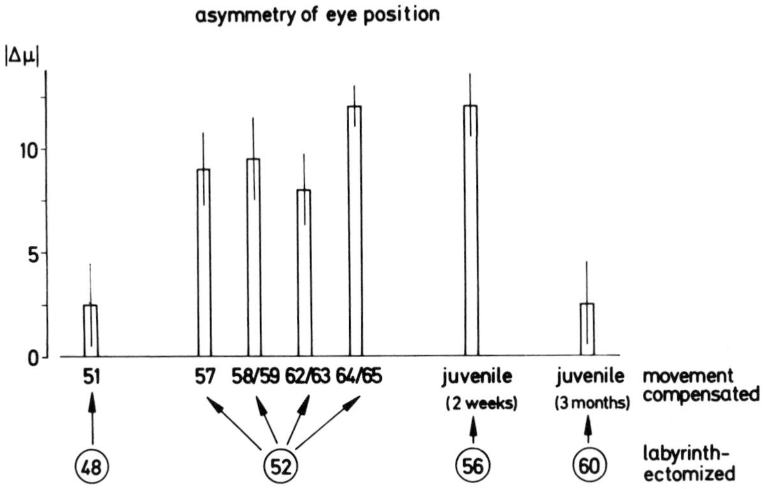

Fig. 4. The relationship between the compensation time of movement and the eye position defects. $|\Delta\mu|$, angular difference between the position of both eyes. *Bottom numbers* indicate the stages at which the left labyrinth was destroyed; *second row numbers* indicate the stages when the animals were movement-compensated

Supposing that the compensation takes place partially in the vestibular nuclei (Precht 1974), this result points to the existence of functionally different complexes within these nuclei of the clawed toad's brain, which were described for the frog's brain recently by Nieuwenhuys and Opdam (1976). On the other hand, it cannot be excluded that motor centers with different plasticity properties participate in this compensation process.

3 Consolidation and Stability of the Compensation Process

Using the method of sucessive labyrinthectomy, it is possible to determine the time between the operation and the initiation of the compensation mechanisms. This time is defined as the period between both operations if the second one induces the mirror-image of the symptoms following the first operation. Thauer and Peters (1935) demonstrated that the compensation started 5 min after the unilateral labyrinthectomy in frogs.

Using this method, the stability of the proceeding compensation can also be studied; especially in the older tadpoles and the metamorphosed animals, which never succeed in compensating for the defects, it must be clarified whether or not there is any compensation process. But although an objective observer never detects changes in the motor behavior, and the eye and body posture, successive bilateral labyrinthectomy proves the existence of a compensation process. So all the symptoms, like rotatory swimming, asymmetrical eye position, or posture of the extremities change their sign

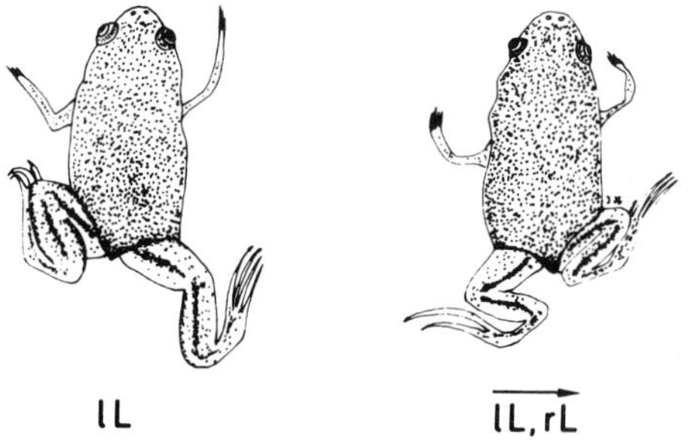

Fig. 5. Asymmetrical limb posture and eye position in a juvenile clawed toad 1 day before and 1 day after the second labyrinthectomy. *lL*, left labyrinth destroyed; $\overrightarrow{lL,rL}$, additionally, the right labyrinth destroyed

after the second operation; for example, the limbs bent after the first operation are now stretched (Fig. 5), and anticlockwise rotation becomes clockwise, etc.

After a time *T(d)*, these asymmmetrical behavioral reactions become indistinguishable from the behavior of animals simultaneously labryrinthectomized. A typical example is demonstrated in Fig. 6. But *T(d)* depends (1) on the period *I(d)* between the first and the second operation, and (2) on the developmental stage at which the first operation was performed (Table 1). In tadpoles, operated for the first time at stage 48, the asymmetries of the eye positions are significant until the 7th to 10th days inde-

Table 1. The stability of the compensation process derived from the time *T(d)* for which the asymmetrical angular position of the eyes caused by the second labyrinthectomy is still significant ($p \leqslant 0.01$). *I(d)* period between the dirst and second operation; – not determined

	First operation at stage			
I(d)	48	52	56	60
5	7	–	–	–
7	–	4	7	22
10	7	–	–	–
14	–	⩾31	22	22
15	10	–	–	–
20	7	–	–	–
21	–	22	48	31
28	–	⩾16	58	⩾42
35	–	25	19	–
42	–	16	⩾42	–

Fig. 6. The eye position μ on day before and 1 to 31 days after the second labyrinthectomy. First operation at stage 52. *lr* = *lL,rL*, simultaneously bilateral-labyrinthectomized tadpoles; *lr* = $\overrightarrow{lL,rL}$, successively bilateral-labyrinthectomized tadpoles. The periods between the leftside labyrinthectomy (*lL*) and the rightside one (*rL*) are 7 days (*upper plot*) and 14 days (*lower plot*). *int*, intact. The frequency distributions of the developmental stages are presented below each plot. *n*, number of experimental animals

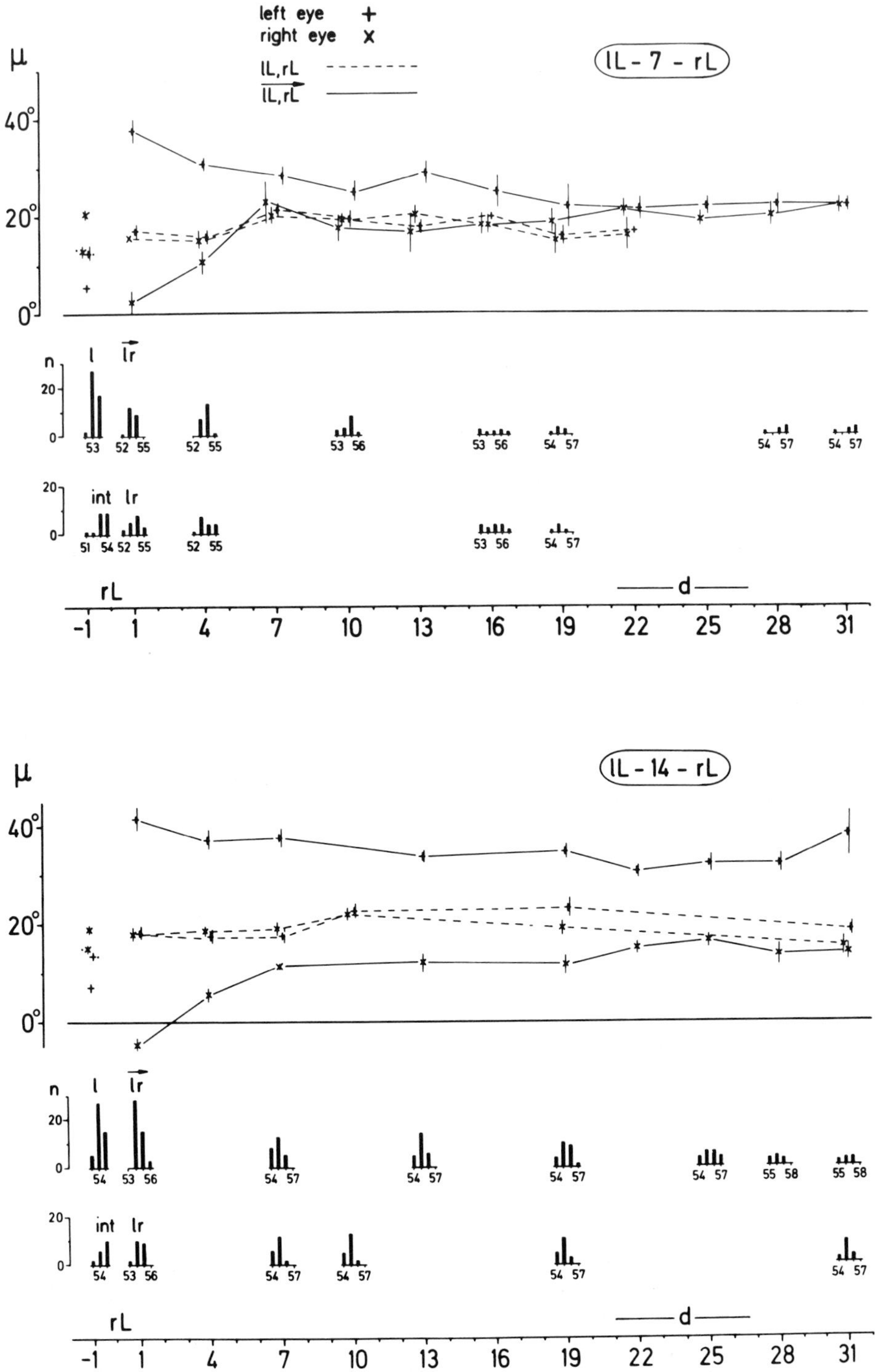
left eye +
right eye x
lL,rL
lL,rL
lL - 7 - rL
µ
40°
20°
0°
n
l
lr
20
0
53
52 55
52 55
53 56
53 56
54 57
54 57
54 57
20
int lr
0
51 54 52 55
52 55
53 56
54 57
rL
d
-1 1 4 7 10 13 16 19 22 25 28 31
lL - 14 - rL
µ
40°
20°
0°
n
l
lr
20
0
54
53 56
54 57
54 57
54 57
54 57
55 58
55 58
20
int lr
0
54
53 56
54 57
54 57
54 57
54 57
rL
d
-1 1 4 7 10 13 16 19 22 25 28 31

Fig. 6

pendent of the period *I(d)* between the first and the second operation. Similar values were obtained for tadpoles of the group L_{52}[3] and L_{56} which lost their asymmetrical eye positions 10 days after the second operation. In contrast, in the L_{60} group the asymmetrical eye position lasts at least 22 days, even if the period between the first and the second operation was only 7 days. *T(d)* increases dramatically in the L_{52}, L_{56}, and L_{60} groups if *I(d)* was longer than 14 days (Table 1; compare the upper and lower plot in Fig. 6). This means that, although the behavioral defects caused by the first unilateral labyrinthectomy are still present without any significant change for a long time, central compensation occurs and becomes remarkably stable. This is valid for the eye positions as well as for the swimming behavior. In the latter case, however, it is difficult to determine the course of temporal changes. Although all the animals eventually swim in an uncoordinated manner like simultaneously bilateral-labyrinthectomized tadpoles (alternating polling, pitching, and zig-zag movements), a typical intermediate type of swimming occurs; it is characterized by alternation of the swimming behavior of a unilateral and of bilateral labyrinthectomized animal. Therefore, a quantitative determination of the modification time is almost impossible (Fig. 7).

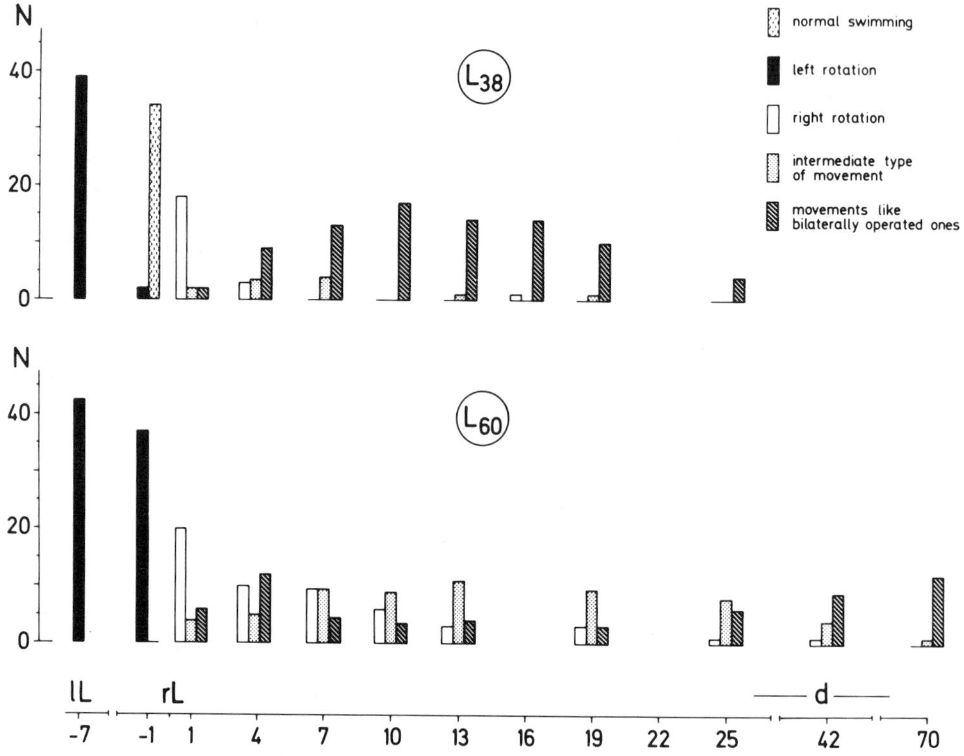

Fig. 7. Swimming behavior of tadpoles before and after the second labyrinthectomy. Period between both operations: 7 days. *lL*, left-side labyrinthectomy performed at stage 38 (L_{38}) and 60 (L_{60}); *rL*, right-side labyrinthectomy. *N*, number of experimental animals

3 L_i labyrinthectomized at stage *i*

The results point to a characteristic change in the plasticity of the CNS in *Xenopus laevis* in relation to the development. Besides the plasticity properties of the very young tadpoles (⩽ 48) mentioned above, there is another factor which influences the plasticity properties of tadpoles at stages 50 to 60. These plasticity properties may not depend only on the neuroanatomical and physiological changes during the period of differentiation of the neurons themselves but also on the possibility that the different vestibular pathways are differentiated independently at first. The older developmental stages (⩾ 60) increasingly lost these plasticity properties; their vestibular pathways became more rigid. Nevertheless, the high stability of the central compensation in older tadpoles (Table 1) demonstrates that they still possess considerable plasticity properties; but that might be due only to the rapid formation of new synapses through sprouting phenomena.

4 Endocrinological Aspects of Central Vestibular Compensation

The most interesting period in the life of a clawed toad with respect to the development of the vestibular pathways is the time between stages 48 and 60. There is not only a remarkable change in the efficiency of the vestibulo-ocular reflex arc (Lang and Horn 1980), but also the differences in the compensation between movement defects and asymmetrical eye position coincide with this period. As pointed out, the differences may be caused by the differentiation processes in the CNS. During development hormones, especially thyroxine, play an essential role in these differentiation processes. In anurans, for example, Mauthner cells increase their volume after thyroxine treatment (Pesetsky 1962), and the development of the cerebellar cortex is specifically influenced by this hormone (Graves 1977). Therefore, the plasticity properties of the vestibular pathways may be influenced by a hormonal component as well as by the vestibular component.

To separate the vestibular component from the hormonal one, hypophysectomized tadpoles were used in the experiments. Because it is generally accepted that this treatment causes extreme retardation in the development (Streb 1967), any compensation within the first 10 weeks following both operations may only be influenced by the vestibular system.

Tadpoles unilaterally labyrinthectomized at stage 54 were additionally hypophysectomized 1 day later. The first normal swimming behavior occurs 6 weeks after operations, whereas in the non-hypophysectomized group this happens 2 weeks after the labyrinthectomy. In contrast, the compensation of the movement defects in thyroxine treated tadpoles, which were labyrinthectomized at stage 54, is remarkably accelerated, especially during the first 2 weeks. This is even the case in older tadpoles (stage 58), but not in younger ones (stage 48). In the L_{48} control group, however, there is an increase in the frequency of rotatory movements, which is never observed in the thyroxine-treated L_{48} group. It may be important that this increase in rotatory movements corresponds with the beginning of the differentiation in the cerebellum (Nieuwkoop and Faber 1975; Fig. 8).

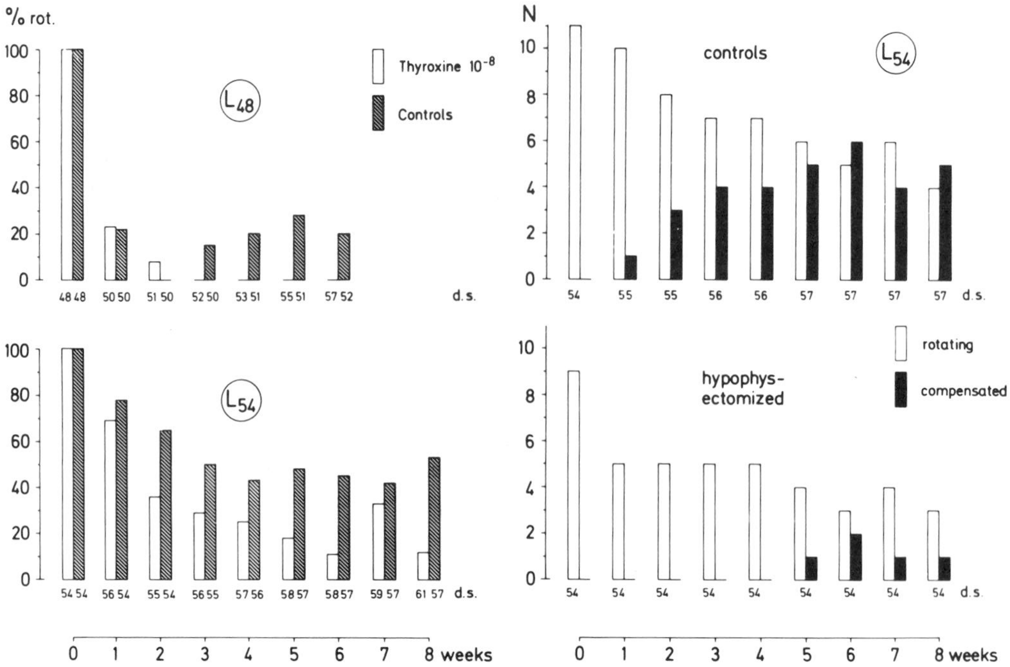

Fig. 8. The influence of thyroxine or hypophysectomy on the compensation of rotatory movements after unilateral labyrinthectomy in tadpoles operated at stage 48 (L_{48}) or 54 (L_{54}). Below each *column*, the developmental stages (*d.s.*) of the experimental animals are indicated. *% rot*, percentage of rotating tadpoles; *N*, number of tadpoles

5 Conclusions

These investigations are a first step in the analysis of central compensation following unilateral labyrinthectomy in *Xenopus laevis* in relation to development. The thyroxine and hypophysectomy experiments are in complete agreement with the suggestion that anatomical changes in the CNS, for instance an increase in the number of synapses through extension of the area of the axonal terminals (Goldberger and Murray 1978), are basic characteritics of stable compensation. Moreover, the plasticity of the CNS is much higher in young than in old tadpoles and in juveniles. It seems that the thyroxine level in the plasma of *Xenopus*, which increases from stage 48 to stages 58/59, and decreases rapidly after reaching the maximal concentration (Schultheiss, pers. comm.; comparable data are presented by Regard et al. 1977, for *Rana catesbeiana*), is important mainly during the stage when the vestibular pathways possess highest plasticity. Other hormones, which are involved in the development and modification of sensory pathways and behavior, may also influence the plasticity properties related to the central vestibular compensation. Prolactin as well as ACTH possibly play a role. It is known that after an injury of the somatomotor cortex or the spinal cord the regeneration of neurons is accelerated by ACTH, possibly through stimulation of protein synthesis (Fertig et al. 1971; McMasters 1962). On the other hand, ACTH modifies behavioral reactions by increasing the state of arousal. In anurans, this mechanism was proposed for the learning behavior in toads (Horn et al. 1979).

References

Fertig A, Kiernan JA, Seyan SSAS (1971) Enhancement of axonal regeneration in the brain of the rat by corticotrophin and triiodothyronine. Exp Neurol 33: 372–385

Goldberger ME, Murray M (1978) Recovery of movement and axonal sprouting may obey some of the same laws. In: Cotman CW (ed) Neuronal plasticity. Raven Press, New York, pp 73–96

Graves GD (1977) Thyroid hormones and brain development. Raven Press, New York

Horn E (1980) Multimodale Konvergenz – ein Verarbeitungsprinzip bei Sinnesleistungen. Naturwiss Rundsch 8: 309–324

Horn E, Rayer B (1978) Compensation of vestibular lesions in relation to development. Naturwissenschaften 65: 441

Horn E, Greiner B, Horn I (1979) The effect of ACTH on habituation of the turning reaction in the toad Bufo bufo L. J Comp Physiol 131: 129–135

Hughes A (1976) Metamorphic changes in the brain and spinal cord. In: Llinas R, Precht W (eds) Frog neurobiology. Springer, Berlin Heidelberg New York, pp 856–863

Jacobson M (1978) Developmental neurobiology. Plenum Press, New York London

Jahn T (1960) Optische Gleichgewichtsregelung und zentrale Kompensation bei Amphibien, insbesondere bei der Erdkröte (Bufo bufo L.). Z Vergl Physiol 43: 119–140

Lang H-G, Horn E (1980) The development of the static vestibulo-ocular reflex in Xenopus. Z. Naturforsch 35c: 1122–1123

Magnus R (1924) Körperstellung. Springer, Berlin

McMasters RE (1962) Regeneration of the spinal cord in the rat. Effects of Piromen and ACTH upon regenerative capacity. J Comp Neurol 119: 113–116

Nieuwenhuys R, Opdam P (1976) Structure of the brain. In: Llinas R, Precht W (eds) Frog neurobiology. Springer, Berlin Heidelberg New York, pp 811–855

Nieuwkoop PD, Faber J (1975) Normal table of Xenopus laevis (DAUDIN). Hubrecht Laboratory, Utrecht

Pesetsky J (1962) The thyroxine-stimulated enlargement of Mauthner's neuron in anurans. Gen Comp Endocrinol 2: 229–235

Precht W (1974) Characteristics of vestibular neurons after acute and chronic labyrinth destruction. In: Kornhuber HH (ed) Handbook of sensory physiology, vol VI/2. Springer, Berlin Heidelberg New York, pp 451–462

Regard E, Taurog A, Nagashima T (1977) Plasma thyroxine and triiodothyronine levels in spontaneously metamorphosing Rana catesbeiana tadpoles and in adult anuran amphibians. Endocrinology 102: 674–684

Streb M (1967) Experimentelle Untersuchungen über die Beziehung zwischen Schilddrüse und Hypophyse während der Larvalentwicklung und Metamorphose von Xenopus laevis DAUDIN. Z Zellforsch 82: 407–433

Thauer P, Peters G (1935) Der Einfluß operativer und pharmakologischer Eingriffe am Labyrinth auf Körperhaltung und Bewegung. Pflügers Arch Ges Physiol 235: 316–329

Functional Restitution of Static and Dynamic Reflexes in the Frog After Hemilabyrinthectomy

N. DIERINGER and W. PRECHT[1]

1 Introduction

Removal of the vestibular end organs on one side results in the degeneration of primary afferent vestibular fibers. Thereby, second order vestibular neurons become partially deafferented on the ipsilateral side. Reactions of these partially deafferented vestibular neurons, such as hypersensitivity to remaining synaptic inputs or reactive synaptogenesis of these intact afferents, may be involved in the recovery of static and dynamic postural reflexes that has been observed in many different species subsequent to the lesion (Schaefer and Meyer 1974). In either case, changes in the response properties of partially deafferented vestibular neurons to their remaining inputs arriving via the vestibular commissure, cerebellum, reticular formation, and spinal cord can be assumed to play an important role in the rebalancing of posture as well as in the recalibration of dynamic reflexes.

In the cat, central canal neurons are connected across the brainstem by a vestibular and a transcerebellar commissure that involves an inhibitory interneuron (Shimazu and Precht 1966; Furuya et al. 1976). After unilateral labyrinthectomy, the potency of this commissurally mediated inhibition increases on the side of the lesion (Precht et al. 1966). Thereby, the recovered resting rate of partially deafferented vestibular neurons is strongly modulated by inhibition and disinhibition. Functionally, these commissural pathways modulate partially deafferented vestibular neurons qualitively in a way similar to that of intact canal inputs.

With respect to the cat and other mammals, in the frog (*Rana temporaria*) several differences are found at the level of the brainstem as also in other parts of the nervous system:

1. Primary afferent vestibular fibers of the frog have about a ten times higher sensitivity (Blanks and Precht 1976) than those in cat or monkey.
2. The sensitivity of central vestibular neurons in frog, cat, and monkey is similar. Thus, in the frog the gain of vestibular inputs drops slightly between first and second order vestibular neurons (Dieringer and Precht, in prep.), whereas in cat and monkey the gain increases (see Precht 1979).

---

1 Max Planck Institut für Hirnforschung, Neurobiologische Abteilung, 6000 Frankfurt, FRG
Present address: Institut für Hirnforschung, August Forel Str. 1, 8029 Zürich, Schweiz

3. This reduction in gain may be related to the fact that commissural brainstem pathways connecting bilateral central vestibular neurons are weakly excitatory in the frog (Ozawa et al. 1974). Suppression of resting discharge or inhibitory postsynaptic potentials are very rarely observed after electrical stimulation of the contralateral eighth nerve (Dieringer and Precht 1979b).

With these differences in mind, one may ask: How does a frog recover from hemilabyrinthectomy? Does a weak inhibitory commissure increase its potency or is the deficient vestibular information substituted by inputs from other sensory organs? To study this problem we investigated the tonic and dynamic postural recovery of the vestibulo-collic reflex as well as the performance of single vestibular neurons in the frog. In the following a brief summary of the data will be given.

2 Recordings from Central Vestibular Neurons

To test the efficacy of axon terminals converging upon partially deafferented vestibular neurons on the lesioned side, technically the best controlled stimulus is an indirect activation of vestibular commissural fibers by means of electrical stimulation of the contralateral eighth nerve. The danger of current spread is thereby reduced and the stimulation intensity, expressed in multiples of threshold of the N_1 field potential recorded in the ipsilateral vestibular nucleus, allows a comparison of the results obtained in different animals. Comparing the results from control and chronically operated animals ($\geqslant$ 60 days), we found that the pattern of evoked activity in vestibular commissural fibers was very similar and that the efficacy of these excitatory commissural fibers was increased on the lesioned side in chronic frogs (Dieringer and Precht 1977, 1979a). In addition, in chronic frogs also the potency of inhibitory pathways was increased on the lesioned side. The onset of most of these inhibitions had a latency that was too long to be attributed to the vestibular commissure and was in part probably mediated via a transcerebellar route (Dieringer and Precht 1979b).

Preliminary experiments employing natural vestibular stimulation gave comparable results. Both in control and in chronically lesioned frogs about half of the central vestibular neurons responding to rotation in the horizontal plane are either spontaneously inactive or have a resting rate below 0.5 Hz (control: 10 out of 20; chronic: intact side 7 out of 18, and lesioned side 14 out of 28). The resting rates of the remaining 50% of neurons had a similar range (1–30 Hz) and similar mean values (control: 8.2 ± 6.5 Hz; chronic intact side 12.4 ± 9.7 Hz, and lesioned side 12.1 ± 9.1 Hz).

The most common responses to rotation in the horizontal plane in the bilateral vestibular nuclei of chronic frogs were a simultaneous increase in activity with rotation to the intact side, i.e., type I activation on the intact side, and type II activation on the lesioned side. So far no type II responses were found on the intact side. Neurons on the lesioned side exhibiting a type II response may have been in part true type II or former type III neurons as they exist in intact animals (about 22% and 12%, respectively). In part, type II responses could also have come from former type I neurons that lost their primary vestibular inputs and were now modulated by the excitatory vestibular commissure. One way to differentiate between these two possibilities would be to observe the responses of these neurons during optokinetic stimulation. Unfortunately, in the frog – unlike in many other vertebrates with an inhibitory vestibular commissure – optokinetic stimuli do not modulate the firing pattern of vestibular neurons (Dieringer and Precht, in prep.). Therefore, a distinction between these vestibular neurons responding in a type II fashion cannot be made on the basis of their response polarity to optokinetic stimuli.

So far in only one out of ten chronically lesioned animals have other than type II responses been recorded in the vestibular nucleus of the lesioned side. Three neurons were activated predominantly during rotation to the lesioned side (i.e., showed a type I response). With increasing levels of acceleration (0.25 Hz, amplitudes ± 10° to ± 20°) the response pattern changed from type I to type III. The type III activation was separated by a period of suppression.

The crossed excitatory output of vestibular neurons activates directly and indirectly extraocular and spinal motoneurons and induces thereby compensatory vestibulo-ocular (VOR) and vestibulo-collic reflexes (VCR). Chronic frogs with vestibular neurons responding only to rotation toward the intact side should have problems – at least in the dark – in producing compensatory eye or head movements directed toward the intact side. Either these dynamic reflexes do not recover, – or recover only in a fraction of animals from which we have not yet recorded, – or the presence of these reflexes in chronic frogs depends upon inputs other than vestibular, such as proprioceptive afferents which were blocked in our recording experiments due to immobilization.

To test these possibilities and to extend our definition of a compensated frog – which relied only on the recovery of static reflexes, i.e., posture of head and body – we began to study, in addition, the dynamic reflexes of intact and hemilabyrinthectomized frogs. To measure head and eye movements we used a magnetic field coil system, developed by Koch (1977). The frog, sitting in a plastic arena (10 cm in diameter), carried a test coil on his head (total weight 0.8–1.0 g) and was free to move. The arena was fixed to the center of a turntable. The turntable was surrounded by a white cylinder with a radius of 60 cm on which black and white vertical stripes (15° period) were projected and could be moved horizontally by a shadow projector. The position of table and shadow projector were recorded simultaneously with the changes in voltage output from the test coil on a chart recorder. Voltage changes from the test coil were later converted into changes of head and body position relative to the turntable.

3 Comparison for Deficits in Tonic Reflexes

Much is known about the acute effects of removal of a labyrinth or even of individual labyrinthine organs on the posture of head, forelimbs, and body owing to the work of McNally and Tait (1933), and Kolb (1955). As a result of the lesion, head and body (up to the pelvic girdle) are tilted mainly along the longitudinal axis toward the side of the lesion. Within the first day the head tilt remains unchanged and amounts to about 30°. Frogs with their eyes covered exhibit a very similar head deviation.

The position of the eyes (measured from single frames recorded by a video camera) is similarly rotated in the orbit, but the degree of deviation is about ten times smaller than that of the head. This relatively small change in eye position is related to the small ocular range of these animals (± 3° to 5°, depending on the size of the animal). No spontaneous eye nystagmus is observed, neither in the light nor in the dark.

In time, the deviation of head and body decreases exponentially ($\tau \approx 20^d$), as observed by Kolb (1955). Chronic frogs ($\geqslant 60^d$) may have a completely normal head position or still a slight deviation of about 5° toward the lesioned side. In about 30%–40% of these animals the head position is not yet very stable. Arousing acoustic or visual stimuli can provoke transient reappearance of acute symptoms.

The tilted head position of an acutely labyrinthectomized frog may be regarded as a new equilibrium that results from tonic reflexes which in part oppose each other. Due to the differences in the resting rates between the bilateral otolithic and semicircular canal inputs and the resulting central vestibular descending outputs the neck would continuously tend to tilt the head towards the lesioned side. Thereby an asymmetry in the reafferent proprioceptive inputs from the neck is induced, which counteracts the vestibularly commanded head torque. This view is supported by several observations:

1. Bilaterally labyrinthectomized frogs exhibit at rest – besides a decreased antigravity tone in their forelimb muscles – a normal head and body posture in the dark. Head and body posture is even normal after a transection of the brainstem at the level of the vagal nerve (Franzisket 1951). Thus, propriospinal networks alone can maintain a normal posture.
2. Tonic neck reflexes can strongly modulate optomotor and vestibulo-collic reflexes of intact frogs (Dieringer and Precht, in prep.).
3. In acutely lesioned animals the head drifts in the dark slowly back toward its lesion-induced new resting position as soon as the head is either tilted more to the side of the lesion or in a position like in an intact animal (see Fig. 1).

The recovered head position of chronic frogs may result from the recovered resting activity of partially deafferented neurons, which might be generated by other inputs still converging on vestibular neurons or by true spontaneous firing. Of these, visual and vestibular commussural inputs may not be as important as proprioceptive afferents for the following reasons:

Blindfolding of a chronic animal does not affect its normal head position, indicating that the recovered head position does not depend on visual information. The prolonged time course of recovery observed in compensating blind frogs (Kolb 1955) might also be explained by a locomotory inactivity, typical of blinded frogs. Removal of the second labyrinth results in a head deviation toward the newly operated side (Bechterew 1883), if the interval between the two operations is longer than 4 days. The amplitude of this new head deviation is in chronic frogs about 15%–20% smaller than that after the first operation and is explained by a lower activity in the vestibular nucleus on the side of the secondary lesion. Thus, the recovered resting activity of vestibular neurons on the side of the first lesion does not depend very strongly on activity mediated by the vestibular commissure.

4 Compensation for Deficits in Dynamic Reflexes

Dynamic reflexes were tested in the horizontal plane. They were evoked by optokinetic stimulation or by rotation of the animal in the dark (vestibular stimulation), or in front of a stationary contrast-rich visual background (combined stimulation). In intact frogs the evoked head movements are smooth and within a range of position changes of ± 10° to 15°, quick phases being very rare. The gain (amplitude of head movement divided by amplitude of drum or table movement) depends on the frequency as well as on the amplitude of stimulation (see Fig. 2C) and becomes position-dependent for lateral head deviations exceeding about 15° from the midline.

4.1 Vestibulo-Collic Responses

In acutely lesioned animals (3^d after labyrinthectomy, which was always performed on the right side), sinusoidal table rotation in the dark initially evokes only head movements directed toward the lesioned side (Fig. 1). The head moves laterally with the lesioned side tilted more downward. Responses can be evoked with accelerations as low as in intact animals (about $1.5°/s^2$), but with low accelerations ($\leqslant 10°/s^2$) responses may be completely or partially suppressed. With higher accelerations the gain of head movements directed to the lesioned side is always lower than in intact animals, and response amplitudes decrease from cycle to cycle with the head position being more and more deviated and tilted towards the lesioned side (Fig. 1). This decrease in amplitude is in part due to a fatigue in responsiveness, and in part due to an influence of the head position on the evoked vestibulo-collic response, as seen in Fig. 1. With the head tilted more towards the lesioned side, small responses directed toward the intact side can be observed (Fig. 1). These responses are similar in velocity to a slow drift (3°–4°/min), which is observed when stimulation is stopped (Fig. 1). This drift is also observed in intact animals in the dark, when their heads are bent by more than 10° laterally. In either case, it may last for 10 min and more until the head has reached its usual, lesion-induced position or, in the case of intact animals, until the head is bent 10 degrees or less to one side. In the lesioned animals this drift is opposite in direction to the vestibularly commanded head position and can be explained, as in intact animals, by the action of neck reflexes induced by proprioceptive inputs. With the head fixed to the table in the normal position, rotation in the dark does not activate neck muscles on the intact side. These muscles are activated, however, by optokinetic stimuli or during rotation in the light. Thus, the lack of vestibulo-collic reflexes of acute animals is not due to the lesion-induced head position and a corresponding misalignment of the semicircular canals on the intact side. Electromyographic activity is observed neither during the slow drift of the head, nor in animals with their head fixed and tilted into a position where this drift would be observed if the head were free to move. The head position, as well as the slow drift, may therefore be maintained by activity of the small-nerve motor system.

In chronically lesioned animals ($\geqslant 60^d$), rotation in the dark evokes responses of a rather variable gain. Some animals can suppress their responses rather strongly. In this case their responses are similar to those of acute animals, i.e., the responses are very

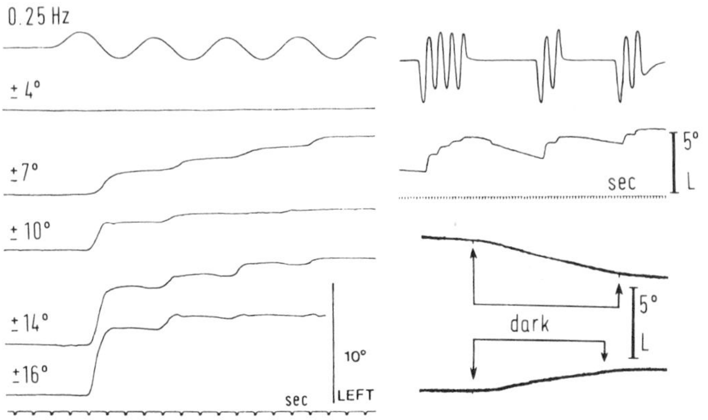

Fig. 1. Vestibulo-collic responses of acutely labyrinthectomized frogs (3^d; lesions on the right side) evoked by sinusoidal table rotation in the dark. *Left:* the table (*top trace*) rotated with amplitudes as indicated. Responses depend on acceleration and are directed toward the right (lesioned) side. Response amplitudes decrease from cycle to cycle. *Right:* At the end of table rotation (0.25 Hz, ± 16°), the head drifts slowly back. Amplitudes of responses depend in part on the head position. *Bottom:* The direction of the slow drift of the head position depends on the side to which the head is deviated. This drift is suppressed when the animal faces an illuminated patterned background

asymmetrical in amplitude (Fig. 2A). However, the same animal may very well also exhibit compensatory responses toward the intact side, even though small in amplitude. If the turntable starts to move first to the lesioned side, often a fast head movement towards the intact side is evoked. After this quick phase in the compensatory direction the animal may continue to exhibit slow compensatory movements of variable symmetry and/or amplitude (Fig. 2A). Head movements directed towards the intact side resemble a sequence of saccades which vary in amplitude and frequency. Typically, motion starts abruptly with a velocity that often remains constant during the later part of the half-cycle, except that it is interrupted by short pauses (Figs. 2A,B and 4A; see Sect 4.4). Thus, compensatory head movements in the dark, directed toward the intact side, do no longer appear sinusoidal in their velocity profile but linear, as if a a sudden tonic drive were turned on that moves the head toward the intact side, and which then decays at the end of the half-cycle. A similarly distorted wave form can also be observed in the eye movements of chronic animals (head fixed). In intact animals distortion occurs whenever the head is bent to one side by more than 10° and the head starts to move toward the midline. In order to evoke a response directed toward the intact side in chronic animals, typically accelerations of about 30° to 50°/s^2 are necessary. With velocity steps and constant accelerations and decelerations in the order of 50° to 100°/s^2, head movements toward the intact side are evoked in all of these animals, even though not in all instances.

In a smaller group of animals (about 25%), symmetrical responses were much more readily obtained (Fig. 2B). The threshold of activation was above 10°/s^2 (and thus higher than in intact animals, Fig. 2C). At higher accelerations responses during the first cycle were asymmetrical. The head thereby shifted more toward the intact side,

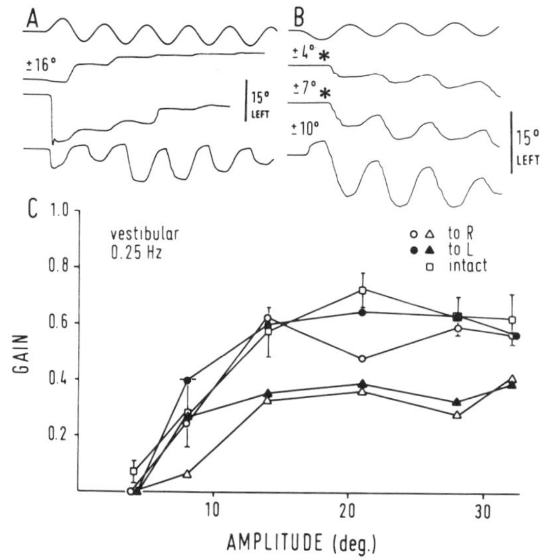

Fig. 2A–C. Compensatory head movements of chronic frogs (⩾ 60^d; lesions on the right side) evoked by sinusoidal table rotation in the dark. **A, B** Head movements from two chronic frogs with a different degree of recovery of their dynamic reflexes in response to table rotations (*top trace*, 0.25 Hz), with amplitudes as indicated. Note the high variability in the responses of animal **A**, the lack of initial responses towards the lesioned (*right*) side at lower stimulus amplitudes in animal **B** (*asterisk*) and the abrupt onset of responses directed toward the left side in **A** and **B**. **C** Comparison of gain values between intact and two well-compensated animals. Note the higher threshold of responses in chronic frogs, the asymmetry at lower and the symmetry at higher stimulus amplitudes. *Squares*, mean values and standard deviation from the means of four intact animals. *Circles* and *triangles*, mean values from two chronic animals

but was then moved to either side with a similar amplitude (Fig. 2B, C). Only at accelerations close to threshold continued an asymmetry in the response amplitude. However, here responses toward the intact side had a larger amplitude (Fig. 2B, C), contrary to the response characteristics of acutely lesioned (Fig. 1), or of the majority of chronically lesioned (Fig. 2A) frogs.

These differences in dynamic behavior in the dark could not always be predicted on the basis of the postural recovery of the animals. Static head position could be good and dynamic reflexes still be poor in the same animal. Recovery of dynamic reflexes started after about 10^d, and could have reached values similar to chronic animals after 30^d or 40^d, even though head posture was not yet fully compensated.

4.2 Responses Evoked by Optokinetic Stimulation

In intact animals, horizontal motion of vertical black and white stripes evokes smooth head movements in the same direction. The gain of these head movements decreases from 0.69 to 0.22 and the phase lag increases from 3.7° to 67° with higher stimulation frequencies (from 0.025 to 0.25 Hz; Dieringer and Precht 1979c). Responses to sinusoidal or constant velocity stimulation become asymmetrical in gain as soon as the head is bent to one side by more than 10°. In this case, the velocity of head movements is increased for movements directed toward the midline, and decreased for movements directed further away from the midline.

In acute animals, due to the lesion-induced head tilt, the evoked optomotor responses are asymmetrical in gain and occur in an oblique plane, i.e., during head movements directed toward the intact side, the head becomes increasingly less tilted in the roll axis and approaches the position exhibited by an intact animal. At the end of stimulation, in the dark the head drifts back to its lesion-induced position and in the light (in front of a patterned background) the head position is maintained (Fig. 1), indicating that visual fixation suppression is not severely affected by hemilabyrinthectomy. In acute animals, with their heads in such a "corrected" position, brief constant velocity stimulation evokes optomotor responses that are symmetrical in their velocity to either side and similar to those of intact animals. During sinusoidal stimulation the amplitudes of the head movements are asymmetrical at the onset of stimulation. After a few cycles they become symmetrical. Then the head oscillates around a position that is always shifted toward the intact side with respect to its resting position. Symmetrical responses may have phase and gain relationships that are very similar to those of intact animals.

In chronic animals, optomotor responses directed toward the intact side are interrupted by short-lasting pauses (Fig. 4B), as they also occur during pure vestibular stimulation and are described in Sect. 4.4. Otherwise, the amplitudes of these responses are quite symmetrical after the head position has shifted more to the intact side during the first few cycles. Their gain and phase relationships are either similar to those of intact animals or slightly improved at higher frequencies. Thus, optomotor responses of the frog's head are basically unimpaired by hemilabyrinthectomy and may be even improved at higher frequencies in chronic animals. Preliminary observations from bilaterally labyrinthectomized animals indicate similar results. As far as the optomotor responses of the frog's eyes are concerned, we have yet too few data to compare phase and gain values between intact and lesioned animals. However, it is clear that chronic animals have eye movements that are symmetrical in their amplitude to either side.

4.3 Responses Evoked by Combined Stimulation

In intact frogs, head movements evoked by rotation of the animal in front of a stationary, patterned background depend similarly on the acceleration as those evoked by rotating the animal in the dark (Fig. 2C). However, with higher accelerations the gain reaches a value of about 0.9 and the phase is shifted by 180° with respect to the table.

In acute frogs, responses are asymmetrical; the gain of head movements toward the intact side is initially larger than toward the lesioned side. Thereby the head position gradually shifts toward the intact side as is the case for optomotor responses. The gain of these responses to either side is much smaller than in intact animals and exceeds the gain of optomotor responses (about 0.3–0.4 at 0.25 Hz) only little.

In chronic animals, the gain of head movements evoked by rotation of the animal in the light can be predicted from the results obtained by rotation of the animal in the dark. Animals with compensatory head movements of small and variable amplitudes (Fig. 2A) have a gain of up to 0.5, which is about half of the gain of intact animals and which corresponds with the maximal gain of their optomotor responses. In these animals many short pauses in their head movements directed toward the intact side occur (Fig. 3I, see Sect. 4.4). Their low gain in response to rotation in the light indicates that these animals did not just suppress their vestibular reflexes during rotation in the dark, but that these reflexes are still deficient. Therefore, these animals can be considered as having poorly compensated for deficits in their dynamic reflex behavior, even though their posture may be as good as it is in other animals. Chronic frogs with a normal or only slightly reduced gain in the dark (Fig. 2B, C) exhibit compensatory head movements in the light, with gain and phase values very similar to those of intact animals.

4.4 Interactions Between Fast Eye and Slow Head Movements

In all lesioned frogs, from about 10 days on after the lesion, head movements directed toward the intact side are more or less frequently interrupted by short-lasting pauses (Figs. 2, 3 and 4). During these periods the activity of neck muscles on the intact side is suppressed and on the lesioned side no activation of the antagonistic muscles occurs (Fig. 3). Occasionally, fast eye movements can be observed to occur during these periods, observation is, however, difficult due to their small amplitudes (2°–5°) and the simultaneous table and head movements. With the head fixed to the turntable (and the radial and sciatic nerves cut bilaterally), similar pauses in the activity of neck muscles on the intact side are still observed, even though much less frequently. Recordings of eye movements show that, with each resetting quick phase, the activity in the neck muscles is suppressed (Fig. 3II). We therefore assume that the pauses in head movements and in neck electromyogram, observed in freely moving animals, are associated with resetting quick phases of the eyes.

The occurrence of these quick phases depends both in intact and in lesioned frogs on eye velocity, eye position, retinal image slip velocity, and other parameters, such as position of the head relative to the body. However, the number of evoked quick phases is typically very small. In chronic frogs, the occurrence of quick phases of the eyes is unilaterally facilitated. With the head fixed, in a chronic frog resetting quick phases are observed more often during rotation of the animal toward the lesioned side than toward the intact side. This basic asymmetry is also seen when the body is positioned to the one or the other side relative to the head fixed to the table (Fig. 3II). During such a static neck bias, more resetting quick phases are evoked during table rotation both in intact and in lesioned frogs.

In chronic frogs, these quick phases are not unilaterally facilitated due to retinal slip (they also occur in the dark), nor due to an extraocular proprioceptive feedback. Head pauses continue to occur after the cranial nerves III, IV, VI are cut bilaterally; and they develop in animals when these nerves were cut prior to hemilabyrinthectomy. After removal of the remaining labyrinth, animals continue to show pauses in head movements directed to the previously intact side for at least 4 days when tested with optokinetic stimulation (Fig. 4). Therefore, the unilateral facilitation may be due to an asymmetry in the effects exerted by proprioceptive spinal inputs (from neck, trunk, forelimbs), resulting in a change of "collico"-ocular reflexes, and of the threshold for resetting quick phases of the eyes. In bilaterally labyrinthectomized monkeys,

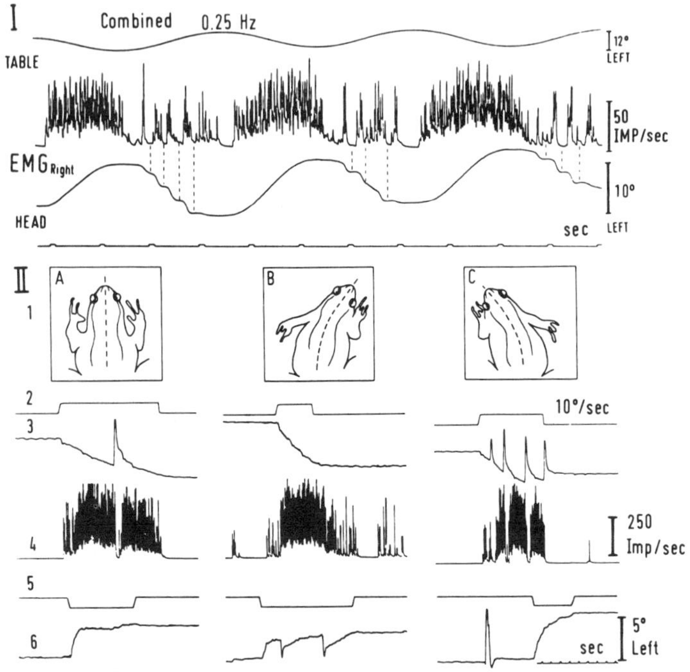

Fig. 3. Interaction between resetting quick phases of the eyes and slow compensatory head movements. **I** Head movements of a chronic frog directed to the left (intact) side are interrupted by short periods of reduced velocity. In the electromyogram of neck muscle activity, recorded monopolarly on the right side, activity originating on the left side is also picked up. Note the suppression of activity associated with periods of reduced head velocity. **II** with the head fixed to the table, combined constant velocity stimulation (10°/s in *2* to the right, in *5* to the left) evokes compensatory eye movements and few resetting quick phases (left eye in *3, 6*). The amplitude of slow eye movements and the number of quick phases depends on the position of the body relative to the fixed head (or, as shown here in **II** *1 A–C,* on the position of the head relative to the body). Note the suppression of activity in the simultaneously recorded electromyogram of a neck muscle on the left side (*4*) following the onset of an eye quick phase. In 6_C prior to the onset of stimulation a blink occurred

as well as in humans with absent labyrinthine function, a symmetrical increase in the gain of collico-ocular reflexes was observed (Dichgans et al. 1973; Kasai and Zee 1978).

5 Conclusions and Discussion

After hemilabyrinthectomy static deviation of head, trunk, limb, and eye positions of the frog is compensated within ca. 2–3 months. Contrary to optokinetically evoked head movements, vestibulo-collic reflexes are impaired by the lesion but gradually recover. The degree of recovery of static and dynamic reflexes is not necessarily correlated in each animal and may differ. This difference may be related to the different functional contributions of the two motor systems of the frog: The postural tone at rest is

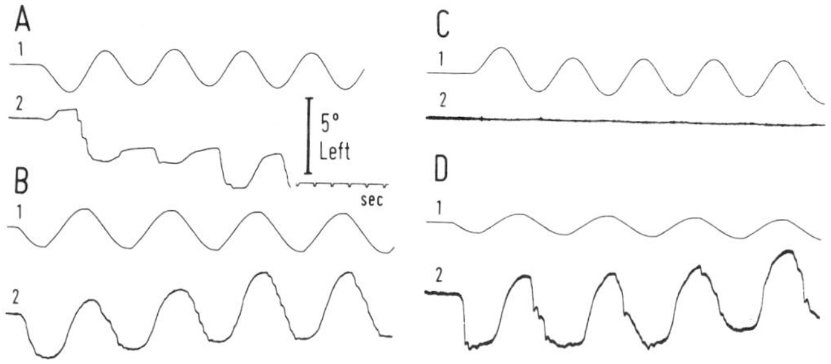

Fig. 4A–D. Responses of a chronic frog to vestibular and optokinetic stimulation before and 1 day after removal of the remaining (*left*) labyrinth. **A, C** Rotation of the body in the dark (0.25 Hz, ± 16°) evokes compensatory head movements (**A**) that are no longer present after removal of the second labyrinth (**C**). **B, D** Optomotor responses evoked by movements of a shadow projector (0.25 Hz, ± 16° in **B** and ± 8° in **D**). Leftward directed head movements are superimposed by short periods of reduced velocity that remain after removal of the second labyrinth (**D**). Traces *1* indicate the position of the table (**A, C**) or of the shadow projector (**B, D**), traces *2* the position of the head relative to the body

probably exclusively produced by the action of the small-nerve motor system, whereas for the generation of dynamic reflexes the twitch motor system has to be activated in addition (see Simpson 1976).

In intact frogs, vestibulo-collic reflexes evoked by sinusoidal rotation of the animal are influenced in amplitude and wave form by the position of the head relative to the body. This influence can be explained by an interaction between labyrinthine and proprioceptive inputs. Chronic frogs with a normal head position (lesioned on the right side) exhibit dynamic responses similar to intact animals that have their heads bent to the right side. The similarities include a slow drift in the dark at rest, an asymmetry in the response amplitude during the first few cycles of sinusoidal rotation, directional-dependent differences in the wave forms of head and eye movements, and a unilateral facilitation of resetting quick phases of the eyes.

In the chronic frog, these symptoms could be due to an asymmetry in the potency of proprioceptive inputs. The significance of these inputs for the compensation of deficits in static and dynamic spinal reflexes was already stressed by several investigators (Kolb 1955; Schaefer and Meyer 1973; Lacour et al. 1976; Jensen 1979a,b). The potency of ascending proprioceptive inputs projecting to partially deafferented vestibular neurons on the lesioned side could have increased with time, as suggested by Azzena et al. (1976) and Jensen (1979a,b), and could thereby substitute for part of the eliminated excitatory input at rest. During rotation of the animal in the dark toward the lesioned side, these inputs could, together with the silencing of most of the type I vestibular neurons on the intact side, participate in the initiation of a compensatory head movement directed toward the intact side. In this case, the discrepancy between the results of our behavioral study (in the dark, chronic animals can produce compensatory head movements directed toward the intact side), and the results of our single unit study (in chronic frogs only very few vestibular neurons on the lesioned side responded with a type I pattern), could be explained by the fact that in the latter study proprioceptive inputs were almost entirely abolished due to immobilization of the animals.

Acknowledgment. Supported by Deutsche Forschungsgemeinschaft (Pr. 158/2).

Note Added in Proof

Trabal et al. (1980) analysed the dynamics of the rightening reflex of the toad after hemilabyrinthectomy and came to a conclusion very similar to ours concerning the role of optokinetic, vestibular and proprioceptive inputs in compensation for the lesion-induced deficits.

Trabal I, Macadar O, Cibilis D, Pereda A (1980) Dynamic analysis of the rightening reflex in the toad; the effects of hemilabyrinthectomy. Neurosci Lett Suppl 5: 282

References

Azzena GB, Mameli O, Tolu E (1976) Vestibular nuclei of hemilabyrinthectomized guinea pigs during decompensation. Arch Ital Biol 114: 389–398

Bechterew W von (1883) Ergebnisse der Durchschneidung des N. acusticus nebst Erörterung der Bedeutung der semicirculären Kanäle für das Körpergleichgewicht. Pflügers Arch Ges Physiol 30: 312–347

Blanks RHI, Precht W (1976) Functional characterisation of primary vestibular afferents in the frog. Exp Brain Res 25: 369–390

Dichgans J, Bizzi E, Morasso P, Tagliasco W (1973) Mechanisms underlying recovery of eye-head coordination following bilateral labyrinthectomy in monkeys. Exp Brain Res 18: 548–562

Dieringer N, Precht W (1977) Modification of synaptic input following unilateral labyrinthectomy. Nature (London) 269: 431–433

Dieringer N, Precht W (1979a) Mechanisms of compensation for vestibular deficits in the frog. I. Modification of the excitatory commissural system. Exp Brain Res 36: 311–328

Dieringer N, Precht W (1979b) Mechanisms of compensation for vestibular deficits in the frog. II. Modification of the inhibitory pathways. Exp Brain Res 36: 329–341

Dieringer N, Precht W (1979c) Analysis of head movements in the frog during optokinetic, vestibular and combined optokinetic and vestibular stimulation. Neurosci Lett Suppl 3: 281

Franzisket L (1951) Gewohnheitsbildung und bedingte Reflexe bei Rückenmarksfröschen. Z Vergl Physiol 33: 142–178

Furuya N, Kawano K, Shimazu H (1976) Transcerebellar inhibitory interaction between the bilateral vestibular nuclei and its modulation by cerebellocortical activity. Exp Brain Res 25: 447–463

Jensen DW (1979a) Reflex control of acute postural asymmetry and compensatory symmetry after a unilateral vestibular lesion. Neuroscience 4: 1059–1073

Jensen DW (1979b) Vestibular compensation: tonic spinal influence upon spontaneous descending vestibular nuclear activity. Neuroscience 4: 1075–1084

Kasai T, Zee DB (1978) Eye-head coordination in labyrinthinedefective human beings. Brain Res 144: 123–141

Koch UT (1977) A miniature movement detector applied to recording of wingbeat in Locusta. Physiology of movement–Biomechanics. Fortschritte der Zoologie, vol 24. Fischer, Stuttgart p 327

Kolb E (1955) Untersuchungen über zentrale Kompensation und Kompensationsbewegungen einseitig entstateter Frösche. Z Vergl Physiol 37: 136–160

Lacour M, Roll JP, Appaix M (1976) Modifications and development of spinal reflexes in the alert baboon (Papio papio) following an unilateral vestibular neurotomy. Brain Res 113: 255–269

McNally WJ, Tait J (1933) Some results of section of particular nerve branches to the ampullae of the four vertical semicircular canals of the frog. Q J Exp Physiol 23: 147–196

Ozawa S, Precht W, Shimazu H (1974) Crossed effects on central vestibular neurons in the horizontal canal system of the frog. Exp Brain Res 19: 394–405

Precht W (1979) Labyrinthine influences on the vestibular nuclei. In: Granit R, Pompeiano O (eds) Progress in brain research, vol 50. Reflex control of posture and locomotion. Elsevier, Amsterdam New York Oxford, p 369

Precht W, Shimazu H, Markham CH (1966) A mechanism of central compensation of vestibular function following hemilabyrinthectomy. J Neurophysiol 29: 996–1010

Schaefer K-P, Meyer DL (1973) Compensatory mechanisms following labyrinthine lesions in the guinea pig. A simple model of learning. In: Zippel HP (ed) Memory and transfer of information. Plenum Press, New York London, p 203

Schaefer K-P, Meyer DL (1974) Compensation of vestibular lesions. In: Kornhuber H (ed) Handbook of sensory physiology, vol VI/I. Vestibular system, part 2. Psychophysics, applied aspects and general interpretations. Springer, Berlin Heidelberg New York, p 463

Shimazu H, Precht W (1966) Inhibition of central vestibular neurons from the contralateral labyrinth and its mediating pathway. J Neurophysiol 29: 467–492

Simpson JI (1976) Functional synaptology of the spinal cord. In: Llinás R, Precht W (eds) Frog neurobiology. A handbook. Springer, Berlin Heidelberg New York, p 728

Aspects of Vestibular Compensation in Guinea Pigs

K.-P. SCHAEFER[1] and D.L. MEYER[2]

1 Introduction

This contribution will give an overview of our studies on compensatory CNS phenomena occurring after labyrinthine lesions in guinea pigs (Dal Ri and Schaefer 1956, 1957; Schaefer and Wehner 1966; Schaefer and Meyer 1973, 1974; Schaefer et al. 1978, 1979; Meyer et al. 1981). It attempts to combine various aspects of seemingly heterogeneous studies which were performed under different experimental conditions, such as cortical and cerebellar ablations, spinal transection, and under the influence of several types of drugs. From these investigations a somewhat more advanced picture of the compensatory phenomena following unilateral as well as bilateral vestibular lesions has evolved. Furthermore, information has been gained with respect to more fundamental aspects of how parts of the CNS work and interact, e.g., insights obtained into mechanisms of multisensory convergence relevant in the context of vestibular compensation may eventually lead to a new definition of cerebellar functions.

In order to allow a clear presentation of the aspects considered important, we shall concentrate on integrative processes; in particular those that deal with afferents from the cortex, from the somatosensory system, and from vestibular circuits. Hence, we shall neither attempt to review individual findings in detail, nor shall we try to discuss thoroughly the data of other researches. For this, we refer to reviews published elsewhere (Schaefer and Meyer 1974).

Labyrinthectomy in guinea pigs was performed by an injection of chloroform into the middle ear (Simonelli 1923; Magnus 1924; Schaefer and Meyer 1973). The simplicity of this procedure rendered studies of labyrinthectomy symptoms possible in a large number of specimens. For a quantitative description three labyrinthectomy symptoms were found to be suitable: Firstly, the deviation of the head in the horizontal plane toward the side of the lesioned labyrinth (Fig. 1); secondly, the ocular nystagmus toward the contralateral side; and thirdly, the torsion of head and body about the animal's longitudinal axis toward the eliminated labyrinth. The latter symptom can best be studied by lifting the animals off the ground and holding them by their backs while

1 Neurobiologisches Laboratorium, Psychiatrische Klinik, Universität Göttingen, 3400 Göttingen, FRG
2 Institut für Histologie und Neuroanatomie, Universität Göttingen, 3400 Göttingen, FRG, and Department of Neurosciences, University of California, San Diego, La Jolla, CA, USA

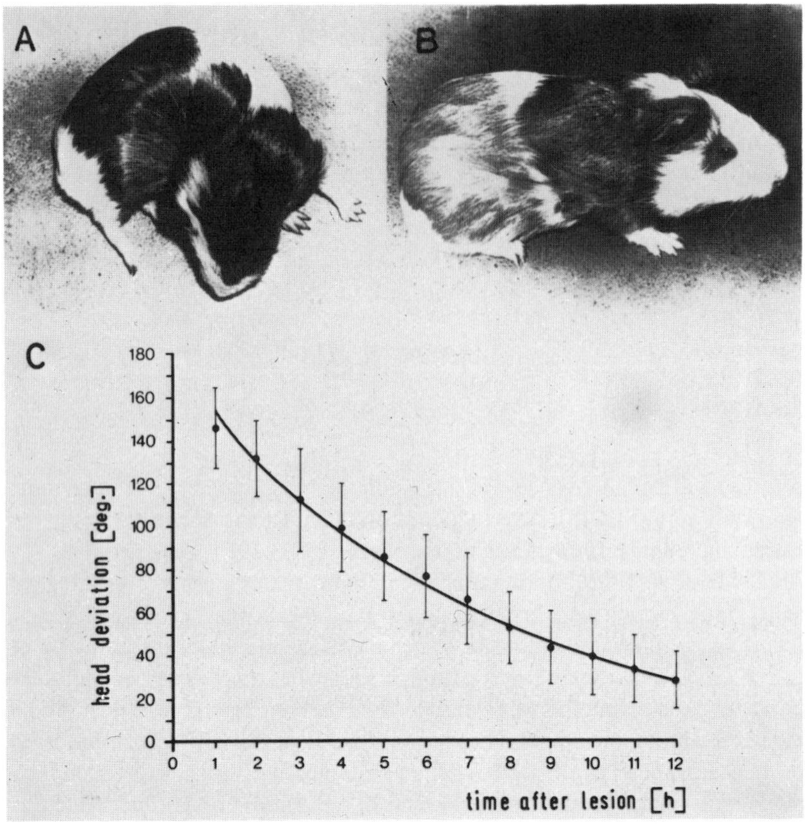

Fig. 1A–C. Compensation of head deviation after unilateral labyrinthecomy. One hour after unilateral labyrinthectomy (right side lesioned), a strongly asymmetrical body posture including a distinct head deviation is displayed (**A**). Twelve hours after lesioning, head deviation is almost compensated (**B**). C shows a plot of the compensation curve, given by the regression line. In these coordinates this is an exponential function (n = 47)

the heads are hanging down freely. This symptom is not compensated for, even after long periods of time, and can only be influenced by certain experimental procedures. In contrast, the symptom of head deviation in the horizontal plane toward the side of the lesioned labyrinth and the ocular nystagmus diminish slowly due to compensatory CNS processes.

Our experiments on successive bilateral labyrinthectomies (Bechterew 1883) were usually performed with a 7-day interval between the two lesions. In these cases, the symptoms observed after the second labyrinthectomy were toward the side of the labyrinth eliminated last (with the exception of nystagmus, the direction of which is defined by its fast phase). Under the conditions existing during the experiments on successive bilateral labyrinthine lesions, compensation was significantly faster after the second labyrinthectomy than that observed after unilateral lesioning. Head deviation in the horizontal plane and ocular nystagmus were down to half of their original values already after about 3 h. In contrast to the observations after unilateral labyrinthectomy, also the symptom of head torsion about the longitudinal body axis diminished and disappeared after a few hours.

2 Results

2.1 Influence of the Cortical Hemispheres

Inflicting a unilateral hemispherectomy on an otherwise intact guinea pig leads to asymmetrical head and body postures which resemble the ones seen after a contralateral labyrinthectomy (Giretti 1971; Schaefer and Meyer 1973, 1974). After *ablation of the left hemisphere* a head deviation toward the right occurs, which is compensated within about 3 days. Neither ocular nystagmus nor head nystagmus was noted in our experiments. The symptoms present instantaneously increase if the specimens are lifted off the ground and thus loose somatosensory input from their extremities.

If a unilateral hemispherectomy is carried out several days *after a bilateral labyrinthectomy,* one first notes a head deviation toward the side ipsilateral to the ablated hemisphere. This diminishes and disappears within ca. 3 days. Thereafter, a head deviation toward the contralateral side is displayed. Already during the first 3 days such a head deviation toward the side contralateral to the lost hemisphere can be elicited if the specimens are lifted off the ground. In contrast to animals with intact labyrinths, bilaterally labyrinthectomized guinea pigs display a vived ocular nystagmus as well as a head nystagmus after unilateral hemispheral lesions. It seems noteworthy that the ocular nystagmus and the head nystagmus are dissociated during the initial 3 days: while the head nystagmus has then its slow phase toward the side of the hemispherectomy (and only later changes direction), the slow phase of the ocular nystagmus is directed to the contralateral side all the time.

The *symptoms resulting from a unilateral labyrinthectomy* in animals that have previously lost one of their cerebral hemispheres depend upon the sides on which both lesions are inflicted. For example, after a hemispherectomy on the left side and a later performed labyrinthectomy on the right side, the symptoms of both lesions are added up and thus a strong head deviation is noted for which compensation is markedly retarded. This observation also holds for specimens that have already compensated for the symptoms resulting from the unilateral hemispherectomy at the time the labyrinthine lesion is inflicted (Schaefer and Meyer 1973). In contrast to the above mentioned observations on head deviation, compensation of ocular nystagmus due to unilateral labyrinthectomy is only insignificantly affected by lesions of the cerebral hemispheres.

A later performed additional lesioning of the ipsilateral labyrinth (that is the left labyrinth in the case of the example given) does not result in an abnormally slow compensation of head deviation or Bechterew nystagmus. It is just the symptom of head- and body torsion about the longitudinal axis caused by the second labyrinthectomy that diminishes more slowly than in specimens subjected only to successive bilateral labyrinthine lesions, but are not hemispherectomized. Contrary to what has been described, a unilateral lesion of the left (ipsilateral) labyrinth after a previous left hemispherectomy does not show any influence of the hemisphere ablation. It is only after the second (contralateral to hemispherectomy) labyrinth is destroyed that a difference between such subjects and control animals becomes obvious. Head deviation and torsion about the longitudinal body axis are compensated very slowly in such cases.

In conclusion one may state that it is the *loss of the contralateral hemisphere* that affects compensation of a labyrinthine lesion. Experiments with both unilateral and successive bilateral labyrinthectomies point in this direction.

2.2 Influences of Spinal Cord and Somatosensory Systems

Compensation of labyrinthectomy symptoms has been demonstrated to be influenced by the spinal cord and somatosensory afferents in three types of experiments: Firstly, animals were suspended in the air after labyrinthectomy; secondly, the animals' heads were restrained in various positions for several hours after a labyrinthine lesion; and thirdly, vestibular compensation has been studied after transection of the spinal cord.

Compensation of head deviation and ocular nystagmus is only insignificantly retarded when the *specimens are suspended in the air.* Putting the animals back on the ground 10h after the unilateral labyrinthectomy results in a drastic increase of head deviation and ocular nystagmus (Fig. 2A). Head deviation then reaches values almost as high as the ones noted briefly after the lesion. Compensation takes another 8 h counting from the time the animals have been allowed ground contact again. Head nystagmus and circulatory movements also reappear as soon as the specimens are put on the ground after 10 h in suspension.

Retardation of compensation by loss of ground contact becomes more clearly visible *after elimination of the second labyrinth* (Bechterew compensation). Compensa-

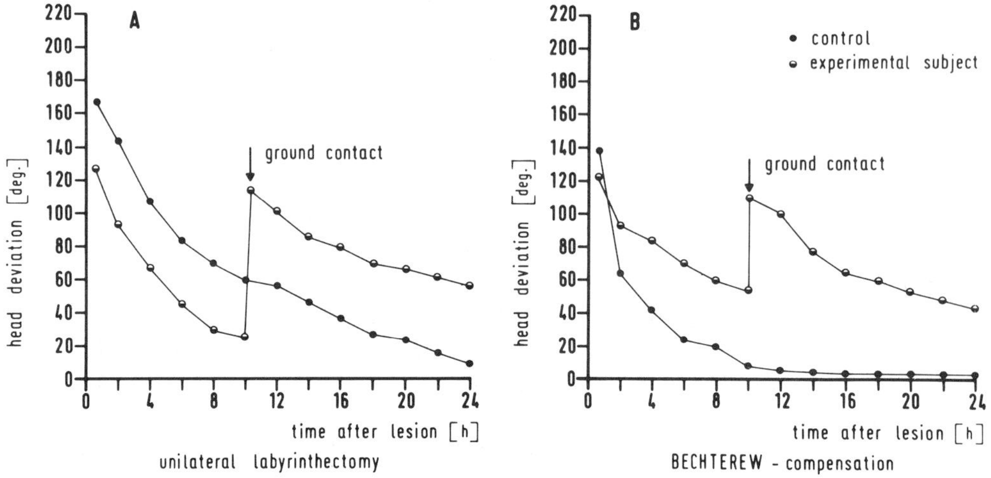

Fig. 2A, B. Somatosensory influences on vestibular compensation. Compensation of head deviation after unilateral (**A**) and successive bilateral (**B**) labyrinthectomy in guinea pigs, suspended in air for the first 10h after lesioning. When ground contact is reestablished, head deviation increases significantly (note *arrow*). The new value of head deviation is also subject to compensation. During the time of suspension Bechterew compensation is more distinctly affected than compensation after unilateral labyrinthectomy tion is now significantly slower than in the controls and half of the initial values for head deviation is reached after ca. 10 h instead of after ca. 2 h. Furthermore, the compensation curve does not have its characteristic asymptotical time course any more. As in the above experiments, putting the animals on the ground after 10 h in the air leads to a strong increase of symptoms (Fig. 2B). Obviously, the compensatory processes depend even more on somatosensory afferents after the loss of both labyrinths, as compared with the situation after unilateral labyrinthectomy.

Since neck-proprioceptive afferents are known to be of extreme significance for the vestibular system, the role of these in compensation for labyrinthine lesions has been studied (Schaefer et al. 1979). For this purpose the *animals' heads were restrained in different positions* for 5 h, starting immediately after unilateral labyrinthectomy. If the head has been restrained in a position 45° to the left in animals that have previously been labyrinthectomized on the right side, a distinct acceleration of compensation can be noted when the head is released after 5 h. The head deviation is already compensated then, whereas it still amounts to almost 90° in control specimens at this time.

Restraining the head in a position toward the right in animals that have previously been labyrinthectomized on the right side does not exert an influence on compensation of either the head deviation in the horizontal plane or the ocular nystagmus. Nevertheless, an interesting observation can be made: when restraining of the head is terminated after 5 h, a general restlessness of the animals, as well as a rolling about the longitudinal body axis and circulatory movements are displayed. This is in clear contrast to the behavior of control specimens at this time. Fixation of the head in a position ipsilateral to the lesioned labyrinth obviously diminishes the more *"dynamic" components of compensation,* although it leaves the normally investigated labyrinthectomy symptoms uninfluenced.

Most dramatically, the significance of somatosensory afferents and spinal circuits for vestibular compensation can be demonstrated in animals that have been subjected to *spinal transection before labyrinthectomy* is carried out (Schaefer and Meyer 1973). The following observations may be obtained from animals with a 5-day interval between the spinal lesion (level of first thoracic segment) and the labyrinthectomy. Compensation of head deviation is significantly retarded: 10 h after the labyrinthine lesion it amounts to 160° and only diminishes to 140° during the following 3 days. Compensation of ocular nystagmus is also retarded. This symptom reaches values of 100 beats/min 10 h after labyrinthectomy.

As described above, the symptom of *torsion about the longitudinal body axis* disappears after the second lesion in animals subjected to successive bilateral labyrinthectomy. In specimens that have an additional previously performed spinal transection, the time course of compensation of this phenomenon too is retarded. The torsion amounts 10 h after the second labyrinthine lesion to 50° and can still be noted after 9 months.

2.3 Influence of the Cerebellum

Before reporting some experimental findings on *labyrinthectomies performed on previously cerebellectomized guinea pigs,* we shall first describe the main effects induced by exclusive cerebellectomy: During the first days after such a lesion most of the mechanisms for postural adjustment are seriously disturbed. It takes several days after cerebellectomy before righting reflexes on the head and on the body can be elicited again. The same holds for the regaining of the ability to right during free fall. Sitting in upright positions takes about 5 days to occur again. Although the reflexes mentioned can be elicited clearly and in a reproducible fashion after 12–14 days, the animals are still significantly impaired after 9 months. Accordingly, compensation of symptoms due to a unilateral labyrinthectomy performed 5 days after cerebellectomy is clearly retarded. This holds for both the ocular nystagmus and the head deviation. With a 4-week and a 9-month interval between both lesions, somewhat different results are obtained. Ocular nystagmus is now compensated at about the same rate as in control animals, whereas compensation of head deviation is still almost as slow as it is with a 5-day interval. Head deviation in the horizontal plane has 10 h after labyrinthectomy, diminished from 180° only to 120°–140°.

In order to further differentiate these findings, compensation has been studied after partial cerebellar ablations. Our assumption that lesions of the vestibulo-cerebellum might be the most effective ones has turned out to be wrong. Instead, such experiments reveal that *ablation of the lobus flocculo nodularis* does not abolish or significantly diminish righting reflexes. Also, compensation of labyrinthectomy symptoms is not dramatically impaired; in particular, ocular nystagmus compensation is hardly influenced. The latter observation is in contrast to the conclusion of other authors with respect to the significance of the flocculus for plasticity in the oculomotor system.

An obvious retardation of vestibular compensation is present after *extirpation of the anterior or the posterior vermis.* After ablation of the posterior vermis including the folium vermis, the tuber vermis, the pyramis, and the cranial uvula, this retardation is almost as pronounced as the one seen after complete cerebellectomy. Also, these experiments reveal that compensation of head deviation is influenced more distinctly than compensation of ocular nystagmus. Similar results are obtained if successive bilateral labyrinthectomies are performed in combination with cerebellar lesions.

Ablation of single lobuli results in the conclusion that folium vermis, tuber vermis (lobulus VI and VII), and pyramis (lobulus VIII) are relatively insignificant for the time course of vestibular compensation. Instead, *destruction of the culmen* (lobulus IV and V), which receives strong projections from the neck region and contains multimodal cells in large number, has an extremely pronounced effect on compensation of labyrinthectomy symptoms. This holds for compensation of both head deviation and ocular nystagmus. The effect is especially strong during the later phases (after 5 h) of compensation (Fig. 3).

2.4 Pharmacological Aspects of Vestibular Compensation

The influence of drugs on functions of the vestibular system has been studied by several investigators since the pioneering work of Magnus (1924). Our own investigations (Fig. 4) have revealed that substances with a narcotic or a sedative action component (such as alcohol, phenobarbital, chlorpromazine, and diazepam) can slow down vestibular compensation significantly (Schaefer and Meyer 1973; Schaefer et al. 1978; Meyer et al. 1981). In contrast, drugs with an excitatory action component (such as

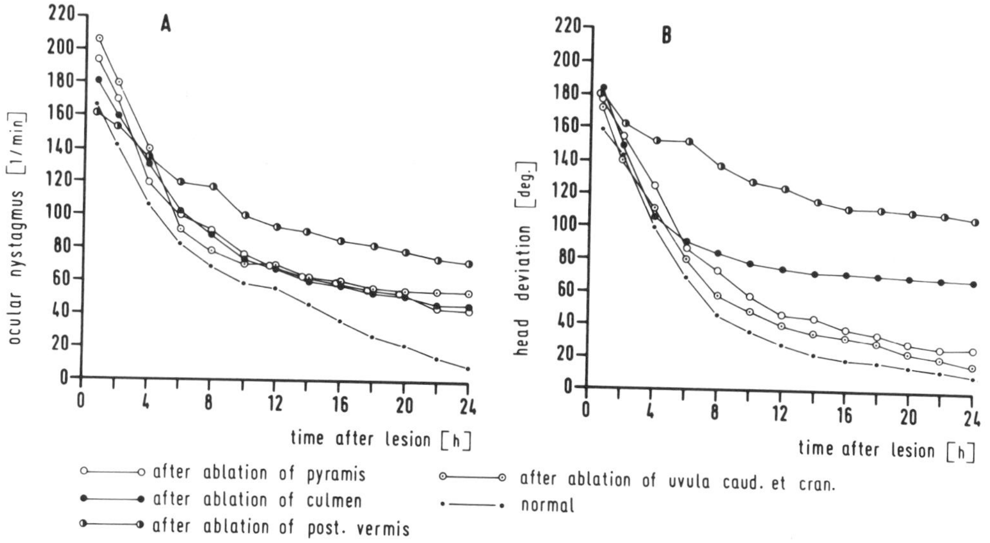

Fig. 3A, B. Influence of various cerebellar lesions on compensation of labyrinthectomy-induced ocular nystagmus and head deviation. Compensation of ocular nystagmus (**A**) is only slightly affected by cerebellar lesions, whereas compensation of head deviation (**B**) is dramatically retarded after lesioning of the posterior vermis. To a lesser degree, this also holds for the situation after lesioning of the culmen (lob. IV and V). Interval between cerebellar lesions and labyrinthectomy is 14 days for the cases shown

caffeine, pentetrazole, metamphetamine, strychnine and paraoxon) exert facilitatory effects on compensation of labyrinthine lesions (Schaefer and Meyer 1974; Meyer et al. 1981). A particularly interesting observation has been obtained with respect to the head and body torsion about the longitudinal body axis. This symptom is not spontaneously compensated for by the CNS after unilateral labyrinthectomy. Under the influence of, e.g., E 600 (paraoxon) this symptom temporarily disappears (Schaefer and Wehner 1966).

In analogy to the findings of Russel (1894/95) on hemispherectomized animals, we noted that labyrinthectomy symptoms, which have already been compensated for, can be re-elicited by the application of certain drugs (Schaefer et al. 1978). Ether and alcohol show this effect for several days after the apparent completion of compensation. E 600 (paraoxon), administered in a dose of 1 mg/kg and in combination with PAM, will do the same for many months, possibly even for the rest of an animal's life. Similar findings have been obtained by Bienhold and Flohr (1980).

3 Discussion

Before discussing the results of labyrinthectomy experiments, one may first consider the *animals' behavior after hemispherectomy, cerebellectomy, and spinal transection.* Disinhibition of lift reactions after lesions of the anterior vermis and temporary loss of

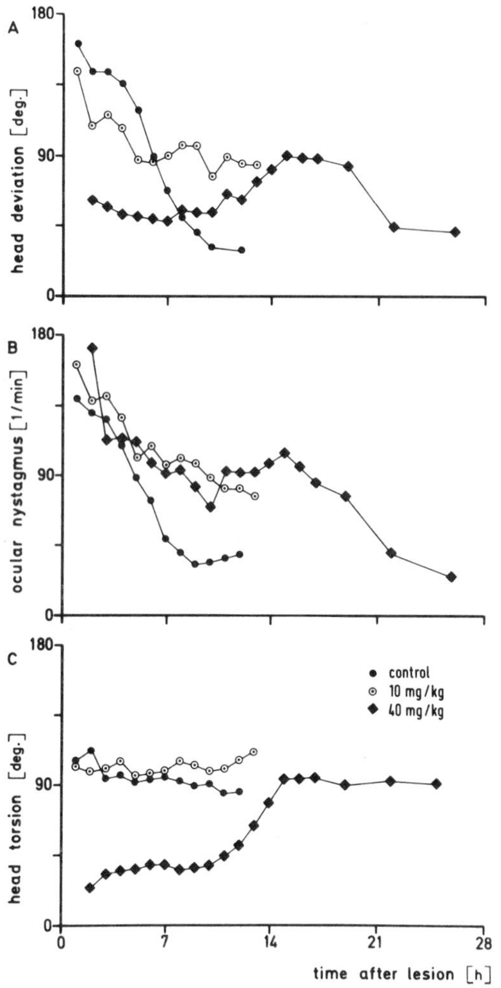

Fig. 4A–C. Effects of chlorpromazine on compensation of symptoms resulting from unilateral labyrinthectomy. Mean values are given from a total of eight specimens tested per condition. Dosis of 10 mg/kg is sufficient to induce a retardation of compensation of head deviation (**A**) and ocular nystagmus (**B**), while 40 mg/kg cause a strong initial decrease of values for head deviation (**A**) and torsion of head and body about the longitudinal axis (**C**). After 10 h the values increase (**A–C**) and later decrease (**A, B**) due to compensation. Time course of compensation is retarded. The torsion of head and body is not compensated for

head nystagmus or righting reflexes after various cerebellar lesions have not attracted much attention so far. Studying these one realizes that symptoms resulting from hemispherectomy, cerebellectomy, or spinal transection are also subject to compensatory processes. Hence, it is important to consider whether a labyrinthectomy is carried out shortly after such a lesion or days to weeks later. The compensation of ocular nystagmus due to a labyrinthectomy, for example, is only slowed down by a previous cerebellectomy, if the vestibular lesion is inflicted shortly thereafter. This is in contrast to the behavior of the symptom of head deviation, whose compensation is still retarded if an interval of 9 months between lesions is allowed.

With increasingly more sophisticated experiments on vestibular compensation – including studies on the effects of drugs – one eventually reaches the conclusion that *the neural basis of this phenomenon involves almost the entire CNS.* The fact that labyrinthine lesion compensation does not originate in the remaining labyrinth alone is already demonstrated by the existence of the Bechterew compensation. Furthermore, vestibular compensation cannot be treated as a homogeneous process, since the different labyrinthectomy symptoms are not affected in identical manner. Compensation for each of these may be achieved to different degrees and with different time courses. Under certain circumstances one may even observe a dissociation of the direction of head deviation and the direction of the slow phase of ocular nystagmus; Bechterew compensation after unilateral hemispherectomy is the example described above. The data presented are in favor of the interpretation that compensation of head deviation depends on compensation of ocular nystagmus. In contrast, compensation of the latter labyrinthectomy symptom appears to be facilitated by the remaining labyrinth, which exerts its influences via pathways that cross the midline (Sanchez-Robles and Anderson 1978; Dieringer and Precht 1979). The complexity of these findings cannot be disregarded when attempting to gain insights into the neuronal mechanisms of vestibular compensation (Precht et al. 1966; Azzena 1969; McCabe and Ryu 1969; Azzena et al. 1979; Dieringer and Precht 1979).

The *complexity of compensatory mechanisms* is further emphasized by interactions between the vestibular system and other sensory modalities or brain structures, as demonstrated by the effects of labyrinthectomy in animals also subjected to CNS lesions. The behavior of the specimens after an exclusive hemispherectomy indicates the presence of a close functional relationship between cortical, vestibular, and somatosensory afferents, as discussed also by Kolb (1955). Head deviation and torsion about the longitudinal body axis elicited resemble the symptoms of a contralateral labyrinthectomy. These symptoms are enhanced if the animals are lifted off the ground. In cases in which hemispherectomy is performed after bilateral labyrinthectomy, one first sees a head deviation toward the side ipsilateral with respect to the hemispheral lesion, which changes into a head deviation toward the contralateral side as soon as the animals are lifted off the ground. In addition, ocular nystagmus is to be noted under such circumstances. From this, one may conclude that the intact labyrinths exert a stabilizing effect on the oculomotor system.

A distinct significance for compensatory mechanisms and for maintaining a symmetrical body posture has to be attributed to somatosensory afferents activated by ground contact. These systems help to eliminate the asymmetrical body posture induced by hemispherectomy and particularly facilitate the progress of compensation for labyrinthine lesions. Accordingly, compensation is retarded after transection of the spinal cord, and asymmetrical body postures are re-elicited if the spinal cord is lesioned after vestibular compensation has already been completed (Azzena 1969). In cases of vestibular compensation occurring without ground contact, asymmetrical body postures reappear once the animals are put on the ground (Schaefer and Meyer 1973). Thus compensation is achieved against a certain functional state of the CNS. If this state changes, compensation has to come into play again. Such changes of the functional state of the CNS can also be induced by various drugs (Schaefer and Meyer 1973; Schaefer et al. 1978). It is for this reason that "release phenomena" may still be observed for months after labyrinthectomy under the influence of appropriate drugs. This way of reasoning offers a probable explanation for the well-established clinical experience that many patients with CNS lesions are extremely sensitive in their response to several drugs, including alcohol.

During the extreme condition present after labyrinthectomy some of the cerebellum's normal functions – our understanding of which is still somewhat limited – may be more easily recognized than otherwise.

After cerebellectomy vestibular compensation is significantly retarded and, again, it is the head deviation that is affected more strongly than the ocular nystagmus. Head and body torsion about the longitudinal body axis resulting from unilateral labyrinthectomy is present under such circumstances, when the animals are lifted off the ground and held by their backs. It seems extraordinarily important that this symptom does not significantly diminish in cerebellectomized specimens, if these are put on the ground. Obviously, the cortical and spinal effects on vestibular compensation processes are mediated mainly via the cerebellum. Remaining cortico-vestibular, spino-reticular, and spino-vestibular connections appear to be unable to substitute completely for the cerebellar connections destroyed by cerebellectomy.

Partial lesions of the cerebellum reveal that it is the loss of cortical and spinal projection areas that is significant for vestibular compensation, rather than a loss of the vestibulo-cerebellum. From this we conclude that the cerebellum with its close relationship to the olive should not be treated as some kind of "plasticity center" (Llinás et al. 1975, 1977) but should be looked upon as a *potent center for multimodal integration.* Hence, with an intact cerebellum a relatively quick "recharging" of vestibular circuits can be achieved after a tonus asymmetry inducing vestibular lesion has occurred.

Acknowledgment. This research was supported by DFG grants to K.-P.S. (SFB 33) and D.L.M. (ME 526, 6–9), and by NIH, NSF and NASA grants to Dr. T.H. Bullock.

References

Azzena GB (1969) Role of the spinal cord in compensating the effects of hemilabyrinthectomy. Arch Ital Biol 107: 43–53

Azzena GB, Mameli O, Tolu E (1979) Cerebellar contribution in compensating the vestibular function. In: Granit R, Pompeiano O (eds) Reflex control of posture and movement. Progress in brain research, vol 50. Elsevier, Amsterdam New York Oxford, pp 599–606

Bechterew W von (1883) Ergebnisse der Durchschneidung des N. acusticus, nebst Erörterung der Bedeutung der semicirculären Kanäle für das Gleichgewicht. Arch Ges Phys 30: 312–347

Bienhold H, Flohr H (1980) Role of cholinergic synapsis in vestibular compensation. Brain Res in press

Dal Ri H, Schaefer K-P (1956) Pharmakologische Untersuchungen am artifiziellen Dauernystagmus des Meerschweinchens. Naunyn-Schmiedebergs Arch Exp Pathol Pharmakol 234: 79–90

Dal Ri H, Schaefer K-P (1957) Beeinflussing des Nystagmus durch Stell- und Haltereflexe am nichtfixierten Meerschweinchen. Pflügers Arch 265: 125–137

Dieringer N, Precht W (1979) Synaptic mechanisms involved in compensation of vestibular function following hemilabyrinthectomy. In: Granit R, Pompeiano O (eds) Reflex control of posture and movement. Progress in brain research, vol 50. Elsevier, Amsterdam New York Oxford, pp 607–615

Giretti ML (1971) Spinal compensation of the cerebral release phenomena. Exp Neurol 30: 459–466

Kolb E (1955) Untersuchungen über zentrale Kompensation und Kompensationsbewegungen einseitig entstateter Frösche. Z Vergl Physiol 37: 136–160

Llinás R, Walton K (1977) Significance of the olivo-cerebellar system in compensation of ocular position following unilateral labyrinthectomy. In: Baker R, Berthoz A (eds) Control of gaze in brain stem neurons. Elsevier, Amsterdam New York Oxford, pp 399–408

Llinás R, Walton K, Hillman DE, Sotelo C (1975) Inferior olive: its role in motor learning. Science 190: 1230–1231

Magnus R (1924) Körperstellung. Springer, Berlin

McCabe BF, Ryu JH (1969) Experiments on vestibular compensation. Laryngoscope 79: 1728–1736

Menzio P (1949) Rapporti fra la corteccia cerebral ed i fenomeni di emislabirintazione. Arch Frisiol 49: 97–104

Meyer DL, Maurer K, Schaefer K-P (1981) Pharmacological influence on vestibular compensation. Submitted

Precht W, Shimazu H, Markham CH (1966) A mechanism of central compensation of vestibular function following hemilabyrinthectomy. J Neurophysiol 29: 996–1010

Russel LSR (1894/95) An experimental investigation of eye-movements. J Physiol (London) 17: 1–26

Sanchez-Robles S, Anderson JH (1978) Compensation of vestibular deficits in the cat. Brain Res 147: 183–197

Schaefer K-P, Meyer DL (1973) Compensatory mechanisms following labyrinthine lesions in the guinea pig. A simple model of learning. In: Zippel HP (ed) Memory and transfer of information. Plenum Press, New York London, pp 203–332

Schaefer K-P, Meyer DL (1974) Compensation of vestibular lesions. In: Kornhuber H (ed) Handbook of sensory physiology, vol VIII. Vestibular system, part 2. Psychophysics. Applied aspects and general interpretation. Springer, Berlin Heidelberg New York, pp 463–490

Schaefer K-P, Wehner H (1966) Zur pharmakologischen Beeinflussung zentralnervöser Kompensationsvorgänge nach einseitiger Labyrinthausschaltung durch Krampfgifte und andere erregende Substanzen. Naunyn-Schmiedebergs Arch Pharmakol Exp Pathol 254: 1–17

Schaefer K-P, Wilhelms G, Meyer DL (1978) Der Einfluß von Alkohol auf die zentralnervösen Ausgleichsvorgänge nach Labyrinthausschaltung. Z Rechtsmed 81: 249–260

Schaefer K-P, Meyer DL, Wilhelms G (1979) Somatosensory and cerebellar influences on compensation of labyrinthine lesions. In: Granit R, Pompeiano O (eds) Reflex control of posture and movement. Progress in brain research, vol 50. Elsevier, Amsterdam New York Oxford, pp 591–598

Simonelli G (1923) Un metodo di distruzione chemica del labirinto. Arch Fisiol 21: 231–233

Spiegel EA, Demetriades TD (1925) Die zentrale Kompensation des Labyrinthverlustes. Pflügers Arch 210: 215–222

Supravestibular Control of Vestibular Compensation After Hemilabyrinthectomy in the Cat

M. JEANNEROD[1], J.H. COURJON[1], J.M. FLANDRIN[1], and R. SCHMID[2]

Compensation of the effects of hemilabyrinthectomy is a good model for the study of central rearrangements which occur after a lesion. Firstly, the pattern of the labyrinthine connections to the vestibular nuclei and of the commissural connections between the two groups of nuclei begins to be extensively known. Secondly, the state of the vestibular system can be easily tested through its well identified responses for the control of gaze and posture. Finally, the existence of many extralabyrinthine afferents to this system raises the possibility of an extrinsic control of its activity.

The part of the vestibular system which controls the eye position in response to head movements operates "open-loop", i.e., it generates ocular responses without being able to evaluate their accuracy. This particularity requires that signals derived from the retina be introduced at the vestibular level, in order to improve and to adapt the dynamic characteristics of the response to the needs of visual stabilization during head/body movements. The role of visual afferences in the control of vestibulo-ocular responses (VOR) has been the subject of many recent studies, both at the anatomical and at the physiological level. A number of pathways have been described, involving several different relays between the retina and the vestibulo-ocular system, including subcortical visual structures and the cerebellar flocculus (Maekawa and Takeda 1976).

The problem discussed in this paper is, to what extent these structures which normally control the VOR might also intervene during the process of compensation in order to re-equilibrate the VOR asymmetry produced by a hemilabyrinthectomy. We will examine the effects, both on the normal VOR and on VOR compensation, of the lesion of two different structures, cerebellar flocculus and superior colliculus. Floccular lesions will be used to determine whether a given aspect of the compensation process (i.e., acquisition or retention) might be preferentially influenced by a supravestibular, cerebellar control. Collicular lesions will be used to determine whether the involvement of the cerebellum in this process is unique, or whether a structure placed at the input level of the visual system, like the superior colliculus, might also play a similar role.

---

1 Laboratoire de Neuropsychologie Experimentale, I.N.S.E.R.M. – Unite 94, 16, avenue du Doyen Lepine, 69500 Bron, France

2 Istituto di Informatica e Sistemistica, Universita di Pavia, Pavia, Italia

1 Methods

The experiments were carried out in adult cats. They were chronically implanted under Nembutal anesthesia with silver silver-chloride EOG electrodes for recording eye movements in the horizontal plane.

Animals underwent either a lesion of the left flocculus or of the left superior colliculus. In both cases, the lesion was made by the way of a suction pipette, via a posterior surgical approach. A dissecting microscope was used during surgery and the lesions were verified histologically at the end of the experiments.

Prior to or after the central lesion (as will be specified in the Results section) animals underwent a right hemilabyrinthectomy. This was made through a ventral approach, by destroying the labyrinth after opening the bulla.

Spontaneous oculomotor activity and VOR were tested preoperatively and at different postoperative stages. During recording the animals were placed in a hammock, with their heads secured at the center of rotation of a horizontal servo-controlled turntable. Eye position was monitored on a polygraph and stored on magnetic tape. VOR was tested in the dark. Velocity functions were applied to the turntable: velocity steps of 160 degrees per second directed clockwise (CW) or counterclockwise (CCW), and sinusoidal oscillations with a peak velocity of $70^\circ/s$. Sinusoidal stimulation was made at frequencies of 0.01, 0.03, 0.05, 0.07, 0.1 Hz, with corresponding peak-to-peak amplitudes of 1150, 849, 509, 364, 255 degrees, respectively.

Vestibular nystagmus was analyzed by constructing manually the slow cumulative eye position (SCEP, Meiry 1965). In the case of step responses the parameters Cm (peak value of SCEP) and t_o (time to SCEP peak) were computed (see Jeannerod et al. 1976, for a more detailed definition of these parameters). In the case of responses to sinuoidal oscillations, the average peak-to-peak values of SCEP during CW and CCW rotations, Cm(R) and Cm(L), were computed. The ratio Cm(R)/Cm(L) gives a measure of VOR symmetry. Since no calibration of eye movements was available, Cm, Cm(R), and Cm(L) were expressed in arbitrary units. The phase shift between the peaks of SCEP and the corresponding peaks of table position during responses to sinusoidal oscillations were measured and averaged.

2 Results

2.1 Effects of Lesions of the Flocculus

At the histological control, the flocculus on the left side was found to be severely damaged in six of the seven cats used for this experiment (Fig. 1). In all cases the lesion also involved other cerebellar structures adjacent to the flocculus. The left dorsal and ventral paraflocculus was completely destroyed in two cats, and partially in the other five. The left lateral cerebellar nucleus was partially damaged in two cases, as also small parts of the vermian lobules.

In one animal, not represented on Fig. 1, the lesion spared the flocculus, although it destroyed the anterior part of the left paraflocculus.

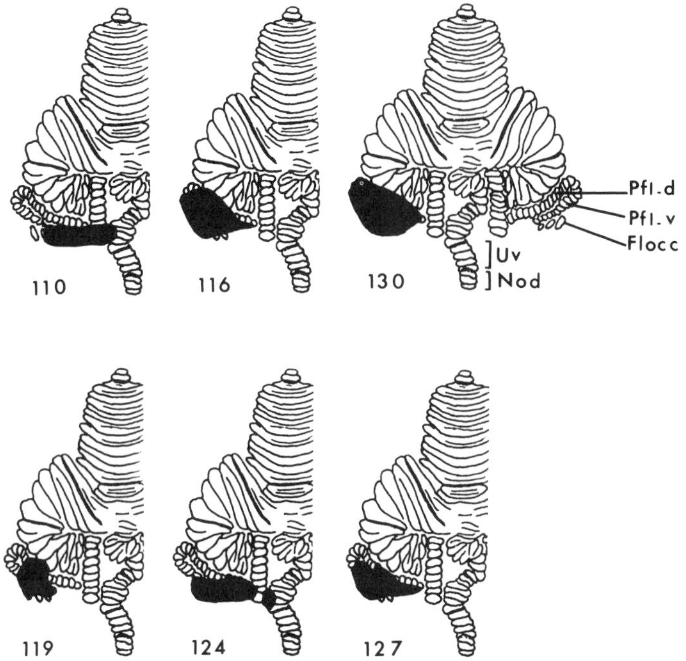

Fig. 1. Histological reconstruction of left floccular lesions (*black area*). *Pfl d, Pfl v,* dorsal, ventral paraflocculus; *Flocc,* flocculus; *Uv,* uvula; *Nod,* nodulus. The planar representation of the cerebellum is redrawn from Brodal and Hoivik (1964)

2.1.1 Effects of Unilateral Flocculectomy on VOR

A clear spontaneous nystagmus could be observed in the dark after the lesion. The fast phase was directed toward the left (lesioned side). However, the direction of the fast phase reverted after some time, i.e., around the 8th postoperative day. Finally, spontaneous nystagmus tended to decrease and to disappear around the 10th postoperative day, in the cats 110, 116, 130.

VOR was found to be highly asymmetrical in the dark. Asymmetry was due to an increase of responses to rotational stimulations directed toward the lesioned side, and to a decrease of responses to stimulations in the opposite direction. Figure 2 exemplifies this effect in one cat where the responses to velocity steps in both directions are represented before (A), and two days after (B) the left flocculectomy. Computation of parameter Cm on that day showed an increase by a factor of 2.5 of the CCW response with respect to the preoperative value. A parallel decrease of Cm (although of a smaller amplitude) was observed in CW responses (Fig. 2C). Parameter t_0 was changed in the same direction as parameter Cm, i.e., it was lenghtened in CCW responses and shortened in CW responses.

Postoperative evolution of the resulting asymmetry, also shown in Fig. 2C, was marked by a maximum on the 2nd and 3rd postoperative days, and by a progressive return to symmetrical responses within about 20 days.

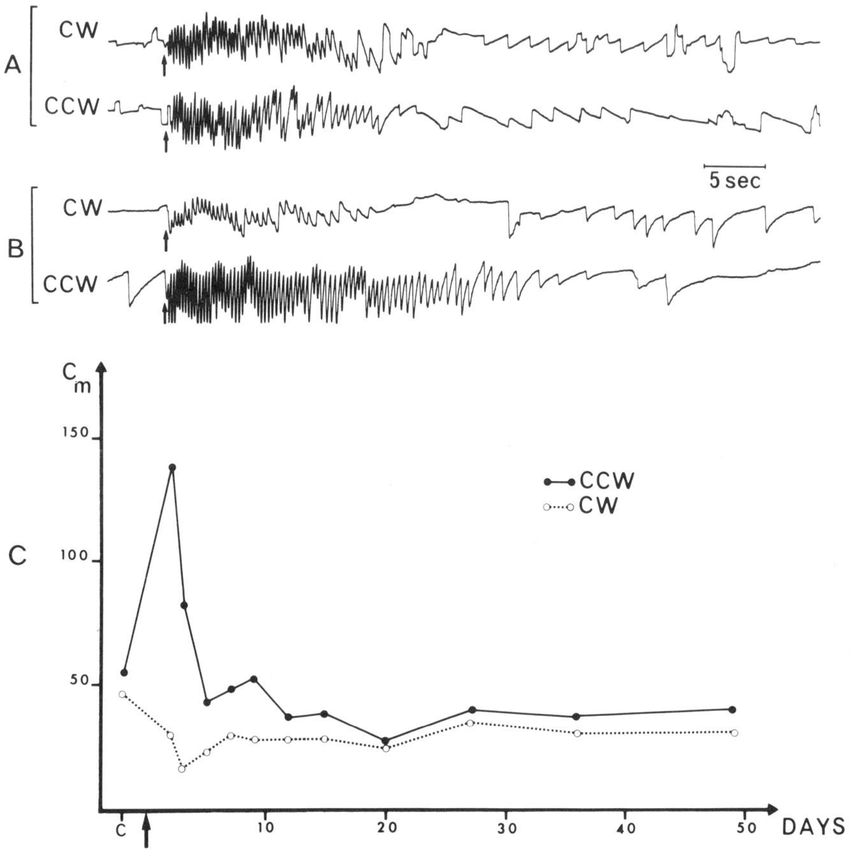

Fig. 2A–C. Vestibulo-ocular responses to velocity steps (160°/s, *arrows*), **A** before, **B** 2 days after a left flocculectomy. **C** Postoperative evolution of parameter C_m in responses to velocity steps directed toward the lesioned side (*CCW*) and toward the normal side (*CW*). *c*, control preoperative values. *Arrow*, time of the operation. Values of C_m are in arbitrary units

Responses to sine wave stimulation in the dark also showed a clear asymmetry after unilateral floccular lesion. Figure 3A compares pre- and postoperative (2 days after the lesion) responses of one cat to a 0.03 Hz sinusoidal oscillation. Amplitude and frequency of nystagmus are clearly increased when the animal is rotated CCW, and decreased when it is rotated CW. In addition, the amount of resulting asymmetry was found to be dependent on the frequency of sinusoidal oscillations. The effect was more pronounced at lower frequencies. As shown in Fig. 3B from the same animal, the Cm(R)/Cm(L) ratio (which takes account of both the increase of Cm in CCW responses and the decrease of Cm in CW responses) indicates a greater asymmetry for a stimulation at 0.01 Hz than at 0.05 Hz and 0.1 Hz. It can be seen, however, that the three curves follow a parallel evolution toward a Cm(R)/Cm(L) ratio equal to one (i.e., toward symmetrical CCW and CW responses) within about two weeks.

A clear asymmetry also occurred in the phase shifts of postoperative responses to sinusoidal oscillations. An increase of the phase lead during rotations toward the intact

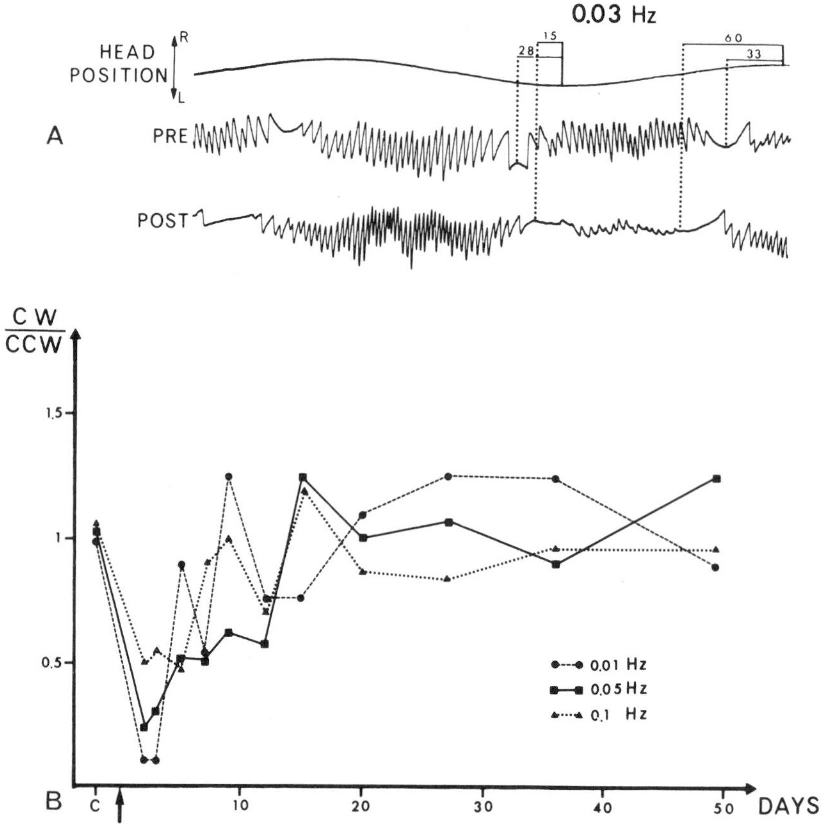

Fig. 3A, B. Vestibulo-ocular responses to sine wave stimulation. **A** *Pre,* symmetrical response to a 0.03 Hz oscillation, before the operation. *Post,* 2 days after left flocculectomy. Note values of phase lead (in degrees) compared before and after operation. **B** Postoperative evolution of responses to sine wave stimulation at different frequencies. Legend as in Fig. 2. The ratio *CW/CCW* indicates the degree of symmetry of VOR during CW and CCW rotations, as computed from parameters C_m(R) and C_m(L). A value of 1 indicates a symmetrical VOR, values below 1 indicate a larger CCW response

side (CW), and a less marked decrease in the opposite direction could be observed. In the same way as for the changes in the "gain" of the responses (reflected by parameter Cm), the changes in phase shift were frequency-dependent, i.e., were more marked at low frequencies than at high frequencies of oscillation. They also disappeared with the same time course.

2.1.2 Effects of Unilateral Flocculectomy in Hemilabyrinthectomized Animals

Three cats (cat 119, 124, 127) had undergone a right hemilabyrinthectomy 27 months, 16 months, and 20 months, respectively, before being implanted for the present study. When they were first tested in the dark, they exhibited a remarkable degree of com-

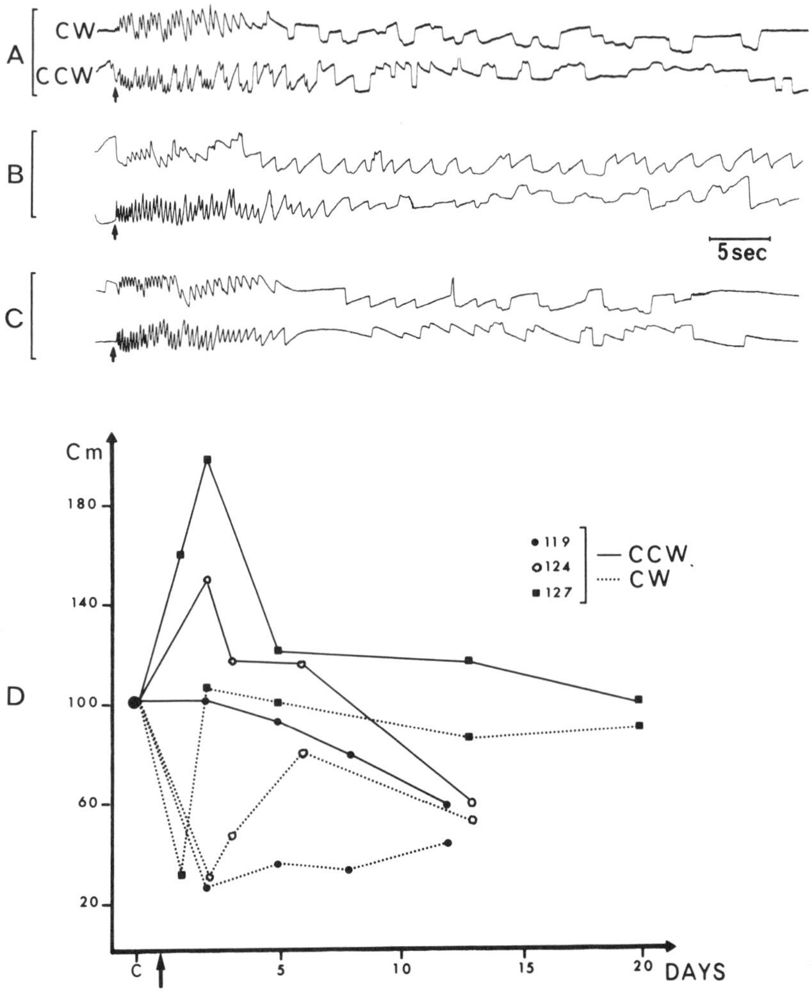

Fig. 4A–D. Effect of a left flocculectomy in compensated animals, after a right hemilabyrinthectomy. **A** Symmetrical responses to velocity steps in CW and CCW directions (*arrows*) in cat 124, 16 months after a right hemilabyrinthectomy. **B** Transient decompensation 2 days after a left flocculectomy. **C** Complete re-compensation 6 days after the left flocculectomy. **D** Postflocculectomy evolution of parameter Cm in responses to CW and CCW velocity steps, in three animals. Legend as in Fig. 2

pensation. No spontaneous nystagmus was present in the dark. Responses to velocity steps were symmetrical for both directions of stimulation, as shown in Fig. 4A, from cat 124. Particularly, the symmetrical reversal of the postrotatory nystagmus in both CW and CCW responses is indicative of a high degree of recovery. Responses to sinusoidal oscillations in the dark were also symmetrical, in the three animals, for what concerns both gain and phase lead.

After left hemiflocculectomy (i.e., on the side opposite to the hemilabyrinthectomy) a strong but transient asymmetry of VOR reappeared. A regular permanent spontaneous nystagmus was observed, with the fast phase directed to the left side. Although this nystagmus also tended to decrease and to disappear around the 4th or 5th day postflocculectomy, it was in many respects different from that observed after flocculectomy in normal cats. Spontaneous nystagmus in the group of hemilabyrinthectomized animals was much stronger, and the direction of the fast phase was never seen to revert.

Vestibular stimulation with velocity steps produced highly asymmetrical responses (Fig. 4B). Cm in responses to steps directed CW (i.e., toward the labyrinthectomized side) was decreased by 70% to 75% after the left flocculectomy, in the three animals. Responses to steps directed CCW (i.e., toward the flocculectomized side) were increased in two animals (124, 127), and unchanged in the other (119) (Fig. 4D). Parameter t_0 was decreased in CW responses, and increased in CCW responses. In responses to sinusoidal oscillations in the dark, the same asymmetry was found, i.e., it was mainly due to a decrease of CW responses. In concordance with this result, the change in phase lead affected both the CCW responses (where phase lead was decreased) and the CW responses (where it was increased).

These effects of hemiflocculectomy were transient. After about one week, CCW responses were back to preoperative levels. Similarly, CW responses tended to reincrease, at least for two animals. In cat 124, and to a lesser degree in cat 127, a high degree of symmetry was restored as early as the 6th day postflocculectomy (Fig. 4C). In the other animal (cat 119), however, the CW responses remained at a low level throughout the time of postoperative testing.

The control animal, with a partial destruction of the left paraflocculus performed 10 months after a right hemilabyrinthectomy, was tested in the same way as the other animals. No spontaneous nystagmus could be observed at the postoperative stage. Responses to velocity steps remained symmetrical for both directions of stimulation. Responses to sinusoidal oscillations in the dark remained symmetrical throughout postoperative evolution.

2.1.3 Effects of Hemilabyrinthectomy Following Unilateral Flocculectomy

In order to test the influence of the serial order of the lesions in the process of vestibular compensation, a right hemilabyrinthectomy was made in one cat (cat 116) 50 days after the left flocculectomy. As described in Sect. 2.1.1, this animal had completely recovered from the effects of the left flocculectomy within about 20 days.

After right hemilabyrinthectomy, the classical syndrome was observed. A strong spontaneous nystagmus with the fast phase directed to the left was present in the light as well as in the dark. During CW stimulation a lack of response contrasted with exaggerated response during CCW stimulation (Courjon et al. 1977).

However, the evolution of the syndrome contrasted markedly with what is usually observed after hemilabyrinthectomy in previously normal animals. Spontaneous nystagmus persisted in the light for 8 days, and was still present in the dark after the 50th day when the recordings were discontinued. No reversal of the fast phase could be observed. VOR asymmetry was also abnormaly prolonged (Fig. 5). The lack of responses during CW stimulation persisted up to the 9th day for the velocity steps, and up to the 7th–9th day for sinusoidal oscillations. After that time, responses during CW stimula-

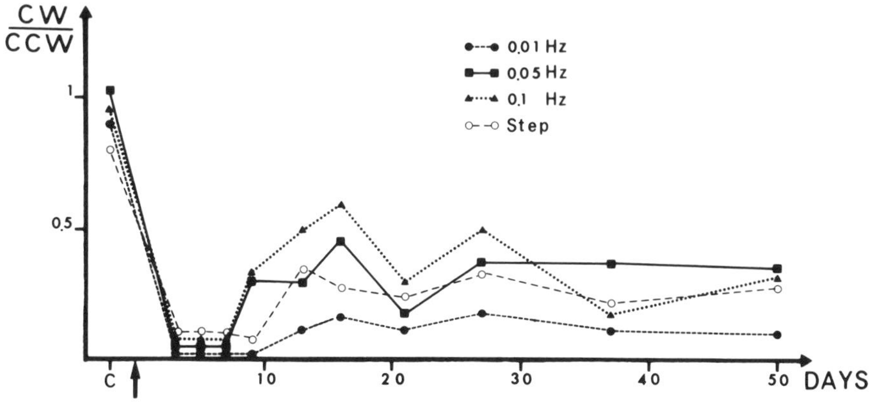

Fig. 5. Evolution of compensation after a right hemilabyrinthectomy in our animal with a previous left flocculectomy. The *CW/CCW ratio* indicates the degree of asymmetry of parameters $C_m(R)$ and $C_m(L)$ obtained from responses to sine wave stimulation at different frequencies and from responses to velocity steps

tion reappeared but remained with a very low gain, thus accounting for a persisting asymmetry up to the end of the observation period (50 days). This effect was verified for what concerns both responses to velocity steps and responses to sinusoidal oscillations.

2.2 Effects of Lesions of the Superior Colliculus

As represented on Fig. 6, the left superior colliculus (SC) was largely damaged in the five animals used for this experiment. The amount of tissue destroyed has been evaluated at 45% of the whole SC in cat C 9, 85% in cat C 10, 60% in Cat C 11, 20% in cat C 12, and 76% in cat C 13. In two cats (C 10, C 13) part of the pretectum was also involved by the lesion.

2.2.1 Effects of Unilateral SC Lesion on VOR

A clear spontaneous nystagmus with the fast phase oriented toward the left lesioned side was present in two animals (cats C 11, C 13) after the operation (Fig. 7).

All cats exhibited a noticeable asymmetry of their vestibulo-ocular response to velocity steps. As a rule, the CCW response (i.e., to steps directed to the side ipsilateral to the lesion) was markedly enhanced with respect to preoperative controls (Fig. 7). Comparison of pre- and postoperative values of parameter Cm showed an average increase of 27% in CCW responses. By contrast, CW responses (i.e., to steps directed to the side contralateral to the lesion) were only slightly decreased or unchanged. The overall asymmetry of VOR (postoperative CW response/postoperative CCW response) was also evaluated by using parameter Cm: the CCW response was 21% to 35% larger than the CW response.

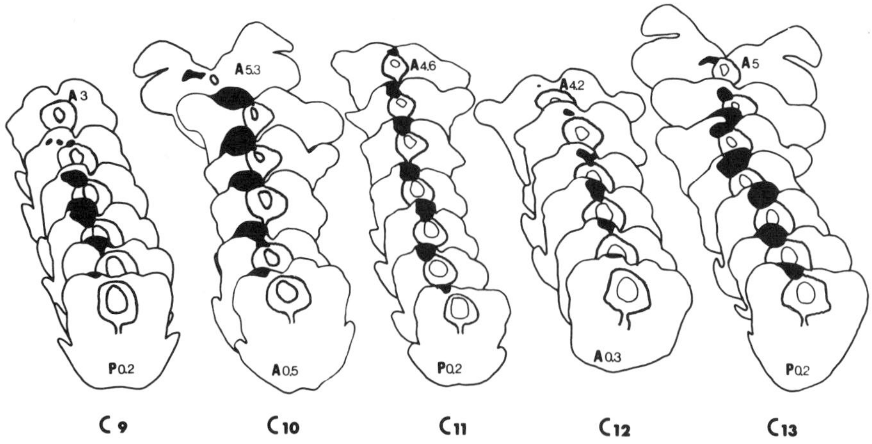

Fig. 6. Histological reconstruction of left superior colliculus lesions in the five animals (*C 9–C 13*). Stereotaxic planes are indicated on the rostralmost and the caudalmost sections for each animal

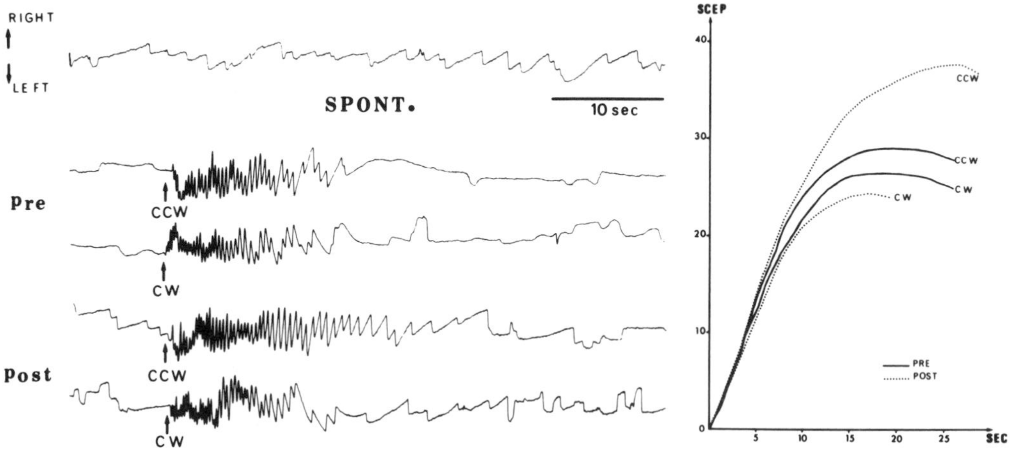

Fig. 7. Spontaneous nystagmus and asymmetrical postrotatory VOR 2 days after a left colliculectomy in cat 11. ***Spont,*** spontaneous nystagmus in the dark. ***Pre, post,*** pre- and postoperative responses to 160°/s velocity steps directed CW and CCW. The ***arrow*** indicates reversal of table rotation. On the postoperative recordings, note asymmetry due to an increase in the CCW response. ***Diagram on the right*** shows the curves of slow cumulative eye position (*SCEP*) as a function of time (in seconds) after stimulation, for the four responses considered in the figure. Note the large increase of the CCW response and the slight decrease of the CW response (*dotted lines*) after operation

Parameter t_0 was also changed in the same direction, showing an average increase of 25% in CCW responses with respect to preoperative controls. By comparing t_0 in responses to both directions of stimulation after the operation, it appeared to be about 40% longer in CCW responses than in CW responses.

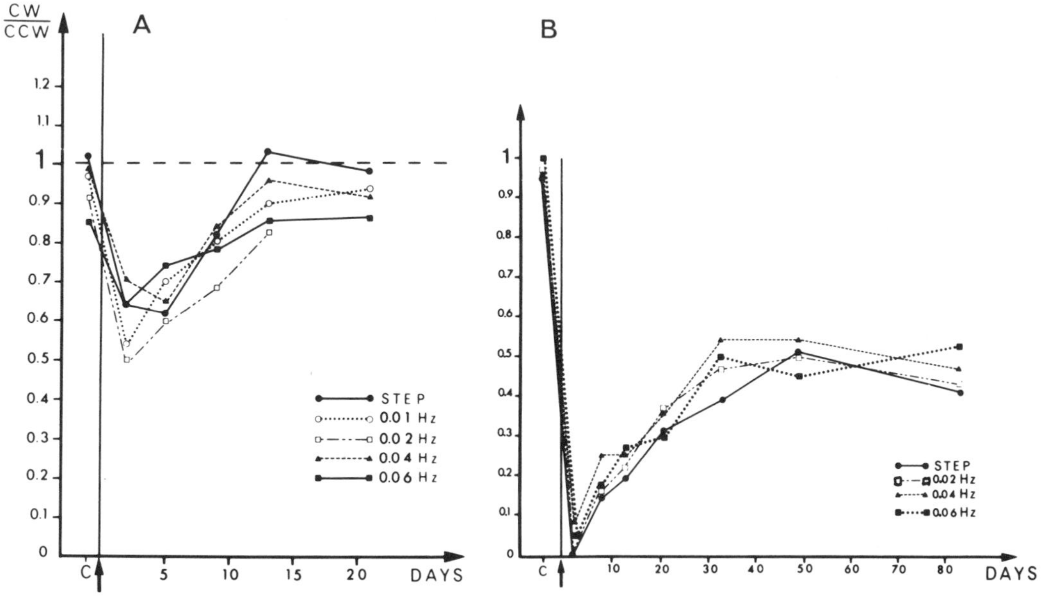

Fig. 8. A Postoperative evolution of VOR asymmetry following left colliculectomy in cat C 13. VOR in the dark. *Abscissae,* postoperative time; *c,* preoperative control. *Arrow* indicates the day of operation. *Ordinates,* gain of VOR in the CCW direction of rotation with respect to gain in the CW rotation. Unit 1 indicates symmetrical gain, values below 1 indicate larger gain in CCW responses. **B** Effect of a right hemilabyrinthectomy several months after a left colliculectomy. VOR asymmetry has been displayed in cat C 10 for responses to velocity steps and to sinusoidal oscillation at various frequencies, as a function of time after hemilabyrinthectomy. *c* indicates the values recorded the day before the operation, i.e., 90 days after left colliculectomy. Note full recovery. After labyrinthine lesion (*arrow*) VOR asymmetry first decreased slowly and then persisted at the same value for up to 83 days

Responses to sine wave stimulation in the dark also showed the same asymmetry after collicular lesion. VOR was increased with respect to preoperative control when the animal was rotated CCW, and decreased when it was rotated CW. The amount of asymmetry was found, however, to be dependent on the frequency of sinusoidal oscillations; the lower the frequency, the larger the asymmetry. VOR asymmetry during sinusoidal stimulation was confirmed by phase changes. As expected from the gain changes, phase lead was decreased in CCW responses and increased in CW responses.

Spontaneous nystagmus in cats C 11 and C 13 disappeared within 3 days after the operation. VOR obtained by vestibular stimulation in the dark showed a definite trend toward a symmetrical gain, due to a reduction of the gain in responses to CCW stimulation. Symmetry was achieved within about 3 weeks (Fig. 8A). This evolution was parallel for responses to velocity steps and to sinusoidal oscillations at different frequencies. In addition to becoming more and more symmetrical, VOR gain also decreased progressively over time for responses to both directions of stimulation.

2.2.2 Effects of a Subsequent Right Hemilabyrinthectomy

A right hemilabyrinthectomy was made in cats C 9, C 10, C 12, 3 to 4 months after they had undergone the left colliculectomy. Immediately after the end of the anesthesia, a strong spontaneous nystagmus with the fast phase to the left was present. This spontaneous nystagmus persisted for a long time. In the light, it persisted for more than 6 days in cat C 12, and up to 22 days in cat C 10. In the dark, it remained at a high level during the first 10 postoperative days, and did not disappear before 1 month. No reversal of the fast phase was observed.

VOR asymmetry was pronounced, and its compensation was delayed. Animals never reached a symmetrical VOR, at least during the observation period (up to 3 months in cat C 10). This was due to a persistent loss of gain in the CW responses, although the gain in CCW responses, which was first exaggerated, became normal again within about 10 days. This was true for responses to velocity steps as well as to sinusoidal oscillations at all frequencies (Fig. 8B). Note that the plateau reached by the compensation process at the end of the first month corresponds to the disappearance of spontaneous nystagmus.

3 Discussion

Involvement of neural structures, such as the cerebellum, in vestibular compensation is a well-known fact. Cerebellar ablation prevents vestibular compensation (Magnus 1924). Lesions restricted to the fastigial nuclei also delay or abolish compensation whether they are made in the same operation as the labyrinthectomy or at the compensated stage (Carpenter et al. 1959). Accordingly, the cerebellar activity is modified during the process of compensation. Blomstrand et al. (1965) have found an increased RNA content of Purkinje cells on the side opposite to a VIIIth nerve section. This finding substantiates the results of McCabe and Ryu (1969) showing that cerebellar neurons are actively involved in inhibiting vestibular nuclei (VN) contralateral to the nerve section. The 2-deoxyglucose study of Walton and Llinás (1978) also shows a cerebellar involvement in compensation, although it shows an increased activity in cerebellar nuclei ipsilateral to the labyrinthine lesion, at variance with previous authors using other techniques.

The influence of flocculus on VOR in the cat is exerted both on the static component of the vestibulo-ocular system (which maintains a symmetrical gaze posture) and on its dynamic component (which produces responses with a symmmetrical gain on head rotations in both directions). This influence is mediated by ipsilateral inhibitory connections to the VN. Accordingly, unilateral floccular destruction produces a deviation of the "gaze posture" toward the contralateral side and an increase in the ipsilateral dynamic vestibulo-ocular response, both of which can be explained by an enhanced (disinhibited) activity of the VN ipsilateral to the lesion. The fact that these effects of flocculectomy compensate rapidly indicates, however, that the flocculus is certainly not the only structures exerting a tonic influence on VN (see below).

The inhibitory role of the flocculus on ipsilateral VN seems well adapted for reducing at least part of the disequilibrium produced in the vestibular system by a unilateral labyrinthectomy. This structure is part of a parallel pathway between the vestibular receptors and the VN; a situation which should allow it to recognize the abnormal increase of spontaneous activity in the VN on the normal side (i.e., in the absence of a peripheral stimulus), and to reduce it by increasing its inhibitory action on that side. This reduction seems to be a prerequisite for restoring spontaneous activity in the deafferented nuclei, by turning down the (increased) commissural inhibition exerted by the normal side.

Such a model of vestibular compensation fits our experimental results. Vestibular compensation cannot be acquired after hemilabyrinthectomy if the flocculus has been previously removed. This is mainly true for compensation of the dynamic component of VOR, which seems to remain impaired for a long time, although the imbalance in gaze posture tends to decrease spontaneously. It might be that in the absence of flocculus, other cues, like static visual cues for instance, could act directly on the VN to reduce this imbalance.

By contrast to the effects of flocculectomy on the acquisition of compensation, this lesion does not seem to affect retention of a previously acquired compensation. When the effects of unilateral flocculectomy were tested in our compensated hemilabyrinthectomized animals, only a transient return of the imbalance and of the asymmetry was observed. In fact, the effect of the flocculectomy in these animals was not greater than that produced by the same lesion in otherwise normal animals.

The difference in the effect of flocculectomy on compensation, whether it precedes or follows the labyrinthine lesion, leads forcibly to the logical conclusion that there are at least two different processes in vestibular compensation. The final process, by which compensation is maintained, might rely on structural changes within the vestibular system itself. The synaptic sites deafferented after the degeneration of the primary afferents in the VN on one side could be reoccupied by synaptic contacts coming from the VN on the normal side. This effect would enhance the action of the commissural pathway (Dieringer and Precht 1977). These newly formed synapses, however, would remain permanently "weak", which would explain incompleteness of compensation and would account for the transient decompensation observed in compensated animals after a short-term anesthesia (Llinás and Walton 1977) or after alcohol injection (Berthoz et al. 1977).

However, before the structural changes can take place (this is a process growing slowly over time, see Jeannerod and Hecaen 1979), some urgent action is needed. The cerebellum is certainly well suited for this role, via its ipsilateral inhibitory output to the VN as previously mentioned, and in concordance with the concept of the "first line of defence" postulated by McCabe and Ryu (1969).

The supravestibular control of VOR seems, in fact, widely distributed in a number of structures. This corresponds to the fact that, in normal conditions, many different cues are used to regulate and to adapt VOR to the needs of visual fixation, e.g., visual cues, such as visual motion signals (retinal slip), or oculomotor cues, such as eye position in the orbit. Such information is transmitted to the VN and to the vestibulo-cerebellum via different specialized visual structures. It is thus not surprising that unilateral ablation of superior colliculus produces at least a transient imbalance of gaze posture and a transient VOR asymmetry. Lesions located in other visual structures (e.g., pretectum, accessory optic tract) would probably produce similar effects. Relative redundancy of visual control of vestibular functions, together with control by other sensory modalities, explain the rapid recovery which can be observed after collicular lesion. The fact that the effects of a subsequent hemilabyrinthectomy will remain permanently uncompensated indicates that compensation requires a fully balanced supravestibular control. In the same way as already shown for floccular lesions, acquisition of compensation becomes impossible if the overall vicariant input, which is now used to reduce VOR imbalance, is no longer symmetrical.

References

Berthoz A, Young L, Oliveras F (1977) Action of alcohol on vestibular compensation and habituation in the cat. Acta Otolaryngol 84: 317–327

Blomstrand O, Mallen A, Hamberger A, Jarlstedt J (1965) Quantitative cytochemical aspects on the mechanism of central compensation after unilateral vestibular neurotomy. Acta Otolaryngol 61: 113–120

Brodal A, Hoivik B (1964) Site and mode of termination of primary vestibulocerebellar fibres in the cat. An experimental study with silver impregnation methods. Arch Ital Biol 102: 1–21

Carpenter MB, Fabrega M, Glinsmann W (1959) Physiological deficits ocurring with lesions of labyrinth and fastigial nuclei. J Neurophysiol 22: 222–234

Courjon JH, Jeannerod M, Ossuzio I, Schmid R (1977) The role of vision in compensation of vestibulo ocular reflex after hemilabyrinthectomy in the cat. Exp Brain Res 28: 235–248

Dieringer N, Precht W (1977) Modification of synaptic input following unilateral labyrinthectomy. Nature (London) 269: 431–433

Jeannerod M, Hecaen H (1979) Adaptation et restauration des fonctions nerveuses. Simep, Lyon

Jeannerod M, Magnin M, Schmid R, Stefanelli M (1976) Vestibular habituation to angular velocity steps in cat. Biol Cybern 22: 39–48

Llinás R, Walton K (1977) Significance of the olivocerebellar system in compensation of ocular position following unilateral labyrinthectomy. In: Baker R, Berthoz A (eds) Control of gaze by brain stem neurons. Developments in neuroscience. Elsevier Biomedical Press, North-Holland, pp 399–408

Maekawa K, Takeda T (1976) Electrophysiological identification of the climbing and mossy fiber pathways from the rabbit's retina to the contralateral cerebellar flocculus. Brain Res 109: 169–174

Magnus R (1924) Körperstellung. Springer, Berlin

McCabe BF, Ryu JM (1969) Experiments on vestibular compensation. Laryngoscope 79: 1728–1736

Meiry JL (1965) The vestibular system and human dynamic space orientation. Sci Dr Thesis, MIT

Walton K, Llinás R (1978) The role of cerebellar and brain stem nuclei in vestibular compensation in rats: a 2-deoxy-D-glucose study. Soc Neurosci Abstr 4: 70

Mechanisms of Compensation of the Vestibulo-Ocular Reflex After Vestibular Neurotomy

W. PRECHT[1,2], C. MAIOLI[1], N. DIERINGER[1], and S. COCHRAN[1]

1 Introduction

The term "compensation" is often used to describe partial or complete restoration of function after lesion of structures causing behavioral deficits. Thus, the widely used term "vestibular compensation" implies that vestibular reflexes are disturbed following lesion of the labyrinth or the 8th nerve and gradually recover in the post-lesion period to control levels or, at least, approximate normal reflex behavior.

There exists ample experimental documentation that normal head, body, and eye posture almost fully recover in all species studied though not necessarily in each experimental individual of a given species (for ref., see Schaefer and Meyer 1974). Furthermore, vestibular reflexes initiated by stimulation of the semicircular canals or the macular organ by active or passive head or body movements have been studied during the process of vestibular compensation but mostly at qualitative levels. On the other hand, quantitative studies of the dynamic reflex behavior are rare. Nevertheless, a few studies dealt with the recovery of cat horizontal vestibulo-ocular reflexes (VOR), in the time domain (Money and Scott 1962; Precht et al. 1966; Courjon et al. 1977) and frequency domain (Moran 1974).

The results obtained in these studies are not uniform and, in many ways, fragmentary, so that we decided to study the recovery of the VOR more systematically in the time and frequency domains. Since previous investigations were performed in cats neurotomized in the adult age, we not only repeated the study with adult animals but, in addition, studied animals which were operated at the age of 6 weeks and investigated more than one year after neurotomy. In addition to the VOR, the horizontal optokinetic reflex (OKN) was measured in both experimental groups.

The present paper describes some of the first results obtained in this series of studies.

1 Max Planck Institut für Hirnforschung, 6000 Frankfurt, FRG
2 Present address: Institut für Hirnforschung der Universität Zürich, August Forel-Strasse 1, 8029 Zürich, Schweiz

2 Material and Methods

Two groups of cats were used in this study: (1) a short-term recovery group consisted of cats operated at *adult* ages. The VOR in these animals was studied at various time periods after the neurotomy starting from 3–4 days to one month post-operatively; (2) a long-term recovery group containing four cats operated at the age of 6 weeks and analyzed 15–19 months after the operation. During this period animals were allowed to move freely in a large room (ca. 15 m^2) and, for the most part, were kept together as a group in this room.

Unilateral section of the right VIIIth nerve was performed under Nembutal anesthesia through a ventral approach in all animals: the bulla tympanica was opened and the vestibulum enlarged to gain access to the ganglion Scarpae which then was destroyed by electrocauterization leaving only the short proximal stump of the VIIIth nerve in the internal acoustic meatus. In the first group of animals silver-silver chloride electro-oculogram (EOG) eloctrodes were permanently implanted before the neurotomy into the lateral bony orbit in order to obtain the controls of the horizontal eye movements. A fixation device was mounted on the head. In the second group EOG electodes and head fixation devices were implanted 3–4 days prior to the first recording session. For recording, animals were placed in a restraining box, which was then placed on a Toennies turntable in such a way as to stimulate mainly the horizontal canals when rotated about a vertical axis (for details, see Keller and Precht 1979).

The EOG was calibrated by rotating the animals (0.25 Hz ± 10°) in normal room illumination before a fixed visual background. The peak velocity of the head was, therefore, 15.7°/s, and the assumption was made that peak compensatory slow-phase eye velocity was equal to head velocity in the alert cat at this frequency and velocity of vestibular stimulation. An independent calibration was also obtained once in each animal by rotating the animal with constant velocity (10°/s) in front of a large-field pattern until eye velocity reached its steady state. The assymption was made that the velocity of steady state, optokinetic slow phase velocity was equal to background velocity. The eye position signal was differentiated to obtain slow phase eye velocity.

Vestibular stimulation consisted of sinusoidal, horizontal rotation in dark and light, and velocity steps of various magnitudes and in both directions in the dark. Optokinetic stimuli were applied by table rotations at various constant velocities in front of an earth-fixed, structured pattern. This stimulus was much more effective than a moving visual scene produced by a shadow projector. During the recording session animals were kept alert by injecting amphetamine ca. 5 min before the recording period (0.5 mg/kg). EOG signals, i.e., eye position and eye velocity were displayed on a Brush recorder together with table position or velocity. Recordings were analyzed by hand as described previously (Keller and Precht 1979).

3 Results and Discussion

3.1 VOR Responses Evoked by Velocity Steps in the Dark

It is well known that in intact animals sudden arrest of the turntable after prolonged horizontal rotation in the dark at constant velocity evokes postrotatory nystagmus of about the same magnitude in either direction; the velocity and displacement of the slow phase is maximal shortly after the stop, then slowly decays to prestimulus levels and often shows one or several reversals in sign thereafter (Precht et al. 1966; Courjon et al. 1977).

Money and Scott (1962) have shown that when one horizontal canal was plugged the responses evoked by stops after rotations to the left and right were still symmetrical. When one labyrinth has been surgically removed, thereby abolishing the resting rate in the VIIIth nerve on that side, responses were apparently different immediately after surgery: a stimulus causing utriculopetal endolymph flow (rotation to the intact side) in the remaining horizontal canal produces strong responses and utriculofugal stimulation gave apparently weak or no responses since it had to counteract the ongoing spotaneous nystagmus.

If one substracted the velocity of the slow phase of this spontaneous nystagmus it was found that both directions of weak stimulations gave similar results, i.e., responses were symmetrical as in the canal-plugged paradigm. There was, however, a very important difference of the responses in both canal-plugged and neurotomized animals when compared to controls, namely that the gain (maximum eye velocity/stimulus velocity) was strongly reduced, i.e., it dropped to values less than controls.

This effect is illustrated in Fig. 1A. It can be seen that 4 days postoperatively the VOR gain was reduced to about one half in this animal. Also there was a particularly strong reduction in gain after utriculofugal stimuli of high magnitudes which was just the opposite behavior to that seen in the control measurements. When the measurements were made 7 days postoperatively (Fig. 1B) the gain values following stops after left and right rotations gave more symmetrical values (even at high velocities). Also, the gains were significantly higher than those measured on day 4 and already approached control values.

Figure 1C shows representative measurements of VOR gain obtained in an animal operated at the age of 6 weeks and recorded 18 months after vestibular neurotomy. The results obtained in the other three animals were similar. It can be seen that the responses obtained in this long-term group were very much the same as those obtained in the short-term group about 7 days postoperatively.

In summary we found that few days after the neurotomy the gain of the VOR on stimuli in either direction decreased and it gradually recovered to reach control values by about the end of the first postoperative week. With high stimulus magnitudes there existed always some asymmetry caused by a lower gain of the responses occurring on utriculofugal stimulus directions.

How can one explain the lower gain of the VOR in either direction during the first postoperative days? It is important to realize that vestibular nuclear neurons of the horizontal canal system (Vn) are not only under the influence of the ipsilateral labyrinth but are also controlled – via the vestibular commissure – from the contralateral

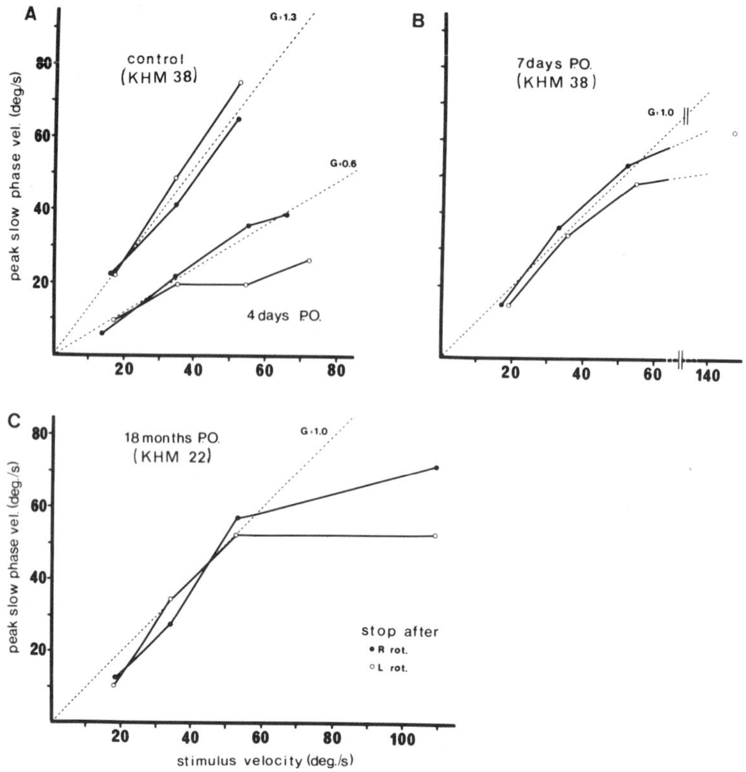

Fig. 1A–C. Relationship between peak slow phase velocity of postrotatory horizontal nystagmus (*ordinate*) and constant table velocity before a sudden stop (*abscissa*). All measurements were taken from the same animal in the dark (**A**) prior to and 4 days after a vestibular neurotomy on the right-hand side and 7 days postoperatively (**B**). **C** same measurements obtained from an animal 18 months after the section of the right VIIIth nerve (performed at the age of 6 weeks). When present the velocity of the spontaneous nystagmus was subtracted. The *dashed lines* in the diagram indicate gain values (indicated by *numbers*) for reference

horizontal canal (Shimazu and Precht 1966). Thus during ipsilateral rotation the main secondary neurons, type I, are excited from the ipsilateral and disinhibited from the contralateral side. When disinhibition is reduced or abolished the gain is expected to drop. Accordingly, type I Vn recorded on the side of the acute hemilabyrinthectomy showed a reduction in gain of ca 50% (Shimazu and Precht 1966; Markham et al. 1977). Furthermore, Abend (1978) has shown that Vn in unilaterally canal-plugged animals also have low sensitivities on either side.

In chronically hemilabyrinthectomized cats the efficacy of the commissural inhibition increases compared to control values (Precht et al. 1966; Shimazu and Precht 1966) and it may be this increased inhibitory/disinhibitory mechanism at the level of the vestibular nuclei which leads to or, at least, supports a recovery of the gain of the VOR.

Single unit work has shown that Vn on the deafferented side not only regain their resting rate but also show type I responses (Precht et al. 1966). These responses were only qualitatively similar to those of intact animals. At the quantitative level clear differences were present. Thus, the frequency increase was limited and the threshold somewhat higher than in control animals. Since frequency increase can only occur through disinhibition, a saturation of firing increase would be expected. This saturation effect may also explain the asymmetry in VOR gain obtained with high stimulus amplitudes.

3.2 VOR Evoked by Sinusoidal Rotation in Dark and Light

The same four cats belonging to the long-term recovery group were also analyzed in the frequency domain, first in the dark and then in the light. The results obtained for gains and phases of VOR's in these four animals are illustrated in Fig. 2A–D. In the light all animals showed a gain of 1 and the VOR phases were perfectly compensatory at all frequencies tested. This finding is also compatible with the normal static and locomotor behavior the animals exhibited in the cage. They were able to move or jump fast and hit their targets with high precision, so that a naive observer was unable to recognize any differences from a normal control group.

In the dark, however, when only the semicircular canals dictate the VOR, clear deficiencies were observed even 18 months after the operation. The gain and phase measurements depicted in Fig. 2A were obtained from a cat which apparently had best recovered from the lesion. Even this animal showed a low gain and large phase lead below frequencies of 0.5 Hz on untriculofugal stimulations (filled triangles). For a comparison control animals showed only a slight reduction in gain and a small increase in phase lead when rotated even at 0.1 Hz in the dark (Keller and Precht 1979). The remaining three animals whose response curves are shown in Fig. 2B–D revealed much more dramatic deficiencies when tested in the dark. Apparently, there exists a wide variation in the adaptive capacities in different individuals. Some compensate for vestibular lesions with "vestibular plasticity" alone quite well, others so poorly that only the presence of a structured world, i.e., an additional visual input, can produce a compensatory VOR.

The frequency domain analysis has shown that the higher the stimulus frequency the better the compensation of gain and phase. This finding is in agreement with the data obtained in the time domain. Since the latter stimuli test predominantly the high frequency performance of the system. At lower frequencies all animals showed severe deficiencies in VOR gain and phase particularly on utriculofugal stimulation.

How can one explain the low gain and large phase lead at low frequency of stimulation? One reason might be the deficiency of the postulated central position integrator converting a velocity signal into an eye position signal (Robinson 1974). If this integrator became more leaky its time constant would drop and one would expect lowering of gain and a larger phase lead. Furthermore, one would expect a deviation of the rectilinear trajectory of the eye position trace during slow phases of vestibular nystagmus into a curvilinear shape.

That this change in trajectory indeed occurred is illustrated in Fig. 3. In Fig. 3A a period of spontaneous nystagmus is shown in an animal before operation. Such episodes of spontaneous nystagmus are occasionally seen when measured in the dark. The slow phase trajectories are rectilinear before (A) and turned into curvilinear (B) after a

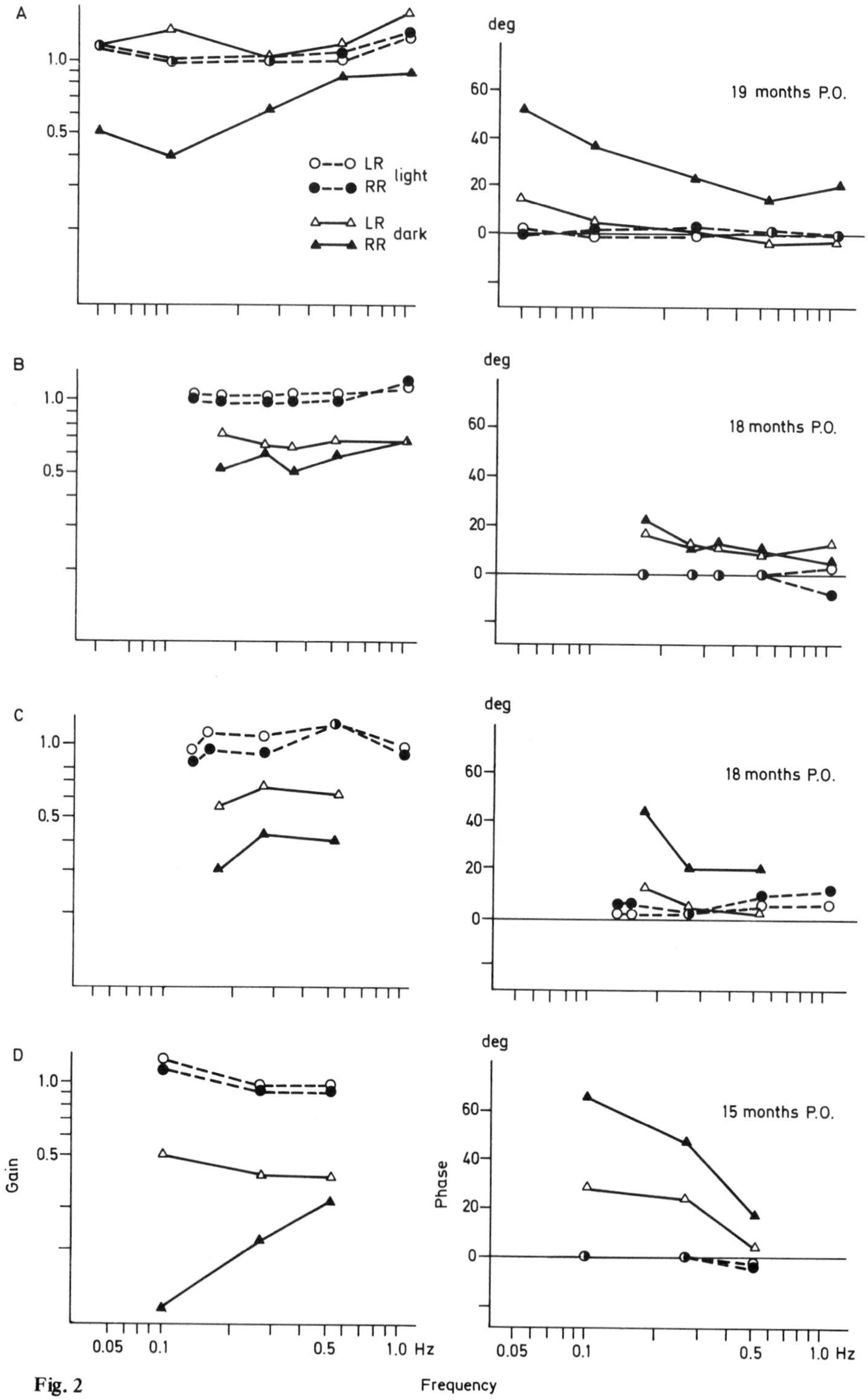
A
B
C
D
1.0
0.5
Gain
deg
60
40
20
0
Phase
19 months P.O.
18 months P.O.
18 months P.O.
15 months P.O.
LR
RR
light
LR
RR
dark
0.05
0.1
0.5
1.0 Hz
Frequency

Fig. 2

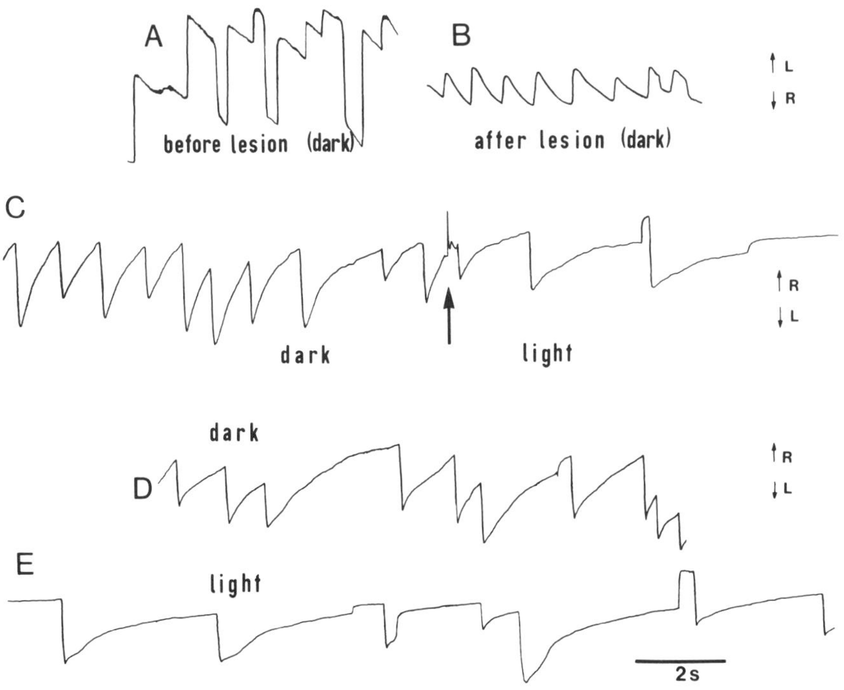

Fig. 3A–E. Sample recording of horizontal EOG's demonstrating curvilinear rather than rectilinear eye position trajectories in hemilabyrinthectomized animals. **A** Spontaneous nystagmus in control animal before (**A**) and after (**B**) lesion of the right eight nerve. **C–E** lesion-evoked vestibular nystagmus recorded in dark and light. Note gaze-holding failure for eye saccades to the left-hand side and curvilinear eye position traces in the dark

vestibular neurotomy on the right side. Figure 3C shows a lesion-evoked nystagmus recorded from a cat in the dark and its suppression in the light. When the animal attempted saccades to the left the eyes always drifted back to the right, i.e., there existed a gaze-holding failure. However, saccades to the right were properly maintained in their new positions. A similar sample is given for another animal in Fig. 3D, E.

These results are taken as evidence that the position integrator became deficient especially for eye movements directed toward the intact side or driven by utriculofugal stimuli. The mechanisms leading to this deficiency remain to be studied. It is interesting to note that this gaze failure was never fully compensated, particularly in those animals which performed poorly in the frequency domain test.

Fig. 2A–D. Measurements of VOR gain and phase in dark (*solid lines*) and light (*broken lines*) performed in four cats of the long-term survival group at postoperative time intervals as indicated. Vestibular neurotomy was performed on the right-hand side. The amplitude of stimulation was always ± 10°. *LR* and *RR* left- and rightward table rotation; *corresponding symbols* give phase and gain values measured for different stimulus directions

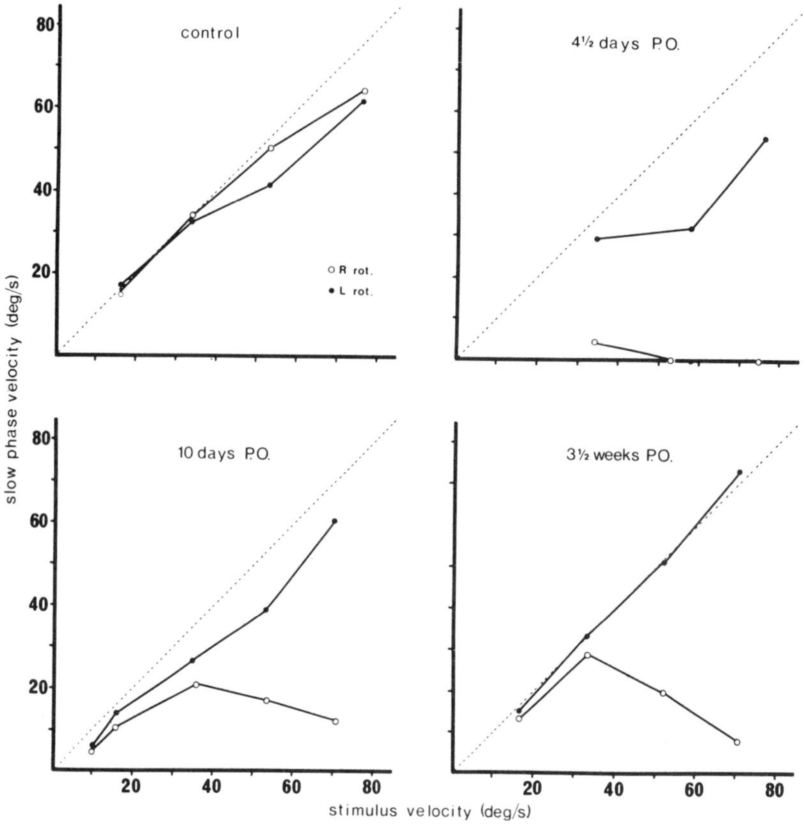

Fig. 4. Relationship between velocity of slow phase of OKN and stimulus velocity recorded in one animal before and at different times after lesion of the right eight nerve. The values for the slow phase velocities are mean values measured in steady-state conditions. Stimulus consisted of constant velocity table rotation in front of an earth-fixed, patterned background. Constant velocities were reached in the dark and lights were turned on after all signs of vestibular nystagmus had disappeared. Symbols: 0 = rightward rotation (visual scene moving to the left); ϕ = leftward rotation (visual scene moving to the right). The *dashed lines* indicate a gain slope of 1

Finally, it should be mentioned that we observed gaze-holding failure in both horizontal directions when both labyrinths were removed.

3.3 Horizontal Optokinetic Nystagmus in Hemilabyrinthectomized Animals

There have been reports showing that bilateral removal of the labyrinths severely affected optokinetic mechanisms (Cohen et al. 1973; Collewijn 1976). We have, therefore, investigated the OKN in the acutely and chronically neurotomized animals.

Figure 4 shows plots of the OKN slow phase velocity versus stimulus velocity taken prior to the hemilabyrinthectomy (control), 4 1/2 days, 10 days and 3 1/2 weeks post-

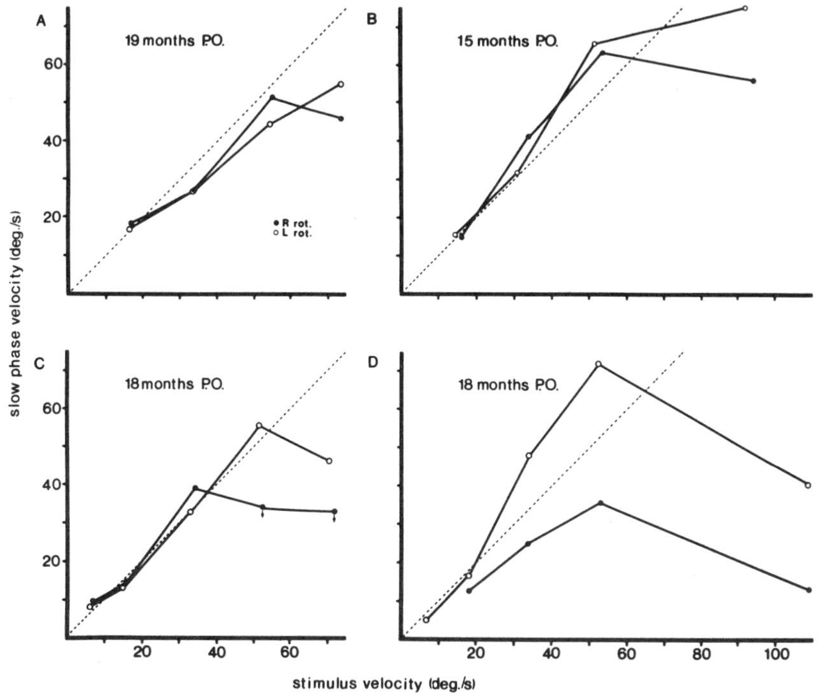

Fig. 5A–D. Relationship between OKN slow phase velocity and stimulus velocity measured in four animals operated at the age of 6 weeks and recorded at the age indicated in the *insets*. Arrangement same as that for Fig. 4. *Arrows* indicate that these values could not be maintained for longer time periods

operatively. It can be seen in the acute postoperative state when the visual surround was moving to the left OKN was extremely poor or absent, whereas responses obtained with rightward movements were only slightly impaired. Ten days after the lesions slight recovery of OKN was noted and after 3 1/2 weeks responses to rightward movements were normal, whereas OKN generated by leftward movements was compensatory only with low stimulus velocity.

In Fig. 5 are shown the stimulus-response curves of OKN obtained in four animals of the long-term recovery group. All animals had their right VIIIth nerve cut at the age of 6 weeks. Clearly, the OKN in these animals showed that three out of four animals had recovered their OKN gain. In the animal whose stimulus-response curve is shown in Fig. 5D the response asymmetry was caused by a somewhat higher gain obtained with rightward surround motion.

In summary we can state that the slow phase velocity of the OKN was strongly impaired when directed away from the lesion and that this deficit compensated with time after lesion. Since Vn on the right side (lesioned side) would normally participate in generating optokinetically driven leftward eye movements by an increase in firing of type I neurons, it is understandable that the strong reduction in resting rate of these neurons on the lesioned side in the acute state (Precht et al. 1966) also leads to a smaller sensitivity of Vn to optokinetic stimuli and thereby to a poorer OKN.

4 Conclusion

The present study so far has revealed that the horizontal VOR in some cats shows a good recovery after hemilabyrinthectomy when measured in the high frequency range (above 0.5 Hz). At low frequencies even the best compensated animals show severe deficiencies more than a year after the operation performed at young age (6 weeks). The low frequency deficiencies were explained – at least in part – by lesion-induced deterioration of the position integrator which also led to gaze-holding failure. All animals studied showed a well-recovered VOR when measured in the light. Apparently optokinetic mechanisms were able to substitute for the vestibular defects still persisting although the optokinetic system per se was also strongly impaired in the acute stage after the lesion.

References

Abend WK (1978) Response to constant angular accelerations of neurons in the monkey superior vestibular nucleus. Exp Brain Res 31: 459–473

Cohen B, Uemura T, Takemori S (1973) Effects of labyrinthectomy on optokinetic nystagmus (OKN) and optokinetic after-nystagmus (OKAN). Equilibrium Res 3: 88–93

Collewijn H (1976) Impairment of optokinetic (after-) nystagmus by labyrinthectomy in the rabbit. Exp Neurol 52: 146–156

Courjon JH, Jeannerod M, Ossuzio I, Schmid R (1977) The role of vision in compensation of vestibulo ocular reflex after hemilabyrinthectomy in the cat. Exp Brain Res 28: 235–248

Keller EL, Precht W (1979) Visual-vestibular responses in vestibular nuclear neurons in intact and cerebellectomized, alert cat. Neuroscience 4: 1599–1613

Markham ChH, Yagi T, Curthoys IS (1977) The contribution of the contralateral labyrinth to second order vestibular neuronal activity in the cat. Brain Res 138: 99–109

Money KE, Scott JW (1962) Functions of separate sensory receptors of non-auditory labyrinth of the cat. Am J Physiol 202: 1211–1220

Moran WB Jr (1974) The changes in phase lag during sinusoidal angular rotation following labyrinthectomy in the cat. Laryngoscope 84: 1707–1728

Precht W, Shimazu H, Markham CH (1966) A mechanism of central compensation of vestibular function following hemilabyrinthectomy. J Neurophysiol 29: 996–1010

Robinson DA (1974) The effect of cerebellectomy on the cat's vestibuloocular integrator. Brain Res 71: 195–207

Schaefer KP, Meyer DL (1974) Compensation of vestibular lesions. In: Kornhuber HH (ed) Handbook of sensory physiology, vol VI. Springer, Berlin Heidelberg New York, pp 463–490

Shimazu H, Precht W (1966) Inhibition of central vestibular neurons from the contralateral labyrinth and its mediating pathway. J Neurophysiol 29: 467–492

The Influence of Unilateral Horizontal Semicircular Canal Plugs on the Horizontal Vestibulo-Ocular Reflex of the Rabbit

N.H. BARMACK[1] and V.E. PETTOROSSI[1,2]

1 Introduction

Vestibulo-ocular reflexes provide a sensitive and convenient means of assaying the normal functions of the peripheral vestibular apparatus and for assaying damage to the central nervous system. The horizontal vestibulo-ocular reflex (HVOR) is ordinarily evoked by reciprocally modulated signals originating from the ampullae of the horizontal semicircular canals. The activity originating from each ampulla is increased by ipsilateral angular acceleration of the head and decreased by contralateral angular acceleration. This stimulus-modulated activity directly excites the ipsilateral medial and superior vestibular nuclei and indirectly inhibits contralateral medial and superior vestibular nuclei via a GABA-ergic commissural pathway (Kasahara and Uchino 1971; Precht et al. 1973) (Fig. 1). The vestibular nuclei send both excitatory and inhibitory projections to the oculomotor (III) and abducens (VI) nuclei (for review see Barmack and Hess 1980). This reciprocal organization is maintained from the peripheral vestibular apparatus to the peripheral oculomotor apparatus and, as a consequence, conjugate compensatory eye movements are evoked by head movements over a wide range of frequencies. This reciprocal organization can be drastically altered by unilateral labyrinthectomy or unilateral vestibular neurectomy. Such operations cause a nystagmus in which the slow phase is directed towards the damaged side (Dow 1938; Precht et al. 1966; McCabe et al. 1973; Schaefer and Meyer 1973; Baarsma and Collewijn 1975; Azzena et al. 1976). The spontaneous nystagmus which is caused by unilateral damage to the vestibular system can be attributed to a tonic imbalance of primary afferent activity. This tonic imbalance, documented at the level of the secondary vestibular neurons by single unit recordings following unilateral labyrinthectomy (Precht et al. 1966; Azzena et al. 1976; Jensen 1979), disrupts not only vestibulo-ocular reflexes, but also horizontal optokinetic reflexes which are mediated in part by the vestibular nuclei (Barmack et al. 1980). The nystagmus caused by hemilabyrinthectomy disappears over a period of several days or weeks (Dow 1938; Baarsma and Collewijn 1975; Schaefer and Meyer 1973). In addition to altering the *tonic balance* of primary afferent activity

1 Department of Ophthalmology, Neurological Sciences Institute, Good Samaritan Hospital and Medical Center, Portland, Oregon 97210, USA
2 Present address: Istituto di Fisiologia Umana, Universita Cattolica Del Sacro Cuore, Roma, Italia

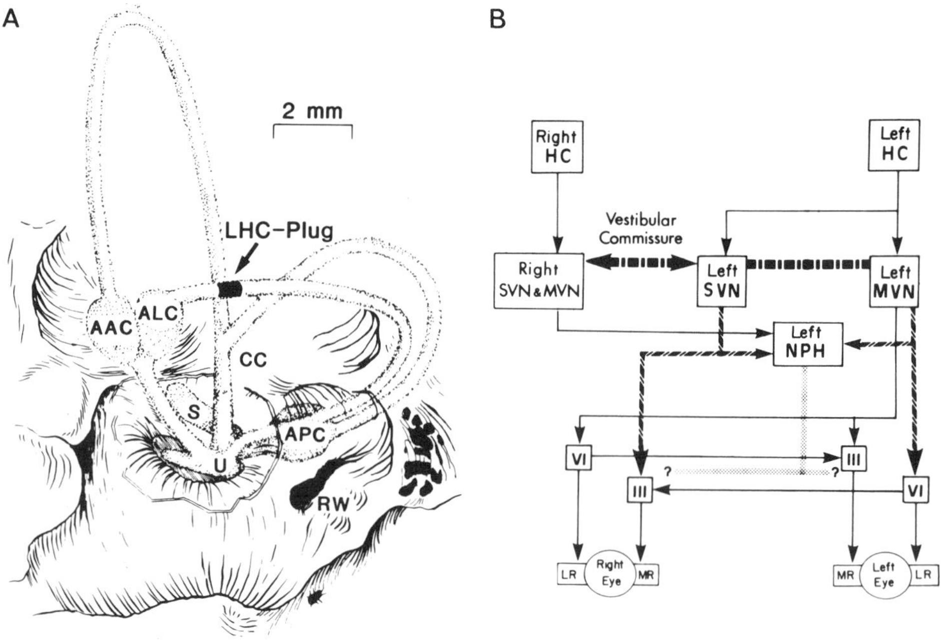

Fig. 1A, B. Location of the LHC-plugs and of the functional peripheral anatomical connections between the vestibular system and oculomotor system. **A** Plugs of the left horizontal semicircular canal (*LHC-plugs*) were placed approximately 2 mm from the ampulla of the left horizontal semicircular canal of the rabbit. **B** Each horizontal semicircular canal directly excites the ipsilateral medial vestibular nucleus and indirectly inhibits the contralateral medial vestibular nucleus via a GABA-ergic commissural pathway. Excitatory pathways are illustrated by *solid lines.* Inhibitory pathways are illustrated by ***interrupted lines.*** Pathways of unknown functional polarity are illustrated by ***dotted lines.*** *HC,* horizontal semicurcular canal; *SVN,* superior vestibular nucleus; *MVN,* medial vestibular nucleus; *NPH,* nucleus prepositus hypoglossi; *VI,* abducens nucleus; *III,* oculomotor nucleus; *LR,* lateral rectus muscle; *MR,* medial rectus muscle; *S,* sacculus; *U,* utriculus; *AAC,* ampulla of anterior semicircular canal; *ALC,* ampulla of lateral (horizontal) semicircular canal; *APC,* ampulla of the posterior semicircular canal; *CC,* common crus; *RW,* round window

originating from the peripheral vestibular apparatus, a unilateral labyrinthectomy also deprives the ipsilateral vestibular nuclei of a *stimulus-modulated* excitatory input, and deprives the contralateral vestibular nuclei of a *stimulus-modulated,* commissurally mediated, inhibitory input.

We have attempted to study the effects on the HVOR caused by a loss of a stimulus-modulated afferent input, as distinct from the effects caused by a loss of tonic vestibular primary afferent activity, by unilaterally plugging the horizontal semicircular canals rather than destroying them. Such unilateral canal plugs leave intact the spontaneous activity originating from the plugged canal, but deprive the vestibular nuclei ipsilateral to the plugged canal of a stimulus-modulated excitatory input, and deprive the vestibular nuclei contralateral to the plugged canal of a stimulus-modulated inhibitory input. Since a plug of the horizontal semicircular canal should not alter the spontaneous primary afferent discharge which originates from the plugged canal, we would expect that this technique would be especially useful in evaluating the relative importance of stimulus-modulated reciprocal signals to central vestibular function.

2 Methods

Surgical Procedures. Fourteen rabbits were anesthetized with ketamine hydrochloride (50 mg/kg intramuscular) and halothane. Two stainless steel screws were anchored to the calvarium with smaller screws and dental cement. The two larger screws mated with a steel rod which restrained the rabbit's head during experiments and supported an eye position monitor. Plugs were made in the left horizontal semicircular canal. The middle ear was approached by a preauricular route. After removing the tympanic membrane and the malleus, the bony surfaces of the horizontal and anterior semicircular canals were partially visible. A small opening approximately 2 mm from the ampulla was made in the bony wall of the left horizontal semicircular canal with a dental burr, leaving the membranous canal intact (Fig. 1A). A silver wire was heated and formed to the shape of a spindle about 0.5–1.0 mm in length and 0.150–0.200 mm in maximum diameter. This spindle was coated with a thin latex polymer and inserted into the opened bony canal compressing the membranous canal. The opening was then sealed with a combination of dental cement and cyanoacrylate.

Vestibular Stimulation and Eye Position Recordings. Rabbits were mounted with head fixed at the center of rotation of a servo-controlled rate table. This rate table was oscillated sinusoidally about an earth-vertical axis at a constant amplitude of $\pm 10^\circ$ over a frequency range of 0.01–0.80 Hz. Eye positions was measured with an infrared light projection technique. The positions of both eyes were monitored. The eye position signal was differentiated electronically with respect to time to obtain eye velocity. The *gain* (G) of the HVOR was determined from measurements of the peak eye velocities attained during each half-cycle of sinusoidal rotation; $G_R = V_R/V_T$, and $G_L = V_L/V_T$, where V_R = peak compensatory eye velocity to the right, V_L = peak compensatory eye velocity to the left, and V_T = peak table velocity. The *phase* of the HVOR (eye position + 180° re: head position) was measured at each half-cycle of rotation.

3 Results

Immediately following a unilateral horizontal semicircular canal plugging operation, the gain of the HVOR was reduced and the phase lead of eye position relative to table position was increased over the entire range of frequencies examined (Figs. 2A, B and 3). The immediate postoperative reduction in the gain of the HVOR was symmetrical (1–10 h, post-LHC-plug), i.e., both G_L and G_R were reduced. However, if post-LHC-plug vestibular stimulation was maintained following the plugging operation, an asymmetry appeared to represent an increase in G_L relative to G_R (Figs. 2C and 4). This apparent increase in the gain of the HVOR toward the side of the plugged canal was

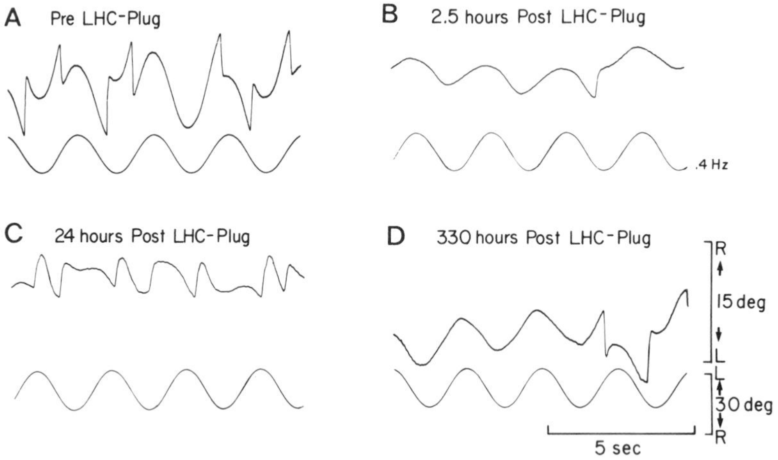

Fig. 2A–D. Influence of a plug of the left horizontal semicircular canal on the horizontal vestibuloocular reflex (HVOR). **A** The HVOR was evoked by sinusoidal horizontal stimulation (± 10°, 0.4 Hz) prior to plugging the left horizontal semicircular canal (LHC-plug). The HVOR was evoked by the same stimulus 2.5 h (**B**), 24 h (**C**), and 330 h (**D**) after LHC-plug. Note that the eye movements evoked in **A**, **B**, and **D** are symmetric but that the eye movements evoked 24 h following the LHC-plug (**C**) are asymmetric with a marked leftward bias

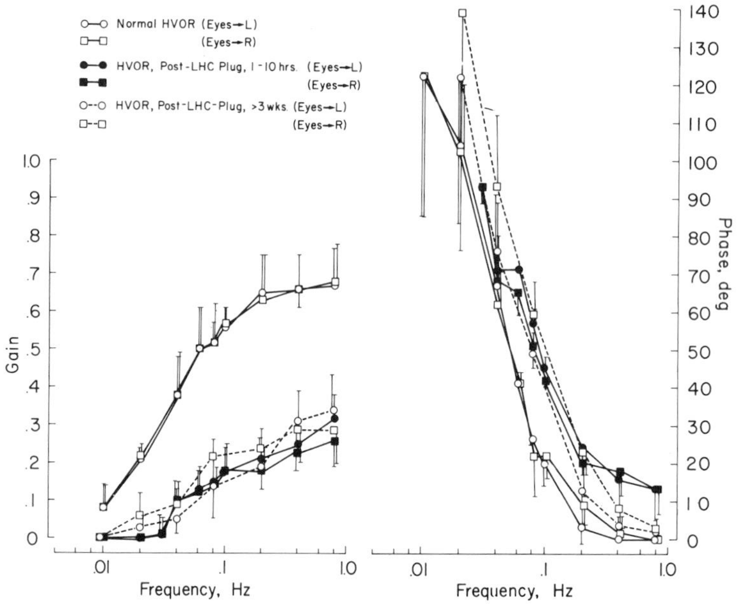

Fig. 3. Comparison of the effects of a left horizontal semicircular canal plug on the HVOR recorded at different times following the plugging operation. The gain and phase of the HVOR were measured in four rabbits before the left horizontal semicircular canal was plugged (*open symbols* connected by *solid lines*), and remeasured in the same group of rabbits 1–10 h after the plugging operation (*filled circles* connected by *solid lines*). The gain and phase of the HVOR were remeasured again in each rabbit at least 3 weeks following the plugging operation (*open circles* connected by *dashed lines*). Note the absence of asymmetry of the HVOR during both measurement intervals

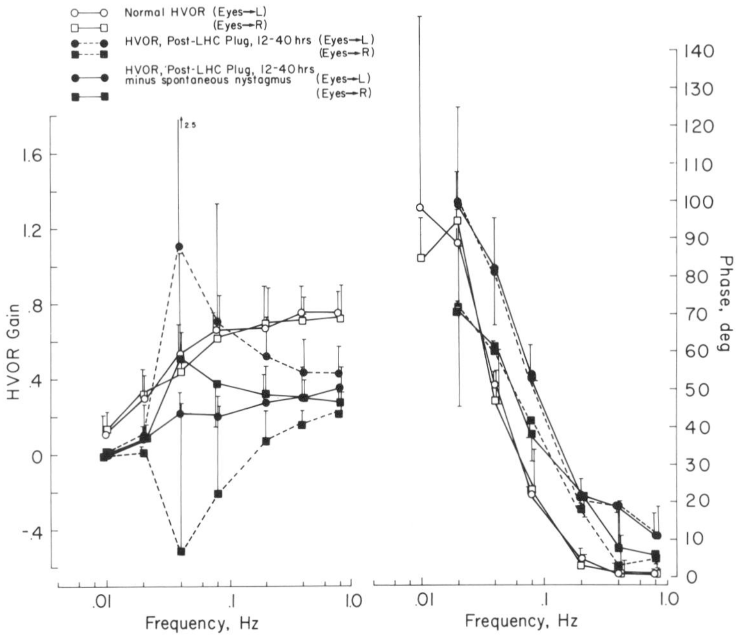

Fig. 4. The influence of left horizontal semicircular canal plugs on the HVOR, recorded 12–40 h following the LHC-plug. The gain and phase of the HVOR were measured for both leftward (*circles*) and rightward (*squares*) eye movements. These preoperative measurements of the HVOR for a group of four rabbits are illustrated by the *open symbols* connected by *solid lines.* The HVOR of the same group of rabbits was remeasured 12–40 h following the plugging operation (*filled symbols* connected by *dashed lines*). During this period each rabbit evinced a spontaneous nystagmus in the dark. The mean spontaneous eye velocity was subtracted from the HVOR-evoked eye velocities. The results of this subtraction are illustrated by *filled symbols* connected by *solid lines.* Standard deviations (+ or –) are illustrated for each data point in this and subsequent figures

often, but not invariably, accompanied by a spontaneous nystagmus which had a slow phase toward the side of the plugged canal. This nystagmus was responsible for the apparent increase in G_L and for the concomitant reduction in G_R. If the spontaneous nystagmus was subtracted from the compensatory eye movements of the HVOR, then the gain of the HVOR toward the side of the plugged canal, G_L, was *reduced,* not enhanced, relative to G_R (Fig. 4). The change in neural activity which causes this spontaneous nystagmus may be influenced by concomitant vestibular stimulation. In our experience with normal rabbits, vestibular stimulation at higher frequencies tends to increase the velocity of a spontaneous drift of the eyes. Therefore, at higher stimulus frequencies subtraction of the spontaneous nystagmus velocity from the compensatory eye velocities of the HVOR may actually lead to an underestimate of the contribution of the spontaneous nystagmus to our measurements of the HVOR gain. Maximum asymmetry in the G_L and G_R, not corrected for by subtraction of the spontaneous nystagmus, occurs in 24–48 h.

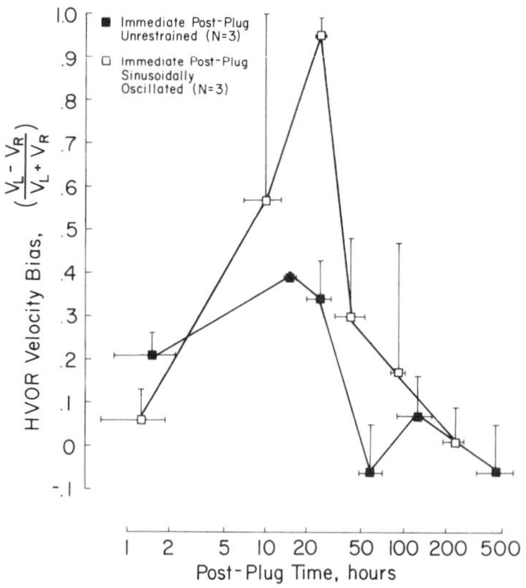

Fig. 5. A comparison of the effects of vestibular stimulation on the HVOR velocity bias evoked at different times following horizontal semicircular canal plugs. The HVOR velocity bias, $(V_L - V_R)/(V_L + V_R)$ was measured at 0.4 Hz, ± 10°. One group of rabbits (*filled squares*) received sinusoidal vestibular stimulation only during the HVOR testing in the first 24 h following the plugging operation. Between testing sessions these rabbits were returned to their own cages. A second group of rabbits (*open squares*) received 24 h of continuous sinusoidal oscillation following the plugging operation, after which they were returned to their cages between test sessions. The horizontal standard deviations indicate the extent of variability caused by combining measurements taken from different rabbits at different postoperative times

Time Course of the Development and Compensation of Asymmetry of the HVOR Following a LHC-Plug. The development of the post-LHC-plug asymmetry was studied in separate groups of animals exposed to different regimens of vestibular stimulation. The asymmetry (or velocity bias) of the HVOR was defined as: $(V_L - V_R)/V_L + V_R)$. For perfectly symmetrical eye movements, this ratio would be equal to zero. For eye movements in which the uncorrected compensatory eye velocity toward the side of the plug was twice the velocity of the eye movements toward the side of the intact canal, an HVOR velocity bias equal to one-third would be obtained. Figure 5 compares the HVOR velocity bias of two groups of rabbits which were stimulated at a frequency of 0.4 Hz at various times following placement of an LHC-plug. One group (*open squares*) received 24 h of continuous vestibular stimulation in the rate table immediately following the plugging operation. After this continuous 24 h of stimulation these rabbits were returned to their home cages during the intervals between HVOR testing. A second group of rabbits did not receive continuous postoperative vestibular stimulation and were returned to their home cages after each test session. A slightly greater asymmetry in the HVOR was obtained in the rabbits which received 24 h of continuous vestibular stimulation following the plugging operation (Fig. 5). After 200 h both groups of rabbits had an essentially symmetric HVOR.

The effect of postoperative vestibular experience was further examined in a group of rabbits which were deprived of all vestibular stimulation, except during test sessions.

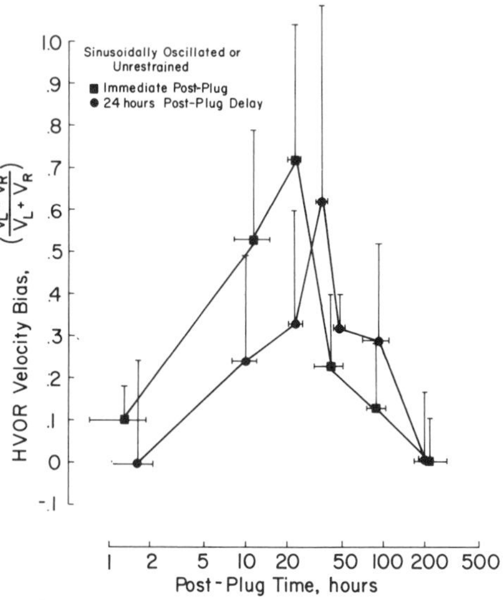

Fig. 6. The influence of 24 h of deprivation of vestibular experience on the HVOR velocity bias evoked at different times following LHC-plugs. The HVOR velocity bias was measured postoperatively in two groups of rabbits. One group of rabbits (N=6) received either sinusoidal vestibular stimulation continuously or were allowed to return to their cages during non-test intervals (*filled squares*). A second group of rabbits (N=6) (*filled circles*) were deprived of postoperative vestibular stimulation for 24 h. Except for brief (1 h) sessions, these animals were maintained for the first 24 h after the LHC-plug in the experimental apparatus, with their heads held rigidly, preventing either passive and active stimulation of the vestibular system. Note that in this group of animals the development of maximal asymmetry was delayed by about 24 h

This vestibular deprivation was achieved by maintaining the rabbit's head fixed for a period of 24 h following the plugging operation, thereby depriving the animal of both passive and active postoperative vestibular experience, except during test sessions. These rabbits were compared with a group of rabbits which were either stimulated continuously for 12–24 h following the plugging operation, or which were allowed to return to their home cages and move about freely. The deprived group developed an asymmetry of the HVOR which reached its peak approximately 24 h after the peak of the asymmetry attained by the nondeprived rabbits (Fig. 6). The asymmetry in the HVOR of the deprived and nondeprived rabbits was fully compensated 200 h after the plugging operation (Fig. 6).

4 Discussion

Unilateral horizontal semicircular canal plugs have several interesting effects on the HVOR. First, such plugs cause an immediate and permanent reduction in the gain of the HVOR (Figs. 2 and 4). Second, such plugs cause an asymmetry in the HVOR to develop over a period of hours. Third, the development of this asymmetry is dependent upon vestibular experience. Fourth, after the asymmetry is developed, it is compensated over a period of days. These data suggest that the disruption of a reciprocally organized and stimulus-modulated signal causes a tonic imbalance of central vestibular function. This central imbalance does not reflect the same imbalance in spontaneous afferent discharge from the two semicircular canals which is observed following hemilabyrinthectomy. In the present experiment, vestibular experience after the LHC-plug was made was necessary for the spontaneous nystagmus to fully develop. This nystagmus was not present immediately postoperatively, and its onset was delayed when the LHC-plugged rabbits were deprived of active and passive vestibular experience following the plugging operation (Fig. 6).

The plugging operation caused an interesting departure from the normal functioning of secondary vestibular neurons. Ordinarily, secondary vestibular neurons receive reciprocally modulated excitatory and inhibitory signals originating from the ipsilateral and contralateral semicircular canals, respectively. However, in the LHC-plugged rabbits the vestibular nuclei on the plugged side received only an inhibitory (GABA-ergic) stimulus-modulated input through the vestibular commissure, whereas the vestibular nuclei on the intact side received only an excitatory input conveyed from the intact horizontal semicircular canal. It is tempting to speculate that the secondary vestibular neurons ipsilateral to the LHC-plug might develop over a period of hours a greater sensitivity to the inhibitory transmitter of the commissural system. If this were the case, then systemically administered GABA-ergic agents which cross the blood–brain barrier (e.g., diazepam) should potentiate the asymmetry of the HVOR in rabbits with unilateral semicircular canal plugs (Barmack and Pettorossi 1979).

Although head movement (active or passive) in LHC-plugged animals is essential for the asymmetry of the HVOR to become manifest, we do not know what behavioral conditions are optimal for the subsequent compensation of this asymmetry. It would seem likely that central neuronal circuits, especially those involving the cerebellum, would contribute to this compensatory process.

Acknowledgments. This research was supported by the National Institutes of Health Grant EY00848 and the Oregon Lions Sight and Hearing Foundation.

References

Azzena GB, Mameli O, Tolu E (1976) Vestibular nuclei of hemilabyrinthectomized guinea pigs during decompensation. Arch Ital Biol 114: 389–398

Baarsma EA, Collewijn H (1975) Changes in compensatory eye movements after unilateral labyrinthectomy in the rabbit. Arch Oto-Rhino-Laryngol 211: 219–230

Barmack NH, Hess DT (1980) Eye movements evoked by microstimulation of dorsal cap of inferior olive in the rabbit. J Neurophysiol 43: 165–181

Barmack NH, Pettorossi VE (1979) Effects of unilateral horizontal semicircular canal plugs and the intravenous administration of diazepam on the development and compensation of asymmetry of the horizontal vestibulo-ocular reflex of the rabbit. Soc Neurosci Abstr 5: 621

Barmack NH, Pettorossi VE, Erickson RG (1980) The influence of bilateral labyrinthectomy on horizontal and vertical optokinetic reflexes in the rabbit. Brain Res 196: 520–524

Dow R (1938) The effects of unilateral and bilateral labyrinthectomy in monkey, baboon and chimpanzee. Am J Physiol 121: 392–399

Jensen DW (1979) Reflex control of acute postural asymmetry and compensatory symmetry after a unilateral vestibular lesion. Neuroscience 4: 1059–1073

Kasahara M, Uchino Y (1971) Selective mode of commissural inhibition induced by semicircular canal afferents on secondary vestibular neurones in the cat. Brain Res 34: 366–369

McCabe BF, Ryu JH, Sekitani T (1973) Further experiments on vestibular compensation. Adv Oto-Rhino-Laryngol 19: 195–205

Precht W, Shimazu H, Markham CH (1966) A mechanism of central compensation of vestibular function following hemilabyrinthectomy. J Neurophysiol 29: 996–1010

Precht W, Baker R, Okada Y (1973) Evidence for GABA as the synaptic transmitter of the inhibitory vestibulo-ocular pathway. Exp Brain Res 18: 415–428

Schaefer K-P, Meyer DL (1973) Compensatory mechanisms following labyrinthine lesions in the guinea-pig. A simple model of learning. In: Zippel HP (ed) Memory and transfer of information. Plenum Press, New York, pp 203–232

Vestibular Compensation: New Perspectives

M. LACOUR and C. XERRI[1]

1 Introduction

The question which arises is: what basic mechanisms are involved, what nervous structures are implicated and what sensory information is needed to attain and maintain vestibular compensation?

Five main points emerge from the literature, which must be considered for a better understanding of vestibular compensation. (1) The recovery process does not involve a single nervous structure, but several brain stem and cerebellar structures. Many well-argued papers support the contribution of the cerebellum (McCabe and Ryu 1969; Azzena et al. 1979; Schaefer et al. 1979), the inferior olive (Llinas et al. 1975; Llinas and Walton 1977), the vestibular nuclei (Precht et al. 1966; Precht 1974); others point to the role of the cerebral cortex (Kolb 1955) and of the spinal cord (Kolb 1955; Azzena 1969; Jensen 1979a,b). A recent study (Llinas and Walton 1979) nicely synthetizes all these previous investigations on single structures. Llinas and Walton concluded that vestibular compensation "is a distributed property of the nervous system". (2) The second point indicates that many sensory inputs intervene in the recovery process. The role of vision (Ewald 1892; Magnus 1924; Kolb 1955; Courjon et al. 1977; Putkonen et al. 1977), of somatosensory afferents (Kolb 1955; Azzena 1969; Schaefer and Meyer 1974; Lacour et al. 1976; Schaefer et al. 1979; Xerri and Lacour 1980) and of the remaining contralateral labyrinthine input (Rademaker 1935; Dieringer and Precht 1979a; Lacour et al. 1979) has been recognized. (3) The so-called Bechterew compensation (Bechterew 1883), observed when the second labyrinth is destroyed following a sufficient time interval after the first lesion. Bechterew hypothetized that the deafferented vestibular nuclei had reestablished a background of activity counterbalancing the vestibular nuclei activity of the opposite side. This view is now confirmed by microrecordings from the partially deafferented vestibular units during the course of compensation (Precht et al. 1966; McCabe and Ryu 1969; McCabe et al. 1972; Precht 1974). (4) The decompensation phenomenon found in already compensated animals when submitted either to various nervous structure lesions, sensory restrictions, or to drug administration (narcotics, alcohol; see Schaefer and Meyer 1974). This suggests

1 Laboratoire de Psychophysiologie, Universite de Provence, Centre de St-Jerome, 13397–Marseille Cedex 4, France

that many structures and sensory inputs intervene not only in establishing but in maintaining compensation, and therefore that vestibular compensation is a continuous dynamic process. (5) The last point concerns the description of functional changes at a cellular level. Dieringer and Precht (1979a,b,c) found electrophysiological signs of functional modifications in the properties of neurons in the deafferented vestibular nuclei of hemilabyrinthectomized frogs. They observed both an increase in the efficiency of the excitatory (from commissural fibers) and inhibitory (via a vestibulocerebello-vestibular loop and the brain stem) inputs to these neurons. They assumed that one possible mechanism is a reactive synaptogenesis leading to new synapses formation.

Assuming that vestibular compensation needs the functional integration of various sensory inputs, we analyzed the role of the remaining labyrinthine afferents, of somatosensory inputs and of visual information in establishing and maintaining compensation. Our own investigations were specifically focused on the recovery of the vestibulospinal functions in awake monkeys and cats. In the monkey, we studied the recovery of spinal reflexes and the compensation of postural reactions to fall. In the cat, we investigated the recovery of posture, locomotion and equilibrium. From these studies, the following conclusions were drawn.

All the sensory inputs involved in perception of space, body posture and body locomotion in space intervene in the recovery process. Vestibular compensation develops in active animals only, i.e., when they can use all available information elicited by an active sensorimotor exploration. These multisensory inputs tonically and dynamically substitute in permanence for the missing labyrinthine afferents. In this process, the remaining labyrinth appears particularly involved in recreating the dynamic counterpart. The earlier all information is provided, the better-adapted the recalibration will be and the better the final compensation.

2 Methods

The vestibular neurectomy was unilateral (U.N.) or bilateral (B.N.). The time-course and the level of compensation was studied both in normally recovering animals and in others which underwent supplementary sensory privation. The relative role of these inputs in establishing and maintaining compensation was taken up by applying the sensory privations at different post-operative periods.

2.1 In the monkey (*Papio papio*), we studied the modifications and the development of spinal reflexes and we examined the compensation of postural reactions to fall (Lacour et al. 1978a, 1979; Lacour and Xerri 1980). The basic experimental set up for this study is illustrated in Fig. 1A. The role of the remaining labyrinthine afferences was inferred by comparing the recovery of muscle responses to fall (EMG) and of spinal reflexes (H and T-reflexes) in U.N. and B.N. baboons. The role of the visual information was demonstrated by modifying the visual environment during fall. Five visual conditions were used: (1) normal vision (NV), (2) visual stabilization (SV), (3) enhanced vision (EV), (4) reduced vision (RV), (5) total darkness (D). In each condition

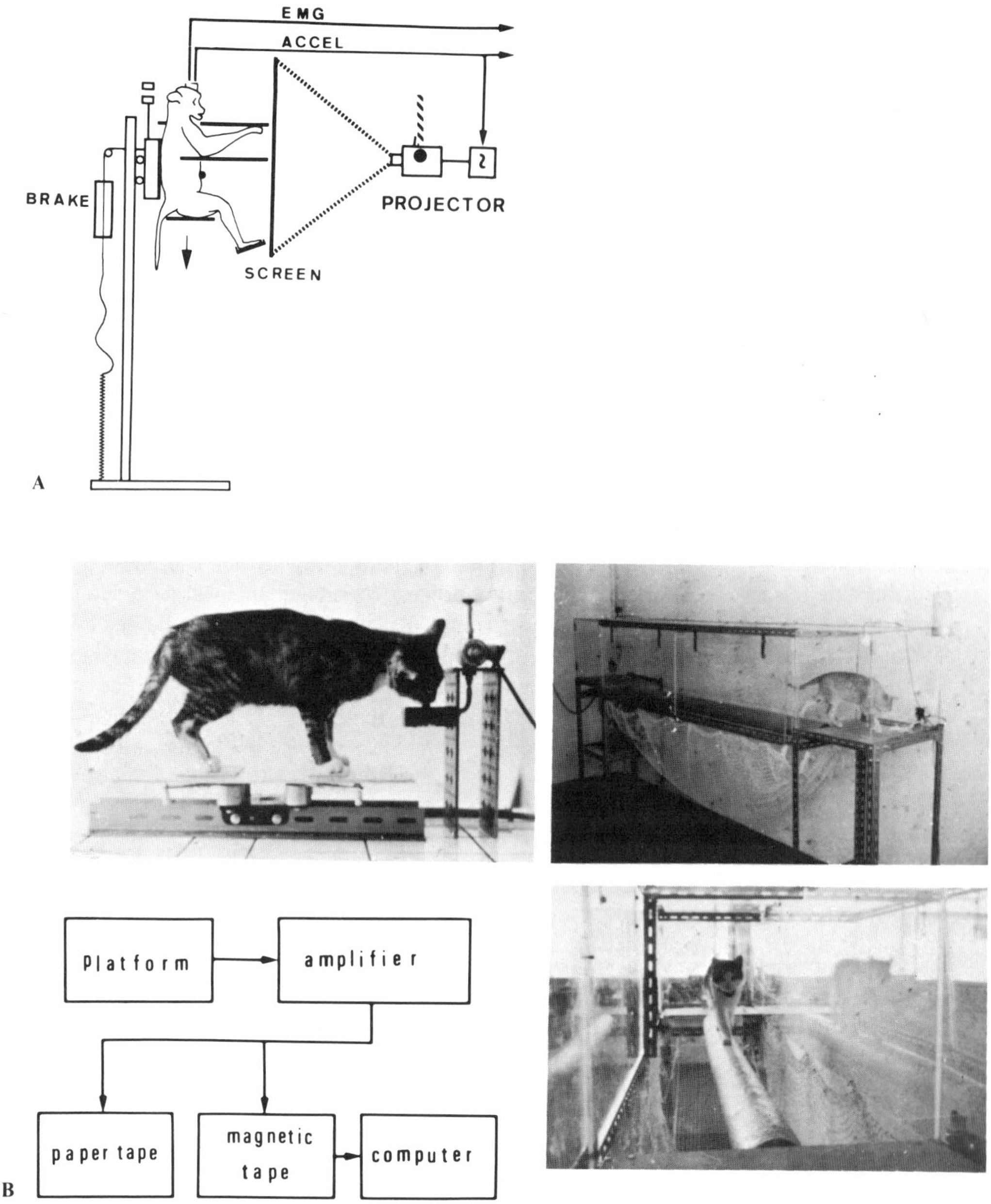

Fig. 1A, B. Experimental sets-up.
A Experimental set-up for study of compensation of postural reactions to fall in the monkey. The baboon is seated on a chair which can slide along a vertical axis. The total height of the free-fall was 0.9 m. Three profiles of acceleration were used: 8.8 m/s^2, 4.4 m/s^2 and 2.2 m/s^2 (peaks of vertical linear acceleration). A V-shaped special screen is placed in front of the baboon; it covers all the peripheral retinal fields of the baboon on its lateral parts and the whole of the height of fall. A visual scene, consisting of a high spatial frequency black and white pattern is projected onto it.

we analyzed the visually induced modifications of muscle responses to fall as a function of the post-operative time. The method used here is the opposite of the visual deprivation method. While not falling, the monkey was maintained in a normal visual environment; while falling, it experienced either normal vision (NV), or total visual restriction (D), or total exclusion of visual motion cues (SV), or enhanced (EV) or reduced visual motion cues (RV). Various vertical linear accelerations were also combined with the various velocities of the visual scene relative to the monkey's head so as to favor either the visual input (low velocity of fall) or the labyrinthine input (high velocity of fall).

2.2 In the cat we studied the recovery of posture and locomotor equilibrium (see Xerri and Lacour 1980) using behavioral tests (Fig. 1B). The degree of postural symmetry was quantified by means of a four-strain gauges platform. Postural symmetry was expressed by ratios between the force exerted by each forelimb and by each hindlimb. The locomotor equilibrium test consisted of two compartments connected by a cylindric beam which could be rotated along its longitudinal axis with a variable speed. The maximum performance of each cat corresponds to the highest speed of rotation of the beam which did not lead to a fall for four consecutive trials. The cats were submitted to vestibular neurectomy and divided in two groups. The first group was composed of cats which remained free after surgery in their usual environment; they had normal vision. The second group was made up of cats that underwent a 7-days' sensorimotor restriction (SMR). They also had normal vision. SMR was applied during either the first, or the third, or the eight postoperative week in order to determine if the level and the time-course of recovery was dependent on the postoperative delay before application of the SMR. Some U.N. cats were submitted to a second vestibular neurectomy performed 1 year after the first section (B.N. cats) in order to test the influence of the remaining labyrinth in recovering these functions.

Motion of the visual scene was performed using a servo-system which had input consisting of the integral of the vertical acceleration record (velocity signal) and output that controlled the film motion in the projector, with a 1 ms delay. Five visual conditions were used: (*a*) normal vision (*NV*): the visual scene was kept stationary on the screen; (*b*) total darkness (*D*); (*c*) visual stabilization (*SV*): the visual scene was moving together with the monkey, in the same direction and with the same velocity as velocity of the falling monkey; (*d*) enhanced vision (*EV*): the visual scene was moving upward; (*e*) reduced vision (*RV*): the visual scene was moving downward with lower velocity than velocity of the falling monkey. The EMG responses to fall were recorded in neck muscles (splenius capitis), soleus and tibialis anterior muscles. The EMG_S were rectified and summated. EMG values resulted from measurement of muscular energy developed in the 20–120 ms interval after release of fall.
B Experimental set-up for study of posture (*left*) and locomotor equilibrium (*right*) recovery in the cat. The degree of postural symmetry is measured using a four-strain gauges platform. Postural symmetry is expressed by the ratios between the force exerted by each forelimb (*left* FL/*right* FL × 100) and by each hindlimb (*left* Hl/*right* Hl × 100). The locomotor equilibrium test consists of two compartments connected by a cylindric beam (3 m long, 12 cm diameter, 1.2 m above ground) which could be rotated along its longitudinal axis with a variable linear speed (0 to 25 m/min). Maximum performance of the cats corresponds to the highest speed of rotation of the beam which did not lead to a fall for four consecutive trials. Data obtained after surgery were expressed in percent of preoperative values

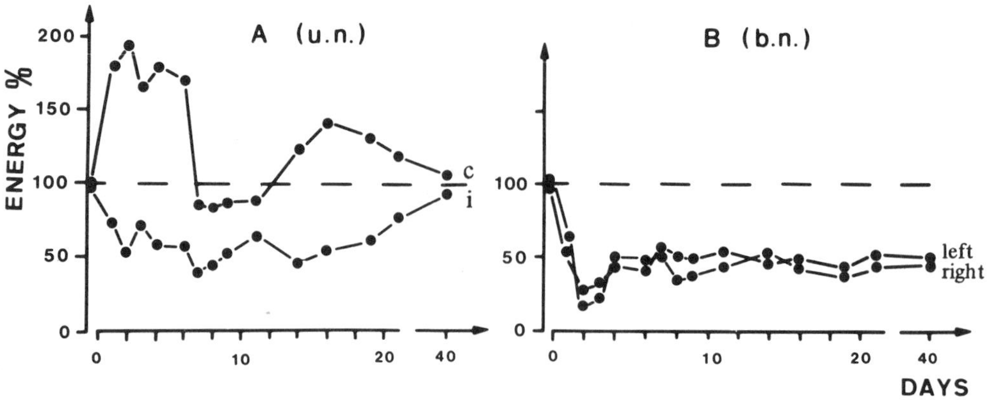

Fig. 2A, B. Role of the remaining labyrinth in compensating soleus muscle responses to fall. **A** Mean evolution recorded from 4 U.N. baboons on the ipsilateral side (i) and on the contralateral side (c). Mean values of energy after surgery are plotted as a function of the postoperative time in days (*abscissa*) and expressed in percent of control values (*ordinate*). Each point is the average of 40 values. **B** Mean evolution recorded from 2 B.N. baboons in left and right soleus muscles. Same presentation as in **A.** In **A** and **B**, muscle responses were recorded during free-fall (acceleration peak: 8.8 m/s^2) with normal vision (NV). Note that recovery is total in the U.N. baboons but remains partial in the B.N. baboons

3 Results

We have shown in a previous report (Lacour et al. 1976) that spinal reflexes are strongly modified in the U.N. baboons and that recovery of normal and symmetrical spinal reflexes, which parallels recovery of posture and locomotion, is accomplished in three stages. A similar time-course with globally identical temporal characteristics is found when recording the H and T-reflexes during fall, and when recording muscle responses to fall. During the first stage (0 to 4–6 days), the EMG responses present a significant decrease on the ipsilateral side and a significant increase on the opposite side in the soleus muscle (Fig. 2A). Crossed effects and opposite effects are found in neck muscles and tibialis anterior flexor muscles, respectively. The second stage (6–14 days) is characterized by a reduction of the initial asymmetries, and the third stage leads to recovery of normal and symmetrical EMG responses to fall in all muscles tested.

In the cat, the postural deficits follow again a three-phases time-course (Fig. 3A) similar to that found in the baboon. Interestingly, recovery of locomotor equilibrium develops fast as postural deficits are fully compensated, i.e., around 40 days (Fig. 3B, left part). This delay corresponds to the necessary period of time for a fully achieved recovery of spinal reflexes and EMG responses to fall in the baboon.

3.1 Role of the Remaining Labyrinthine Afferents

In the baboon, a bilateral vestibular neurectomy performed in one-stage results in markedly depressed H an T-spinal reflexes, and in strongly depressed EMG responses

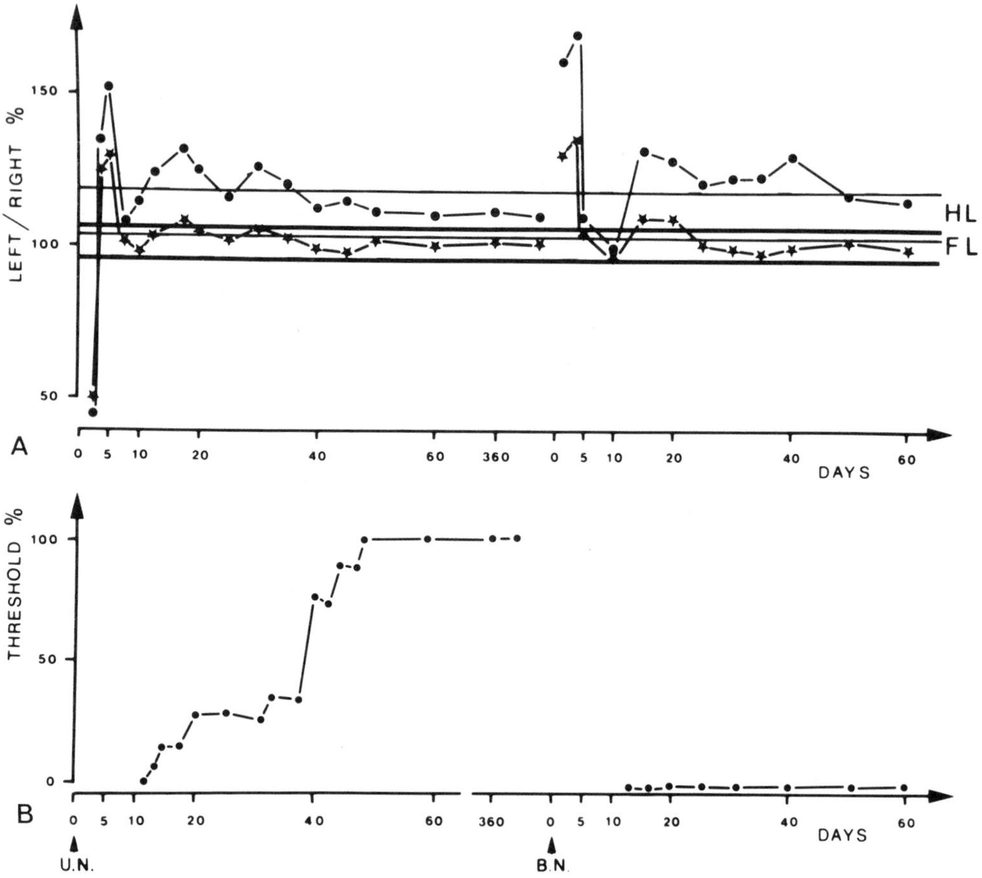

Fig. 3A, B. Role of the remaining labyrinth in compensating posture and locomotor equilibrium in the cat. **A** Mean evolution of the degree of postural asymmetry in the forelimbs (*FL, stars*) and the hindlimbs (*HL, filled circles*) as a function of the postoperative time in days (*abscissae*). Postural asymmetry is expressed in percent of control values recorded before surgery. The *horizontal thick and thin lines* are the confidence intervals ($P < 0.01$) of control values in Fl and HL, respectively. Vestibular neurectomy is performed on the right side (U.N.) and on the left side (B.N.) one year later. Note the Bechterew's phenomenon when lesioning the second labyrinth, and the full recovery of postural symmetry in both U.N. and B.N. cats. **B** Locomotor equilibrium recovery as testified by the maximum performance on the rotating beam. In *ordinate* maximum performance in percent of control maximum performance. In *abscissae* postoperative time in days. Note that equilibrium recovery develops fast as postural deficits are fully compensated (40 days) and is complete at around 50 days in U.N. cats. But all cats failed to recover following the second vestibular nerve section (B.N. cats)

to fall (Fig. 2B), on both sides. The recovery during postoperative days of normal spinal reflex activity relates closely to the compensation of postural and locomotor disorders. But while recovery of these functions is complete, the compensation of postural reactions to fall remains partial with a mean energy representing about 50% of control in the soleus muscle even 6 weeks post-surgery. In B.N. baboons following a two-stages surgery, postural and locomotor deficits, spinal reflex activity and EMG patterns to fall are first the mirror-images of the asymmetries resulting from the first lesion. This stage is followed by a period of bilateral depression in spinal activity and muscle responses to fall. Recovery of posture is complete and spinal activity returns toward normal values at about 40 days post-surgery, a period of time which is shorter than in B.N. baboons following one-stage surgery but similar to that found in U.N. baboons. The compensation of postural reactions to fall remains again partial in these animals.

Similar results were observed in the cat. The Bechterew phenomenon is illustrated in Fig. 3A: the postural asymmetries found after the second vestibular nerve section are the mirror-images of those seen after the first lesion. Recovery of posture develops in an identical way in both U.N. and B.N. two-stages cats. But all the B.N. cats (in one-stage or in two-stages) failed to return to a pre-operative level of performance with the locomotor equilibrium test (Fig. 3B). They remained unable to traverse the rotating beam, even in the lowest range of rotation and even at around 2 months post-operative. This latter observation confirms the results from the squirrel monkey rail test (Igarashi et al. 1970).

The remaining labyrinth appears therefore to play a major role in compensation of the dynamic functions in both cats and monkeys, but it does not constitute a necessary condition for full recovery of the static ones.

3.2 Role of the Visual Cues

Our results in the intact monkey (Lacour and Vidal 1978b; Vidal et al. 1979) have demonstrated that visual information concerning motion intervenes in the genesis of the early postural reactions to free-fall, suggesting that the visual motion cues could play an important role in compensating these postural reactions in U.N. and B.N. baboons.

Figure 4 presents these results by comparing the recovery of muscle responses during fall in the NV and SV conditions. In the U.N. baboon (Fig. 4A), one can observe a strong decrease of the responses in the SV condition as compared to the energy recorded in the NV condition. These significantly depressed EMG activities occur during the first two stages of compensation only (0–2 weeks). Later, the responses recorded in both NV and SV conditions do not differ from those found in intact baboons. In the B.N. baboons (Fig. 4B), the results show that the SV condition is always accompanied by a very strong motor depression during the entire test period. At 40 days post-surgery, the average response in both splenius muscles is 5% and 55% in the SV and NV condition, respectively. We also recorded the muscle responses in U.N. baboons when submitted to different vertical linear accelerations combined with various velocities of visual scene relative to the monkey's head. Figure 5 illustrates these results when the velocity of the visual scene is 0.6 times the velocity of the falling monkey and when the motion of the images is directed downward (reduced visual input: RV condition) or upward (enhanced visual input: EV condition). A visually induced modulation of the EMG responses is found which is (1) direction-specific: the muscle response energy increases in the EV condition and decreases in the RV condition, (2) acceleration amplitude-dependent: the EMG activity modulation increases as the acceleration amplitude decreases, (3) post-operative time-dependent: the most striking modulations are found during the first two stages of compensation and particularly during the second

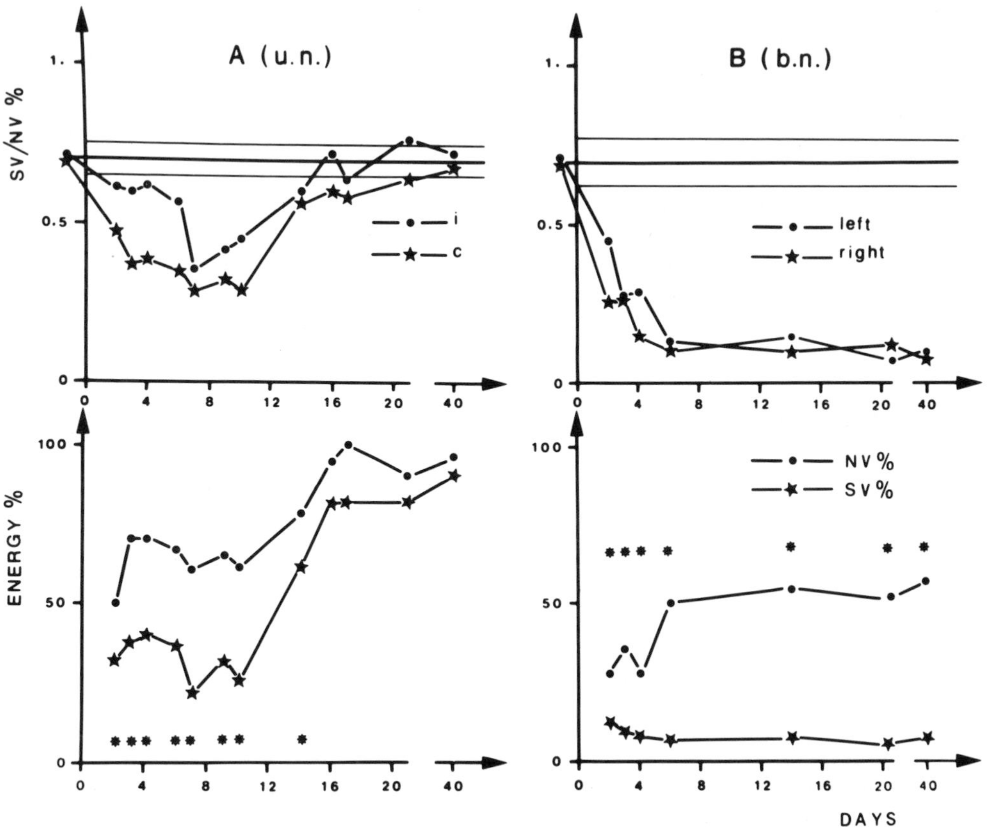

Fig. 4A, B. Role of the visual motion cues in compensating muscle responses to fall in U.N. and B.N. baboons. The average energy of splenius muscles responses are calculated during free-falls (acceleration peak = 8.8 m/s^2) with normal vision (NV) and with visual stabilization (SV). **A** Mean results from 5 U.N. baboons. *Upper graph* mean evolution of ratio SV/NV in ipsilateral (i) and contralateral (c) splenius muscles as a function of postoperative time in days (*abscissae*) and in percent of the control SV/NV ratio (*ordinate;* 25 values per point). The *thick* and the *thin horizontal lines* represent the mean value of SV/NV before surgery and its confidence interval ($P < 0.01$), respectively (n = 125 simples). *Lower graph* mean energy of contralateral splenius muscle recorded in NV and SV conditions. The energy is here expressed in percent of the control values in NV (NV %, *filled circles*) and SV (SV %, *stars*). Significant differences ($P < 0.01$) are indicated by *asterisks*. **B** Mean results from 3 B.N. baboons. Same presentation as in **A**

stage. This latter point confirms our results in the SV condition (cf. Fig. 4A). Moreover, a greater visually induced modulation is observed in the EV condition in the contralateral splenius muscle which is mainly related to the deafferented vestibular nuclei. This greater enhancement was also found in the ipsilateral soleus muscle, which is again related to the deafferented nuclei.

It is concluded that the partial recovery of EMG responses to fall in the B.N. baboons in the N.V. condition is mainly due to visual information concerning motion,

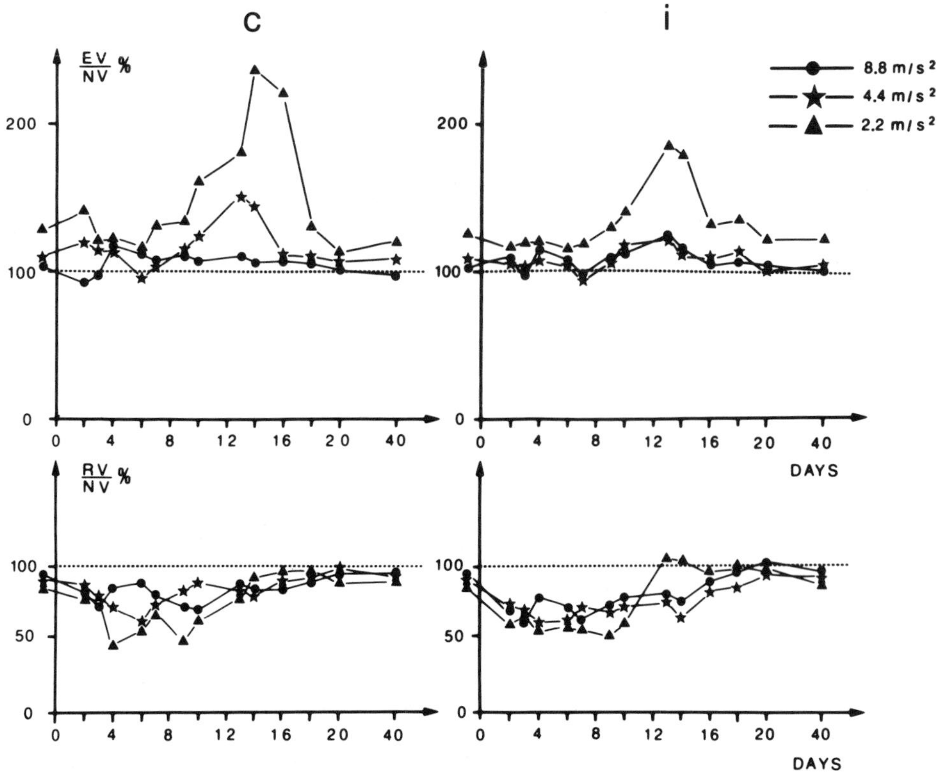

Fig. 5. Role of the visual motion cues in U.N. baboons. The muscle responses from ipsilateral (*i*) and contralateral (*c*) splenius capitis muscles were recorded during falls at different accelerations (8.8 m/s^2, 4.4 m/s^2 and 2.2 m/s^2) and with enhanced (EV) and reduced vision (RV). The velocity of the visual scene was 0.6 times the velocity of the falling monkey and motion of the images was either upward (EV condition) or downward (RV condition). We measured the ratios between energy recorded in EV and NV condition (*upper graphs*) and energy recorded in RV and NV condition (*lower graphs*). These ratios are expressed in percent of the control values (*ordinate*) and plotted as a function of the postoperative time in days (*abscissae*) (see text)

which replaces to the labyrinthine afferents. The visual motion cues fulfil only a transitory substitution function in the U.N. baboons, by supplying the decrease of neuronal activity in the vestibular nuclei. Once a background of activity is restored, the full compensation seems to be carried out by way of the intact labyrinth.

3.3 Role of the Sensorimotor Activity

This experiment was performed in cats by applying a sensorimotor restriction (SMR) at different postoperative periods.

When SMR is applied in the first postoperative week (Fig. 6A), postural symmetry recovery is blocked. The degree of postural asymmetry is similar before SMR application (2 days post-surgery) and just after release (9 days post-surgery). Later on, postu-

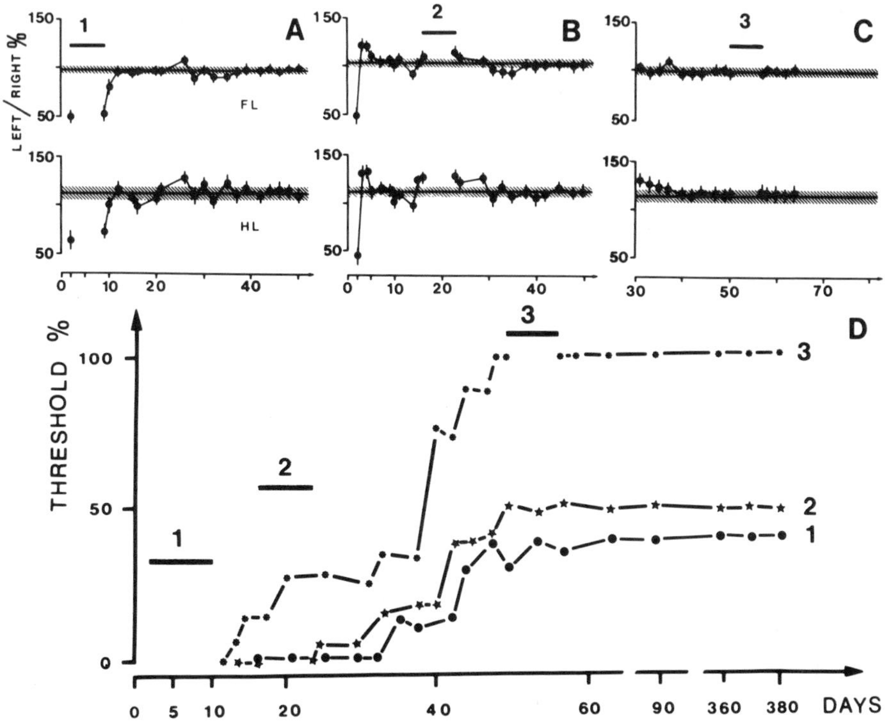

Fig. 6A–D. Role of the sensorimotor activity in compensating postural deficits and locomotor equilibium in U.N. cats. The sensorimotor restriction is applied either during the first postoperative week (*1* from 2nd to 9th day), or during the third week (*2* from 16th to 23rd days), or during the eight week when postural deficits are totally compensated (*3* from 50th to 57th day). **A B C** the degree of postural symmetry in the forelimbs (*FL, upper graphs*) and in the hindlimbs (*HL, lower graphs*) is expressed as in Fig. 3. Note that the recovery process is blocked when restriction is applied in the first week (**A**), is suspended when it is applied in the third week (**B**), and that there is no effect when it is performed in already compensated cats (**C**). *Each point* is represented with its 1% confidence interval; *the hatched area* is the confidence interval of control values ($P < 0.01$). **D** maximum performance of the U.N. cats on the rotating beam expressed in percent of the control maximum performance and plotted as a function of postoperative time. Note that the most striking effects are again found when restriction is applied early after surgery (*1* and *2*) and that locomotor equilibrium recovery remains incomplete even one year later. A restriction applied in already compensated cats (*3*) has no effect

ral deficits compensation is fully achieved and appears to develop faster, at least initially (cf. Fig. 3A). When SMR is applied in the third week (Fig. 6B) the recovery process is suspended: the postural asymmetry values are identical before and after restriction, but posture recovery develops normally later on. SMR applied in already compensated cats (Fig. 6C) does not affect the maintenance of compensation: no decompensation is observed. On the other hand, SMR applied in the first and third week prevented and delayed locomotor equilibrium recovery (Fig. 6D), with the earlier SMR producing again the most striking effects. The recovery process is blocked and develops only after release. But whereas posture recovery is fully achieved whatever the time of sensorimotor restriction application, locomotor equilibrium recovery remains incomplete. One year after unilateral vestibular nerve section, the maximum performance is about 40% (SMR in first week) and 50% (SMR in third week) of controls. SMR applied at a later time in already compensated cats has not effect.

It is interesting to see that recovery of dynamic functions such as locomotor equilibrium on the rotating beam is more affected by the sensorimotor restriction than recovery of static functions such as posture. One explanation is that the former requires multisensory inputs and a fast processing of information, the latter not needing such requirements.

4 Discussion

The spinal activity results from the integration at the spinal motoneuron level of both peripheral (proprioceptive and exteroceptive) and supra-spinal influences. This activity is adapted to the maintenance of posture and governs locomotion. The unilateral vestibular nerve section induces a strong imbalance between the vestibular nuclei activity on both sides (Gernandt and Thulin 1952; Shimazu and Precht 1966; Precht 1974) which leads to asymmetrical tonic and phasic vestibular influences on the spinal neurons. An asymmetrical spinal activity is thus created, which results in the impairment of the postural and locomotor progams. This first stage represents the immediate post-operative state of a system functionally disorganized by the sudden loss of a sensory input; it does not constitute a step in vestibular compensation. The compensation of postural and locomotor disorders parallels the recovery of tonic and dynamic vestibulospinal influences. This strongly suggests that recovery of a symmetrical and normal resting rate in the vestibular nuclei is a basic process in vestibular compensation.

Compensation starts at the second or acute stage with a fast but incomplete reduction of the initial asymmetries. This stage of reduction of the asymmetries is seen when testing the spinal activity or the EMG responses to fall of sensorimotor restrained baboons. It is again found when blind-folding the monkey during the first ten post-operative days, an observation which confirms the findings of Courjon et al. (1977) and Putkonen et al. (1977) in the cat. These results indicate that neither vision nor sensorimotor activity constitute major factors conditioning the appearance of the second stage of vestibular compensation. McCabe and Ryu (1972) reported a shutdown of resting activity in the vestibular nuclei on the intact side, occurring in animals with intact cerebellum only. They suggested that this fast-acting mechanism, tending to restore a new balance between the vestibular nuclei, constitutes a "first line of defense" against the initial imbalance and would be due to the adaptative function of the cerebellum. We suggest to compare this stage to the phenomenon variously known in the 19th century literature as central shock, diaschisis, asynapsia, depression, protective inhibition. It is for us a general adaptative reaction of the whole system which would use a reset to zero as a preliminary requirement to the recalibration process.

The recalibration process consists in disinhibiting the vestibular nuclei and, therefore, in restoring a balanced activity between nuclei on both sides as shown by Precht et al. (1966) and McCabe and Ryu (1969). This restored activity can continuously and tonically exert balanced influences on the spinal neurons and can be modulated in a reciprocal fashion by the intact labyrinth, resulting in restored functions which are qualitatively similar to those observed when both labyrinths are intact. Tonic and dynamic vestibular reflexes can be compensated for. The Putkonen assumption that static visual input represents a primary factor conditioning disinhibition of vestibular nuclei appears invalid. In our conditions, the sensorimotor restrained cats experienced normal static vision, but they failed to compensate postural and locomotor disorders until they became active. We do not mean that vision does not intervene at all: we have found that visual motion cues act as a transitory substitution process in the U.N. baboons, probably by improving the amount of activity in the deafferented vestibular nuclei. Instead, we believe that all available information experienced by active exploration is needed to restore an adequate resting rate in the vestibular nuclei. No one piece is sufficient alone, all are necessary for achieving a normally developing, well-adapted compensation. These multisensory inputs tonically and dynamically substitute in permanence for the missing labyrinthine afferents. In this process, the remaining labyrinth appears to be the most effective for recreating the dynamic counterpart: muscle responses to fall as well as locomotor equilibrium on the beam fail to recover totally in B.N. animals. Furthermore, our studies suggest that recovery will be maximum (fast and complete) only if all available information is actively used in the early stages of compensation. This is illustrated by the incomplete and delayed locomotor equilibrium recovery when cats were submitted to sensorimotor restriction applied in the first and third post-operative weeks. It is also shown by the predominant role played by the visual motion cues during this period in the U.N. baboons. These results suggest that a C.N.S. "sensitive period" probably exists for functional recovery, which may be crucial for achieving functionally well- or mal-adapted recovery. But its real existence, which would be of great importance in human pathology, should be fully investigated.

As in the intact subject, the concerted activity of many central nervous structures is required to integrate the various sensory inputs involved in the regulation of motor programs. The vestibular nuclei, the reticular formation, the cerebellum, the cerebellar nuclei and the inferior olive are now known to be such integrative structures where labyrinthine, visual and somatosensory afferents converge. In the U.N. animals, these structures cooperate to forward to the deafferented vestibular nuclei the most appropriate substituted signals. It is interesting to note that all these structures show increased activity in compensated rats and a return to normal activity in decompensated rats (Llinas and Walton 1979), except the vestibular nuclei which present in the latter case a strong imbalance similar to that recorded in the uncompensated rats. Furthermore, they are highly interelated anatomically and functionally, and they all play a significanct role in motor control, posture and equilibrium. Any defect in any sensory input or central nervous structure implicated in the readjustment of the motor programs and in the development of the new automatisms will result in decompensation, i.e., reappearance of some vestibular deficits. Synaptic mechanisms in the partially deafferented vestibular nuclei can improve the efficiency of such a central processing. Electrophysiological signs of functional changes were found in the properties of these neurons (Dieringer and Precht 1979a,b,c). The first signs were observed as soon as 3 to 4 days post-operative. This time interval is sufficient for degeneration of vestibular afferent terminals (2 to 3 days: see Hillman 1972) and, in the frog, it corresponds globally to the necessary minimal time period for occurrence of Bechterew's phenomenon. It appears thus that denervation supersensitivity and collateral sprouting can play a positive role. But we believe that neural plasticity has a complementary rather than a leading role in vestibular compensation in adult subjects.

Finally, it is concluded that vestibular compensation is achieved by means of a multisensory substitution process requiring the activity of the subject. It resembles a sensorimotor relearning process which demonstrates plasticity within the functioning C.N.S. and which is aided by neural plasticity at the cellular level.

References

Azzena CB (1969) Role of the spinal cord in compensating the effects of hemilabyrinthectomy. Arch Ital Biol 107: 43–53

Azzena GB, Mameli O, Tolu E (1979) Cerebellar contribution in compensating the vestibular function. In: Granit R, Pompeiano O (eds) Reflex control of posture and movement. Prog in Brain Res, vol 50. Elsevier/North-Holland Biomed Press, Amsterdam New York, pp 599–606

Bechterew W von (1883) Ergebnisse der Durchschneidung des N. acusticus nebst Erörterung der Bedeutung der semicirculären für das Körpergleichgewicht. Pflügers Arch Ges Physiol 30: 312–347

Berthoz A, Lacour M, Soechtering J, Vidal PP (1979) The role of vision in the control of posture during linear motion. In: Granit R, Pompeiano O (eds) Reflex control of posture and movement. Prog in Brain Res, vol 50. Elsevier/North-Holland Biomed Press, Amsterdam New York, pp 197–209

Courjon JH, Jeannerod M, Ossuzio I, Schmidt R (1977) The role of vision in compensation of vestibulo-occular reflex after hemilabyrinthectomy in the cat. Exp Brain Res 28: 235–248

Dieringer N, Precht W (1979a) Mechanisms of compensation for vestibular deficits in the frog. I. Modification of the excitatory commissural system. Exp Brain Res 36: 311–328

Dieringer N, Precht W (1979b) Mechanisms of compensation for vestibular deficits in the frog. II. Modification of the inhibitory pathways. Exp Brain Res 36: 329–341

Dieringer N, Precht W (1979c) Synaptic mechanisms involved in compensation of vestibular function following hemilabyrinthectomy. In: Granit R, Pompeiano O (eds) Reflex control of posture and movement. Prog Brain Res, vol 50. Elsevier/North-Holland and Biomed Press, Amsterdam New York, pp 607–615

Ewald JR (1892) Physiologische Untersuchungen über das Endorgan des nervus octavus. Bergmann, Wiesbaden, p 325

Gernandt BE, Thulin CA (1952) Vestibular mechanism of facilitation and inhibition of cord reflexes. Am J Physiol 172: 653–660

Hillman DE (1972) Vestibulocerebellar input in the frog: Anatomy. In: Brodal A, Pompeiano O (eds) Basic aspects of central vestibular mechanisms. Prog Brain Res, vol 37. Elsevier/North-Holland, Amsterdam, pp 329–339

Igarashi M, Watanabe T, Maxian PM (1970) Dynamic equilibrium in squirrel monkeys after unilateral and bilateral labyrinthectomy. Acta Otolaryngol 69: 247–253

Jensen DW (1979a) Reflex control of acute postural asymmetry and compensatory symmetry after a unilateral vestibular lesion. Neuroscience 4: 1059–1073

Jensen DW (1979b) Vestibular compensation: tonic spinal influence upon spontaneous descending vestibular nuclear activity. Neuroscience 4: 1075–1084

Kolb G (1955) Untersuchungen über zentrale Kompensation und Kompensationsbewegungen einseitig enstateter Frösche. Z Vergl Physiol 37: 136–160

Lacour M, Vidal PP (1978b) Influence de l'environnement visuel sur les réponses musculaires précoces du Singe (Papio papio) en chute libre. J Physiol 74: 9A

Lacour M, Xerri C (1980) Compensation of postural reactions to fall in the vestibular neurectomized monkey. Role of the visual motion cues. Exp Brain Res 40: 103–110
Lacour M, Roll JP, Appaix M (1976) Modifications and development of spinal reflexes in the alert baboon (Papio papio) following a unilateral vestibular neurotomy. Brain Res 113: 255–269
Lacour M, Xerri C, Hugon M (1978a) Muscle responses and monosynaptic reflexes in falling monkey. Role of the vestibular system. J Physiol 74: 427–438
Lacour M, Xerri C, Hugon M (1979) Compensation of postural reactions to fall in the vestibular neurectomized monkey. Role of the remaining labyrinthine afferences. Exp Brain Res 37: 563–580
Llinas R, Walton R (1977) Significance of the olivo-cerebellar system in compensation of ocular position following unilateral labyrinthectomy. In: Baker R, Berthoz A (eds) Control of gaze by brain stem neurons. Developments in neuroscience, vol 1. Elsevier/North-Holland Biomed Press, Amsterdam new York, pp 399–408
Llinas R, Walton K (1979) Vestibular compensation: a distributed property of the central nervous system. In: Asanuma H, Wilson VJ (eds) Integration in the nervous system. Igaku-Shoin, Tokyo New York, pp 145–166
Llinas R, Walton R, Hillman DE, Sotelo C (1975) Inferior olive: its role in motor learning. Science 190: 1230–1231
Magnus R (1924) Körperstellung. Springer, Berlin
McCabe BF, Ryu JH (1969) Experiments on vestibular compensation. Laryngoscope (St. Louis) 79: 1728–1736
McCabe BF, Ryu JH, Sekitani T (1972) Further experiments on vestibular compensation. Laryngoscope (St. Louis) 82: 381–396
Precht W (1974) Characteristics of vestibular neurons after acute and chronic labyrinthine destruction. In: Kornhuber HH (ed) Vestibular system, Part II, Handbook of sensory physiology. Springer, Berlin Heidelberg New York, pp 451–462
Precht W, Shimazu H, Markham CH (1966) A mechanism of central compensation of vestibular function following hemilabyrinthectomy. J Neurophysiol 29: 996–1010
Putkonen PTS, Courjon JH, Jeannerod M (1977) Compensation of postural effects of hemilabyrinthectomy in the cat. A sensory substitution process. Exp Brain Res 28: 249–257
Rademaker CGJ (1935) Réactions labyrinthiques et équilibre. Masson, Paris
Schaefer KP, Meyer DL (1974) Compensation of vestibular lesions. In: Kornhuber HH (ed) Vestibular system, Part II. Handbook of sensory physiology. Springer, Berlin Heidelberg New York, pp 463–490
Schaefer KP, Meyer DL, Wilhelms G (1979) Somatosensory and cerebellar influences on compensation of labyrinthine lesions. In: Granit R, Pompeiano O (eds) Reflex control of posture and movement. Prog Brain Res, vol 50. Elsevier/North-Holland Biomed Press, Amsterdam New York, pp 591–598
Shimazu H, Precht W (1966) Inhibition of central vestibular neurons from the contralateral labyrinth and its mediating pathway. J Neurophysiol 29: 467–492
Vidal PP, Lacour M, Barthoz A (1979) Contribution of vision to muscle responses in monkey during free-fall: visual stabilization decreases vestibular-dependent responses. Exp Brain Res 37: 241–252
Xerri C, Lacour M (1980) Compensation des déficits posturaux et cinétiques après neurectomie vestibulaire unilatérale chez le chat. Rôle de l'activité sensorimotrice. Acta Otolaryngol 90: 414–424

The Lateral Reticular Nucleus. Role in Vestibular Compensation

G.B. AZZENA, E. TOLU, and O. MAMELI[1]

1 Introduction

These experiments were performed to verify an assumption resulting from previous researches. It was, in fact, observed that compensation of defects provoked by unilateral lesion of the labyrinth could be impaired by removal of spinal afferents. This spinal decompensation was followed by the reappearance of all the symptoms elicited by previous vestibular deafferentation (Azzena 1969). Furthermore, the balance of electrical activity between the vestibular nuclear complexes of both sides was upset by spinal decompensation and was found to be similar to that recorded in the acute stage of unilateral labyrinthectomy (Azzena et al. 1976, 1977). Thus, the release of vestibular symptoms depended upon the different level of excitability of the vestibular nuclei. According to these results, the vestibular compensation could be considered as a substitution process in which the spinal cord is involved. Since the effects of unilateral lesion of the labyrinth result in a dramatic alteration of postural tone and of oculomotor control, it was assumed that the role of the spinal cord in compensation could take place through the influence of the spino-reticular pathways. In fact, the ascending spino-reticular neurons must be deeply modified by the postural asymmetries which follow unilateral vestibular deafferentation. Since these neurons receive signals arising from the bilateral cutaneous and high threshold afferents (components of flexor reflex afferents, FRA; Eccles and Lundberg 1959; Grant et al. 1966; Lundberg and Oscarsson 1962; Oscarsson 1973; Oscarsson and Rosén 1966), the lesion of one labyrinth should be followed by an asymmetrical projection on the spino-reticular neurons. Furthermore, the same neurons are modulated by descending signals from ipsilateral Deiters' nucleus and contralateral somatosensory cortex (Brodal et al. 1967; Clendenin et al. 1974; Coulter et al. 1974, 1976; Grillner et al. 1968; Hoshino and Pompeiano 1977; Künzle and Wiesendanger 1974; Kuypers 1958a,b,c; Pompeiano 1975, 1977; Pompeiano and Hoshino 1977; Rosén and Scheid 1973b).

The output of spino-reticular neurons, resulting from the integration of descending and ascending messages, is forwarded to the contralateral lateral reticular nucleus (LRN) through the bilateral ventral flexor reflex tract (b VFRT) (Grant et al. 1966; Lundberg and Oscarsson 1962; Oscarsson 1973; Rosén and Scheid 1973a,b). As a con-

1 Institute of Human Physiology, University of Sassari, Via Muroni 23, 07100 Sassari, Italy

sequence, the lateral reticular nucleus is situated in a crucial position for controlling the posture and reflex movements, since its tonic discharge also activates the cerebellar cortex (Azzena and Ohno 1973; Eccles et al. 1967; Sasaki and Strata 1967). We have, therefore, studied in hemilabyrinthectomized and compensated guinea pigs both the effects of LRN lesions and the modifications to the electrical activity of LRN neurons, before and after spinal decompensation. In addition, the effects produced by LRN lesions were compared with those elicited by lesions of the inferior olives (IO). Previous researches showed that chemical lesion of inferior olive neurons resulted in vestibular decompensation (Azzena et al. 1979; Llinàs et al. 1975).

2 Methods

The experiments were performed on 90 guinea pigs. Each was anesthetized with ether and subjected to destruction of the left labyrinth by drilling the internal ear. The animals were allowed to compensate the symptoms elicited by the unilateral vestibular lesion and were subdivided in two groups. The animals of the first group (36 guinea pigs) were then anesthetized by Ketamine plus Valium. Out of 36 animals 24 were submitted to electrolytic lesion of one LRN, ipsilateral or contralateral to the vestibular deafferentation. These lesions were made by passing positive dc between a monopolar, stereotaxically driven, electrode and a reference electrode fixed to the ipsilateral temporal muscle. In 12 animals the electrolytic lesion was aimed at the inferior olive of one side. Since no stereotaxic coordinates of these central areas are available, preliminary lesions were performed in 10 normal guinea pigs. Different degrees of lesions were obtained by varying the intensity and duration of the dc between 1.2 and 2.5 mA and 10–25 s. The animals were examined only for changes in posture, motility, and eye movements, observations starting when the effects of anesthesia faded away. Electro-oculograms were in some cases recorded through bipolar electrodes placed in the external canti and connected to dc amplifiers and to a Grass model 7 polygraph. The position, as well as the extent of electrolytic lesion, was examined by histological control in serial sections stained by the Nissl method. Postmortem controls were also performed for lesions of the VIII nerve. The animals of the second group (54 guinea pigs) were utilized for recording the electrical activity from neurons of lateral reticular nuclei. The animals were anesthetized with Ketamine plus Valium, placed in the stereotaxic apparatus, immobilized with Flaxedil and artificially respired. Body temperature was maintained at 37°C throughout the experiments and ECG was continuously monitored. Additional doses of anesthetic drug were administered at 30 min intervals. The lateral reticular nuclei were approached from the dorsal side by exposing the brainstem at the obex level and employing the same stereotaxic coordinates as for electrolytic lesions. Extracellular unitary discharge in the LRN was recorded by tungsten microelectrodes (resistance 700–900 kΩ). During the first ten experiments the LRN neurons were identified by antidromic stimulation through stainless steel electrodes inserted in the cerebellar white matter. A laminectomy between T3 and T4 exposed the spinal cord, which was then protected by warm mineral oil. Both common radial nerves were dissected and mounted on bipolar electrodes connected to an insulated stimulator (Digitimer). Intensities of 5–10 times the threshold were usually employed for nerve stimulation. Analyses of LRN neurons were performed by converting single spikes to standard pulses, which were fed to a microprocessor for construction of post-stimulus-time-histograms (PSTH) and cumulative frequency distributions (CFD) following 100 stimuli to each radial nerve and using 1 ms address. The spontaneous discharge rate of the LRN cells was also measured together with the evoked potentials elicited by the radial nerve stimulations. Recordings were carried out before and after spinal transection at T3–T4 level. Position of the microelectrode was checked by histological control.

3 Results

Effects of Lesions. The first observations of the effects provoked by chronic lesions of the LRN and inferior olive started after the anesthesia had completely worn off. Figures 1A–D display the effects provoked by unilateral lesion of LRN. A normal guinea pig is shown in Fig. 1A, and following lesion of the left labyrinth in Fig. 1B. The same animal recovered from vestibular deafferentation, and compensation was complete after 25 days (Fig. 1C). After right LRN lesion (Fig. 1D) the curvature of the trunk and torsion of the head toward the labyrinthine lesion reappeared, together with circling movements toward the operated side. However, the main aspect of decompensation provoked by LRN lesion is represented by asymmetries of muscle tone, particularly of the forelimbs. The effects of LRN lesion are superimposed on those elicited by previous contralateral vestibular deafferentation, thus resulting an increased tonic contraction of the extensor muscles of the forelimb, contralateral to the vestibular deafferentation and ipsilateral to LRN lesion. Contrarily, the forelimb ipsilateral to the vestibular deafferentation and contralateral to the LRN lesion showed a tonic increase of flexor muscle. The lesion of the LRN ipsilateral to the vestibular deafferentation was less effective. Only moderate torsion of the trunk and of the head was observed. In any case, lesion of LRN was followed by alterations of oculomotor control. These effects were more marked when the LRN lesion was located in the ventrocaudal part of the nucleus (Fig. 2), while lesions were ineffective when areas of the reticular formation around the LRN were affected. Figure 3 illustrates the position of a lesion placed in the dorsal cap of the left inferior olive in a left hemilabyrinthectomized and compensated guinea pig (Fig. 3A, B). Figure 3C and D show the specific feature of the inferior olive lesion. In this case, decompensation was characterized by the reappearance of the ocular nystagmus, lacking after LRN lesion. The direction of the nystagmus was independent of lesion laterality, but it was not so for the frequency of eye jerks. In fact, the direction was similar to that elicited by the labyrinthine lesion, while the frequency was higher following lesion of the left inferior olive.

Effects of Spinal Decompensation on LRN. Twentyeight units were recorded from left and 26 from right lateral reticular nuclei of left hemilabyrinthectomized and compensated animals, before and after spinal decompensation. The great majority of these cells were recorded from the ventral-caudal part of the LRN and responded to elec-

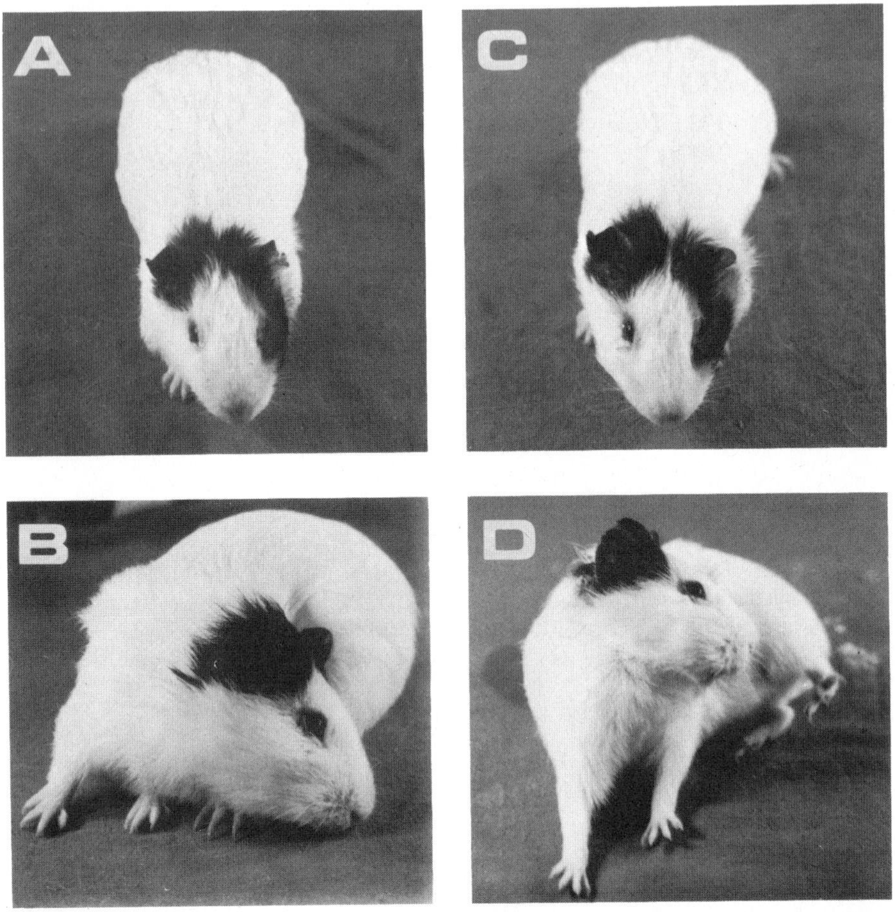

Fig. 1A–D. Compensation and decompensation following lesion of right LRN of asymmetries elicited by left hemilabyrinthectomy. **A** normal; **B** 60 min after labyrinthine lesion; **C** compensation after 45 days; **D** decompensation following right LRN lesion

trical stimulation of radial nerves of both sides. Therefore, these neurons can be attributed to that part of the LRN which receives bilateral projections of spino-reticular neurons, whose axons ascend within the bVFRT (Ekerot et al. 1979; Grant et al. 1966; Lundberg and Oscarsson 1962; Oscarsson 1973; Oscarsson and Rosén 1966). Figure 4 illustrates the response of a cell recorded from the left LRN to stimulation of the contralateral radial nerve, before spinal decompensation (**A** and **B**) and after (**C** and **D**). As shown by PSTH and CFD, the response of the cell was increased by spinal transection. During compensation the response consisted of 1.54 spikes/stimulus and of 2.43 spikes/stimulus after removal of spinal afferents. Figure 5 reports the effects of spinal decompensation on the response of a right LRN neuron to stimulation of the ipsilateral radial nerve. Figures 5A and B are the PSTH and CFD obtained during compensation. The response was characterized by 2.34 spikes/stimulus. Figures 5C and D

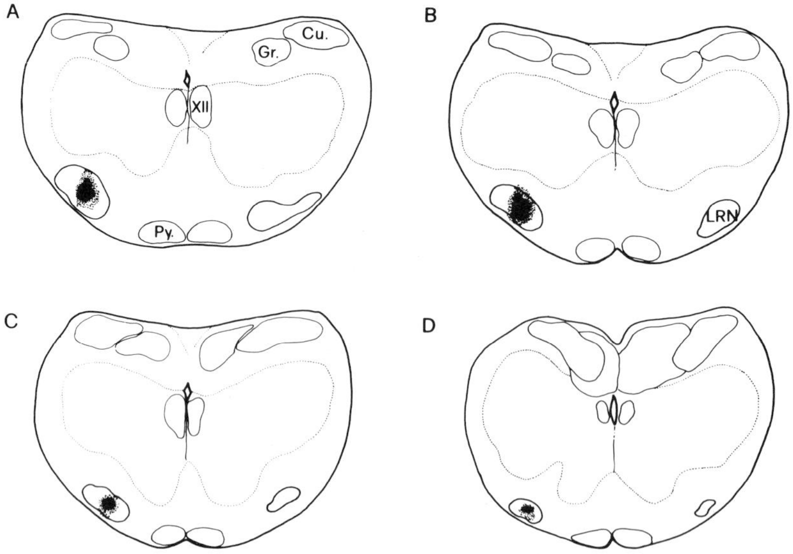

Fig. 2A–D. Anatomical localization of lesion of the LRN in the guinea pig reported in Fig. 1. The extent of lesion is shown by *black* and *stippled areas* indicating complete lesion and glial processes. Schematic drawings taken from histological serial sections. *Gr,* gracile nucleus; *Cu,* cuneate nucleus; *XII,* hypoglossal nerve nucleus; *Py,* pyramidal tract; *LRN,* lateral reticular nucleus

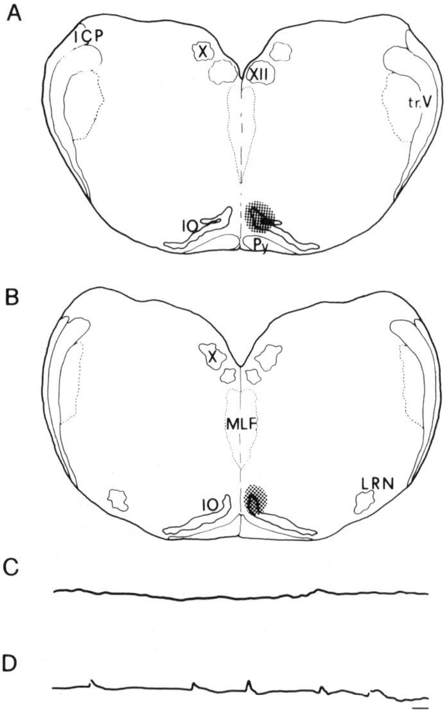

Fig. 3. A,B Schematic drawings taken from histological sections of brainstem of a hemilabyrinthectomized and compensated guinea pig showing the localization of the electrolytic lesion (*dotted areas*) in the dorsal cap of the left inferior olive. **C, D** Electro-oculograms recorded during compensation stage and after the inferior olive lesion as reported in **A** and **B**. *ICP,* inferior cerebellar peduncle; *tr.v,* nucleus and tract of the fifth nerve; *X,* dorsal nucleus of vagus nerve; *XII,* hypoglossal nucleus; *LRN,* lateral reticular nucleus; *Py,* pyramidal tract; *MLF,* medial longitudinal fasciculus. Horizontal calibration for **C** and **D**: 1 s

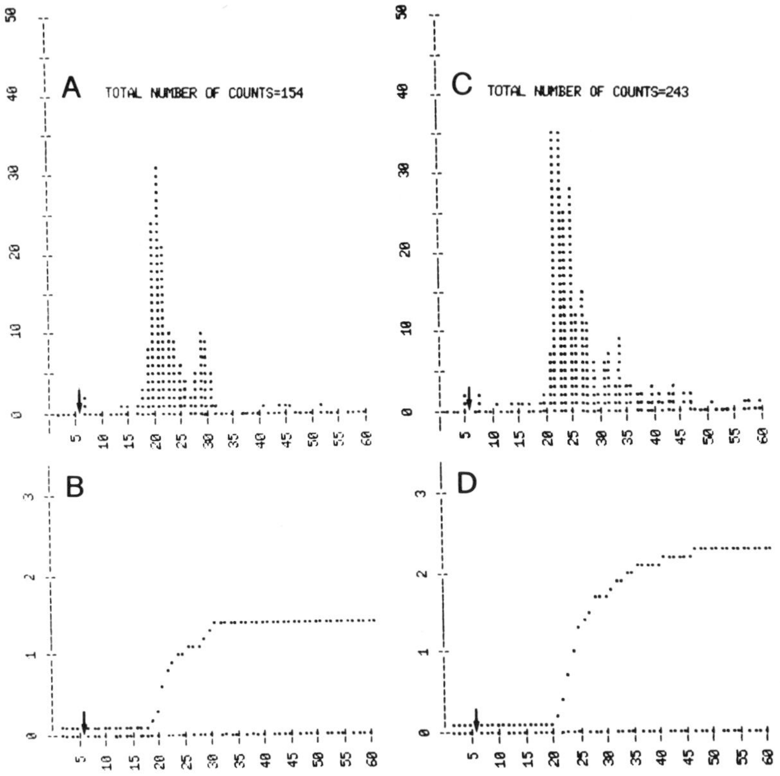

Fig. 4A–D. PSTHs and CFDs of response of a left LRN neuron to 100 stimuli to right radial nerve during compensation (**A, B**), and following spinal decompensation (**C, D**). Stimulation consisted in double shock at 500 Hz. *Ordinate,* for PSTH, number of counts; for CFD, counts added per stimulus. *Abscissa,* for PSTH and CFD, 5 ms/division. The *arrows* mark the moment of stimulus

show, following spinalization, a decrease of the response which consisted of 1.51 spikes/stimulus. Therefore, following spinal decompensation the response of LRN neurons is reduced during stimulation of the ipsilateral radial nerve and increased during stimulation of the contralateral radial nerve.

4 Discussion

Compensation of the vestibular syndrome is a particular aspect of the labyrinthine physiology at present under intensive investigation. The unilateral lesion of the labyrinth is followed by a series of defects which gradually disappear. Thus, the study of vestibular compensation leads to the investigation of the mechanisms underlying the gradual readjustment of the posture. According to the results of Courjon et al. (1977) and of Putkonen et al. (1977), the visual input is a valid candidate for the generation of vestibular compensation. In hemilabyrinthectomized kittens, the deprivation of visual input delays the compensation which proceeds faster after allowing the animals to

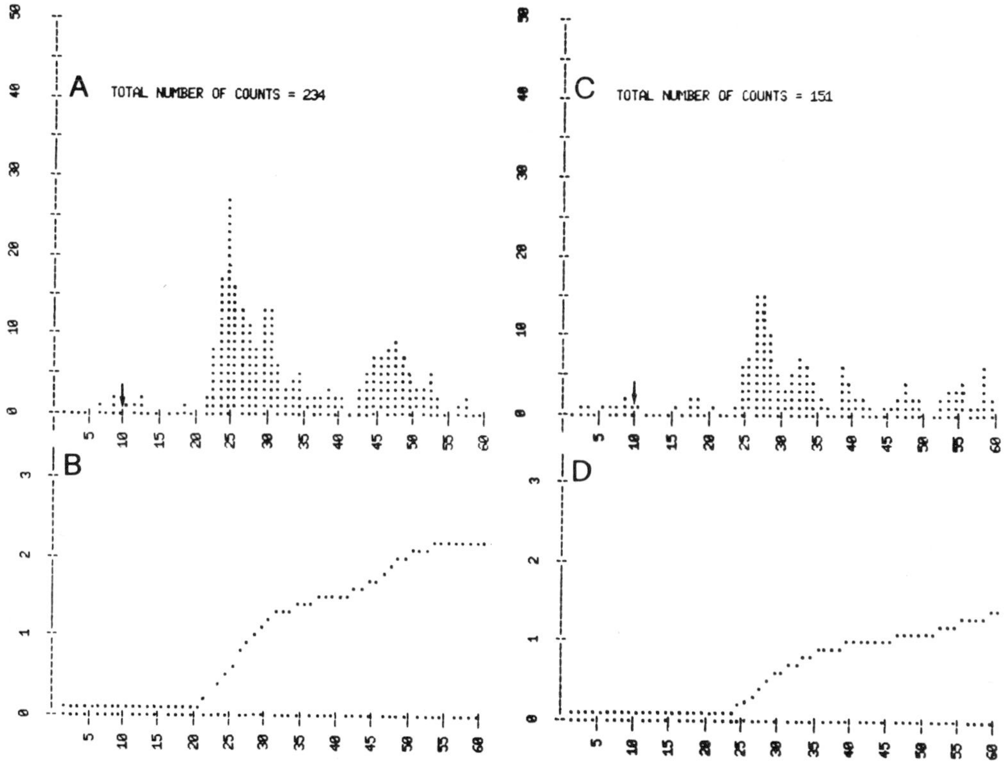

Fig. 5A–D. PSTHs and CFDs of response of a right LRN neuron to 100 stimuli to right radial nerve during compensation (**A, B**), and after spinal decompensation (**C, D**). Calibrations as in Fig. 4

behave in a normally lighted environment. This observation agrees with the results which indicate that visual input impinges upon cells of vestibular nuclei modulating their unitary discharge (Azzena et al. 1978, 1980). Furthermore, responses of vestibular neurons to optokinetic stimulation were also found (Azzena et al. 1974; Waespe and Henn 1977). In our laboratory we ascribed the vestibular compensation to the influence of the spinal cord. Section of the spinal cord not only induced the reappearance of all the symptoms elicited by previous hemilabyrinthectomy, but disrupted the balance of the electrical activity between the vestibular nuclear complexes which was restored during the compensation stage (Azzena et al. 1976, 1977). The unitary discharge of Deiters' cells following spinalization is similar to that observed by Precht et al. (1966) in cats during the acute stage of vestibular deafferentation. Both the acute and decompensated stages are characterized by a decrease in electrical activity of the deafferented vestibular cells and by an increase in those of the intact side. In both conditions the different level in excitability of vestibular neurons is the basis of changes in posture and oculomotor control. The spinal afferents should then participate in vestibular compensation by providing an excitatory input to the vestibular neurons of the lesioned side and exert an inhibitory effect on those of the intact side. Since the acute stage of unilateral labyrinthectomy is characterized by an intense alteration of the posture (Azzena 1969), we suggested that the influence of the spinal cord could take place through the asymmetrical activation of spinal neurons which are connected with cutaneous and high threshold receptors, these being particularly influenced by muscle tone and postural asymmetries (Eccles and Lundberg 1959; Ekerot et al. 1979). Since the central connections of these neurons act on a control system which involves the LRN, the lateral vestibular nucleus and the cerebellar cortex, these experiments were performed to verify whether the LRN participates in compensation. The results of this research showed that lesions of the LRN, particularly when the nucleus contralateral to the labyrinthine lesion was destroyed, induced the reappearance of the labyrinthine syndrome. The postural behavior of the animal indicated an increase of the extensor tonus in the forelimb ipsilateral to the LRN lesion and contralateral to the vestibular deafferentation. This is justified by the conditions established by both lesion. The LRN lesion, in fact, is followed by ipsilateral extensor tonus due to disinhibition of the neurons of the lateral vestibular nucleus and disfacilitation of the fastigial nucleus (Corvaja et al. 1977; Pompeiano 1979). This effect augment that elicited by previous contralateral hemilabyrinthectomy (Azzena 1969). When the lesion affects the LRN ipsilateral to the labyrinthine lesion, the effects are less pronounced owing to the opposite sign. Furthermore, it must be stressed that lesion of the LRN misses the reappearance of the eye nystagmus, but influences only the posture. Proof that the LRN neurons exert an asymmetrical control arises from the modifications in their responses to electrical stimulation of the peripheral nerves following spinal decompensation. If we assume that the stimulation of the nerves, in animals previously paralized, replaces to a certain extent the influence of peripheral afferents in the normally behaving animal, the spinal decompensation can be said to provoke a reduction of the response following ipsilateral nerve stimulation, and opposite pattern following contralateral nerve stimulation. Since, in the present research, the responses of the LRN neurons were analyzed with a bilateral receptive field, it means that the nerve stimulations influenced the neurons of the LRN through receiving afferents from spinal neurons whose axons ascend through the bVFRT (Clendenin et al. 1974; Grant et al. 1966; Lundberg and Oscarsson 1962; Oscarsson and Rosén 1966; Rosén and Scheid 1973a,b). Therefore, the spinal transection provokes an asymmetrical response of the LRN, in that this asymmetry actually arises within the motor spinal centers where interneurons are present which connect the FRA with the bVFRT neurons (Ekerot et al. 1979). On the other hand, the cervical asymmetry could well depend upon the propriospinal connections deriving from the thoracic and lumbar segments (Ekerot et al. 1979; Gernand and Megirian 1961). Thus, it could be assumed that, at cervical level, following spinal transection the interneurons of the motor center, which receive signals from the forelimb ipsilateral to the NRL, are disfacilitated, while those receiving signals from the contralateral forelimb are disinhibited. The presence of a spinal asymmetry is shown also by the fact that hemisection of the spinal cord is able to revive the vestibular syndrome (Azzena 1969). The results obtained by lesions of the inferior olive deserve comment, particularly in order to stress the reappearance of the eye nystagmus that was lacking after LRN lesions. It has been recently shown by recording, lesion, and microstimulation experiments that the dorsal cap of the inferior olive receives visual information, which is in turn forwarded to the contralateral cerebellar flocculus (Barmack and Hess 1980a,b; Barmack and Simpson 1980;

Maekawa and Simpson 1973). Since floccular Purkinje cells control the ocular motoneurons through their influence on vestibular nuclei (Ito 1977), it is likely that lesion of the dorsal cap of the inferior olive is followed by a vestibular decompensation characterized by the reappearance of the eye nystagmus. Similar results were obtained in hemilabyrinthectomized and compensated rats and guinea pigs following injection of 3-acetyl-pyridine (Azzena et al. 1979; Llinàs et al. 1975). The only difference was represented by a complete labyrinthine syndrome, since in these cases the drug provoked a complete lesion of all neurons of both inferior olives.

5 Summary

In hemilabyrinthectomized and compensated guinea pigs the effects of lesions of the lateral reticular nucleus and of the inferior olives are studied. Both lesions provoke the revival of the labyrinthine syndrome, the only difference being represented by the fact that LRN lesions mainly concern the postural asymmetries, while those of inferior olives provoke the reappearance of the eye nystagmus as well. In a second group of similarly prepared animals the recordings of the electrical activity of LRN neurons show that spinal decompensation provokes an asymmetrical modification of their responses to electrical stimulation of forelimb nerves. It is concluded that spinal decompensation is brought about by removal of afferents to the LRN from spino-reticular neurons connected with the cutaneous and high threshold receptors.

Acknowledgment. This research was supported by grants of CNR and Ministero Pubblica Istruzione.

References

Azzena GB (1969) Role of the spinal cord in compensating the effects of hemilabyrinthectomy. Arch Ital Biol 107: 43–53

Azzena GB, Ohno T (1973) Influence of spino-reticulo-cerebellar pathway on Purkinje cells of the paramedian lobule. Exp Brain Res 17: 63–74

Azzena GB, Azzena MT, Marini R (1974) Optokinetic nystagmus and vestibular nuclei. Exp Neurol 42: 158–168

Azzena GB, Mameli O, Tolu E (1976) Vestibular nuclei of hemilabyrinthectomized guinea pigs during decompensation. Arch Ital Biol 114: 389–398

Azzena GB, Mameli O, Tolu E (1977) Vestibular units during decompensation. Experientia 33: 234–235

Azzena GB, Tolu E, Mameli O (1978) Responses of vestibular units to visual input. Arch Ital Biol 116: 120–129

Azzena GB, Mameli O, Tolu E (1979) Cerebellar contribution in compensating the vestibular function. In: Granit R, Pompeiano O (eds) Reflex control of posture and movement. Progress in brain research, vol 50. Elsevier/North-Holland Biomedical Press, Amsterdam New York Oxford, p 599

Azzena GB, Mameli O, Tolu E (1980) Distribution of visual input to the vestibular nuclei. Arch Ital Biol 118: 196–204

Barmack NH, Hess DT (1980a) Multiple-unit activity evoked in dorsal cap of inferior olive of the rabbit by visual stimulation. J Neurophysiol 43: 151–164

Barmack NH, Hess DT (1980b) Eye movements evoked by microstimulation of dorsal cap of inferior olive in the rabbit. J Neurophysiol 43: 165–181

Barmack NH, Simpson JI (1980) Effects of microlesions of dorsal cap of inferior olive of rabbits on optokinetic and vestibuloocular reflexes. J Neurophysiol 43: 182–206

Brodal P, Marsala J, Brodal A (1967) The cerebral cortical projection to the lateral reticular nucleus in the cat with special reference to sensorimotor cortical areas. Brain Res 6: 252–274

Clendenin M, Ekerot CF, Oscarson O, Rosén I (1974) The lateral reticular nucleus in the cat. I. Mossy fiber distribution in cerebellar cortex. Exp Brain Res 21: 473–486

Corvaja N, Grofova I, Pompeiano O, Walberg F (1977) The lateral reticular nucleus in the cat. II. Effects of lateral reticular lesions on posture and reflex movements. Neuroscience 2: 929–943

Coulter JD, Mergner T, Pompeiano O (1974) Macular influences on ascending spino-reticular neurons located in the cervical cord. Brain Res 82: 322–327

Coulter JD, Mergner T, Pompeiano O (1976) Effects of static tilt on cervical spino-reticular tract neurons. J Neurophysiol 39: 45–62

Courjon JH, Jeannerod M, Ossuzio I, Schmid R (1977) The role of vision in compensation of vestibulo-ocular reflex after hemilabyrinthectomy in the cat. Exp Brain Res 28: 235–248

Eccles RM, Lundberg A (1959) Synaptic actions in motoneurones by afferents which may evoke the flexion reflex. Arch Ital Biol 97: 199–221

Eccles JC, Ito M, Szentagothai J (1967) The cerebellum as a neuronal machine. Springer, Berlin Heidelberg New York

Ekerot CF, Larson B, Oscarsson O (1979) Information carried by the spino cerebellar paths. In: Granit R, Pompeiano O (eds) Reflex control of posture and movement. Progress in brain research, vol 50. Elsevier/North-Holland Biomedical Press, Amsterdam New York Oxford, p 79

Gernandt BE, Megirian D (1961) Ascending propriospinal mechanisms. J Neurophysiol 24: 364–376

Grant G, Oscarsson O, Rosén I (1966) Functional organization of the spinoreticulocerebellar path with identification of its spinal component. Exp Brain Res 1: 306–319

Grillner S, Hongo T, Lund S (1968) The origin of descending fibres monosynaptically activating spino-reticular neurones. Brain Res 10: 259–262

Hoshino K, Pompeiano O (1977) Responses of lateral vestibular neurons to stimulation of contralateral macular labyrinthine receptors. Arch Ital Biol 115: 237–261

Ito M (1977) Functional specialization of flocculus Purkinje cells and their differential localization determined in connection with the vestibulo-ocular reflex. In: Baker R, Berthoz A (eds) Control of gaze by brain stem neurons. Elsevier, Amsterdam New York Oxford, p 177

Künzle H, Wiesendanger M (1974) Pyramidal connections to the lateral reticular nucleus in the cat: a degeneration study. Acta Anat 88: 105–114

Kuypers HGJM (1958a) An anatomical analysis of cortico-bulbar connexions to the pons and lower brain stem in the cat. J Anat 92: 198–218

Kuypers HGJM (1958b) Some projections from the peri-central cortex to the pons and lower brain stem in monkey and chimpanzee. J Comp Neurol 111: 221–251

Kuypers HGJM (1958c) Corticobulbar connexions to the pons and lower brain stem in man. An anatomical study. Brain 81: 364–388

Llinàs R, Walton K, Hillman DE, Sotelo C (1975) Inferior olive: its role in motor learning. Science 190: 1230–1231

Lundberg A, Oscarsson O (1962) Two ascending spinal pathways in the ventral part of the cord. Acta Physiol Scand 54: 270–286

Maekawa K, Simpson J (1973) Climbing fiber responses evoked in vestibulo-cerebellum of rabbit from visual system. J Neurophysiol 36: 649–666

Oscarsson O (1973) Functional organization of spino cerebellar paths. In: Iggo A (ed) Somatosensory system. Handbook of sensory physiology, vol II. Springer, Berlin Heidelberg New York, p 339

Oscarsson O, Rosén I (1966) Response characteristics of reticulocerebellar neurones activated from spinal afferents. Exp Brain Res 1: 320–328

Pompeiano O (1975) Macular input to neurons of the spinoreticulocerebellar pathway. Brain Res 95: 351–368

Pompeiano O (1977) Macular influences of somatosensory transmission through the spinoreticulocerebellar pathway. J Physiol 73: 387–400

Pompeiano O (1979) Neck and macular labyrinthine influences on the cervical spino-reticulocerebellar pathway. In: Granit R, Pompeiano O (eds) Reflex control of posture and movement. Progress in brain research, vol 50. Elsevier/North-Holland Biomedical Press, Amsterdam New York Oxford, p 501

Pompeiano O, Hoshino K (1977) Responses to static tilts of lateral reticular neurons mediated by contralateral labyrinthine receptors. Arch Ital Biol 115: 211–236

Precht W, Shimazu H, Markham CH (1966) A mechanism of central compensation of vestibular function following hemilabyrinthectomy. J Neurophysiol 29: 996–1010

Putkonen PTS, Courjon JH, Jeannerod M (1977) Compensation of postural effects of hemilabyrinthectomy in the cat. A sensory substitution process? Exp Brain Res 28: 249–257

Rosén I, Scheid P (1973a) Responses to nerve stimulation in the bilateral ventral flexor reflex tract (bVFRT) of the cat. Exp Brain Res 18: 256–267

Rosén I, Scheid P (1973b) Responses in the spino-reticulocerebellar pathway to stimulation of cutaneous mechanoreceptors. Exp Brain Res 18: 268–278

Sasaki K, Strata P (1967) Responses evoked in the cerebellar cortex by stimulating mossy fiber pathways to the cerebellum. Exp Brain Res 3: 95–120

Waespe W, Henn V (1977) Neuronal activity in the vestibular nuclei of the alert monkey during vestibular and optokinetic stimulation. Exp Brain Res 27: 523–538

Drug Effects on Vestibular Compensation

H. BIENHOLD, W. ABELN, and H. FLOHR[1]

1 Introduction

Since the investigations of Flourens (1842), Goltz (1870), and Ewald (1892) it has been known that unilateral labyrinthectomy results in characteristic deficits of posture and locomotion. Bechterew (1883) observed that all symptoms subside with time and normal function is restored.

Magnus (1924) realized that as the vestibular end organ does not regenerate, the compensation process requires an extensive, adaptive reorganization of the remaining central structures involved in the control of posture and locomotion.

Since then vestibular compensation has been regarded as an attractive model for the investigation of the plastic process involved in motor learning. It was recognized early that this process could be influenced pharmacologically. Both the acquisition and the retention of the compensated stage can be affected by drugs (cf. Schaefer and Meyer 1973).

Systematic pharmacological studies could therefore be an important approach in understanding the basic cellular mechanisms involved in this plastic process.

2 Drug Effects on Vestibular Compensation

2.1 Drugs Delaying Compensation

Pharmacologically, the process of the compensation can be both accelerated and delayed. Dietl (1966) and Schaefer and Meyer (1973) observed a marked inhibition of the compensatory process with sedating agents. Phenobarbital administered to guinea pigs, both in a single injection given shortly after labyrinthectomy and repeatedly during the compensation process, retarded recovery.

The time for recovery from the postural symptoms, taken as a measure for compensation velocity, was approximately tripled.

This effect of barbiturates can also be observed in *Rana.* Figure 1 shows the result of an experiment in the frog. Following hemilabyrinthectomy the animals received

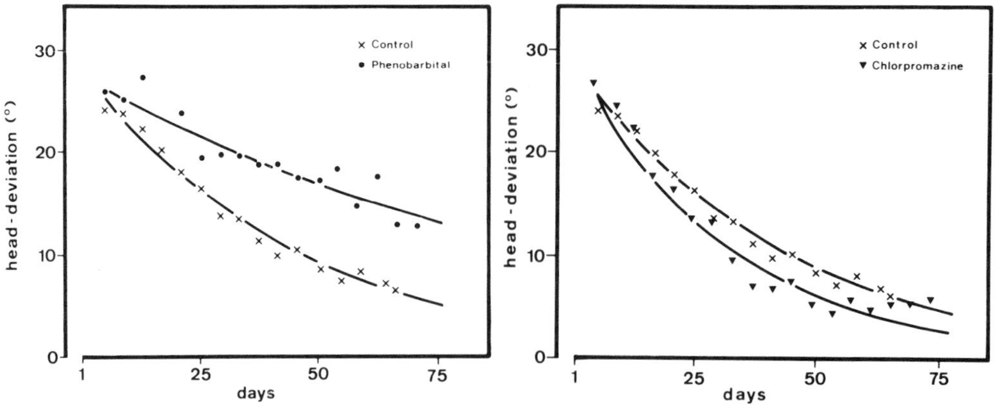

Fig. 1. Effects of phenobarbital (50 mg/kg every second day after hemilabyrinthectomy) and chlorpromazine (10 mg/kg every second day after hemilabyrinthectomy) on the time course of compensation in frogs. The symbols indicate the mean values for the head tilt symptom. Phenobarbital: n = 14; chlorpromazine: n = 16; control: n = 15

50 mg/kg phenobarbital, every second day. As can be seen, there is a significant delay in the compensation of the head deviation.

Chlorpromazine administered intraperitoneally in doses of 5–10 mg/kg had a strong delaying effect in guinea pigs. The same was observed for other neuroleptics with high sedative effects, e.g., chlorprothixen and perazine (Schaefer and Meyer 1973).

This effect, however, could not be reproduced in the frog. Figure 1 shows an experiment with chlorpromazine (10 mg/kg injected intralamyphatically every second day). As compared to the control group there is no delaying effect.

Neuroleptic drugs with marked neuroleptic potencies and with strong antipsychotic effects exerted little influence on the compensation velocity.

The same is true for diazepam which suppresses the acute effects of labyrinthectomy in the cat (Bernstein et al. 1974) and in guinea pigs (Altkemper 1966).

2.2 Drugs Accelerating Compensation

Acceleration of the compensation process is observed with excitants. In the guinea pig marked effects were observed with strychnine, metamphetamine, pentetrazole and caffeine. Different deficits were influenced to various degrees, for example head deviation was found to be more strongly affected than spontaneous eye nystagmus.

E 600, a cholinesterase inhibitor, exerted strong accelerating effects in guinea pigs. With this drug body rotation about the animals' longitudinal axis, a symptom which does not compensate spontaneously, was brought to full compensation.

In *Rana temporaria* chronic application of E 600 (1 mg/kg every fourth day after hemilabyrinthectomy) had a comparable effect. Compensation of the head tilt was markedly accelerated (Fig. 2). The same was true for all other symptoms.

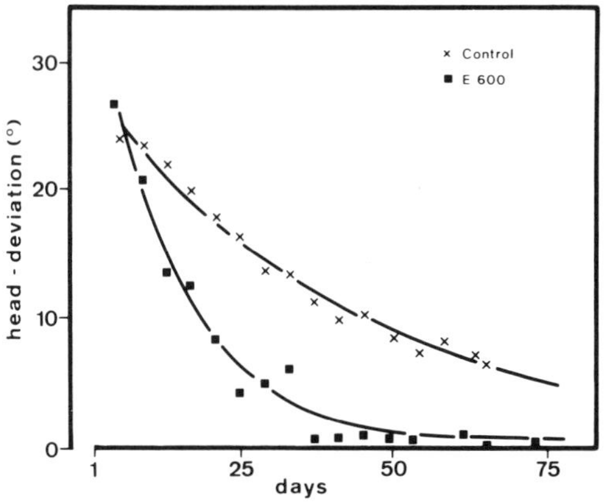

Fig. 2. Effect of E 600 (1 mg/kg every fourth day after hemilabyrinthectomy) on the time course of compensation in frogs. The symbols indicate the mean values for the head tilt symptom. E 600: n = 15; control: n = 15

3 Drug Effects Following Complete Compensation

3.1 Effects of Acetylcholine-Agonists

Recent investigations have shown that the compensated state can be strongly influenced by acetylcholine-agonists (ACh-agonists) and acetylcholine-antagonists (ACh-antagonists) (Bienhold and Flohr 1980).

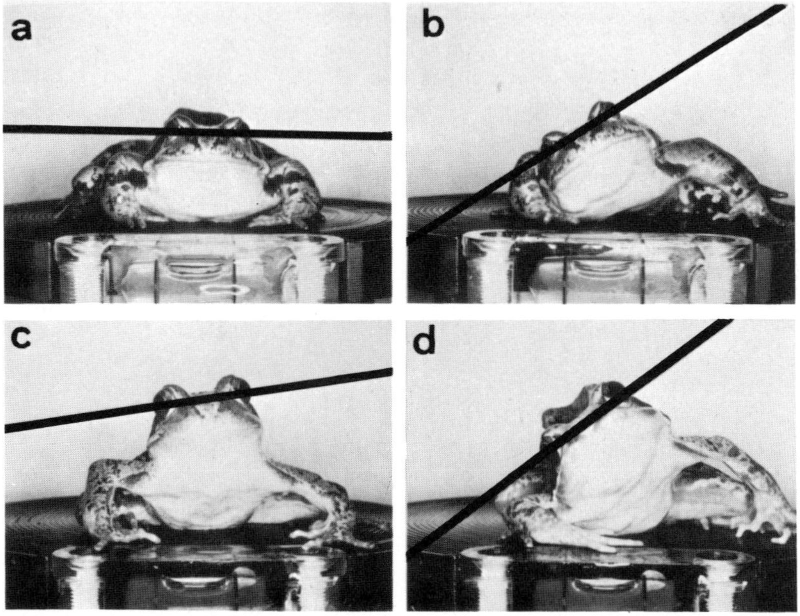

Fig. 3a–d. Postural effects of intralymphatic application of 6 mg/kg E 600. The photographs show the same animal (**a**) before unilateral labyrinthectomy, (**b**) 30 min after right hemilabyrinthectomy, (**c**) after complete compensation (70 days after hemilabyrinthectomy), (**d**) 60 min after application of E 600

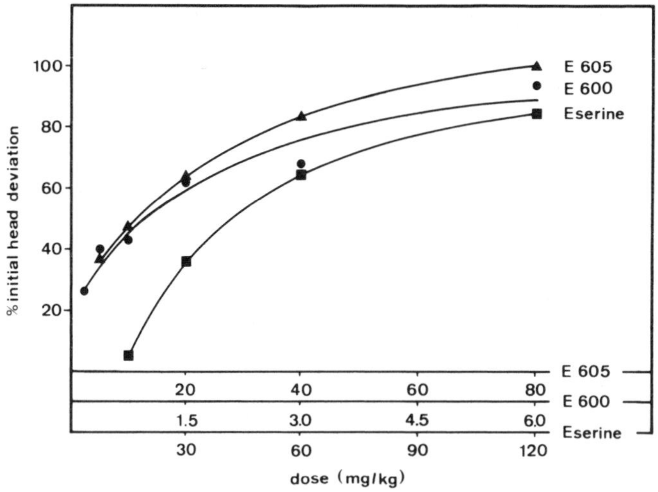

Fig. 4. Dose-dependence of the decompensatory effect of three different anticholinesterases. *Ordinate,* Mean values for head deviation in percent of initial head deviation after hemilabyrinthectomy (n = 8). *Abscissa,* Doses applied in mg/kg

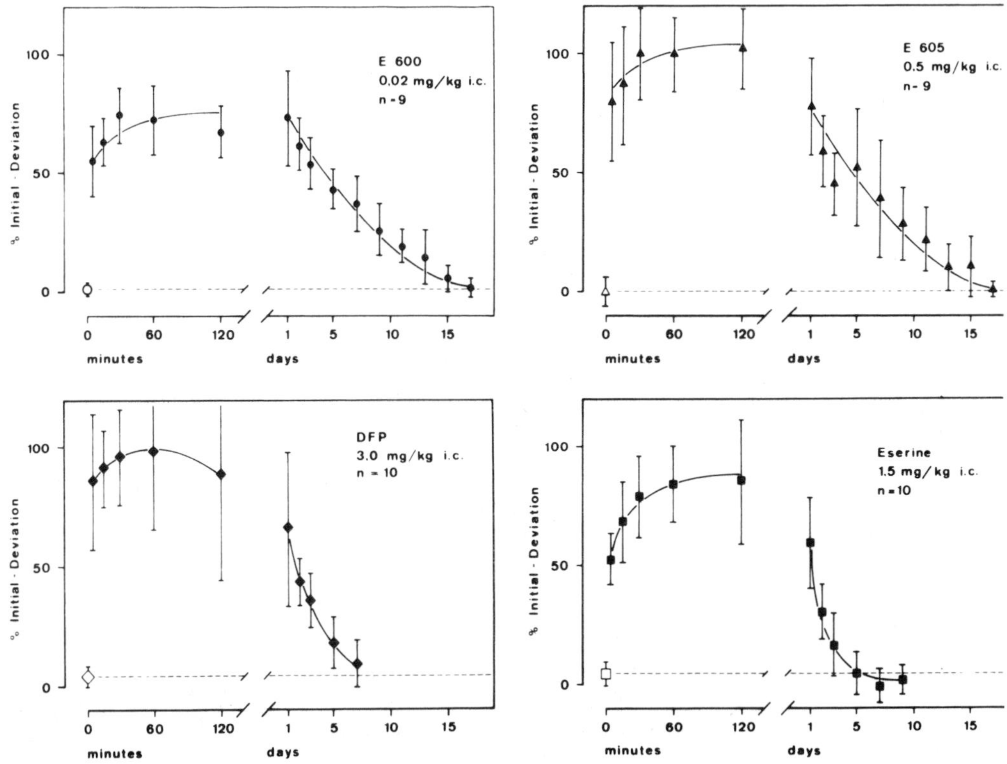

Fig. 5. Time course of decompensatory effect of anticholinesterases following an intracisternal injection at time zero. *Filled symbols,* Mean values (± SD) for head tilt in percent of initial head deviation after hemilabyrinthectomy. *Open symbols,* Head angle before drug administration. Drugs, doses, and number of the animals are indicated in the figures

In hemilabyrinthectomized and completely compensated frogs intralymphatic application of 6 mg/kg E 600 is followed by an immediate and total reappearance of the head tilt to the deafferented side (Fig. 3). All other postural and locomotor symptoms are also restored. This effect is independent of the time interval between hemilabyrinthectomy and drug injection. The same decompensatory effect was obtained by the systemic application of E 605 and eserine.

The effects are dose-dependent (Fig. 4) and reversible. There was no clear effect with diisopropyl fluorophosphonate (DFP) injected intralymphatically (1.0–200.0 mg/kg) since a pronounced peripheral paralysis occured.

The lipid insoluble drugs, neostigmine (0.10–3.0 mg/kg) and pyridostigmine (10.0–200.0 mg/kg), were ineffective.

When given intracisternally into the fourth ventricle, E 600, E 605, eserine, and DFP all led to an immediate and reversible decompensation including all postural and locomotor symptoms (Fig. 5). The equi-effective doses for intracranial injection were considerably lower than for systemic application. For this reason it could be assumed that the drug effect has a central origin.

Intracisternal applications of cholinomimetics, such as arecoline, carbachol, nicotine, muscarine, and oxotremorine also led to an immediate decompensation. With bethanechol and methacholine no complete decompensation could be observed, because with high doses peripheral paralysis occured. With doses which had no marked peripheral effects a decompensation of approximately 50% of the initial head deviation was obtained (Fig. 6).

With excessive doses of intracisternally applied eserine (5 mg/kg) and oxotremorine (1–2 mg/kg) the reverse effect with head tilt to the intact side was obtained.

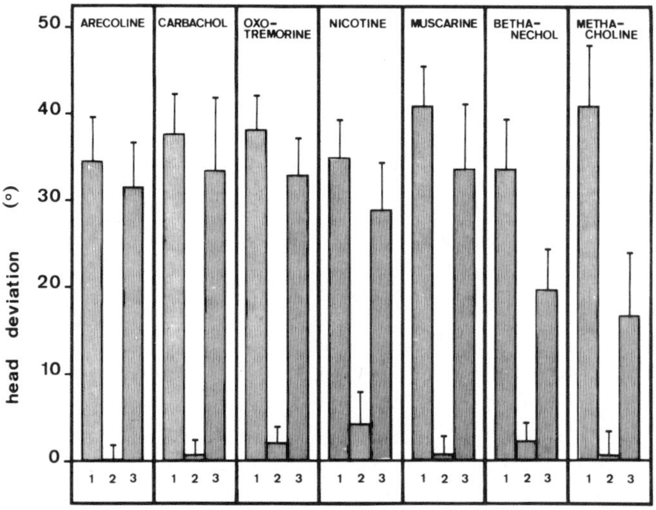

Fig. 6. Decompensatory effect of cholinomimetics after intracisternal application. The columns show head tilt *1*, after hemilabyrinthectomy, *2*, after complete compensation, and *3*, after drug administration following complete compensation (mean values + SD). Doses and number of animals: *arecoline*, 3 mg/kg (n = 9); *carbachol*, 0.25 mg/kg (n = 6); *oxotremorine*, 0.25 mg/kg (n = 8); *nicotine*, 2 mg/kg (n = 10); *muscarine*, 0.25 mg/kg (n = 11); *bethanechol*, 2 mg/kg (n = 8); *methacholine*, 2 mg/kg (n = 8)

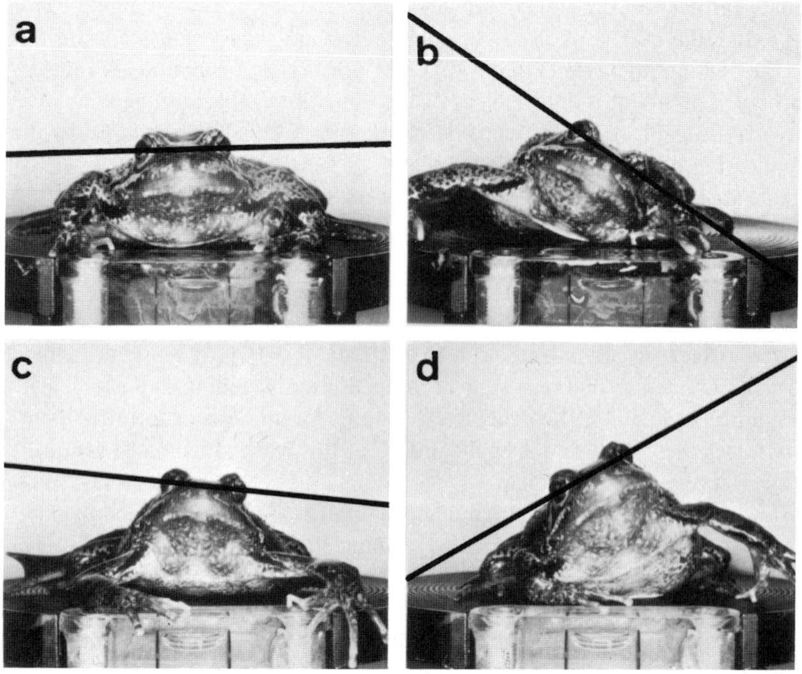

Fig. 7a–d. Postural effects of intracisternal application of 1 mg/kg atropine. The photographs show the same animal (**a**) before unilateral labyrinthectomy, (**b**) 30 min after left hemilabyrinthectomy, (**c**) after compensation (70 days after hemilabyrinthectomy), (**d**) 30 min after application of atropine

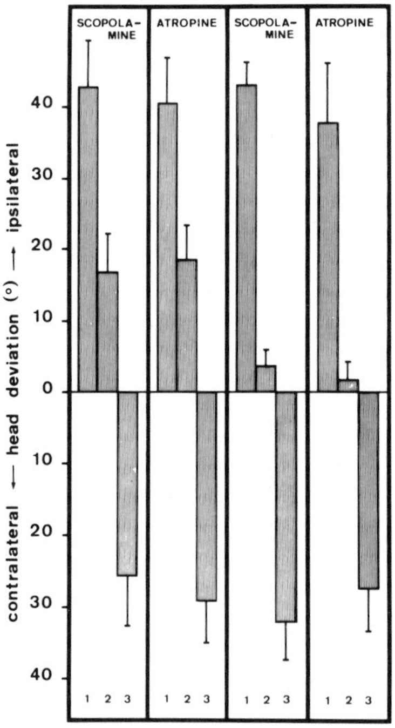

Fig. 8. Effect of cholinolytics after intracisternal application. The columns show head tilt *1*, after hemilabyrinthectomy, *2*, after partial and complete compensation, and *3*, to the contralateral side after drug administration (mean values + SD). Doses and number of animals: *scopolamine*, partially compensated, 3 mg/kg (n = 9); *atropine*, partially compensated, 1 mg/kg (n = 12); *scopolamine*, completely compensated, 3 mg/kg (n = 9); and *atropine*, completely compensated, 1 mg/kg (n = 10)

3.2 Effects of Acetylcholine-Antagonists

Cholinolytics, such as atropine (1 mg/kg) and scopolamine (3 mg/kg) had the expected antagonistic effects. Following complete compensation a head deviation was induced to the intact side. Figure 7 shows this effect for atropine applied intracisternally in an animal labyrinthectomized on the left side. The effect could also be observed in partly compensated animals as can be seen in the first two sections in Fig. 8.

4 Summary and Conclusions

The compensation process following unilateral labyrinthine lesions can be affected by drugs in different ways. Firstly, the velocity of the process and the ultimate degree of recovery can be influenced. In general, excitants accelerate and improve compensation, whereas sedating agents have the reverse effect, that is, retard recovery. Secondly, the state of the compensated system as compared with that of the intact system is characterized by an altered sensitivity toward drugs.

As far as known at present, this is primarily true of drugs which act on the central cholinergic synapses. Obviously, the compensated vestibular system is distinguished from the intact one by an asymmetrical distribution in the number and/or efficacy of cholinergic synapses. This indicates that changes in cholinergic pathways of the brainstem have a definite and probably specific role in the compensation process.

The exact physiological role of cholinergic pathways within the vestibular complex is not known. Investigations of Diamant (1954), Yamamoto (1967), and Épshtein and Shipov (1970) indicate, however, that cholinergic transmitter systems are present and probably involved in normal function. There exists a large body of evidence from human and animal studies that central cholinergic systems have a definite relationship to acquisition, storage, and retrieval of information. This has been confirmed in different species, such as invertebrates, e.g., snails and insects (Kerkut et al. 1971, 1972), and in vertebrates, e.g., mice, rats, rabbits, cats, and man (cf. DeFeudis 1974), and in different learning tasks such as habituation, active and passive avoidance, maze learning, instrumental conditioning, discrimination learning, and verbal learning in man (cf. DeFeudis 1974; Drachman 1978; Zornetzer 1978). The exact role of the cholinergic transmitter system in learning and memory is still poorly understood. However, one conclusion seems possible, namely that a common mechanism underlies different plastic processes, of which vestibular compensation is one.

The symptoms following unilateral labyrinthectomy reflect an imbalance in the activity of the vestibular nuclei on the two sides, which is initially depressed on the deafferented side. During compensation, activity on the deafferented side regenerates and is raised until a new equilibirum with its intact counterpart is attained. The source of this regained activity is not known.

One often discussed assumption is that denervation supersensitivity develops on the deafferented side (Spiegel and Démétriades 1925; Schön 1950; McCabe et al. 1972; Dieringer and Precht 1979). The present observations, however, are not compatible with the assumption that a denervation-induced supersensitivity in cholinergic neurons develops in the deafferented nucleus. In true supersensitivity the effects of agonists of the presumed transmitter should be greater within the supersensitive locus. By contrast the supersensitive neurons should become less responsive to antagonists of the presumed transmitter because of an increase in transmitter receptor sensitivity.

If this were the case in vestibular compensation, ACh-agonists in the compensated state should have a greater effect on the deafferented side, and ACh-antagonists would have the opposite effect.

The actual effects observed indicate the contrary. Hence, the present results do not support the assumption that a true supersensitivity in the deafferented nucleus underlies the recovery of spontaneous activity in that nucleus.

References

Altkemper R (1966) Zur Wirkung von Phenothiazinen und anderen Psychopharmaka auf zentralnervöse Kompensationsvorgänge nach Labyrinthausschaltung. Doct Diss, Göttingen

Bechterew W (1883) Ergebnisse der Durchschneidung des N. acusticus, nebst Erörterung der Bedeutung der semicirculären Canäle für das Körpergleichgewicht. Pflügers Arch 3: 312–347

Bernstein P, McCabe BF, Ryu JH (1974) The effect of diazepam on vestibular compensation. Laryngoscope 84: 267–272

Bienhold H, Flohr H (1980) Role of cholinergic synapses in vestibular compensation. Brain Res 195: 476–478

DeFeudis FV (1974) Central cholinergic systems and behavior. Academic Press, London New York

Diamant H (1954) Cholinesterase inhibitors and vestibular function. Acta Otolaryngol Suppl 111

Dieringer N, Precht W (1979) Mechanisms of compensation for vestibular deficits in the frog. I. Modification of the excitatory commissural system. Exp Brain Res 36: 311–328

Dietl G (1966) Zur Wirkung von Luminal, Megaphen and Pervitin auf kompensatorische Vorgänge nach Labyrinthausschaltung. Doct Diss, Göttingen

Drachman DA (1978) Central cholinergic systems and memory. In: Lipton MA, DiMascio A, Killam KF (eds) Psychopharmacology: A generation of progress. Raven Press, New York, pp 651–662

Épshtein EL, Shipov AA (1970) Unilateral labyrinthectomy as a model for assessing effect of drugs on vestibular function. Environ Space Sci 4: 339–341

Essig CF, Hampson JL, Bales PD, Himwich HE (1949) Biochemically induced forced circling behavior. Trans Am Neurol Assoc 74: 154

Essig CF, Hampson JL, McCauley A, Himwich HE (1950) An experimental analysis of biochemically induced circling behavior. J Neurophysiol 13: 269

Ewald JR (1892) Physiologische Untersuchungen über das Endorgan des Nervus octavus. J.F. Bergmann, Wiesbaden

Flourens JPN (1842) Recherches expérimentales sur les propriétés et les fonctions du système nerveux dans les animaux vertébrés. Baillère, Paris

Goltz F (1870) Über die physiologische Bedeutung der Bogengänge des Ohrlabyrinths. Pflügers Arch 3: 172–192

Hampson JL, Essig CF, McCauley A, Himwich HE (1950) Effects of di-isopropylfluorophosphate (DFP) on electroencephalogram and cholinesterase activity. Electroencephalogr Clin Neurophysiol 2: 41

Kerkut GA, Oliver GWO, Rick JT, Walker RJ (1971) The effects of drugs on learning in a simple preparation. Comp Gen Pharmacol 1: 437–484

Kerkut GA, Emson PC, Brimblecombe RW, Breesley P, Oliver GW, Walker RJ (1972) Changes in the properties of acetylcholinesterase in the invertebrate central nervous system. Prog Brain Res 36: 65–78

Magnus R (1924) Körperstellung. Springer, Berlin
McCabe BF, Ryu GH, Sekitani T (1972) Further experiments on vestibular compensation. Laryngoscope 82: 381
Schaefer KP, Meyer DL (1973) Compensatory mechanisms following labyrinthine lesions in guinea-pigs. A simple model of learning. In: Zippel H-P (ed) Memory and transfer of information. Plenum Press, New York London, pp 203–232
Schön L (1950) Quantitative Untersuchungen über die zentrale Kompensation nach einseitiger Utriculusausschaltung bei Fischen. Z Vergl Physiol 32: 121–150
Spiegel EA, Démétriades TD (1925) Die zentrale Kompensation des Labyrinthverlustes. Pflügers Arch 210: 215–222
Yamamoto C (1967) Pharmacologic studies of norepinephrine, acetylcholine and related compounds on neurons in Deiters' nucleus and the cerebellum. J Pharmacol Exp Ther 156: 39–47
Zornetzer SF (1978) Neurotransmitter modulation and memory: A new pharmacological phrenology? In: Lipton MA, DiMascio A, Killam KF (eds) Psychopharmacology: A generation of progress. Raven Press, New York, pp 637–649

IIc. Plasticity in the Oculomotor System and Cerebellum

Long-Term Effects of Dove Prism Vision on Torsional VOR and Head-Eye Coordination

A. BERTHOZ, G. MELVILL JONES, and A. BÉGUÉ[1]

Previous experiments with both human (Gonshor and Melvill Jones 1971, 1976a,b; Gauthier and Robinson 1975; Melvill Jones 1977) and animal (Ito et al. 1974; Miles and Fuller 1974; Melvill Jones and Davies 1976; Robinson 1976; Miles and Eighmy 1980) subjects have demonstrated profound effects of optically modified vision upon the *horizontal* vestibulo-ocular reflex (HVOR) and associated neural pathways (Ito 1979; Keller and Precht 1979; Miles et al. 1980). However, modified vision calls for adaptive changes in sensory motor mechanisms other than the HVOR. For example, since horizontally reversing dove prisms also produce reversal of image movement during head rotation in the frontal, or roll, plane, the question arises whether adaptive changes occur in the torsional vestibulo-ocular reflex (TVOR). As will appear later, this question has important theoretical implications. Again, vision reversal would be expected to disorganize visuo-spinal reflexes associated with posture and head movement control. Indeed marked adaptive effects on postural control have already been reported (Gonshor and Melvill Jones 1980).

The present account briefly reports preliminary results of experiments which examine the effect of dove prism vision on TVOR (see also Berthoz et al. 1981) and the coordination of head and eye movements during rapid changes of head position.

1 Methods

Using methods described in detail elsewhere (Gonshor and Melvill Jones 1976b), horizontally reversing dove prisms were mounted in close fitting goggles which were worn continually by the subject over a 19-day period of adaption. During and after this period of adaption, measurements were made of horizontal and torsional eye movement reflexly induced by sinusoidal rotation in the appropriate plane, and of various forms of coordinated head and eye movements as described below.

---

1 Laboratoire de Physiologie Neurosensorielle, CNRS, Paris, France and
Aviation Medical Research Unit, Department of Physiology, McGill University, Montreal, Canada

1.1 Measurement of Eye Movement

Horizontal eye movements were recorded by conventional dc electro-oculography (EOG), with EOG calibrations performed before and after each relevant test run, care being taken to avoid changes of EOG sensitivity due to changes of light/dark adaptation in the retina (Gonshor and Malcolm 1971). Torsional eye movements were recorded using a modified version of a previously described cine-photographic method (Melvill Jones 1963). In the present experiments infrared (IR) video photography was employed to avoid visual influences on oculomotor control during TVOR testing. As in earlier experiments referred to above, torsional eye rotation was measured by means of a transparent disc, attached through a miniature parallel arm system (akin to that of a drawing board) to a rotary potentiometer clamped to the bench. With this arrangement the potentiometer responds *only* to rotation of the disc about its own axis and not at all to linear displacements of the disc. Hence, by sketching the pupil and appropriate radially oriented marks of the iris on the disc, and matching the sketched disc to stationary video images of the eye, the potentiometer can be made to follow "frame by frame" the angular movement of the eye in the frontal plane of the skull.

1.2 Measurement of Head–Eye Coordination

Head movements were measured by means of a flexible cable, stiff in torsion, attached at one end to a lightweight structure fitted tightly to the skull and at the other end to a rotary potentiometer. Simultaneous measurements of head and eye movements were then made, with head free, during rapid horizontal head rotations through small angles in the following conditions: (1) passively generated horizontal head rotation in the dark, and (2) active change of gaze between two stationary, normally lit, visual targets separated by 15°.

1.3 Sinusoidal Stimulation of VOR

For routine stimulation of HVOR, the servo-driven turntable was oscillated as in previous human experiments (Gonshor and Melvill Jones 1976b), at 1/6 Hz and a peak-to-peak amplitude of 120°. Oscillatory stimulation of TVOR was conducted at the same frequency, but with a lower peak-to-peak amplitude of 70° owing to limitations of the servomotor when driving the turntable loaded with accessory equipment for IR video photography and blackout of the subject. During all such stimuli the subject's head was tilted backward through 90° to bring the frontal plane of the skull into an earth-horizontal plane, thus avoiding the complication of dynamic stimulation of the otolith organ due to relative movement of the gravity vector.

1.4 Comparison of HVOR and SVOR After Adaptation

Adpative effects in HVOR and the vertical VOR activated by head movements in the saggital plane (SVOR) were compared by means of a sensitive qualitative test extensively employed for this purpose in previous experiments (Melvill Jones and Drazin

1962; Gonshor 1974). The objective of the test is to estimate visual blur whilst oscillating the head at a frequency too high for visual following (3 Hz) in either the horizontal or the saggital plane of the skull. The previous experiments referred to above have established a consistent relationship between the degree of VOR adequacy for reflex ocular stabilization and the degree of blur seen in these circumstances.

2 Results

2.1 Torsional Vestibulo-Ocular Reflex

Figure 1 *top trace* illustrates a segment of a normal control record of compensatory torsional eye movement, resulting from standard sinusoidal rotation (head fixed relative to body) in the frontal plane of the head. Since these records were obtained in infrared light with only a small central fixation point, they are considered to represent specifically TVOR without significant optokinetic influence. Since head rotation was conducted about an axis parallel to the gravitational field, vestibular stimulation was confined to the canals (especially the four vertical canals).

It can be seen that quite large torsional eye angles, up to 20° peak-to-peak, were induced, having a sinusoidal pattern interspersed with occasional well-marked saccades. Aligning successive smooth eye movements to generate curves of cumulative eye position (CEP; after the method of Meiry 1966) allows an estimate of TVOR gain (eye ang. vel./head ang. vel.) by measurement of peak-to-peak amplitude of the CEP curve. Relating this value to the corresponding amplitude of turntable rotation produced a mean control TVOR gain of 0.27 (SE = 0.02; n = 9) from the preliminary data so far available. Evidently an active and functionally meaningful TVOR is normally present under these stimulus conditions, although with a rather low reflex gain compared to a mean control HVOR gain of 0.55 (SE = 0.02; n = 10) obtained from this subject on the same day.

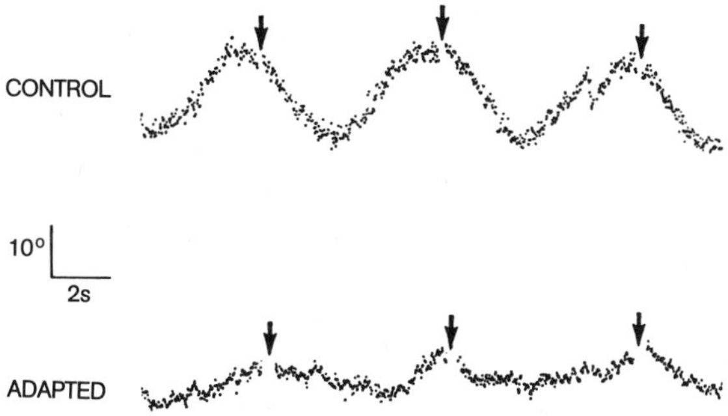

Fig. 1. Torsional eye rotation induced by sinusoidal rotation in the frontal plane of the head while turning about an axis parallel to the gravitational field. The control record was obtained 31 days after return to normal vision. The adapted record was obtained at the end of 19-days continuous exposure to dove prism vision. Both records were obtained in infrared light. The sinusoidal stimulus was of 70° peak-to-peak amplitude at 1/6 Hz in both cases. Each *dot* represents torsional eye angle measured from a single "frame" of stationary video tape record, with 20 ms between dots. *Arrows* indicate the moments of peak clockwise (as seen from above) displacement of the turntable

The *lower trace* of Fig. 1 illustrates a similar record of TVOR obtained after 19 days of continual adaptation to dove prism vision. Simple visual inspection shows that the adapted response is substantially modified compared with the control curves. Thus, from the available data the mean *adapted* TVOR gain was only 0.13 (SE = 0.0093; n = 13), which represents a highly significant ($P < 0.001$) attenuation of some 55% relative to the corresponding control value. Interestingly, on the same day the same percentage adaptive attenuation of 55% was found in the HVOR of this subject. It seems that similar adaptive processes were active in HVOR and TVOR, that is in the two degrees of freedom in which vision reversal occurs with the horizontally oriented dove prisms.

Most significantly, as in all previous experiments (Gonshor and Melvill Jones 1976b), there was no evidence of any adaptive change in SVOR as determined by the blur tests described and referred to in Methods. Bearing in mind that there was no optical vision reversal in the saggittal plane, the general conclusion may therefore be drawn that such adaptive changes as occured in the vestibulo-ocular reflex system as a whole proved to be strictly specific to the functional requirements imposed by the optical system employed.

Of equal, if not greater, physiological significance are the differential adaptive effects found in TVOR and SVOR, since these two reflexes employ the same sensory, neural, and motor elements. Important theoretical implications stem from this finding, as discussed later.

A noteworthy additional feature of Fig. 1 is the variability in *form* of the adapted response. Owing to this variability no attempt has been made to estimate TVOR phase from presently available data.

2.2 Head–Eye Coordination

Figure 2 shows tracings from five samples of head–eye coordination in the normal and adapted subject. The control response to *passive head movement in the dark (top left)* demonstrates HVOR compensation with (or in some cases without) the presence of small repositioning saccades. The gain of the HVOR, measured by comparison of initial curves of head and eye movements, was in these circumstances close to unity, so that good occular compensation was achieved even in the absence of vision.

In the adapted state the HVOR was much reduced, as demonstrated by the relatively slow initial "compensatory" eye movement which starts synchronously with that of the head. Such HVOR attenuation is certainly appropriate for improvement of vision with the prisms on. But for ideal fixation on the reversed moving image seen during head rotation with the prisms on, a *reversed* compensatory eye movement would be required. Not infrequently something akin to such a response was observed, as in the middle set of adapted records. However, since this type of movement usually occurred after an initial presumed HVOR in the *normal* compensatory direction (see Fig. 2), the reversed movement is unlikely to represent simple reflex reversal. Possibly it might derive from superposition of an attenuated HVOR and a modified (i.e., slowed) saccade in the "leading" direction, positioned as in the clear-cut saccade of the upper adapted records. Possibly, in view of its latency relative to initiation of head movement, the reversed slow movement might represent a centrally programed re-

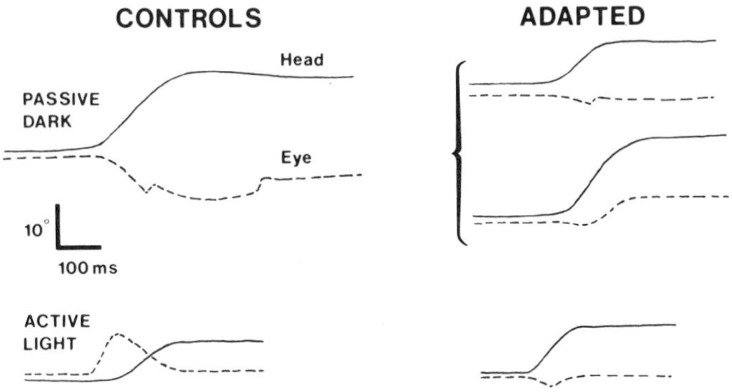

Fig. 2. Head–Eye coordination under normal conditions (*control*) and after 19 days of continuous dove prism vision (*adapted*). All lines are traced from original records of head and eye movement obtained during passive head movement in the dark and active head movement in the light with no prisms (*control*) and with prisms on, after adaptation (*adapted*)

sponse; possibly an adaptively enhanced form of neck-generated oculomotor reflex. Whatever its origin, it appears as a smooth movement in the appropriate direction and of approximately the required speed for tracking the reversed image movement which occurs during rotation of the head; even though there was in this instance no vision.

The *lower left record* in Fig. 2 illustrates a normal combination of head and eye movements associated with *rapid gaze change between two targets with eyes open in the light.* First a normal ocular saccade shifts the gaze quickly from one target to the other. Then a rapid head movment begins, generating a normal compensatory HVOR at approximately unity gain, which therefore holds the eye on the new target during the remaining head movement (Morasso et al. 1973). This sequence of events would, however, be quite inappropriate for fixating the new target with the reversing prisms in place. Ideally, the initial saccade should then be in the opposite direction to the ensuing head rotation, whilst for subsequent target fixation during head movement there should be a reversed HVOR. In practice, such an ideal pattern was never seen. Rather a great variety of eye movements were observed. One of these is shown in the *bottom right* set of records. As in the adapted response with eyes closed, there was an initial, attenuated HVOR in the normal direction. Again, this was followed by a reversal of eye movement at about the mid point of the head rotation. The overall sequence represents a fair compromise solution, in which the direction of gaze eventually becomes aligned with the new target after the cessation of head movement. The penalty is one of delayed target acquisition, rather than failure of eventual target fixation.

Another pattern of eye movements consists in a complete blockage of eye position in the orbit, and a third one of a saccade made towards the target, before the eye movement, followed by a "slowed saccade" having the same direction, amplitude, and velocity as the head movement.

3 Comments

Earlier investigation of behavioral adaption to dove prism vision has demonstrated large changes in HVOR and in visually guided postural control, as described and referred to in the Introduction. The present experiments demonstrate that adaptive effects can also be induced in TVOR. In previous human experiments conducted with the same dove prism orientation (Gonshor and Melvill Jones 1976b) it was conclusively shown that in these circumstances there is no change of SVOR measured in the orthogonal saggittal plane, in which there was no optical reversal of vision. That differential adaptive effects can be simultaneously induced in frontal and saggital planes is particularly interesting, since vestibulo-ocular responses in *each* of these planes employ all four vertical semicircular canals and all four corresponding disynaptically innervated pairs of extraocular muscles. It would therefore seem that *any* adaptive change in these short synaptic pathways should inevitably induce modification of both the TVOR and the SVOR. The findings would thus appear to argue strongly against long-term changes of synaptic efficacy in any of the disynaptic pathways driving the combined vertical VOR system. Presumably more complex mechanisms must be at play in the adaptive process, perhaps involving some kind of neural transform of information from the diagonal coordinates of the canals and muscles to the saggital and frontal planes of the skull.

With regard to head–eye coordination it is clear that some form of adaptive modification takes place in response to dove prism vision, as has been noted in monkey by Miles and Eighmy (1980). In line with their findings, there was however great variability in the adapted pattern of response, with no evidence of overt HVOR reversal despite marked phase change in the sinusoidally tested reflex ($-110°$, SE = $8°$; n = 10 cycles, on the last day of prism vision). Probably this variability stems from the considerable variety of potential contributing factors: For example modified HVOR, modified neck–eye reflexes (Morasso et al. 1973); modified saccades; modified optokinetic response (Melvill Jones et al. 1980); adaptive generation of central programs (Collewijn and Grootendorst 1979). Evidently there is scope for a wide range of adaptive strategies in coordinated movements of this nature (Davies and Melvill Jones 1977).

References

Berthoz A, Melvill Jones G, Bégué A (1981) Differential visual adaptation of vertical canal dependant vestibulo-ocular reflexes. Exp Brain Res in press

Collewijn H, Grootendorst AF (1979) Adaptation of optokinetic and vestibular reflexes to modified visual input in the rabbit. Prog Brain Res 50: 771–781

Davies PRT, Melvill Jones G (1977) Adaptive "strategy" in cats exposed to long term optical reversal of vision. XXVII Int Cong Physiol Sci, Paris

Gauthier AM, Robinson DA (1975) Adaptation of humans' vestibulo-ocular reflex to magnifying lenses. Brain Res 92: 331–335

Gonshor A (1974) An investigation of plasticity in the human vestibuloocular reflex arc. PhD Thesis Dept Physiol, McGill Univ

Gonshor A, Malcolm R (1971) Effects of changes in illumination level on electro-oculography (EOG). Aeroscape Med 42: 138–140

Gonshor A, Melvill Jones G (1971) Plasticity in the adult human vestibulo-ocular reflex arc. Proc Can Fed Biol Soc 14: 11
Gonshor A, Melvill Jones G (1976a) Short term adaptive changes in the human vestibulo-ocular reflex arc. J Physiol 256: 361–379
Gonshor A, Melvill Jones G (1976b) Extreme vestibulo-ocular adaptation induced by prolonged optical reversal of vision. J Physiol 256: 381–414
Gonshor A, Melvill Jones G (1980) Postural adaptation to prolonged optical reversal of vision in man. Brain Res 192: 239–248
Ito M (1979) Adaptive modification of the vestibulo-ocular reflex in rabbits affected by visual inputs and its possible neuronal mechanisms. Prog Brain Res 50: 757–761
Ito M, Shiida T, Yagi N, Yamamoto M (1974) Visual influence on rabbit's horizontal vestibulo-ocular reflex that presumably is effected via the cerebellar flocculus. Brain Res 75: 170–174
Keller EL, Precht W (1979) Adaptive modification of central vestibular neurons in resppnse to visual stimultion through reversing prisms. J Neurophysiol 42: 896–911
Meiry JL (1966) The vestibular system and human dynamic space orientation. Washington DC, NASA CR-628
Melvill Jones G (1963) Ocular nystagmus recorded simultaneously in three orthogonal planes. Acta Otolaryngol 56: 619–631
Melvill Jones G (1977) Plasticity in the adult vestibulo-ocular reflex arc. Philos Trans R Soc London Ser B 278: 319–334
Melvill Jones G, Davies PRT (1976) Adaptation of cat vestibulo-ocular reflex to 200 days of optically reversed vision. Brain Res 103: 551–554
Melvill Jones G, Drazin DG (1962) Oscillatory motion in flight. In: Barbour and Wittingham (eds) Human problems of supersonic and hypersonic flight. Pergamon Press, London, pp 134–151
Melvill Jones G, Mandl G, Cynader M (1980) Modification of optokinetic tracking (OKN) by maintained vision reversal in normal and strobe reared cats. Neurosci Abstr in press
Miles FA, Eighmy BB (1980) Long-term adaptive changes in primate vestibulo-ocular reflex. I. Behavioural observations. J Neurophysiol 43: 1406–1426
Miles FA, Fuller JH (1974) Adaptive plasticity in the vestibulo-ocular responses of the rhesus monkey. Brain Res 80: 512–516
Miles FA, Fuller JH, Braitman DJ, Dow BM (1980) Long term adaptive changes in primate vestibulo-ocular reflex. III. Electrophysiological observations in flocculus of normal monkeys. J Neurophysiol 43: 1437–1476
Morasso P, Bizzi E, Dichgans J (1973) Adjustment of saccade characteristics during head movements. Exp Brain Res 16: 492–500
Robinson DA (1976) Adaptive gain control of the vestibulo-ocular reflex by the cerebellum J Neurophysiol 39: 954–969

Adaptive Modification in Brainstem Pathways During Vestibulo-Ocular Reflex Recalibration

E.L. KELLER[1] and W. PRECHT[2]

1 Introduction

1.1 Criteria for Neural Models of Plasticity

Studies concerned with elucidating the neuronal mechanisms underlying plasticity in brain function are greatly facilitated if the behavior being modified is simple, reproducible, and capable of being quantitatively measured. Furthermore, in the complex mammalian brain, it is necessary that the anatomical substrates mediating the behavior should have been delimited if progress is to be made in understanding the synaptic modifications involved in the plasticity. On the other hand, the behavior undergoing adaptive modification must be significant and general if one wishes to generate an understanding of plastic mechanisms that can serve as a model for understanding more complex behavior. Because the vestibulo-ocular reflex (VOR) meets all of these ideal criteria, the interest of the neurobiological community in it and its plastic modification has been growing steadily in the expectation that it will serve as just such a model.

1.2 Theoretical Background

The purpose of the VOR, to stabilize gaze during head movements, is clear. The neural organization generating the VOR is an open-loop control system. That is, the semicircular canals transduce angular acceleration of the head into a neural signal propertional to head velocity. This signal, after further central modification, emerges in the form of ocular muscle control signals, which move the eyes to compensate exactly for the head motion. This action leaves gaze fixed in space. Any resultant error in this system, which would take the form of retinal image slip and concomitant visual blur, is not sensed at the canals. In view of the precise calibration of this reflex, which is maintained throughout life, it is obvious that vision must play a role in maintaining this proper calibration. Ito (1970) first pointed out these conclusions and supplied a theoretical framework for understanding the role played by vision by hypothesizing that the floccular lobes of the cerebellum received independent head velocity and retinal image slip signals. He further suggested that this cerebellar network contains modifi-

1 Smith-Kettlewell Institute of Visual Sciences, San Francisco, CA, USA
2 Max-Planck-Institut für Hirnforschung, 6000 Frankfurt, FRG

able synaptic elements that change over a period of time in a direction to produce reduction of the image slip during head movements. In this theory, the reduction is produced by floccular Purkinje cells (P-cells) which directly inhibit vestibular nucleus neurons (Vn). These Vn in turn control oculomotor neurons (Baker et al. 1972; Fukuda et al. 1972).

1.3 Experimental Support for the Theory

This hypothesis is supported by the observation that the VOR can be adaptively modified by optical alteration of the normal visual feedback accompanying head movements (Gonshor and Melvill Jones 1971; Ito et al. 1974; Miles and Fuller 1974). Ablation studies involving the flocculus support the view that the cerebellum is involved in these modifications, since visual recalibration of the VOR can no longer be produced in animals with total lesions in this area (Ito et al. 1974; Robinson 1976). More recent single-unit recording studies designed to pinpoint the exact location of the modified neural elements have produced contradictory results. Ito (1977), recording in the rabbit cerebellum, has reported results consistent with the idea that floccular P-cells contain the modified synapses. However, his results require modification of a certain subset of P-cells and only certain subpopulations of VN, namely the inhibitory side of vestibular nucleus projections to oculomotor neurons. Studies in the alert monkey flocculus have produced further results that cloud such simple interpretations of P-cell data (Lisberger and Fuchs 1978) and directly challenge the notion that the modification has occurred in the cerebellum (Miles et al. 1980). The later study supports the view that the cerebellum receives a modified eye velocity signal indicating that the major change has occurred elsewhere.

1.4 Vestibular Nucleus Studies

Our own work on this problem has centered on studies of the vestibular nucleus. This large nuclear complex contains a variety of neurons related to labyrinthine input and oculomotor and cervicomotor output. Rather circumscribed regions of the nucleus contain the neurons projecting directly to oculomotor neurons (Precht 1978). The floccular projection to vestibular nucleus is also most extensive in this same region of vestibular nucleus. Therefore, our studies of the changes that occur in Vn in cats with adapted VOR may lead to a better understanding of the role played by possible floccular adaptations in this process.

Vestibular neurons also receive an independent optokinetic input in addition to the head velocity signal from the labyrinth (Waespe and Henn 1977). Furthermore, at least in the cat, this visual signal appears to be coding retinal slip velocity and is not dependent on the cerebellum (Keller and Precht 1979b). Therefore, Vn recieve the same mix of head velocity and image slip signals that goes to the flocculus. Thus, vestibular neurons may themselves be the modifiable brainstem element, whose existence is hypothesized on the basis of adaptation studies in the primate (Miles et al. 1980).

Our results have been reported previously in the literature (Keller and Precht 1979a) so we provide here only a brief summary of this work.

1.5 Tests for Concomitant Modifications of the Optokinetic Reflex

The foregoing discussion has dealt with changes in the VOR induced by optical alteration of the normally synergistic optokinetic input. In studies on the rabbit, Collewijn and Kleinschmidt (1975) found the opposite effect. During 24-hour periods of forced vestibular rotation with visual stimulation similar to that provided by left-right reversing prisms, the gain of the VOR was not changed, but instead the gain of the optokinetic (OK) tracking was significantly increased. Similar studies have not been reported in the cat, but Robinson (1976) found some improvement in its visual tracking during rotations with the prisms in agreement with the rabbit results.

The reason for our interest in possible changes induced in the OK reflex can be seen in Fig. 1. The direct brainstem pathway (which includes the vestibular nuclei) mediating the VOR is shown as path 1, while the parallel pathway through the flocculus is shown as route 2. The separate optokinetic (retinal slip) signal input to vestibular neurons is shown. It modulates the same Vn which receive direct vestibular input from the canals. If either Vn or the remainder of the brainstem VOR pathways contain the modifiable neural elements, then they may be modified to the same extent for vestibular and optokinetic inputs. On the other hand, if parallel pathways like those shown through the flocculus contain the modifiable elements, then a change in the gain of the VOR might be detected while none would occur in those tested by optokinetic stimuli. In this respect, it is important to note that the retinal slip signal to the flocculus is not required for the generation of OK tracking (Robinson 1974; Keller and Precht 1979b). Thus, the use of OK stimuli tests the direct brainstem pathway independent of the cerebellum.

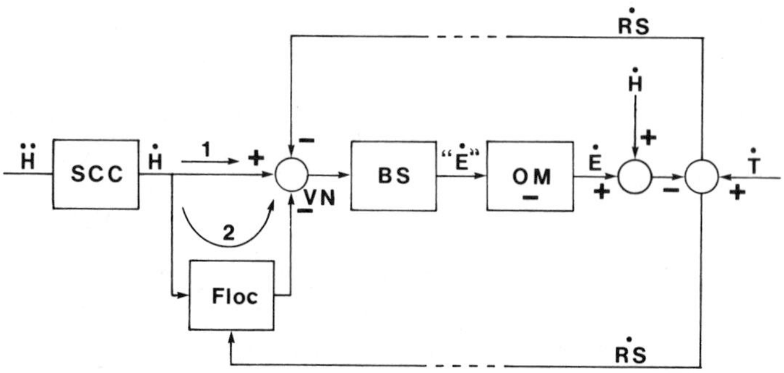

Fig. 1. Schematic view of the basic vestibuloocular and optokinetic neural pathways. For a complete discussion, see text. $\ddot{H}$, head acceleration; *SCC*, semicircular canal; $\dot{H}$, head velocity; *Floc*, flocculus; *VN*, central vestibular neuron; *BS*, additional brain stem pathways; "$\dot{E}$", internal copy of eye velocity command; *OM*, oculomotor plant; $\dot{E}$, eye velocity; $\dot{T}$, velocity of the external visual world; $\dot{RS}$, retinal slip velocity

2 Methods

These experiments were carried out on alert cats implanted chronically with head fixation platforms. The cats utilized for testing single-unit vestibular nucleus responses were also implanted with stereotaxically aimed microelectrode recording cylinders. Eye movements in these animals were measured with implanted silver-silver chloride electrodes. Eye movements in the more recent OK tests were measured with the implanted search-coil technique.

Vestibular stimuli were provided by placing the cats in a loose restraining box with their heads bolted to a framework mounted on the box. The box was then placed on a rate table and the whole animal was rotated in a totally dark room about a vertical axis passing through the center of the head.

Optokinetic stimuli were delivered by lowering a large, full-field drum around the restrained cat. The inner surface and ceiling of the drum contained a pattern of random-width, vertical black stripes on a white background (with spatial frequencies from 0.125 to 1.0 cycles/deg). Motion of this drum was controlled by a servo system. A mirror was placed below the animal's chin to provide OK stimulation from the inferior visual field.

Standard extracellular microelectrode recording techniques were utilized in the Vn study.

Adaptation of the VOR was accomplished by fitting the restrained animal with spectacles containing either left–right reversing prisms or large positive (8X) lens. A mask prevented nonspectacle vision. The prism cats viewed a highly textured earth-fixed pattern through the spectacles. The cats fitted with positive lens viewed a textured pattern placed at the focal distance of the lens and fixed to the rate table so that the field of view rotated with the animal (called the fixed-field condition).

Before the animal had obtained any experience with vision through the optical devices, the gain and phase of the VOR were measured in darkness. The animal was oscillated at 0.25 Hz (peak velocity about 16 deg/s) and the peak velocity and phase of the compensatory eye movements were measured. Gain is defined as the ratio of peak slow-phase eye velocity to peak head velocity. Phase is always with respect to head velocity.

Following this initial measurement the animals were force-rotated at frequencies which were varied from 0.1 to 0.17 Hz, at peak velocities of about 10–15 deg/s with continuous visual input through the spectacles. The gain and phase of the VOR were remeasured every hour or two hours in the dark. After a 4 to 5-h period of head rotation with altered visual input all the cats showed the same consistent pattern of decreasing gain of the VOR without noticeable phase change. The measured VOR gains (which were about one before rotation) decreased to 0.35 to 0.5. We then carried out neural recordings in the vestibular nucleus in one series of adapted animals and measured the gain of the OK reflex in the other cats.

3 Results

3.1 Vestibular Nucleus Responses

In order to provide a data base for comparative purposes, we recorded from a sample of Vn in the normal VOR gain cats. In all these cases the animals had a VOR gain equal to about one at 0.25 Hz. We made 35 electrode penetrations in four cats that passed through the area of the vestibular nuclei and isolated 119 neurons that responded selectively to horizontal accelerations. Thus about 3.4 cells responding selectively to horizontal angular acceleration were isolated per penetration in the normal cat.

From the entire sample of 119 neurons 51 cells were classified as type I and 68 were classified as type II, after the nomenclature of Duensing and Schaefer (1958). In this alert preparation the resting discharge rates were relatively high with an overall average of 35.4 spikes/s (± 39 S.D.) and with no significant difference between type I and II unit resting rates.

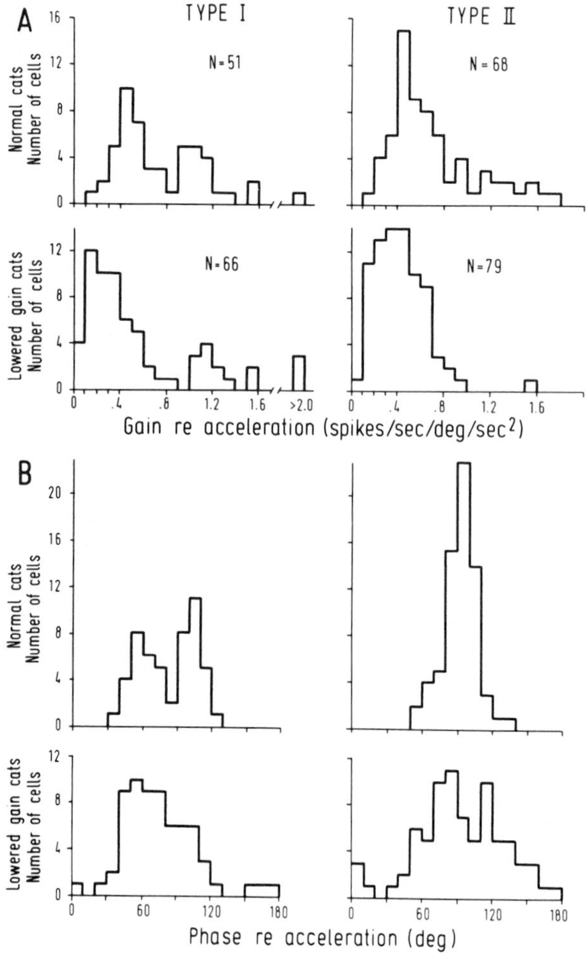

Fig. 2A, B. Histograms of unit responses in vestibular nucleus to horizontal sinusoidal oscillation of the head at 0.25 Hz. **A** Unit gains re head acceleration; units in cats with normal VOR, *upper plates;* units in same animals with lowered-gain VOR, *lower plates.* **B** Unit response phases re acceleration; normal VOR, *upper plates;* lowered gain VOR, *lower plates.* All *plates in left-hand column,* type I responses; all *plates in righthand column,* type II responses (Keller and Precht 1979a)

The gains and phases of these 119 neurons with respect to angular acceleration were calculated by Fourier analysis and the results are shown in Fig. 2 in separate columns for type I and II neurons. For type I neurons the individual unit values of gain (Fig. 2A) show a distribution skewed toward higher values with a mean of 0.75 spikes/s per deg/s^2 (± 1.4 S.D.). Most of the population variance is contributed by the presence of those units with higher gains giving the suggestion of a second peak in the distribution above about 0.9. These cells will arbitrarily be called high-gain units (gain > 0.9 spikes/s per deg/s^2). Such type I units in the normal cat constitute 40% of the sample (20 out of 51 cells).

The histogram of phases for type I units in the normal cat (Fig. 28, upper left) shows a bimodal distribution. Approximately equal numbers of cells are found distributed around the peak of 55° of phase lag re ipsilateral acceleration and around another peak at 105° of phase lag. The mean value of phase for the whole population of type I units was 82.5° lagging ipsilateral acceleration.

For type II cells the histogram of unit gains (Fig. 2A, upper right) is unimodally distributed but skewed toward units with higher gain (mean gain = 0.69 spikes/s per deg/s^2, ± 1.3 S.D.). High-gain type II units are found, but constitute only 25% of the sample (17 out of 68 cells).

The histogram of phases for type II units in the normal cat (Fig. 2B, upper right) is distributed tightly around a single peak at 95° (mean = 91°) close to the same value of the phase lag noted for the larger phase lag type of unit in the type I population.

In the same four cats, having lowered-gain VORs, we made 40 penetrations and isolated 145 Vn that responded selectively to horizontal accelerations. Thus we obtained an almost identical ratio (3.6) of horizontal sensitive neurons per electrode penetration as we found in the cats with normal VOR gain. Therefore, it is apparent that the mechanism which lowers VOR gain does not cause a total inhibition of even a subset of the entire Vn population of horizontal-acceleration sensitive neurons. Morevoer, the mean resting discharge rate (38.3 spikes/s, ± 42 S.D.) of units in the lowered-gain VOR animals was almost identical to that found in the normal animals.

On the other hand, the gains and phases of the horizontal-acceleration sensitive population of Vn were altered clearly and reproducibly by the short-term periods of visual-vestibular conflict caused by the reversing prism vision.

Figure 2A shows that for type I units there is a shift of the lower gain model peak to lower values (overall population mean = 0.57 spikes/s per deg/s^2, ± 1.3 S.D.). This shift is, we believe, rather significant because the most frequently encountered value of neuronal gain was now between 0.1 and 0.2, a value that hardly ever occurs (only 1 cell out of 51) in normal cat vestibular nucleus. High-gain type I cells were still found in the lowered-gain animals, but less frequently (15 out of 66 cells – 23%) than in normal animals.

The histogram of phases for type I units (Fig. 2B) shows a unimodal distribution with a peak at 55° lagging ipsilateral acceleration (population mean = 76°). These two sets of histograms show that a total loss of high-gain type I units with large phase lags has occurred in the lowered-gain VOR animals.

The histogram of unit gain for type II units in the lowered-gain VOR animals (Fig. 2B) shows a similar shift to smaller values (overall population mean = 0.43 spikes/s per deg/s^2, ± 1.3 S.D.).

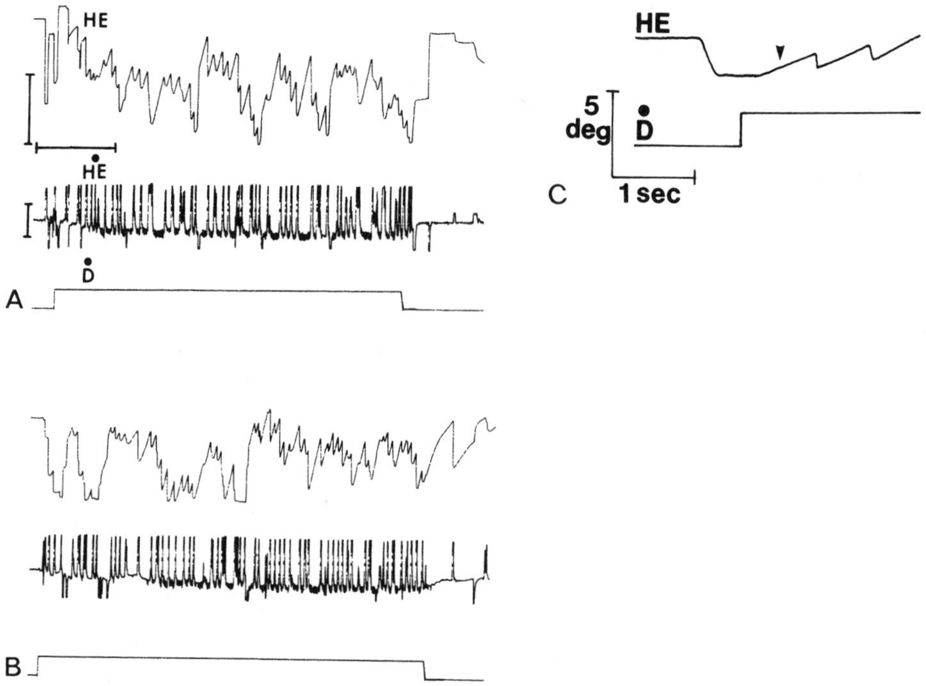

Fig. 3A–C. Constant velocity OK tests in the normal VOR gain cat (**A**) and in the same animal with the lowered VOR gain (**B**). *Upper trace* in each record is horizontal eye position (*HE*), *middle trace* shows eye velocity ($\dot{HE}$), and *lower trace* is OK drum velocity ($\dot{D}$). Calibrations shown in **A** equal 20 deg for *HE*, 20 deg/s for $\dot{HE}$ and $\dot{D}$, and 10 s for time. **C** Higher speed record showing an example of the initial three slow-phase responses in a test similar to those illustrated in **A** and **B**. The slope of the initial phase was measured at the *arrow* to estimate open-loop OK gain

The histogram for phases of type II units in the prism vision cats is widely spread over a range of phases from a value in phase with contralateral acceleration to 180° lagging this acceleration (overall mean = 88°). This wide spread is in marked contrast to the narrowly distributed range of phase lags shown by type II units in normal animals.

3.2 Optokinetic Gain Measurements in Adapted Cats

In this second series of experiments the response of both the VOR (measured in dark) and the OK tracking to pure drum motion were measured before the cats received any combined visual-vestibular experience with the optical devices. The cats were then subjected to 4 to 5 h of forced rotation while viewing the patterned background which rotated with them (fixed-field spectacles). In each of three cats the gain of the VOR (tested at 0.25 Hz) dropped to 0.5 or less (mean = 0.39) by the end of this period. The spectacles were then removed and the response of the OK system to full-field visual motion was remeasured.

The response to constant velocity drum rotations was measured first. Figure 3A shows the response to 10 deg/s drum motion in a normal gain VOR cat, and 3B a similar response to the same drum motion in the cat with VOR gain of 0.4. We tested with several different drum velocities from 5 to 20 deg/s and obtained similar results in all three cats. There was no measurable difference in the steady-state OK gain in the normal and VOR adapted cats. At 10 deg/s the calculated mean values of gain were 0.93 (± 0.5 S.D.) in normal and 0.95 (± 0.7 S.D.) in adapted cats.

However, there is one difficulty in these measurements. The OK system operates as a closed-loop feedback system in contrast to the open-loop VOR. One well-known characteristic of closed-loop feedback systems is that they function in the closed-loop mode to reduce externally measured changes in gain due to internal changes in gain in the forward loop. In our situation we want to measure a possible change in element BS in Fig. 1. We do this with measurements at the input and output. Since the forward-loop steady-state gain must be about 13 to provide the observed approximately 93% of stimulus velocity tracking, we estimate that the gain of BS would have to change by at least 65% for us to reliably detect the decrease with the closed-loop measurements. It is unreasonable to expect that the change would be this big, since the VOR gain only changed by about 50%.

Therefore, we made two additional measurements of the OK gain in these VOR adapted animals. Figure 3 shows that in response to step changes in surround velocity, the OK velocity tracking of the eyes builds up slowly with an approximately exponential time course. Similar behavior has been previously reported in the cat (Evinger and Fuchs 1978) and also in the monkey (Cohen et al. 1977) and the rabbit (Collewijn 1969).

Of particular interest here is the initial slow-phase response following the target step in velocity. A typical response is shown in Fig. 3C. The first response begins at about 180 (± 100) ms following the onset of drum motion. It is a slow-phase movement in the same direction as the drum motion, is about 20% of the final steady-state velocity, and remains at approximately constant velocity for the whole first phase. During the latency period and during the first part of this initial response the OK system is essentially in the open-loop condition until feedback from the retina can be processed through delays in the visual centers and reach the brainstem oculomotor circuits. Thus the slope of this initial slow-phase response approximates the direct pathway gain of the OK system. We measured this initial velocity for ten individual responses in each of the normal and lowered-gain VOR cats and found no difference in the two classes of response. The initial gain was 0.25 (± 0.15 S.D.) in the normal cats and 0.22 (± 0.1 S.D.) in the lowered-gain cats.

Finally we tested the response of the OK system to sinusoidal motions of the drum over the frequency range of 0.01 to 1 Hz in the normal cat. The results are shown in Fig. 4. In the normal cat, even at the lowest frequencies tested, peak eye velocity did not quite equal peak drum velocity, but there was little phase lag even up to 0.1 Hz where gain had fallen off considerably. The gain and phase values in the lowered-gain VOR cats were almost identical. The values of gain at stimulus frequencies of about 1 Hz are particularly interesting for our analysis here. The gain fell to about 20% of normal steady-state response to constant velocity drum rotation. With gain values this low the loop is essentially open, and if a 50% change in any element downstream from

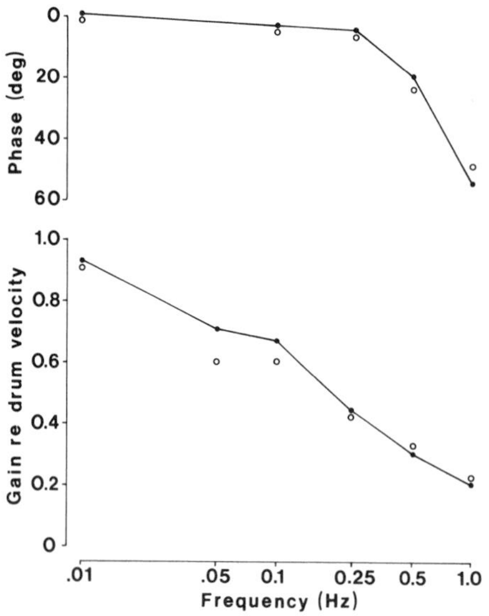

Fig. 4. The gain and phase (both re drum velocity) of the cat OK system in response to sinusoidal motion of the visual surround. The *filled circles* and *interconnecting lines* show the average response (five measurements at each frequency in each of three animals) for the animals in the normal VOR gain state. The *open circles* show corresponding mean values obtained from the same cats in the lowered VOR gain state

Vn has occurred, it could be detected with our measurements. Instead, the gain values in the adapted cats are equal to those in the normal anmals at 1 Hz.

3.3 Conclusions

The gain of the VOR in cat can be consistently modified over a short period of several hours by forced rotation with vision restricted to that seen through reversing prisms or fixed-field spectacles. This short-term modification of the VOR provides a suitable preparation for studying the neuronal elements involved in the VOR recalibration.

Vestibular nucleus neurons seem to participate in this recalibration, but the mean population gain change in type I neurons is not nearly large enough to account for the total decrease observed in VOR gain. However, there are major gain changes in a subset of Vn, namely the high-gain, large phase lag type I neurons which could account for the VOR modifications, if these neurons are more heavily weighted in producing the VOR than the overall population of Vn.

The gain changes observed in Vn are consistent with the hypothesis that this subset of cells receives an in-phase, parallel inhibitory input from the flocculus or elsewhere. The gain in this pathway, if plastically increased by the conflicting visual input during vestibular stimulation, could result in the lowered Vn gain observed.

The direct OK pathways, which are probably shared with the VOR pathways from Vn on to the eye velocity output, are not modified during VOR recalibration. Possible gain changes in the hypothesized internal positive feedback loop which provides most of the steady-state gain of the OK response (Cohen et al. 1977; Robinson 1977) were not tested in the present closed-loop experiments. However, they are unlikely to be involved in the gain of the VOR at frequencies of 0.25 Hz where we measured our recalibration. The OK results provide additional evidence that major changes must occur at the level of Vn, if the hypothesis is correct that the OK and VOR pathways peripheral to the vestibular nucleus are shared. Further, they support the concept of a parallel modifying projection to Vn rather than a modification of Vn themselves, because the same Vn receive both the pure head velocity signal and the OK signal. Since a subset of these neurons show a modification for head velocity signals, they would be expected to show the same change for OK inputs, but this would result in an observed change in gain of the OK response contrary to our present results.

Acknowledgments. The authors are indebted to Marla Smith, Jona Countie, and Helen Sullivan. Research was supported by NIH Grants ROl EY-03280-01, 5P 30 Ey-01186, and The Smith-Kettlewell Eye Research Foundation. E.L. Keller was partially supported by a grant from the Alexander von Humboldt Foundation.

References

Baker R, Precht W, Llinas R (1972) Cerebellar modulatory action on the vestibulo-trochlear pathway in the cat. Exp Brain Res 15: 364–385

Cohen B, Matsuo V, Raphan T (1977) Quantitative analysis of the velocity characteristics of optokinetic nystagmus and optokinetic after-nystagmus. J Physiol (London) 270: 321–344

Collewijn H (1969) Optokinetic eye movements in the rabbit: input-output relations. Vision Res 9: 117–132

Collewijn H, Kleinschmidt HJ (1975) Vestibuloocular and optokinetic reactions in the rabbit: changes during 24 hrs. of normal and abnormal interaction. In: Lennerstrand G, Bach-y-Rita P (eds) Basic mechanisms of ocular motility and their clinical implications. Pergamon Press, London, pp 477–483

Duensing F, Schaefer KP (1958) Die Aktivität einzelner Neurone im Bereich der Vestibulariskerne bei Horizontalbeschleunigungen unter besonderer Berücksichtigung des vestibulären Nystagmus. Arch Psyhciatr Nervenkr 198: 225–252

Evinger C, Fuchs AF (1978) Saccadic, smooth pursuit, and optokinetic eye movements of the trained cat. J Physiol (London) 285: 209–229

Fukuda J, Highstein SM, Ito M (1972) Cerebellar inhibitory control of the vestibulo-ocular reflex investigated in rabbit III rd nucleus. Exp Brain Res 14: 511–526

Gonshor A, Melvill Jones G (1971) Plasticity in the adult vestibuloocular reflex arc. Proc Can Fed Biol Soc 14: 11

Ito M (1970) Neurophysiological aspects of the cerebellar motor control system. Int J Neurol 7: 162–176

Ito M (1977) Neuronal events in the cerebellar flocculus associated with an adaptive modification of the vestibulo-ocular reflex of the rabbit. In: Baker R, Berthoz A (eds) Control of gaze by brain stem neurons. Elsevier, Amsterdam, pp 391–398

Ito M, Shiida T, Yagi N, Yamamoto M (1974) The cerebellar modification of rabbit's horizontal vestibulo-ocular reflex induced by sustained head rotation combined with visual stimulation. Proc Jpn Acad 50: 85–89

Keller EL, Precht W (1979a) Adaptive modification of central vestibular neurons in response to visual stimulation through reversing prisms. J Neurophysiol 42: 896–911

Keller EL, Precht W (1979b) Visual-vestibular responses in vestibular nuclear neurons in the intact and cerebellectomized, alert cat. Neuroscience 4: 1599–1613

Lisberger SG, Fuchs AF (1978) Role of the primate flocculus during rapid behavioral modification of vestibuloocular reflex. I. Purkinje cell activity during visually guided horizontal smooth-pursuit eye movements and passive head rotation. J Neurophysiol 41: 733–763

Miles FA, Fuller JH (1974) Adaptive plasticity of the vestibulo-ocular responses of the rhesus monkey. Brain Res 80: 512–516

Miles FA, Braitman DJ, Dow BM (1980) Long-term adaptive changes in primate vestibuloocular reflex. IV. Electrophysiological observations in flocculus and adapted monkeys. J Neurophysiol 43: 1477–1493

Precht W (1978) Neuronal operations in the vestibular system. Springer, Berlin Heidelberg New York

Robinson DA (1974) The effect of cerebellectomy on the cat's vestibulo-ocular integrator. Brain Res 71: 195–207

Robinson DA (1976) Adaptive gain control of vestibuloocular reflex by the cerebellum. J Neurophysiol 39: 954–969

Robinson DA (1977) Vestibular and optokinetic symbiosis: an example of explaining by modelling. In: Baker R, Berthoz A (eds) Control of gaze by brain stem neurons. Elsevier, Amsterdam, pp 49–58

Waespe W, Henn V (1977) Neuronal activity in the vestibular nuclei of the alert monkey during vestibular and optokinetic stimulation. Exp Brain Res 27: 523–538

Adaptive Plasticity in the Oculomotor System

D.A. ROBINSON[1] and L.M. OPTICAN[1,2]

The contents of this symposium bear witness to the importance of the oculomotor system in the study of neuronal plasticity. Part of this recent development is due to a surge of progress in understanding the oculomotor system itself, made possible by the ability to record from the neurons of the brainstem and cerebellar oculomotor pathways in alert animals making normal eye movements. An additional factor is the mechanical simplicity of the eyeball and its muscles that makes the relationship between neural activity in the brain stem and the resulting eye movements relatively direct. A very important factor in using the oculomotor system to study plasticity is that it may be divided into about five major subsystems the functions of which are fairly obvious. Thus, one can speak of dysmetria as a failure to achieve a certain function, and of adaptive plasticity as its restoration.

Seven types of plasticity have been identified and studied so far in the oculomotor system: three of them associated with the vestibulo-ocular reflex and two with the vergence system. These will be mentioned briefly and the last two, associated with the saccadic system, will be described in more detail.

1 Balance Control of the Vestibulo-Ocular Reflex

A lesion of the peripheral vestibular apparatus or nerves upsets the balance between the resting discharge rates of cells in the vestibular nucleus representing a push-pull pair of canals, and creates, among other things, ocular nystagmus. This nystagmus is compensated in a few days or weeks depending on age and species, and eye volocity returns to zero. This process is the subject of several of the contributions to this symposium and needs no further comment here, except to note that there is still controversy over the role of the cerebellum in this recovery process. Removal of the vestibulo-cerebellum in the cat does not affect recovery (Haddad et al. 1977) nor does cerebellar decortication in the rat (Llinás et al. 1975; Llinás and Walton 1977) but destruc-

1 Departments of Ophthalmology and Biomedical Engineering, The Johns Hopkins University, Baltimore, MD, USA

2 Currently at the Laboratory of Sensorimotor Research, The National Eye Institute, Bethesda, MD, USA

tion of the inferior olive does (ibid.). Removal of the entire cerebellum, which includes the deep cerebellar nuclei, gives confusing results: nystagmus is still compensated in the guinea pig (Schaefer and Meyer 1974), but is not in the rat (Llinás et al. 1975).

2 Gain Control of the Vestibulo-Ocular Reflex

The gain of this reflex is defined as the ratio of the compensatory eye velocity to head velocity. Normally the gain is 1.0 so that images do not move on the retina during head movements. If, for example, an animal or human wears 2X telescope lenses chronically, the gain of the reflex must be increased from 1.0 to 2.0 if images are to be kept from slipping on the retina when the head moves and this, in fact, happens. Using other optical devices the gain has been shown capable of increasing, decreasing, and even reversing in man (Gauthier and Robinson 1975; Gonshor and Melvill Jones 1976), monkey (Miles and Fuller 1974), cat (Melvill Jones and Davies 1976; Robinson 1976), rabbit (Ito et al. 1974), chicken (Green and Wallman 1978), and goldfish (Schairer and Bennett 1977).

The purpose of gain control, like that of other forms of plasticity, is obviously not to deal with experimental lenses and prisms but to calibrate the gain at birth, maintain calibration through the changes associated with growth and aging, and repair the dysmetria created by lesions throughout life. Removing the vestibulo-cerebellum or inferior olive abolishes this form of plasticity (Robinson 1976; Haddad et al. 1980).

3 Direction Control of the Vestibulo-Ocular Reflex

A head rotation may be described by a vector indicating instantaneous, angular head velocity; rotation of the eye by another vector. A vector has both magnitude and direction so that gain control, just described, should include a consideration of both the speed and the direction of the eye. Nevertheless, the two aspects of the movement are sufficiently different, qualitatively, to describe them separately. The direction of the vestibularly induced eye movements is controlled by the relative strengths of the connections between the six semicircular canals and the six extraocular muscles of each eye. These connections may be described by a matrix which converts the head rotation vector from the coordinate system of the canals to that of the eye muscles. A change in the relative strengths of these connections will cause the eye to rotate in a plane that differs from the plane of head rotation. Some system must calibrate and repair this connectivity matrix.

Direction plasticity has been implicated by Hay (1968) in a psychophysical experiment and been confirmed in humans and cat by L.W. Schultheis and D.A. Robinson (unpublished observations). It may be demonstrated by allowing oscillatory, vertical head motion to drive a visual stimulus (e.g., an optokinetic drum) horizontally. After a few minutes to a few hours of such stimulation, a vertical head movement in the dark will create a compensatory eye movement with a horizontal component that can be as large as 20% of the vertical component. Thus, a connection has been established between the vertical canals and the horizontal muscles. This plastic change remains for at least several hours if subjects are kept in the dark.

4 Vergence Tone

When a subject has a base-out prism in front of one eye, it must converge by the prism angle to fuse images binocularly. If that eye is covered, it will swing out by the prism angle plus any idiosynchratic angle of phoria of the subject. If humans wear such a prism for about 1 h during normal activities (reading, walking about, watching television) a tonic vergence angle develops so that the convergence needed for fusion becomes automatic: when the eye is covered, it no longer swings out by the prism angle (G. Milders and R.D. Reinecke, unpublished observations). Evidently, a baseline vergence adjustment has occurred to maintain the needed convergence without extra effort. Patients with cerebellar lesions that interfere with eye movements fail to show this plasticity.

5 Accomodative Vergence

When an eye accommodates by focusing from a far to a near target, the other eye, if under a cover, nevertheless converges. The ratio between the accommodative convergence angle (AC) and the angle appropriate to the accommodative stimulus (A) is called the AC/A ratio. This ratio depends on the interpupillary distance. The latter can be changed if subjects wear periscope glasses that effectively spread their eyes apart by a factor of 2. In this situation, subjects must produce twice the normal amount of convergence for a given accommodative stimulus to fuse the images seen in each eye. After wearing such prisms for 1 h, the AC/A ratio approximately doubles: accommodation by one eye produced twice the normal convergence in the opposite, covered eye (Judge and Miles 1980). The increase in the ratio for such exposure times was not entirely plastic in the sense that the ratio decreased toward the normal value if the subject was subsequently denied binocular vision, although some change was still observable after 24 h.

6 Saccadic Gain Control

Around 1975, when the only types of oculomotor plasticity known were the first two described above, it occurred to us to see if plasticity could be demonstrated in an oculomotor system phylogenetically quite different from the vestibulo-ocular reflex, namely the saccadic system. When we see a target 10° to the left of the line of sight, we execute a 10° saccade to the left which is planned before the event occurs and cannot be corrected in flight because of delays in the visual system (e.g., 55–65 ms). This type of movement is similar to the vestibulo-ocular reflex in that the movement occurs in an open-loop fashion, without the benefit of visual feedback. Consequently, it is necessary to monitor the success of this system from trial to trial, to calibrate the gain (saccade size/retinal error), maintain it during growth and aging, and repair it after damage. Thus, there was little doubt that the saccadic system was plastic, and even as we began our research, Kommerell et al. (1976) demonstrated such plasticity in humans with a palsy of a muscle in one eye by requiring them to view the world for several days through the normal and then the palsied eye. The parameters of the patients' saccades were adjusted so as to optimize the movements in whichever eye was viewing.

Our study (Optican 1978; Optican and Robinson 1980) employed the rhesus monkey because we wanted to observe the effects of cerebellar lesions on saccadic plasticity . The monkeys were trained to follow visual targets; eye movements were recorded by the search coil-magnetic field method. To demonstrate plasticity, the horizontal recti of one eye were tenectomized, the tendons were excised and the muscle allowed to fall back into the orbit. The muscles reattached after several days, but more posteriorly than normal, so that they were weaker. After a few days the eye reached a mechanical steady state in which it moved by only a fraction (20%–60%) of the distance of the normal eye. This produced the saccadic hypometria illustrated at the left in Fig. 1. When the monkey made a 10° saccade with the normal eye, the weak eye, which was covered by a patch during this period, made only a 4° saccade (defined as the amplitude of the rapid, initial part of the movement – the subsequent drifting movement will be described in the next section). The patch was then switched, forcing the monkey to view the world with the dysmetric eye. At first the monkey made a staircase of saccades to get on target (Fig. 1, center), each saccade reducing the remaining error by only 40%. But, within just a few hours the amplitude of the initial saccade to a target jump could be seen to increase and after 3 days spent in the home cage, except for

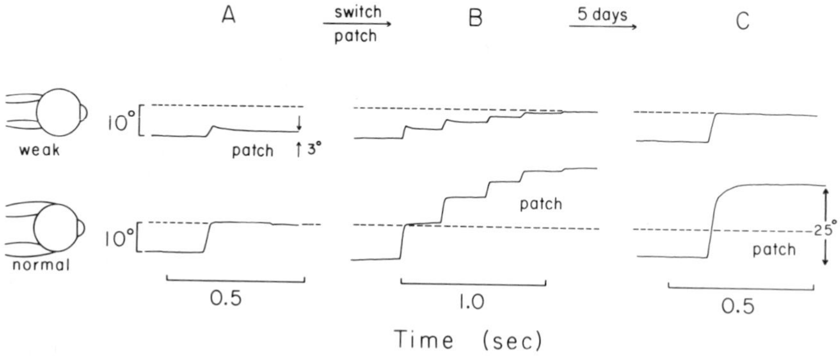

Fig. 1A–C. Saccadic dysmetria and its repair. **A** The saccade made by the surgically weakened eye (*weak*) makes a rapid movement of only 4°, when the normal eye makes a 10° saccade, and then drifts back to a final displacement of 3°. **B** Immediately after switching the patch from the weak to the normal eye, the monkey makes a staircase of hypometric saccades to a 10° target jump (*dashed lines*). **C** After 3 days, the weakness has been compensated by central changes in innervation: the weak eye makes a normal saccade. Data shown was taken 5 days after the patch was switched daily recording sessions, the weak eye made normal saccades and target displacements were followed by a single rapid movement (Fig. 1, right).

These results clearly demonstrate saccadic plasticity. The central nervous system had increased the innervation sent to the muscles to compensate for their weakness and repair the dysmetria. The increased innervation was reflected in the normal eye moving under the patch: after adaptation to the weak eye, the normal eye made a saccade almost twice as large as before. Under our conditions, where viewing was always monocular, plasticity obeyed a sort of Hering's law in that the innervations were altered equally in both eyes. When the patch was moved back to the weak eye after, typically, 5 days of visual experience, the normal eye initially made hypermetric saccades and acquired the target by a series of damped saccadic oscillations. This pattern quickly changed and innervation returned to normal within 1 day.

Total cerebellectomy in two monkeys created saccadic dysmetria and abolished all plastic changes to visual experience. Saccades were hypermetric by factors of 2–3, centripetal saccades being more hypermetric than centrifugal. The dysmetria depended on initial eye position and saccade size and direction, and was enduring. This finding suggests that one role of the cerebellum might be adjusting innervation for initial eye position to compensate for nonlinearities. If the cerebellum maintains calibration, it is necessary to recognize that nonlinearities in the neural networks and muscle and orbital mechanics demand different calibration for saccades in different directions and positions in the orbit. The permanence of the dysmetria already indicated that saccadic plasticity had been abolished so it was not surprising that forcing the monkey to view the world with the weak or the normal eye made no difference at all in the dysmetria.

To try and localize the part of the cerebellum essential for saccadic plasticity, we attempted to remove the vermis, lobes IV–VII, in two monkeys since the results of stimulation (Ron and Robinson 1973), unit recording (Llinás and Wolfe 1977), and lesions (Ritchie 1976) indicate this region to be most involved with saccades. Unfortunately, we also inadvertently removed the fastigial nucleus, thereby disconnecting the entire vermis. This lesion had essentially the same result as total cerebellectomy on the initial, rapid part of saccades: the movements were hypermetric and the dysmetria could not be repaired or modified by visual experience with the weak or normal eye. The rapid part of a saccade is made by a pulse or burst of high-frequency discharges on the part of motoneurons. We concluded that the fastigial nucleus and, perhaps, its overlying cerebellar cortex are necessary for the nervous system to control the size of the pulse and effect saccadic plasticity.

7 Post-Saccadic Drift Control

Figure 1A shows that the tenectomy not only weakened the muscles but upset the ratio between the viscous and elastic components of the net muscle and orbital mechanics which caused the eye to slide back after the saccade from an initial 4° displacement to a final 3° displacement. The pulse of motoneuronal discharge rate, which generates a large momentary force to overcome viscous impedances and get the eye quickly from here to there, is followed by a step change in discharge rate which creates a steady force to counterbalance elastic elements in the orbit and hold the eye in its new position (e.g., Robinson 1970). If the ratio between either the size of the pulse to the step, or the viscosity to elasticity, should change, the position of the eye just after the pulse will differ from that demanded by the step and the eye will drift (exponentially), either backward or onward, to its final position. Again, there is no time for visual feedback to correct such a drift immediately after a saccade and one might suspect, as is the case, that some central mechanism monitors and adjusts the amplitude of the step relative to the pulse to eliminate post-saccadic drift.

Such control is evident in Fig. 1. When the patch was moved to the normal eye, the pulse increased until the saccade size was increased from 4° to 10°, a rise of 2.5. But, to eliminate post-saccadic drift, the step increased until steady-state position rose from 3° to 10°, an increase of 3.3. Thus, innervation was not just increased in a general way, but the pulse and step rose by different amounts suggesting independent control. The increase of the step relative to the pulse is revealed by the normal eye under cover (Fig. 1C) which now drifted onward, after the saccade, to a larger final deviation. Independent control of the pulse and step was confirmed by cerebellar lesions. After removing the fastigial nuclei, saccades were dysmetric, but the eye which normally viewed had no post-saccadic drift. If the weak eye was patched, it drifted; the normal eye did not. If the normal eye was patched, it drifted and the weak eye did not. This lesion abolished control of the pulse but not of the step. The step was always adjusted by visual experience, not to bring the eye to the target but to eliminate post-saccadic drift. Thus, the criteria for this mechanism, unlike that for pulse control, is not whether the eye got on target but whether images slipped on the retina just after a saccade.

Total cerebellectomy not only created saccadic dysmetria but also post-saccadic drift, which was also enduring and failed to respond to visual experience. Consequently, control of drift requires that some portion of the cerebellum be intact, other than the fastigial nucleus and overlying cortex. It has subsequently been shown that the flocculus is essential for the elimination of post-saccadic slip. Optican and Miles (1979) have demonstrated plasticity of this control system in intact monkeys by causing a visual scene to move after each saccade in such a way as to create the same sort of retinal image motion that would be created if the monkeys had a pulse–step mismatch. After several hours of exposure to this situation, the monkeys generated a post-saccadic drift in such a direction as to lessen post-saccadic retinal image motion. This alteration of saccadic behavior could not be induced in monkeys without flocculi (Optican et al. 1980). In retrospect, localization of the control of post-saccadic slip to the flocculus is not especially surprising, since this structure has been shown to be important in controlling several oculomotor functions designed to prevent images from slipping on the retina (e.g., Zee et al. 1978).

8 Discussion

The important question behind all these examples of adaptive motor plasticity is the mechanism and location of the neural circuits which effect the observed changes. Unfortunately, there is still no clear answer to this question. As this symposium shows, there are a variety of mechanisms throughout the nervous system that participate in compensation and plasticity, but the fact that the cerebellum is implicated in all five of the seven examples given, where a cerebellar involvement has been looked for, makes it necessary to consider the hypothesis that, among other functions, the cerebellum may not only coordinate movements but maintain that coordination by correcting dysmetria – a form of motor learning. The problem now is determining whether modifiable synapses, the presumed basis for motor learning, are in the cerebellum or not.

Ito (1972) has proposed that the activity of climbing fibers from the olive may somehow alter the strengths of synapses between parallel T fibers and Purkinje cells. In the vestibulo-ocular reflex the flocculus lies in parallel with the direct projection from the semicircular canals to the vestibular nucleus so that such changes in synaptic strengths would change the gain of the entire reflex. It has also been demonstrated that the error signal for gain control – the velocity of retinal image slip – is relayed to the flocculus on climbing fibers (Maekawa and Takeda 1977; see also Miyashita, this vol.). Thus, all the pieces, pathways and signals required by this theory have been demonstrated, but there is still no firm evidence that synaptic modifications can occur in cerebellar cortex. Although Keller and Precht (1979, and this vol.) have found altered sensitivities of cells in the vestibular nucleus to canal stimulation that could, given certain assumptions, explain the gain changes induced by prisms in the cat, Lisberger and Miles (1980) could find no such changes in the monkey's vestibular nucleus. The latter finding does not rule out the idea that the gain changes might be effected by changes in the flocculus, but certainly complicates the circuitry necessary since it indicates that the projection of the flocculus onto the vestibular nucleus via Purkinje cells does not carry the altered signal by which the gain is changed. Thus, continued research has provided more puzzles than answers, but has neither confirmed or denied the possibility that changes in the gain of the vestibulo-ocular reflex are effected by synaptic modifications in the flocculus.

An alternative theory (Llinás et al. 1975, see also Llinás, this vol.) is that motor learning occurs elsewhere in the nervous system but makes its modifications on motor performance by signals which only pass through the cerebellum. Thus, the cerebellum would be essential for plasticity, but would not contain modifiable synapses. These authors found that destruction of the inferior olive abolished compensation of vestibular imbalance and suggested that the signals for modified behavior passed into the cerebellum on climbing fibers. Ito et al. (1979) found, however, that when Purkinje cells lose their climbing fiber input, they undergo some sort of metabolic change and lose the ability to inhibit their target cells. In that case, destruction of the olive effectively decorticates the entire cerebellum since Purkinje cells, which can still conduct action potentials, no longer have any influence on the rest of the brain and, by the same token, neither does the mossy fiber input to the cerebellum. Thus, the signals which mediate learned behavior could enter on mossy fibers. On the other hand, Llinás and Walton (1977) found that removing cerebellar cortex did not abolish compensation of vestibular imbalance which reemphasizes the climbing fiber input. It is important to note, however, that removing the vestibulo-cerebellum, a purely cortical lesion, does abolish gain control of the vestibulo-ocular reflex so that one cannot generalize from the effects of a lesion on one type of plasticity to its effect on other types (Haddad et al. 1977).

It would seem unlikely that the signal for the learned behavior itself is carried by climbing fibers. Olivary cells discharge at a very low rate (1–4 spikes/s) and project, with a very secure synapse, onto only a few Purkinje cells. This severely limits the bandwidth of any signal carried by one climbing fiber, and increasing the bandwidth by using many climbing fiber-Purkinje cells in parallel would require a very accurately timed multiplexing scheme. Many of the compensatory eye movements during head turns only last for 400 ms and monkey saccades last, typically, 40 ms. It seems unlikely that climbing fibers are guiding such movements on line. And, in fact, there is evidence in the rabbit that climbing fibers which project to the flocculus do not carry a signal proportional to head velocity (Barmack 1977), which they should if they are carrying the learned signal that can change the gain of the vestibulo-ocular reflex. The unusual arborization of a single climbing fiber over the entire dendritic tree of the Purkinje cells would suggest that the climbing fiber had some other function than simply relaying complex spikes through the Purkinje cell, and the fact that the ability of Purkinje cells to inhibit depends on climbing fibers (Ito et al. 1979) certainly reinforces that idea.

On the other hand, climbing fibers could easily act as a control valve, altering the sensitivitiy of Purkinje cells to mossy fiber signals or, perhaps, the effectiveness of Purkinje cells to inhibit. There is certainly evidence suggesting the former: altering the discharge rate of climbing fibers causes a reciprocal change in the simple spike activity of Purkinje cells (Colin et al. 1980). Whether this also causes changes in gain (Purkinje cell firing rate/mossy fiber firing rate) is still not known. The changes in Purkinje cell rate, when climbing fiber activity is changed, occur over periods measured in minutes so that this inhibitory channel also does not work by transmitting high-frequency, learned signals. More important, however, is that these authors could not demonstrate any form of memory in the behavior of Purkinje cells in response to climbing fiber activity. This suggests that while olive cells may set base-line discharge rates of Purkinje cells and possibly cerebellar input–output gains by means of slight alterations of their low discharge rates, they must be instructed to do so by some other neural structure, in which case the latter structure is the one that contains the modifiable synapses. The modifiable synapses could be on the olive cells themselves or could even still be in the cerebellum in the form of an olivo-cerebellar-olivary feedback loop. Obviously, there are many possibilities and, at the rate that new, unsuspected results are being discovered, it is premature, at the moment, the champion any particular theory.

References

Barmack NH (1977) Visually evoked activity of neurons in the dorsal cap of the inferior olive and its relationship to the control of eye movements. In: Baker R, Berthoz A (eds) Control of gaze by brain stem neurons. Elsevier, Amsterdam, p 361

Colin F, Manil J, Desclin JC (1980) The olivocerebellar system. I. Delayed and slow inhibitory effects: an overlooked salient feature of cerebellar climbing fibers. Brain Res 187: 3–27

Gauthier GM, Robinson DA (1975) Adaptation of the human vestibuloocular reflex to magnifying lenses. Brain Res 92: 331–335

Gonshor A, Melvill Jones G (1976) Extreme vestibuloocular adaptation induced by prolonged optical reversal of vision. J Physiol 256: 381–414

Green AE, Wallman J (1978) Rapid change in gain of vestibulo-ocular reflex in chickens. Soc Neurosci Abstr 4: 163

Haddad GM, Friendlich AR, Robinson DA (1977) Compensation of nystagmus after VIIIth nerve lesions in vestibulocerebellectomized cats. Brain Res 135: 192–196

Haddad GM, Demer JL, Robinson DA (1980) The effect of lesions of the dorsal cap of the inferior olive on the vestibulo-ocular and optokinetic systems of the cat. Brain Res 185: 265–275

Hay J (1968) Visual adaptation to an altered correlation between eye movement and head movement. Science 160: 429–430

Ito M (1972) Neural design of the cerebellar motor control system. Brain Res 40: 81–84

Ito M, Shiida T, Yagi N, Yamamoto M (1974) The cerebellar modification of rabbit's horizontal vestibulo-ocular reflex induced by sustained head rotation combined with visual stimulation. Proc Jpn Acad 50: 85–89

Ito M, Nisimaru N, Shibuki K (1979) Destruction of inferior olive induces rapid depression in synaptic action of cerebellar Purkinje cells. Nature (London) 277: 568–569

Judge SJ, Miles FA (1980) Short-term modification of stimulus AC/A induced by spectacles which alter effective interocular separation. Proc Assoc Res Vis Ophthalmol Abstr, Orlando, Fla, p 79

Keller EL, Precht W (1979) Adaptive modification of central vestibular neurons in response to visual stimulation through reversing prisms. J Neurophysiol 42: 896:911

Kommerell G, Olivier D, Theobold H (1976) Adaptive programming of phasic and tonic components in saccadic eye movements. Investigations in patients with abducens palsy. Invest Ophthalmol 15: 657–660

Lisberger SG, Miles FA (1980) Role of primate medial vestibular nucleus in long-term adaptive plasticity of vestibuloocular reflex. J Neurophysiol 43: 1725–1745

Llinás R, Walton K (1977) Place of the cerebellum in motor learning. In: Brazier MA (ed) Brain mechanisms in memory and learning. Raven Press, New York, p 17

Llinás R, Wolfe JW (1977) Functional linkage between the electrical activity in the vermal cerebellar cortex and saccadic eye movements. Exp Brain Res 29: 1–14

Llinás R, Walton K, Hillman DE, Sotelo C (1975) Inferior olive: its role in motor learning. Science 190: 1230–1231

Maekawa K, Takeda T (1977) Afferent pathways from the visual system to the cerebellar flocculus of the rabbit. In: Baker R, Berthoz A (eds) Control of gaze by brain stem neurons. Elsevier, Amsterdam, p 187

Melvill Jones G, Davies P (1976) Adaptation of cat vestibulo-ocular reflex to 200 days of optically reversed vision. Brain Res 103: 551–554

Miles FA, Fuller JH (1974) Adaptive plasticity in the vestibulo-ocular response of the rhesus monkey. Brain Res 80: 512–516

Optican LM (1978) Cerebellar-dependent adaptive control of the saccadic eye movement system. PhD Diss. Johns Hopkins Univ, Baltimore

Optican LM, Miles FA (1979) Visually induced adaptive changes in oculomotor control signals. Soc Neurosci Abstr 5: 380

Optican LM, Robinson DA (1980) Cerebellar-dependent adaptive control of the primate saccadic system. J Neurophysiol 44: 1058–1076

Optican LM, Zee DS, Miles FA, Lisberger SG (1980) Oculomotor deficits in monkeys with floccular lesions. Soc Neurosci Abstr 6: 474

Ritchie L (1976) Effects of cerebellar lesions on saccadic eye movements. J Neurophysiol 39: 1246–1256

Robinson DA (1970) Oculomotor unit behavior in the monkey. J Neurophysiol 33: 393–404

Robinson DA (1976) Adaptive gain control of vestibuloocular reflex by the cerebellum. J Neurophysiol 39: 954–969

Ron S, Robinson DA (1973) Eye movements evoked by cerebellar stimulation in the alert monkey. J Neurophysiol 36: 1004–1022

Schaefer K-P, Meyer DL (1974) Compensation of vestibular lesions. In: Kornhuber HH (ed) Handbook of sensory physiology, vol VI/2. Vestibular system Springer, Berlin Heidelberg New York, p 463

Schairer JO, Bennett WVL (1977) Adaptive gain control in vestibulo-ocular reflex of goldfish. Soc Neurosci Abstr 3: 157

Zee DS, Yamazaki A, Gücer G (1978) Ocular motor abnormalities in trained monkeys with floccular lesions. Soc Neurosci Abstr 4: 168

Differential Roles of the Climbing and Mossy Fiber Visual Pathways in Vision-Guided Modification of the Vestibulo-Ocular Reflex

Y. MIYASHITA[1]

1 Introduction

The hypothesis that the cerebellar flocculus adaptively controls the vestibulo-ocular reflex (VOR) by referring to visual information is based upon the existence of efferent projection from the flocculus to relay cells of the VOR, as well as afferent visual pathways to the flocculus (Ito 1972). However, since two different visual pathways project to the flocculus, one as climbing fiber (Maekawa and Simpson 1973) and the other as mossy fiber afferents (Maekawa and Takeda 1975), they may play different roles in the postulated floccular functions. The purpose of the work to be reported here was to differentiate these roles by interrupting each of the two visual pathways to the flocculus in rabbits.

There are at least three components in the climbing fiber visual pathway to the flocculus, having different courses and relay sites and eventually being connected with different components of the VOR (Ito et al. 1977). For the horizontal component of VOR (HVOR) to one eye, the climbing fiber visual pathway originating from that eye is relayed by the contralateral pretectal area, possibly at dorsal terminal nucleus and/or nucleus of optic tract, and projects to the dorsal cap of the contralateral inferior olive (Fig. 1). From the caudal part of the contralateral dorsal cap climbing fiber afferents project to the flocculus ipsilateral to the eye and activate those Purkinje cells which in turn inhibit relay cells of the HVOR from the ipsilateral horizontal canal to medial rectus and lateral rectus muscles of that eye, but not other components of the HVOR (Fig. 1).

Mossy fiber visual pathways originating from retinae bilaterally are relayed by the pretectum and then by nucleus reticularis tegmenti pontis (NRTP), and eventually project to the flocculus as mossy fiber afferents (Maekawa and Takeda 1979). The mossy fiber visual pathway which is related to the horizontal eye movement appears to be mediated by contralateral NRTP in rabbits (Fig. 1; see Sect. 3).

In the present experiment, the climbing fiber visual pathway was interrupted by placing electrolytic lesions (dc, electrode positive, 1 mA, 60 s) about 3 mm rostral to the right dorsal cap, avoiding direct involvement of the dorsal cap neurons. This last condition is important, because damage of dorsal cap neurons themselves will not only

1 Department of Physiology, Faculty of Medicine, University of Tokyo, Tokyo, Japan

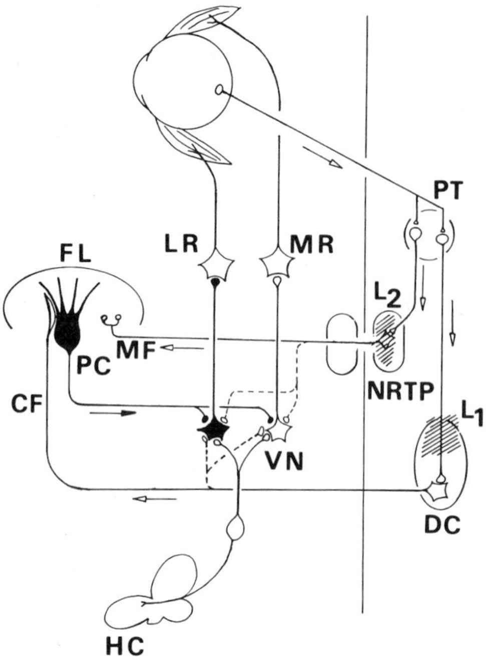

Fig. 1. Schematic neuronal connections for horizontal eye movements. Location of each electric lesion is *hatched*. L_1, pre-olivary lesion (see Fig. 5); L_2, NRTP lesion (see Fig. 4); *PT*, pretectal area; *NRTP*, nucleus reticularis tegmenti pontis; *DC*, dorsal cap of the inferior olive; *FL*, cerebellar flocculus; *PC*, Purkinje cell; *MF*, mossy fiber; *CF*, climbing fiber; *HC*, horizontal canal; *VN*, vestibular nuclei; *MR*, Medial restus; *LR*, lateral rectus; *Dotted lines*, from *DC* to *VN* and from *NRTP* to *VN*, are possible but not yet demonstrated collateral innervations of cerebellar afferents (see Sect. 5)

deprive climbing fiber afferents of the flocculus but also depress the Purkinje inhibition upon vestibular neurons rather rapidly (Ito et al. 1979). To interrupt the mossy fiber visual pathway, lesions were placed unilaterally in NRTP by passage of 1 mA dc for 60 s.

Effects of these lesions were compared with those induced by unilateral destruction of the whole flocculus, either surgical or chemical (see Sect. 2).

All experiments were done with albino rabbits. Surgical operations were performed under anesthesia by pentobarbitone sodium (35–50 mg/kg). Operated rabbits were used for eye movement and microelectrode recording experiments not earlier than 4 days after the operations and used in completely alert state.

2 Effects of Cerebellar Flocculectomy

In order to evaluate how the flocculus utilizes visual information relevant to eye movement, surgical ablation of the flocculus has been widely adopted (Ito et al. 1974; Takemori and Cohen 1974; Robinson 1976). However, it was recently pointed out that surgical flocculectomy reduced the number of cells in the dorsal cap of the inferior olive (Barmack and Simpson 1980). This complication was minimized by use of chemical flocculectomy with kainic acid (Herndon and Coyle 1977; Ito et al. 1980).

For chemical flocculectomy, 2 μl of saline containing 0.1 % of kainic acid was injected into the left flocculus with microsyringe. Two weeks after kainate injections Purkinje cells had disappeared from the entire flocculus, while granule cells appeared

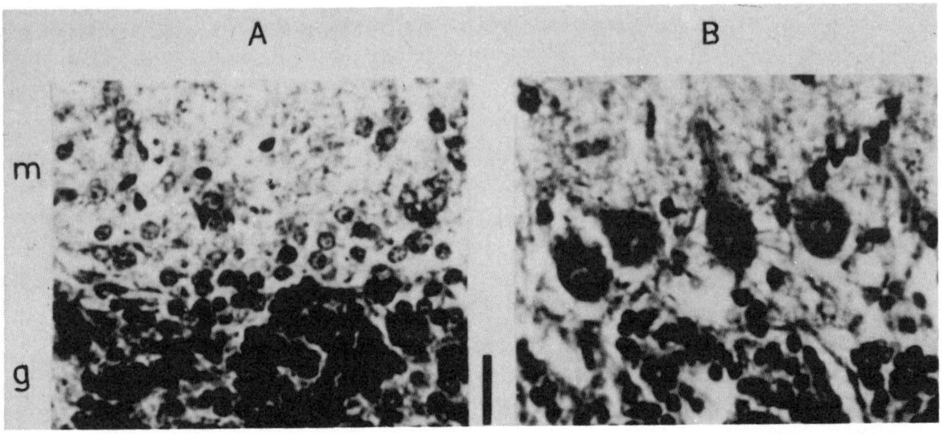

Fig. 2A, B. Photomicrographs of the cortex of the cerebellar flocculus. **A** Kainate-injected, **B** control side (contralateral to injection). Note the absence of Purkinje cells in **A**. *g*, granular layer; *m*, molecular layer (Ito et al. 1980)

normal (Fig. 2). Chemical flocculectomy did not cause any cell loss in the dorsal cap of the inferior olive, while surgical flocculectomy induced a prominent cell loss (41% as compared with the control side) (Ito et al. 1980).

Effects of flocculectomy on eye movements were tested both for the optokinetic response (OKR) and for vision-guided adaptation of the horizontal vestibulo-ocular reflex (HVOR). The OKR was evoked in one eye by moving a vertical slit light sinusoidally by an angular amplitude of 2.5° (peak-to-peak) at four different frequencies (0.17, 0.1, 0.05, and 0.033 Hz), while the opposite eye was kept closed. The OKR gain, defined as the amplitude ratio of eye movement to slit light movement, was depressed in the eye ipsilateral to the flocculectomy at all test frequencies (Fig. 3A) compared to normal controls. The OKR gain in the contralateral eye displayed no appreciable reduction.

The influence of flocculectomy on the ipsi-OKR gain was not exactly the same between the surgical and chemical subgroups. At higher frequencies the ipsi-OKR gain was equally depressed; at 0.17 Hz, 0.04 in both subgroups, and at 0.1 Hz, 0.08 in the surgical group and 0.10 in the chemical group. At lower frequencies, however, the average value of the ipsi-OKR gain was larger in the chemical subgroup than in the surgical one; at 0.05 Hz, 0.22 ± 0.10 (n = 6) for the surgical and 0.39 ± 0.29 (n = 5) for the chemical subgroup. At 0.033 Hz, 0.27 ± 0.11 (n = 6) for the surgical and 0.49 ± 0.29 (n = 5) for the chemical one. Statistical meaning could be attached marginally to the difference at 0.033 Hz ($p = 0.05$), but not at 0.05 Hz ($p > 0.05$).

Vision-guided adaptability of the horizontal vestibulo-ocular reflex (HVOR) was tested by sustained whole-body rotation (5° peak-to-peak) with a fixed slit light presented to one eye for 3 h. The HVOR gain, defined as the amplitude ratio of eye movement to head movement, was measured once every hour in total darkness. In normal control animals, the HVOR gain increases significantly ($p < 0.01$) within the initial hour (Fig. 3D). In flocculectomized rabbits, there was no significant increase of

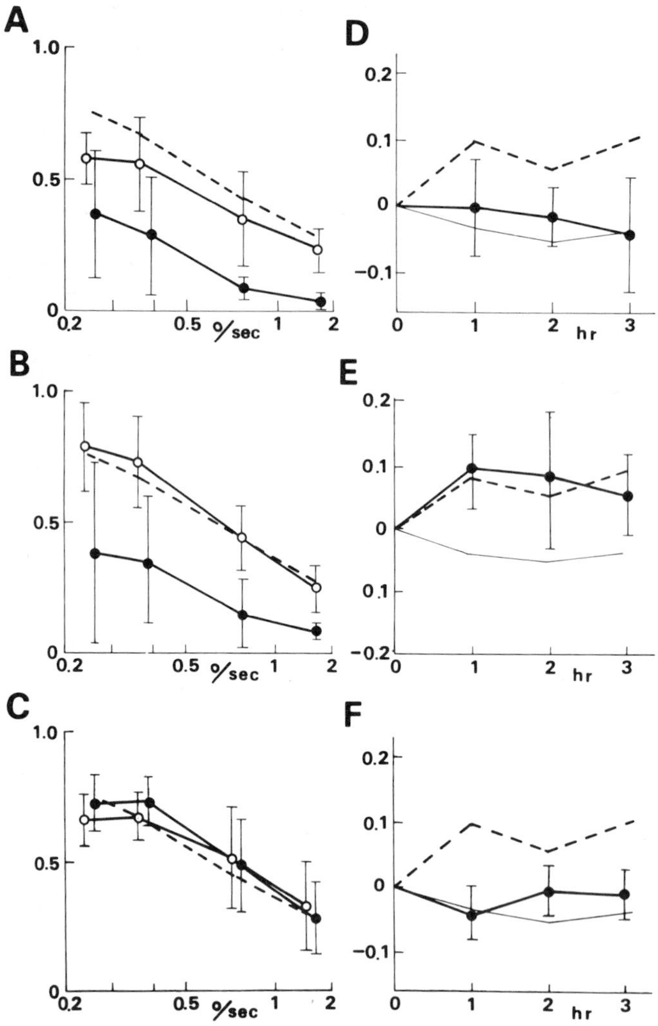

Fig. 3A–F. Effects of lesions on eye movements. **A, D** Flocculectomy, **B, E** NRTP lesions, **C, F** interruption of pretecto-olivary fibers. **A–C** OKR gain, **D–F** gain change in HVOR adaptation. **A** Average values of the OKR gain (*black dots,* ipsi-, *open circles,* contra-lateral to flocculectomized side) in seven rabbits with unilateral flocculectomy as a function of the maximum velocity of slit light movements (see Batini et al. 1979). *Broken line* shows mean values of the OKR in control rabbits for comparison. **B** same as **A**, but in seven rabbits with unilateral NRTP lesions (*black dots,* contra-, *open circles,* ipsi-lateral to NRTP lesions). **C** same as **A**, but in six rabbits whose visual pretecto-olivary fibers were interrupted (*black dots,* contra-, *open circles,* ipsi-lateral to preolivary lesions). **D** Average changes in HVOR gain as a function of time after the onset of continuous rotation with a fixed slit light. The rotation was presented once to each rabbit, and changes of the HVOR gain were measured before and during continuous rotation. Ipsilateral eye to flocculectomy in seven rabbits. *Broken line* shows mean values of the gain change in control rabbits. *Thin line* represents mean values in control rabbits rotated in darkness. **E** same as **D**, but in seven rabbits with unilateral NRTP lesions (*black dots,* contralateral to NRTP lesions). **F** same as **D**, but in six rabbits whose pretecto-olivary fibers were interrupted. *Vertical bars* in figures are standard deviations the HVOR gain when the slit light was presented to the eye ipsilateral to the flocculectomy, whereas the contra-HVOR gain exhibited an appreciable increase ($p < 0.01$) comparable with that of normal control. There was no significant difference between effects of chemical and surgical flocculectomy concerning the HVOR adaptation.

3 Effects of Lesions Placed at the Nucleus Reticularis Tegmenti Pontis (NRTP)

Extent of a lesion of nucleus reticularis tegmenti pontis (NRTP), a relay site of the visual mossy fiber afferent to the flocculus, is exemplified in Fig. 4A, B. Figure 4C summarizes extents of lesions in seven rabbits. Although destruction was only partial in some cases, all lesions involved the middle longitudinal zone of the NRTP, which contains a large number of cells projecting to the flocculus (Maekawa and Takeda 1979). In these seven rabbits, the lesion reduced the OKR gain without affecting the adaptability of the HVOR (Miyashita et al. 1980). The OKR gain of the eye contralateral to the lesion was significantly ($p < 0.01$) lower than that of the ipsilateral eye at all test frequencies (Fig. 3B). The OKR gain in the ipsilateral eye was identical with that of the control rabbits. Adaptability of the HVOR was tested as described in Sect. 2. During rotation under presentation of the fixed slit light, the eye contralateral to the lesion in the seven rabbits exhibited increased HVOR gain (black dots in Fig. 3E) comparable to that in control rabbits. This increase parallels that in control rabbits, and differred statistically significantly from the control curve obtained for rotation in darkness.

In three rabbits, unit spike discharges were recorded extracellularly from flocculus Purkinje cells contralateral to the NRTP lesion (Fig. 1). The flocculus contains at least five different microzones (Yamamoto 1979), only one of which (H-zone) is related to horizontal eye movement. The H-zone was located by observing horizontal eye move-

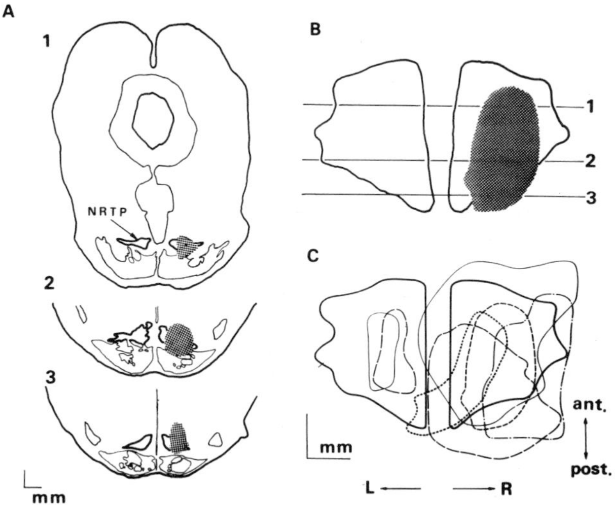

Fig. 4A–C. Lesions of NRTP. **A** Frontal sections of the brainstem of an operated rabbit. The lesioned area is *stippled.* The anterior–posterior levels of the three sections (*1, 2, 3*) are indicated in **B** on the dorsal view of the NRTP, as reconstructed from frontal serial sections. **C** Summary of mapping of lesions, as exemplified in **B**, in seven experimental rabbits. *L,* left; *R,* right; *ant.,* anterior; *post.,* posterior (Miyashita et al. 1980)

ment evoked with electric pulse trains applied through the microelectrode (Dufossé et al. 1977).

In control rabbits, the majority of H-zone cells exhibited a significant modulation of *simple* spikes to sinusoidal movement of slit light (2.5°, 0.1 Hz) (Ito 1977). Amplitude of modulation, relative to the mean discharge frequency, ranged from 3% to 15% (mean 8.1, S.D. 3.8). However, in rabbits with NRTP lesions, *simple* spikes of H-zone Purkinje cells exhibited significant modulation much less frequently (26 cells among 44 H-zone cells) and amplitude of the modulation never exceeded 10%; mean value was 3.38% (S.D. 1.59). By contrast, modulation of *complex* spikes in rabbits with NRTP lesions appeared normal and their amplitude of the modulation ranged from 7% to more than 40%.

4 Effects of Interruption of the Preolivary Visual Pathway

Climbing fiber visual input to the flocculus was interrupted by placing unilateral preolivary lesion, the extent of which is exemplified in Fig. 5A, B.

In order to assure the effect of lesions, the reflex testing method for canal-ocular reflexes (Ito et al. 1977) was used. In operated rabbits, conditioning stimuli to the flocculus evoked a prominent inhibition of the test reflex to the medial rectus muscle (MR), while conditioning stimuli to the retina evoked only slight and late inhibition of the MR reflex. These results show that the visual information to the flocculus through climbing fibers was interrupted at preolivary level, while floccular Purkinje inhibition to secondary vestibular neurons was kept intact.

Eye movements were tested between the 6th and 18th postoperative days in six rabbits with these preolivary lesions. The OKR gain was measured as described in Sect. 2. The eye contralateral to the lesion (Fig. 1) did not exhibit any reduction of the

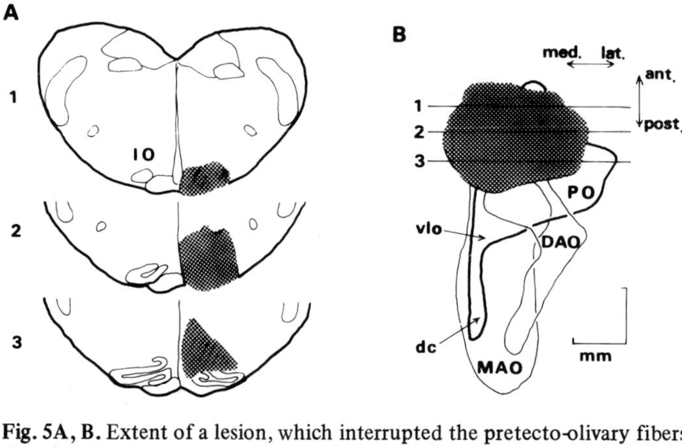

Fig. 5A, B. Extent of a lesion, which interrupted the pretecto-olivary fibers. **A** Frontal sections of the modulla of an operated rabbit. The lesioned area is *stippled.* The anterior–posterior levels of the three sections (*1, 2, 3*) are indicated in **B** on the dorsal view of the inferior olive. *PO,* principal olive; *MAO,* medial accessory olive; *DAO,* dorsal accessory olive; *vlo,* ventro-lateral outgrowth; *dc,* dorsal cap; *med.,* medial; *lat.,* lateral; *ant.,* anterior; *post.,* posterior

OKR gain (Fig. 3C), compared either with the ipsi-OKR gain (open circles) or with normal control. However, adaptability of the HVOR in the contralateral eye was completely abolished. The HVOR gain did not increase when the animal was rotated for 3 h with a fixed slit light presented to the eye contralateral to the lesion (black dots in Fig. 3F). Thus, the adaptation curve for operated rabbits (black dots) was significantly different from the control curve ($p < 0.05$).

In two lesioned rabbits, visual responses of Purkinje cells were recorded from the flocculus contralateral to the lesion as described in Sect. 3. In the majoritiy of H-zone Purkinje cells, *simple* spike exhibited significant modulation (22 among 28 cells) to sinusoidal rotation of the slit light (2.5° peak-to-peak, 0.1 Hz). Their amplitude of modulation ranged from 3% to 13%. As would be expected, *complex* spikes showed no significant modulation.

5 Discussion

The present study with preolivary lesions and lesions of nucleus reticularis tegmenti pontis disclosed that the two vision-related functions of the cerebellar flocculus, optokinetic response (OKR) and vision-guided adaptation of the horizontal vestibulo-ocular reflex (HVOR), can be related differentially to two floccular afferent systems, visual mossy fiber and visual climbing fiber. The results support the hypothesis that *simple* spikes represent the major dynamic characteristics of Purkinje cell output in motor control, whereas *complex* spikes represent a "teacher's signal" to modify this *simple* spike activity (Marr 1969; Albus 1971).

This view is also cinsistent with previously recorded discharge patterns of H-zone Purkinje cells in control rabbits (Ito 1977). With sinusoidal movement of slit light by 2.5° (peak-to-peak) at 0.1 Hz, the majority of H-zone cells increase discharge frequencies of their *simple* spikes during backward movement of the slit light and decrease them during forward movement. Since stimulation of floccular Purkinje cells causes backward movement of the ipsilateral eye (Dufossé et al. 1977), it is suggested that *simple* spike modulations in flocculus Purkinje cells facilitate the OKR and, consequently, that their removal by flocculectomy or NRTP lesions impairs the OKR (see Sect. 3).

Collateralization of mossy and climbing fiber afferents is a matter to be considered in evaluating present results. For example, the difference in the ipsi-OKR gain at relatively low frequencies between chemical and surgical flocculectomy (Sect. 2) might be explained by the fact that in surgically, but not chemically, flocculectomized rabbits not only climbing fiber afferents but also their possible collaterals to vestibular nuclei (Ito et al. 1977) are impaired. Collaterals of visual mossy fiber afferents might impinge on vestibular neurons and thereby contribute to the OKR (Precht and Strata 1980). Under the assumption that chemical flocculectomy spares these collateral innervation, the difference between the OKR gain with chemical flocculectomy and that with NRTP lesion may give an estimate of the net contribution of the postulated NRTP-vestibular nuclei projection. There was little difference at relatively fast velocities, although at slower velocities there may be some difference.

Another matter to be considered in evaluating the present results is the possible eye velocity input postulated from observations on the monkey flocculus (Lisberger and Fuchs 1978; Miles et al. 1980). Their hypothesis is that modulation of flocculus Purkinje cells represents a positive feedback of eye velocity signals rather than visual inputs. The relevance of this pathway to eye movements of rabbits has not been studied in detail. However, recent work by Neverov et al. (1980) demonstrates that during reversed postoptokinetic nystagmus, when eye was moving without visual signal, there was little response of Purkinje cells in rabbit flocculus. This suggests that eye velocity input may not be a major input to rabbit flocculus.

References

Albus JS (1971) A theory of cerebellar function. Math Biosci 10: 26–61

Barmack NH, Simpson JI (1980) Effects of microlesions of dorsal cap of inferior olive of rabbits on optokinetic and vestibulo-ocular reflexes. J Neurophysiol 43: 182–206

Dufossé M, Ito, M, Miyashita Y (1977) Functional localization in the rabbit's cerebellar flocculus determined in relationship with eye movements. Neurosci Lett 5: 273–277

Herndon RM, Coyle JT (1977) Selective destruction of neurons by a transmitter agonist. Science 198: 71–72

Ito M (1972) Neural design of the cerebellar motor control system. Brain Res 40: 81–84

Ito M (1977) Neuronal events in the cerebellar flocculus associated with an adaptive modification of the vestibulo-ocular reflex of rabbit. In: Baker B, Berthoz A (eds) Control of gaze by brain stem neurons. Elsevier, Amsterdam, pp 391–398

Ito M, Miyashita Y (1975) The effects of chronic destruction of the inferior olive upon visual modification of the horizontal vestibulo-ocular reflex of rabbits. Proc Jpn Acad 51: 716–720

Ito M, Shiida T, Yagi N, Yamamoto M (1974) The cerebellar modification of rabbit's horizontal vestibulo-ocular reflex induced by sustained head rotation combined with visual stimulation. Proc Jpn Acad 50: 85–89

Ito M, Nishmaru N, Yamamoto M (1977) Specific patterns of neuronal connexions involved in the control of the rabbit's vestibulo-ocular reflexes by the cerebellar flocculus. J Physiol (London) 265: 833–854

Ito M, Nishmaru N, Shibuki K (1979) Destruction of inferior olive induces rapid depression in synaptic action of cerebellar Purkinje cells. Nature (London) 277: 568–569

Ito M, Jastreboff PJ, Miyashita Y (1980) Retrograde influence of surgical and chemical flocculectomy upon dorsal cap neurons of the inferior olive. Neurosci Lett 20: 45–48

Keller EL, Precht W (1979) Visual-vestibular responses in vestibular nuclear neurons in the intact and cerebellectomized, alert cat. Neuroscience 4: 1599–1613

Lisberger SG, Fuchs AF (1978) Role of primate flocculus during rapid behavioral modification of vestibuloocular reflex. I. Purkinje cell activity during visually guided horizontal smooth-persuit eye movements and passive head rotation. J Neurophysiol 41: 733–778

Maekawa K, Simpson JI (1973) Climbing fiber responses evoked in vestibulo-cerebellum of rabbit from visual system. J Neurophysiol 36: 649–666

Maekawa K, Takeda T (1975) Mossy fiber responses evoked in the cerebellar flocculus of rabbits by stimulation of the optic pathway. Brain Res 98: 590–595

Maekawa K, Takeda T (1979) Origin of the mossy fiber projection to the cerebellar flocculus from the optic nerves in rabbits. In: Ito M, Tsukahara N, Kubota K, Yagi K (eds) Integrative control functions of the brain. Kodansha, Tokyo, Elsevier, Amsterdam, pp 93–95

Marr D (1969) A theory of cerebellar cortex. J Physiol (London) 202: 437–470

Miles FA, Braitman DJ, Dow BM (1980) Long-term adaptive changes in primate vestibuloocular reflex. IV. Electrophysiological observations in flocculus of adapted monkeys. J Neurophysiol 43: 1477–1492

Miyashita Y, Ito M, Jastreboff PJ, Maekawa K, Nagao S (1980) Effect upon eye movements of rabbits induced by severance of mossy fiber visual pathway to the cerebellar flocculus. Brain Res 198: 210–215

Neverov VP, Sterc J Bures J (1980) Electrophysiological correlates of the reversed postoptokinetic nystagmus in the rabbit: Activity of vestibular and floccular neurons. Brain Res 189: 355–367

Precht W, Strata P (1980) On the pathway mediating optokinetic responses of vestibular nuclear neurons. Neuroscience 5: 777–787

Robinson DA (1976) Adaptive gain control of vestibulo-ocular reflex by the cerebellum. J Neurophysiol 39: 954–969

Takemori S, Cohen B (1974) Loss of visual suppression of vestibular nystagmus after flocculus lesions. Brain Res 72: 213–224

Yamamoto M (1979) Topographical representation in rabbit cerebellar flocculus for various afferent inputs from the brainstem investigated by means of retrograde axonal transport of horseradish peroxidase. Neurosci Lett 12: 29–34

Reorganization of the Cerebello-Cerebral Projection Following Hemicerebellectomy or Cerebral Cortical Ablation

S. KAWAGUCHI[1] and T. YAMAMOTO[1,2]

1 Introduction

It is well known that functional deficiencies caused by damage to the cerebellum show remarkable recovery, particularly in children and young animals. Luciani, at the end of the last century, and many investigators later, repeatedly observed in partially decerebellated animals that deficiency signs of a compensated animal reappear following extirpation of the bilateral motor cortex. On the basis of such observations, Luciani conceived the idea that compensation for cerebellar deficiencies occurred through the acquisition of new functions by structures which were not involved previously (organic compensation) as well as through learning and training (functional compensation) (Dow and Moruzzi 1958). Since then, little has been known about the neural basis of compensation either organic or functional, whether they are really different.

Recent morphological (Nakamura et al. 1974; Leong 1977; Castro 1978; Kawaguchi et al. 1979c) and electrophysiological studies (Tsukahara et al. 1975; Kawaguchi et al. 1979a,b) provided evidence for occurrence of a marked reorganization of the neuronal circuitry of the cerebellum and related structures during the compensation period. This article deals with plastic reorganization of the cerebellar output systems following hemicerebellectomy (Kawaguchi et al. 1979b,c) or cerebral cortical ablation (Kawaguchi et al. 1979a), although its functional significance remains unclarified.

2 Cerebello-Cerebral Response in Intact Animals

2.1 Cerebello-Cerebral Response in Cat

Stimulation of the interpositus or the lateral nucleus of the cerebellum in adult cats (Sasaki et al. 1972, 1973) as well as in kittens from newborn period (Kawaguchi et al. 1979b) induces two distinct types of responses contralaterally in the two discrete cor-

1 Department of Physiology, Institute for Brain Research, Faculty of Medicine, Kyoto University, Kyoto 606, Japan

2 Present address: Max-Planck-Institut für Hirnforschung, Deutschordenstraße 46, 6000 Frankfurt 71, FRG

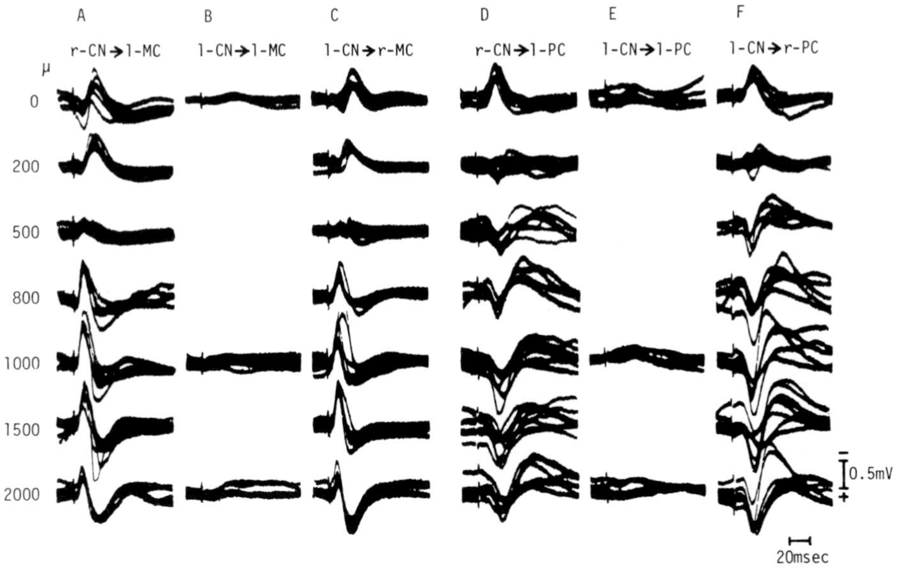

Fig. 1A–F. Cerebello-cerebral response recorded from the cerebral cortex at depths given *in front of traces.* Response in the frontal motor cortex on the left side *(l-MC)* evoked by stimulation of the right cerebellar lateral nucleus *(r-CN)* is indicated by *r-CN→l-MC,* other responses in the same manner. Marked responses were evoked contralaterally in the frontal motor cortex (**A** or **C**) and in the parietal cortex (**D** or **F**). By contrast, no response was evoked ipsilaterally either in the frontal cortex (**B**) or in the parietal cortex (**E**)

tical areas, i.e., the frontal motor cortex (areas 4 and 6) and the parietal association cortex (areas 5 and 7). The response in the frontal cortex, as shown in Fig. 1A or C, is characterized by a positive–negative diphasic potential in the superficial cortical layers and a negative–positive diphasic potential in the deeper cortical layers. The response in the parietal cortex (Fig. 1D or F) is characterized by a negative potential in the superficial cortical layers and a positive potential in the deeper cortical layers. No response is evoked ipsilaterally. A small negative wave in Fig. 1B or E, which was induced ipsilaterally, is merely a reflection of an actual response of remote places, presumably the contralateral cortex, since such a wave remained unchanged through the entire cortical layers and no sites were found in the ipsilateral cortex where polarity of potentials reversed in the deeper cortical layers. When a reversal of potential was employed as a criterion of an actual response, none of 16 normal kittens ranging from 2 to 142 days of age showed an actual response ipsilaterally.

2.2 Cerebello-Cerebral Response in Rat

Stimulation of the cerebellar nucleus (either of the three nuclei) in the rat (Yamamoto et al 1979), unlike in the cat, induces one type of response in a continuous cortical area inclusive of the whole motor cortex and a part of the somatosensory cortex. The responsive area is exclusively contralateral to the cerebellar nucleus for stimulation.

The response is a small positive followed by a large negative potential in the superficial cortical layers, and a small negative followed by a large positive potential in the deeper cortical layers. Potential reversal occurs at a depth between 1,000 and 1,200 μm from the cortical surface, much deeper than a depth of 200 to 300 μm in the cat.

3 Collateral Sprouting of Cerebellothalamic Neurons in Kittens Following Neonatal Hemicerebellectomy

3.1 Electrophysiological Evidence

Bilateral Cerebello-Cerebral Response. In all of 11 kittens, in which one half of the cerebellum had been removed before 11 days of age and which were permitted to survive for more than 16 days after surgery, stimulation of the lateral nucleus of the spared hemicerebellum induced a marked cerebello-cerebral response not only contralaterally, just as in intact animals, but also ipsilaterally. Examples of such a bilateral cerebello-cerebral response are shown in Fig. 2. The bilateral cerebello-frontal cortical response in A and B was recorded from the medial portion of the anterior sigmoid gyrus contralateral (A) and ipsilateral (B) to the cerebellar lateral nucleus stimulated, in a kitten operated on at 4 days of age and kept for 56 days. The bilateral cerebello-

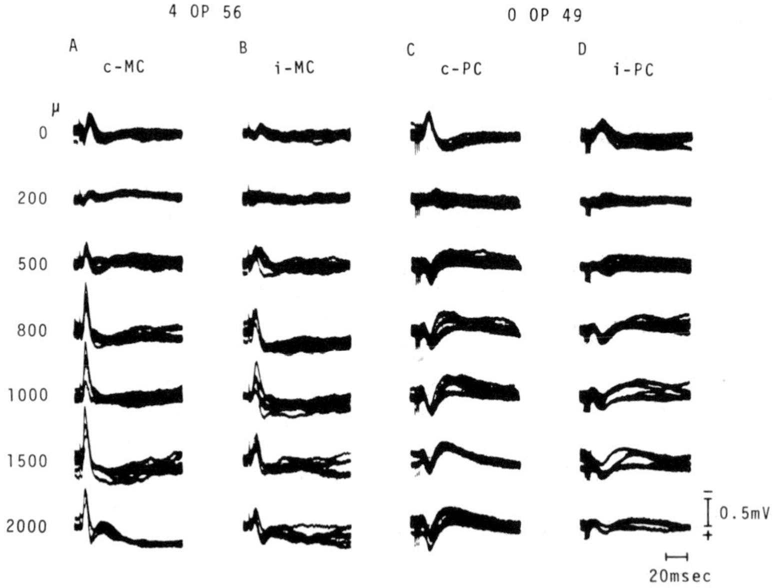

Fig. 2A–D. Bilateral cerebello-cerebral response in hemicerebellectomized kittens. Responses **A** and **B** were recorded from the frontal motor cortex contralateral (*c-MC*) and ipsilateral (*i-MC*) to the spared cerebellar lateral nucleus stimulated, in a kitten 56 days after being operated on at 4 days of age. Responses **C** and **D** were recorded from the parietal association cortex contralateral (*c-PC*) and ipsilateral (*i-PC*) to the spared cerebellar lateral nucleus stimulated, in a kitten 49 days after being operated on at the day of birth parietal cortical response in C and D was recorded from the rostral portion of the middle suprasylvian gyrus contralateral (C) and ipsilateral (D) to the cerebellar lateral nucleus stimulated, in a kitten operated on at the day of birth and kept for 49 days after surgery. Responses were weaker in the ipsilateral cortex than in the contralateral cortex. However, the contour of the depth profile and the level of potential reversal of the bilateral cerebello-cerebral response were identical on both sides of the cortex and were the same as those of the cerebello-cerebral response in intact animals.

The ipsilateral cerebello-cerebral response could evidently be evoked as early as 16 days after surgery but was not detectable in three kittens at 12–14 days after surgery. When the postoperative interval was short (< 30 days), the latency of the response was remarkably longer in the ipsilateral cortex than in the contralateral cortex. Such latency difference became insignificant in 2 months after surgery.

Thalamic Relay Nucleus: Stimulation and Destruction Experiments. The thalamic relay nucleus for the cerebello-frontal cortical response is the lateral ventral (VL) nucleus. Stimulation of the VL nucleus, contralateral to the spared hemicerebellum, induced a marked response in the frontal cortex not only ipsilaterally, just as in intact animals, but also contralaterally. Destruction of the VL nucleus, as expected, abolished the contralateral cerebello-cerebral response, whereas the ipsilateral cerebello-cerebral response remained unchanged. The latter response, thus, appears to be mediated, at least mainly, by ipsilateral branches of cerebello-thalamic neurons projecting bilaterally upon the thalamus. An axon reflex of such a bilateral projection neuron may account for the marked response in the frontal cortex evoked contralaterally by stimulation of the VL nucleus. To test whether such a bilateral projection neuron does really exist in the hemicerebellectomized kittens in a number sufficient to mediate an ipsilateral cerebello-cerebral response, unitary recording of cerebellar nuclear neurons with antidromic activation was attempted.

Bilateral Cerebellothalamic Projection Neuron. In four kittens hemicerebellectomized at 0–2 days of age and kept for 30–40 days, 153 neurons were sampled with antidromic activation on stimulation of the thalamic nucleus mostly from the lateral nucleus and partly from the interpositus nucleus of the spared hemicerebellum. Of the 153 neurons, 121 responded only contralaterally, 21 only ipsilaterally and 11 were activated bilaterally. In control experiments, 150 neurons were sampled in the same manner from four intact kittens of comparable age. Of the 150 sampled neurons, 146 were activated only contralaterally, 3 only ipsilaterally, and 1 was activated bilaterally. In six neonatal kittens ranging from 2 to 9 days of age, 133 neurons were sampled in the same manner, of which 131 responded only contralaterally, 2 only ipsilaterally, and none was activated bilaterally. Statistical significance between the operated animals and the intact animals of comparable age was $P < 0.005$ for the ipsilaterally activated neurons and $P < 0.05$ for the bilaterally activated neurons. In the control animals there was no statistical significance between the older and the neonatal kittens.

Neurons activated only ipsilaterally were assumed mostly, if not exclusively, to be bilateral projection neurons. The reason is, firstly, that the bilateral projection neurons could not be activated always bilaterally but unilaterally since the thalamic relay nucleus is too large for a pair of concentric electrodes to activate fully the entire nucleus.

Secondly, ipsilaterally activated neurons were quite sparse in the intact animals irrespective of age. In this connection, the cerebello-thalamic projection appears to have been established mostly by birth since the cerebello-cerebral response could be evoked in the frontal cortex at birth with a magnitude comparable to an adult's response. Therefore, most of the ipsilaterally activated neurons are neither due to persistence of a connection which may exist in a neonatal period, nor to misrouting of developing cerebello-fugal axons. Thus, the ipsilateral cerebello-thalamic projection in the operated animals must arise mostly from the contralateral cerebello-thalamic projection. Presence of numerous bilateral projection neurons is consistent with the results of stimulation and destruction experiments of the thalamic relay nucleus.

Conclusions. For the abundance of the ipsilateral cerebello-thalamic projection in the hemicerebellectomized kittens four possible explanations can be offered. (1) Ipsilateral cerebello-thalamic fibers, which may exist numerously in a newborn period and normally regress during development, may persist following damage to the cerebellum. (2) Some cerebello-fugal axons which may be developing in a newborn period may change their course to be distributed ipsilaterally. (3) The preexisting ipsilateral cerebello-thalamic fiber terminals, even though quite sparse, may proliferate in the thalamus deafferentated from contralateral cerebello-thalamic fibers. (4) Axon collaterals sprouted from contralateral cerebello-thalamic fibers may be distributed ipsilaterally. The first and the second possibility can obviously be ruled out as stated above. The third possibility may not be excluded, but can hardly account for the presence of so many neurons that are antidromically activated ipsilaterally or bilaterally, since an activation of each axon may not be influenced significantly by terminal proliferation. The reason is that the areas activated with electrical stimulation are uncomparably larger (Jankowska et al. 1972) than the areas which would be expected to be distributed with proliferated terminals of an axon (Raisman 1977). The most plausible explanation is, thus, the fourth one.

3.2 Morphological Evidence

Labeling of Cerebello-Thalamic Projection by Retrograde HRP Method. Horseradish peroxidase (HRP) was injected unilaterally into the anterior ventral-lateral ventral (VA-VL) nuclear complex of the thalamus in three hemicerebellectomized kittens and, for control, in three animals of comparable age and in four neonatal animals. In the operated animals, the enzyme was injected on the side ipsilateral to the spared hemicerebellum. HRP-labeled neurons were distributed through the entire rostrocaudal extent of all three cerebellar nuclei. In the intact animals, the vast majority of neurons in the lateral nucleus contralateral to the HRP-injected thalamus were labeled (Fig. 3A). Numerous neurons were also labeled in the interpositus nucleus, although less than in the lateral nucleus, whereas labeled neurons in the medial nucleus were seen relatively sparse. In the cerebellar nuclei ipsilateral to the HRP-injected thalamus, labeled neurons were always observed, although quite sparsely in the intact animals (Fig. 3B). This pattern of labeling in the intact animals was similar either in the neonatal or in the older animals. Ipsilaterally labeled neurons were seen remarkably more numerous in the hemicerebellectomized animals (Fig. 3C) than in the intact animals. Particularly in the

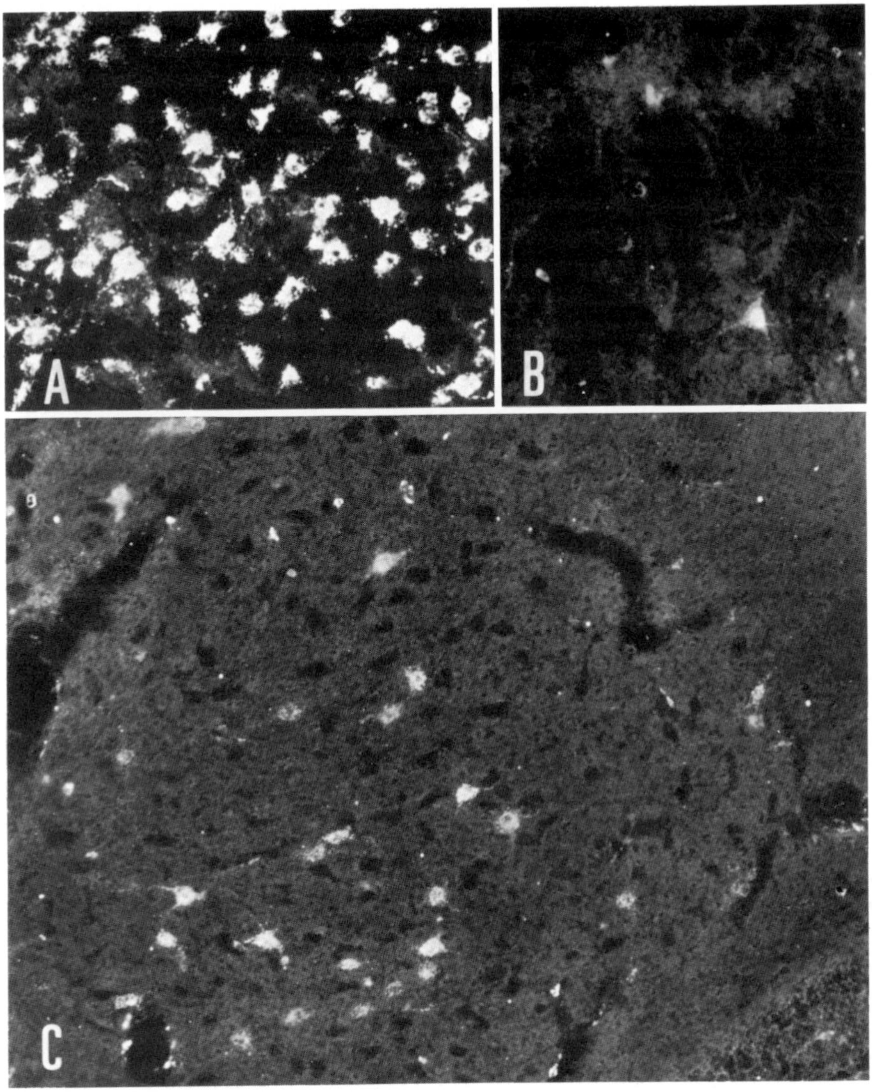

Fig. 3A–C. Neurons labeled with HRP in the lateral nucleus of the cerebellum after a HRP injection into the VA-VL complex of the thalamus, labeled contralaterally (**A**) and ipsilaterally (**B**) in an intact kitten (35-day old), labeled ipsilaterally (**C**) in a hemicerebellectomized kitten (2 OP 41). Ipsilaterally labeled neurons were seen obviously more numerous in the hemicerebellectomized kitten than in the intact kitten. *Dark field,* 160×

lateral nucleus, labeled neurons of the operated kittens were ten times more than those of the control animals.

Labeling of Cerebello-Thalamic Projection by Anterograde HRP Method. After injection of HRP into the cerebellar nucleus, axons and terminals labeled with HRP transported anterogradely from the injection site could be traced in the thalamic areas. The labeled terminals were distributed most numerously in the rostral and the dorsomedial portion of the VA-VL nuclear complex, where neurons projecting onto the rostral portion of the middle suprasylvian gyrus or the medial portion of the anterior sigmoid gyrus have been known to exist (Mizuno et al. 1977; Itoh and Mizuno 1977; Rispal-Padel and Grangetto 1977). No difference could be detected in the distribution pattern and number of contralateral cerebello-thalamic fibers between the intact and the hemicerebellectomized kittens. By contrast, axons and terminals of ipsilateral cerebello-thalamic fibers were apparently more numerous and dense in the hemicerebellectomized kittens than in the intact animals.

Conclusions. The results are consistent in every respect with electrophysiological findings and offer corroborating evidence for collateral sprouting of cerebello-thalamic projection fibers in kittens following neonatal hemicerebellectomy.

4 New Connection of Cerebello-Thalamic Projection in Rat Following Neonatal Hemicerebellectomy

Occurrence of a bilateral cerebello-cerebral response with concomitant increase in the number of cerebellar nuclear neurons projecting bilaterally or ipsilterally upon the thalamus was demonstrated electrophysiologically also in rats following neonatal hemicerebellectomy (Yamamoto et al. 1981). It is consistent with morphological findings (Lim and Leong 1975; Leong 1977; Castro 1978) that destruction of the deep cerebellar nuclei or hemicerebellectomy in rats in an early postnatal period induced an aberrant ipsilateral cerebello-thalamic and cerebello-rubral projection.

A marked bilateral cerebello-cerebral response was evoked in all of five rats hemicerebellectomized before 6 days of age (early hemicerebellectomy), whereas in all of five rats operated on at 8 to 15 days of age (late hemicerebellectomy), and in three rats operated on in adulthood, the cerebello-cerebral response could be evoked only contralaterally, just as in intact animals.

Unitary recording of antidromic response of cerebellar nuclear neurons revealed that bilateral or ipsilateral cerebello-thalamic projection neurons were remarkably ($P < 0.001$) more numerous in the cases of early hemicerebellectomy than in controls. Such neurons were less remarkably but significantly ($P < 0.05$) more numerous in the cases of late hemicerebellectomy than in controls. Absence of an ipsilateral cerebello-cerebral response in the cases of late hemicerebellectomy indicates that bilateral or ipsilateral cerebello-thalamic neurons in these animals may not be sufficient in number, or in efficiency of synaptic transmission, to mediate a detectable response.

Conclusions. From an analogy of the results obtained in kittens, collateral sprouting appears the most likely explanation for the abundance of the ipsilateral cerebello-thalamic projection in the hemicerebellectomized rats. However, we have no evidence to rule out the possibility that there may be numerous developing cerebellofugal axons changing their course to be distributed ipsilaterally or bilaterally. The latter possibility was first speculated upon by Lim and Leong (1975) on the basis of their finding that aberrant ipsilateral cerebellothalamic fibers were uncrossed from the cerebellum through the thalamus. However, their finding was disputed by Castro (1978) who observed recrossed but not uncrossed fibers, the recrossed fibers being crossed once at the decussation of the brachium conjunctivum and recrossed in the thalamic massa intermedia, in agreement with the results in kittens (Kawaguchi et al. 1979c).

5 Reorganization of Cerebello-Cerebral Response in Cat Following Cerebral Cortical Ablation

In kittens, as well as in adult cats, ablation of the cerebral cortical areas receiving the cerebellar projection led to an extensive reorganization of the cerebello-cerebral response, i.e., occurrence of an abnormal response and appearance of ectopic responsive areas.

In 24 kittens ranging from newborn to 196-day old, and in 4 adult cats, the anterior sigmoid gyrus (ASG) and/or the rostral half of the middle suprasylvian gyrus (MSSG) were ablated unilaterally or bilaterally. In other 5 kittens younger than 7 days of age, hemicerebellectomy was performed in addition to cerebral cortical ablation. In these animals, at 7 to 182 days after the operation, the cerebello-cerebral response was investigated by laminar field potential analysis in various portions of the cerebral cortex.

Responses in the decorticate animals whose cerebellum had been kept intact were evoked only contralaterally, whereas bilateral cerebello-cerebral responses were evoked in the kittens subjected to hemicerebellectomy in addition to cerebral cortical ablation. In the latter animals, the following changes occurred in the contralateral as well as ipsilateral cerebello-cerebral response. In the operated animals, the response in the ASG spared from ablation showed an unusual, large surface positive–deep negative wave which followed a wave complex, just as seen in the frontal cortical response of intact animals (Fig. 1A or C) to become a positive–negative–positive triphasic wave in superficial cortical layers and a negative–positive–negative wave in the deeper cortical layers. The parietal cortical response of the operated animals, i.e., the response in the rostral portion of the lateral gyrus and in the rostral half of the MSSG spared from ablation, tended to resemble a frontal cortical response of intact animals.

In the operated animals, normal or abnormal responses were encountered in normally unresponsive cortical regions, such as the posterior sigmoid gyrus (PSG), the anterior suprasylvian gyrus (ASSG), the caudal portion of the MSSG, the posterior suprasylvian gyrus (PSSG) and the posterior ectosylvian gyrus (PEG). Responses in the rostral portion of the PSG were similar to a normal frontal cortical response in some cases, and an abnormal motor cortical response in other cases, while those in the caudal portion of the PSG (around the postcruciate dimple) were similar to a normal parietal cortical response. Responses in the ASSG were a negative wave in the superficial cortical layers, and a small negative followed by a large positive wave in the deeper cortical layers. Responses in the caudal portion of the MSSG and in the PSSG and PEG were similar to a normal parietal cortical response. The degree of alterations in the contour of laminar field potentials and the extent of ectopic responsive areas varied from animal to animal. They can hardly be related to the location and the extent of the cortical area which had been ablated. When the cortex was ablated unilaterally, changes in the cerebello-cerebral response were not restricted to the ablated side, but similar changes were frequently observed on the intact side.

Conclusions. Reorganization of the cerebello-cerebral response induced by cerebral cortical ablation differs in two respects from that induced by hemicerebellectomy: (1) Cerebral cortical ablation at any age from newborn through adulthood induced similar changes in the cerebello-cerebral response, whereas the age of the animal at the time of hemicerebellectomy was a critical factor for occurrence of an ipsilateral cerebello-cerebral response. (2) Of the cerebello-cerebral response in the neonatally hemicerebellectomized animals, no abnormalities were seen either in the contour of potentials or in the responsive area except for the bilaterality of the response. By contrast, the cerebello-cerebral response following cerebral cortical ablation could be evoked only contralaterally, just as in intact animals, but the response showed marked abnormalities either in the contour of potentials or in the responsive area. In the animals subjected to hemicerebellectomy in addition to cerebral cortical ablation, reorganization following hemicerebellectomy coexisted with that following cerebral cortical ablation.

5 Concluding Remarks

Following hemicerebellectomy, the cerebello-thalamic projection shows a great capacity to reconstitute the communication line to the cerebral cortex. It is by collateral sprouting from the remaining cerebellar nuclear neurons, evidently in kittens and presumably in rats. As revealed by unitary recording of cerebellar nuclear neurons with antidromic activation in the cases of late hemicerebellectomy in rats, such a capacity appears, even if decreasingly, to continue much longer than the critical period of surgery for occurrence of an ipsilateral cerebello-cerebral response. A remarkable capacity for reorganization of the cerebello-cerebral projection following cerebral cortical ablation persists from newborn period through adulthood.

In general, the reorganization of the cerebello-thalamo-cerebral connection appears to correspond to a remarkable functional recovery after damage to the cerebellum and related structures. However, such a damage will induce, perhaps, various changes in various structures in the central nervous system simultaneously as well as sequentially. For example, neonatal hemicerebellectomy induces not only collateral sprouting of cerebello-thalamic neurons but also extensive cell loss of the inferior olivary nucleus by retrograde degeneration, cellular hypertrophy and dendritic alterations in Clarke's column (Smith et al. 1979), and probably reorganization of the cerebrorubral and cerebrocerebellar projection. This makes enormously difficult to analyze the functional significance of each change in relation to behavioral recovery.

Acknowledgment. We express our gratitude to Prof. K. Sasaki for his constant encouragement, helpful advice and critical reading of the manuscript.

References

Castro AJ (1978) Projections of superior cerebellar peduncle in rats and the development of new connections in response to neonatal hemicerebellectomy. J Comp Neurol 178: 611–628

Dow RS, Moruzzi G (1958) The physiology and pathology of the cerebellum. Univ of Minnesota Press, Mineapolis

Itoh K, Mizuno N (1977) Topographical arrangement of thalamocortical neurons in the centrolateral nucleus (CL) of the cat, with special reference to a spino-thalamo-motor cortical path through the CL. Exp Brain Res 30: 471–480

Jankowska E, Roberts WJ (1972) An electrophysiological demonstration of the axonal projections of single spinal interneurones in the cat. J Physiol (London) 222: 597–622

Kawaguchi S, Yamamoto T, Samejima A (1979a) Changes in the cerebello-cerebral response in the cat following cerebral cortical ablation with or without hemicerebellectomy. In: Ito M, Tsukahara N, Kubota K, Yagi K (eds) Integrative control functions of the brain, vol II. Kodansha-Elsevier, Tokyo Amsterdam

Kawaguchi S, Yamamoto T, Samejima A (1979b) Electrophysiological evidence for axonal sprouting of cerebellothalamic neurons in kittens after neonatal hemicerebellectomy. Exp Brain Res 36: 21–39

Kawaguchi S, Yamamoto T, Samejima A, Itoh K, Mizuno N (1979c) Morphological evidence for axonal sprouting of cerebellothalamic neurons in kittens after neonatal hemicerebellectomy. Exp Brain Res 35: 511–518

Leong SK (1977) Plasticity of cerebellar efferents after neonatal lesions in albino rats. Neurosci Lett 7: 281–289

Lim KH, Leong SK (1975) Aberrant bilateral projections from the dentate and interposed nuclei in albino rats after neonatal lesions. Brain Res 96: 306–309

Mizuno N, Konishi A, Sato M, Kawaguchi S, Yamamoto I, Kawamura S, Yamawaki M (1975) Thalamic afferents to the rostral portions of the middle suprasylvian gyrus in the cat. Exp Neurol 48: 79–87

Nakamura Y, Mizuno N, Konishi A, Sato M (1974) Synaptic reorganization of the red nucleus after chronic deafferentation from cerebellorubral fibers: an electron microscope study in the cat. Brain Res 82: 298–301

Raisman G, Field P (1973) A quantitative investigation of the development of collateral regeneration after partial deafferentation of the septal nuclei. Brain Res 50: 241–264

Rispal-Padel L, Grangetto A (1977) The cerebello-thalamo-cortical pathway. Topographical investigation at the unitary level in the cat. Exp Brain Res 28: 101–123

Sasaki K, Kawaguchi S, Matsuda Y, Mizuno N (1972) Electrophysiological studies on cerebello-cerebral projections in the cat. Exp Brain Res 16: 75–88

Sasaki K, Matsuda Y, Mizuno N (1973) Distribution of cerebellar-induced responses in the cerebral cortex. Exp Neurol 39: 342–354

Smith DE, Castro AJ (1979) Retrograde changes in Clarke's column following neonatal hemicerebellectomy in the rat. Am J Anat 156: 533–542

Tsukahara N, Hultborn H, Murakami F, Fujito Y (1975) Electrophysiological study of formation of new synapses and collateral sprouting in red nucleus neurons after partial denervation. J Neurophysiol 38: 1359–1372

Yamamoto T, Kawaguchi S, Samejima A (1979) Electrophysiological studies on the cerebellocerebral projection in the rat. Exp Neurol 63: 545–558

Yamamoto T, Kawaguchi S, Samejima A (1981) Electrophysiological studies on plasticity of cerebellothalamic neurons in rats following neonatal hemicerebellectomy. Jpn J Physiol 31: 217–224

Locomotor Behavior After Cerebellar Lesions in the Young Rat

A. GRAMSBERGEN[1]

1 Introduction

Animal experiments have demonstrated frequently that brain damage sustained in early life has less severe behavioral effects than similar lesions in later life (for reviews consult: Stein et al. 1974; Finger 1978). Although the notion that the brain of young animals has a greater compensational capacity than the adult brain has become almost a dogma, critical reading of literature does not support this unequivocally (Johnson and Almli 1978). Results of Di Giorgio (1944), who studied the effects of cerebellar lesions in newborn guinea pigs (born with an almost mature brain) indicate that not the chronological *age* as such but rather the *stage* of brain maturation is the determining factor for recovery.

Another consideration involved is whether the lesions are uni- or bilateral. Kennard (1944) did not find any disturbances of motor development after a unilateral lesion of the motor cortex in newborn rhesus monkeys. However, bilateral lesions led to sustained dysfunction. Several authors have reported that behavioral deficits as a consequence of induced brain damage become manifest only after considerable time has elapsed [e.g., delayed alternation tasks after dorsolateral frontal cortex lesions in monkeys: Goldman (1972, 1974); and the disturbed fine control of finger movement after bilateral pyramidal tract lesions in monkeys: Lawrence and Hopkins (1970, 1976)]. The picture is further complicated by findings of Spear and Barbas (1975), reporting that recovery of function is not necessarily limited to lesions at early ages. Bilateral lesions in the visual cortex of adult rats appeared to be compensated for after long training. In this study a visual discrimination task was applied.

We decided to study the effects of uni- and bilateral cerebellectomy sustained at different ages in rats. The rat was chosen as the experimental animal. Rats are born at an early stage of cerebellar maturation (Altman et al. 1969; Ebels 1970; Altman and Anderson 1971). This provides the opportunity to make surgical cerebellar lesions during early stages of maturation in the rat's postnatal period, which evidently has methodological advantages. We decided to operate rats at the 5th postnatal day (when proliferation and migration of the later granular cells occur), the 10th day (when the ulti-

---

1 Department of Developmental Neurology, University Hospital, Oostersingel 59, Groningen, The Netherlands

mate number of neurons has been formed and migrated), and the 30th day (when cerebellar maturation has been nearly completed).

The present report will be concerned mainly with the effects on locomotion after hemicerebellectomy. The investigation into behavioral deficits after total cerebellar ablation as well as into the relation between behavioral anomalies and neuroanatomical remodelling, as demonstrated by histological techniques, is the subject of ongoing research.

2 Methods

2.1 Housing Conditions

Rats of the white and black hooded Lister strain were housed in cages (38 X 25 X 16 cm high) with excelsior on the floor for nesting. The temperature in the animal room was kept at 20°C, relative humidity at 50%, lighting schedule: 08.00 h until 18.00 h light. Nonsuckling animals were fed a standard food. On the 25th day the young rats were weaned and separated by gender.

2.2 Operations

Both hemi- and total cerebellectomies were performed in rats from the same litter by aspiration under ether anesthesia at 5 days, 10 days, and 30 days of age. After recovery from the anesthesia the surviving rats were replaced in the litter of origin. Altogether 83 animals survived until the age of 360 days.

At this age the animals were killed by perfusion under ether anesthesia. Their brains were dissected, immersed in fixative and photographed. The extent of the lesions was studied in cresyl violet-stained sections. Attention was paid especially to the entireness of the dorsal aspect of the metencephalic brainstem, the presence of the vestibular nuclei and the contralateral cerebellar nuclei in case of hemicerebellectomy. After autopsy the rats were distributed in four groups:

Group A: hemicerebellectomy at the left side; vermis not included.
Group B: hemicerebellectomy at the left side, vermis partially removed.
Group C: hemicerebellectomy at the left side, vermis removed totally.
Group D: complete cerebellectomy.

A total of 66 rats could be classified into one of the groups and the behavioral records were processed accordingly. For a distribution of the individuals over the experimental groups see Fig. 1. Because of the lack of data, rats from the groups B-30 days, C-10 days, and D-5 days were not considered. The data obtained from the groups B-5 days, B-10 days, and D-10 days were employed only to validate the behavioral testing procedure. The material for all groups is in the process of being supplemented.

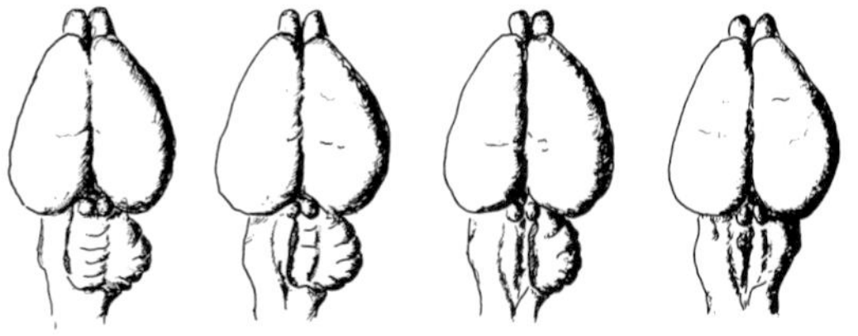

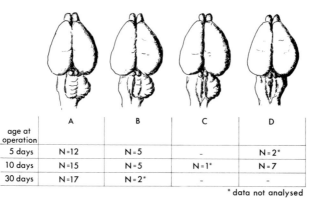

age at operation	A	B	C	D
5 days	N=12	N=5	-	N=2*
10 days	N=15	N=5	N=1*	N=7
30 days	N=17	N=2*	-	-

* data not analysed

Fig. 1A–D. Adult brains that sustained lesions at the age of 5 days, 10 days, and 30 days. **A** Hemicerebellectomy at the left side; **B** hemicerebellectomy at the left side, vermis partially included; **C** hemicerebellectomy at the left side, vermis removed totally; **D** complete cerebellar ablation

2.3 Behavioral Testing and Coding

Rats operated on the 5th and 10 day were tested daily after the operation until their 31st day and with 30-day intervals thereafter until they were 360 days old. Rats operated on the 30th day were tested 3 days after the operation for the first time and with 30-day intervals thereafter. Testing, lasting 10–15 min per rat, occurred between 14.00 and 18.00 h in the animal room. The testing platform consisted of a table (80–120 cm) with a smooth surface.

In a pilot study containing about 110 rats, which were subjected to hemi- and total cerebellectomy on the 5th, 10th, and 30th day, and 30 control rats, an inventory of locomotor abilities was made. For rats younger than 12–13 days, which are not yet able to walk on all fours, a scale of locomotor abilities was applied (derived from the scale described by Almli and Fisher 1977; see also, Altman and Sudarshan 1975).

Category I: Ventral body surface in contact with the testing platform; head motion and uncoordinated swimming movements and pivoting.

Category II: Ventral body surface in contact with the platform; coordinated and directive crawling with the forelimbs only.

Category III: Ventral body surface in contact with the platform; coordinated and directive crawling with all four limbs.

Category IV: Walking on all four limbs with the ventral body surface off the surface of the testing platform.

(Categories I and IV are congruent to Almli and Fisher's categories 1 and 3, respectively; our categories II and III subdivide their category 2.)

For rats aged 12 days and older a scale of six locomotion categories was designed, classifying the locomotor abilities of handicapped rats in comparison with locomotion of normal rats:

Category 1: Ventral or lateral body surface in contact with the testing platform. No effective locomotive movements occurring in fore- or back limbs.
Category 2: Ventral or lateral body surface in contact with the testing platform. Effective goal directed and locomotive movements in forelimbs only.
Category 3: Ventral body surface in contact with the testing platform. Goal directed and locomotive movements occur in all four limbs.
Category 4: Locomotion on all fours with the ventral surface off the testing platform. Lateral sways exceeding half of body diameter occur (due to falling or ataxia). Short-lasting arrests during locomotion.
Category 5: Locomotion on all four limbs with the ventral body surface off the floor. Slight swaying of less than one half body diameter. Clumsy locomotion caused by unsmooth placing of paws, waddling gait, postural tremor, abduction of limbs; eventually a combination of these phenomena.
Category 6: Undisturbed, age-adequate locomotion without any of the abnormalities mentioned above.

Locomotion of rats is documented by the predominant category (or categories, if occurring).

Apart from locomotor patterns, specific motor phenomena may be observed, which are not occurring continuously and are not obligatory for any of the locomotion categories. Per rat and per age studied an inventory of these concomitant locomotor handicaps was made.

1. Corkscrew movement
The rat's body turns over with a corkscrew-like distortion of the body axis from rostral to caudal.
Scoring: turn of 360°: +
incomplete and actively stopped turn: ±

2. Falling
Falling of the rat on its lateral body surface.
Scoring: yes/no.

3. Ataxia
Marked swaying with low, irregular frequency and large amplitude occurring in forward–backward direction and/or left–right direction.
Scoring: yes/no.

4. Postural tremor
High frequency (up to approximately 4 Hz) and low amplitude tremor of the trunk.
Scoring: yes/no.

5. Increased gait width
Abduction of one or both hind limbs.
Scoring: Abduction of one hind limb: +
Abduction of two hind limbs: ++

6. Paw dysmetria ("Goose step")
Locomotion becomes clearly audible due to unduly hard placing of paws.
Scoring: yes/no.

7. Waddling gait
Unstabilized, wobbling pelvis during locomotion due to hampered flexion in one or both hind legs.
Scoring: yes/no.

For a review of motor phenomena occurring in experimental animals with cerebellar lesions, see Dow and Moruzzi (1958). We applied nomenclature proposed by Walker and Botterell (1937) in pertinent instances.

Postural asymmetries appeared to be a common finding in rats with cerebellar lesions. These asymmetries in posture during locomotion and rest are produced by a moderate or marked abduction of the hind leg or by both limbs on the same side.
Scoring: abduction at *left* or *right* side
abduction of the distal part of the leg only: +
abduction of the entire leg from the hip joint or abduction of both homolateral legs: ++

2.4 Quantitative Analysis of the Behavioral Data

In order to compare behavioral data of the same rat at different ages, quantification is essential. Although the numerals attached to the (arbitrarily chosen) locomotion categories (ranging 1–6) are ordinal and far from a proportional representation of functional abilities, the scale provides a reasonable first approximation. With the same objective, the inventory of concomitant motor phenomena has been quantified. In this case abnormal motor phenomena are considered as penalties to be subtracted from the maximum value of "6". Because some motor abnormalities mean a much greater impediment for locomotion than others, they were given a heavier penalty. (These penalties are chosen arbitrarily; see Table 1).

Table 1. Inventory of locomotor handicaps in rats sustaining cerebellar lesions. Scores and penalties as defined in text

		Score	Penalty
Corkscrew movement	360°	+	2.5
	incomplete	±	2
Falling		+	1.5
Ataxia		+	0.5
Postural tremor		+	0.25
Increased gait width		++	0.5
		+	0.25
Paw dysmetria (goose step)		+	0.25
Waddling gait		+	0.25

In the pilot group, some hemicerebellectomized rats showed retarded locomotor development, as indicated by the retarded disappearance of category III. A retardation was rated as follows: III before 13 days: score 6; III at day 13 and 14: score 5; III at day 15: score 4; III after day 15: score 3. The values derived from the locomotion categories and the inventory of locomotor handicaps were analyzed further with non-parametrical statistical tests.

3 Results

3.1 The Postoperative Period

Rats which were either hemicerebellectomized or totally cerebellectomized on the 5th day do not show abnormal locomotion patterns, nor any of the "concomitant locomotor handicaps" until the 12th day. The only symptom to be observed in some of the hemicerebellectomized rats is asymmetrical posture due to abduction of one hind limb. The two rats which were cerebellectomized totally did not show any abnormality nor asymmetry at all until the 13th day. In rats operated on the 10th day, the first symptoms of the lesion emerge, likewise, on the 12th day.

All rats, hemicerebellectomized on the 30th day, show in the immediate postoperative period without exception violent, corkscrew-like body movements, directed "away from the lesion". This condition improves remarkably in the next hours, and 3 days after the operation, at the first testing session, their locomotion and posture are essentially the same as they remain until the age of 360 days.

3.2 Locomotor Behavior from the 12th Day Onwards

3.2.1 Locomotion Categories

Because the locomotion scores per individual appear to be relatively stable over time, we decided to average for each animal the scores obtained from 4 consecutive days in the first 31 days, the scores obtained on the 60th and 90th day, the 120th–180th day, the 210th–270th day, and the 300th–360th day. For rats operated on the 30th day, the locomotion score on the 33rd day is averaged with values on the 60th and 90th day. Between the 12th and 15th day the locomotion scores of the 5-day-old operated group range between 3.5 and 5, resulting in a median score of 4.50 (Fig. 2). These scores increase up to values of 5.16 to 5.30 between the 20th and 30th day, but decrease thereafter to median values between 4.67 and 4.79 from the 60th to the 90th day onwards. The increase between the 12th and 15th day, and the 20th and 23rd day as well as the decrease between the 28th and 31th day, and 60th and 90th day are significant, both at the 0.001 level (Friedman's rank test for correlated samples, 2-tailed test; see Ferguson 1966). The median score for the rats operated on the 10th day is 4.75 between the 12th and 15th day. No particular trend occurs thereafter: the scores remain at this level.

The median of locomotion scores of rats from the group operated at the age of 30 days is remarkably high (5.46) when compared with the values in the other experimental groups of rats of the same age. However, the median score decreases gradually

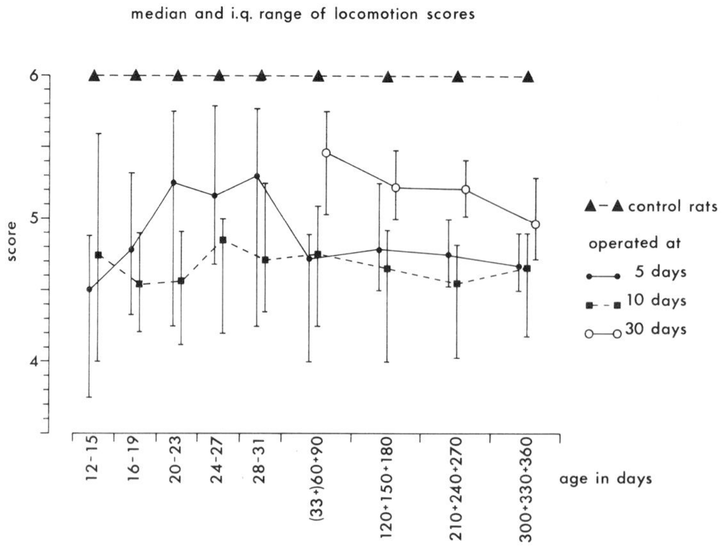

Fig. 2. Median values and interquartile (i.q.) range of locomotion scores in the groups of rats hemicerebellectomized on the 5th, 10th, and 30th day, and age-matched controls. *Vertical scale,* locomotion scores; *horizontal scale,* ages as indicated

to the value of 4.97 at the 300th–360th day. (The decrease is significant at the 0.001 level; Friedman's test.) When comparing the data obtained from the group operated when 30 days old with age-matched data from the other groups, the first appears to differ significantly from the two others (Mann-Whitney U test; significance levels: 0.4–0.006). The groups operated on the 5th and 10th day do not show significant differences in this age span.

3.2.2 Inventory of Concomitant Locomotor Handicaps

The locomotor handicaps in either of the three groups are limited to mild handicaps such as increased gait width, paw dysmetria, waddling gait, and postural tremor and ataxia, in only a few cases. Corkscrew movements and falling have never been observed during any of the test sessions. (These movements do occur in more severely damaged rats.)

When considering the medians of the handicap scores of the group operated on the 5th day, the values appear to increase between the 12th and 15th day and the 24th 27th day, but decrease thereafter (Fig. 3).

Principally the same occurs in rats which were operated on the 10th day: an increase between the 12th and 15th day, and the 28th and 31st day, and a decrease thereafter.

In the group of rats hemicerebellectomized on the 30th day, a (slight) decrease in the scores was observed.

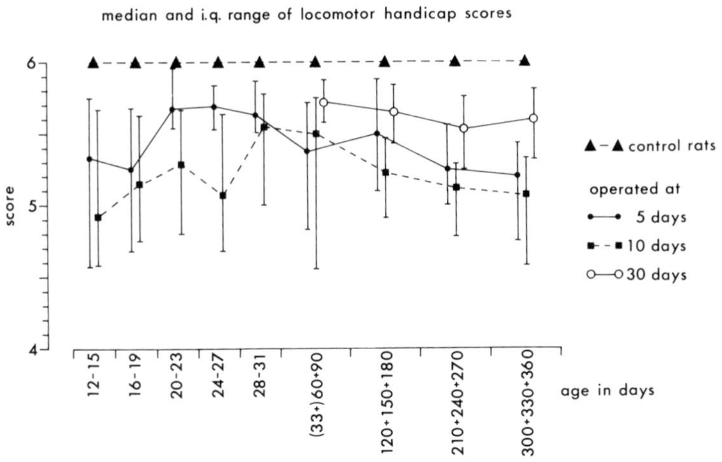

Fig. 3. Median values and interquartile (i.q.) range of locomotor handicap scores in the groups of rats hemicerebellectomized on the 5th, 10th, and 30th day, as well as age-matched control rats. *Vertical scale,* locomotor handicap scores; *horizontal scale,* ages as indicated

3.2.3 Postural Asymmetries

Asymmetries in posture during locomotion as well as during rest are relatively frequently occurring phenomena. Rats operated on the 5th day show a postural asymmetry in 83% of the cases; the group operated on the 10th day in 84%, and the group operated on the 30th day in 74% of the cases. These values indicate no important differences related to the time of operation. In the first 2 postoperative days in rats operated on the 5th day or 10th day, the incidence of asymmetries is still low. Neither an age-specific trend in the occurrence of postural asymmetries nor any trend in the severity of the asymmetry over age or experimental group has been observed.

In the majority of cases abduction is at the side ipsilateral to the cerebellar lesion. However, in the rats operated on the 5th day and the 10th day, 8.4% and 20.2% respectively of all asymmetrical postures observed occur at the side *contralateral* to the lesion (Figs. 4 and 5). In the group of rats operated on the 30th day this percentage of *contralateral* abduction is lower (2.7%; Fig. 6).

The occurrence of contralateral abduction is not limited to a particular age. In certain animals, however, the occurrence of contralateral limb abduction appears to be more consistent than in others.

Note: Rats which were hemicerebellectomized with half of the vermis included appear to rank only slightly lower than rats which were hemicerebellectomized without damage to the vermis. (Group B operated on day 5 – mean values of scores: 4.21–4.99; Group B operated on day 10 – 3.28–4.00.) However, rats in which the cerebellum was ablated totally remain severely handicapped and unable to produce normal or near-normal locomotion. (Mean values of locomotion scores: 2.95–3.67.) In neither of these groups appears improvement of locomotion to occur.

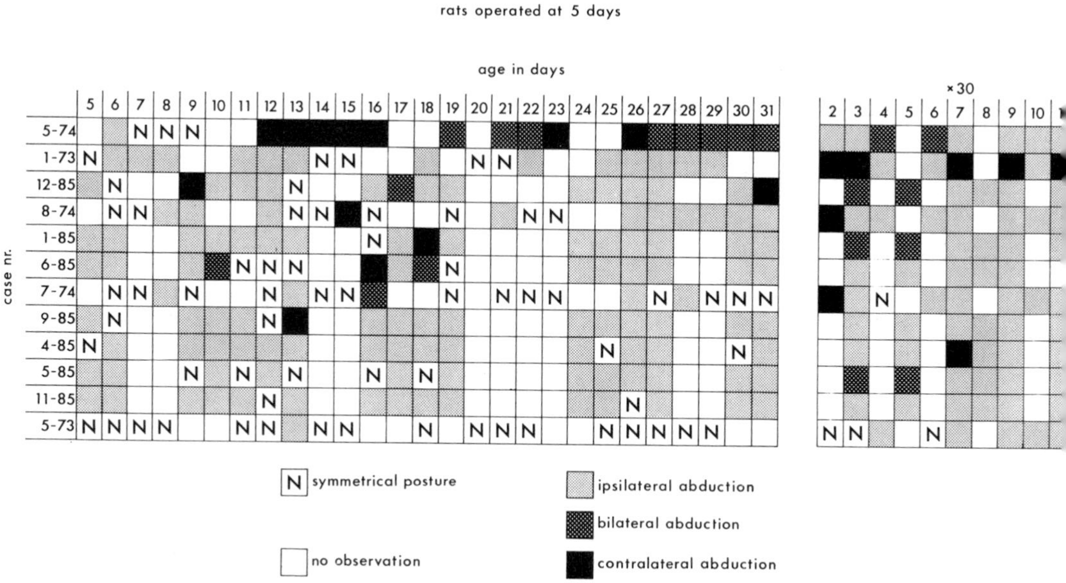

Fig. 4. Limb abduction in rats, hemicerebellectomized on the 5th day. *Vertical axis,* case numbers; *horizontal axis,* ages in days and 30-day periods, respectively

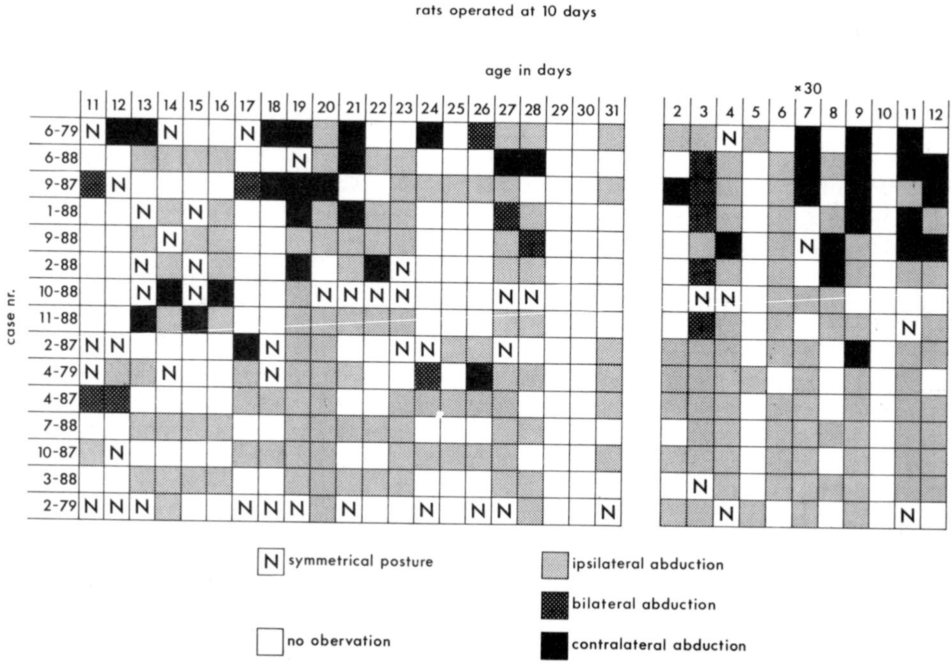

Fig. 5. Limb abduction in rats, hemicerebellectomized on the 10th day. *Vertical axis,* case numbers; *horizontal axis,* ages in days and 30-day periods, respectively

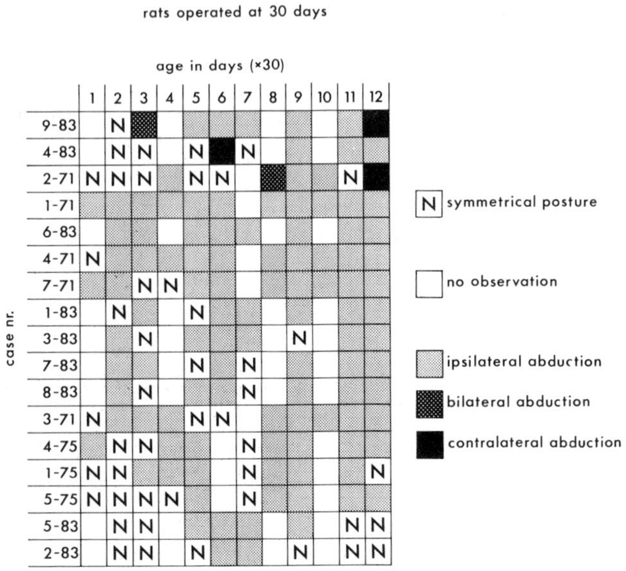

Fig. 6. Limb abduction in rats, hemicerebellectomized on the 30th day. *Vertical axis,* case numbers; *horizontal axis,* ages in 30-day periods

4 Discussion

The long-term effects of hemicerebellectomy and complete cerebellectomy at early and later ages on locomotion in rats have been investigated in the present study. Although much has been revealed in relation to neuroanatomical remodelling, systematic study of the effects on motor behavior has been seemingly neglected.

After hemicerebellectomy on the 5th day and on the 10th day asymmetrical posture develops in the majority of the rats. However, no signs of locomotor handicaps become apparent until the 12th or 13th day in either groups of hemicerebellectomized rats (nor in rats which were lesioned more extensively), but they do thereafter. Di Giorgio (1944, article in Italian; quoted by Dow and Moruzzi 1958) found in newborn kittens and rabbits subjected to a cerebellar lesion that the first symptoms only appeared days after the operation. However, in newborn guinea pigs (animals which are born at a mature state of brain development) the first symptoms become apparent immediately after recovery from the operation. (It has to be taken into account that Di Giorgio's experimental animals were decerebrated in addition.) These results as well as the time lag between the operation and the occurrence of disturbed locomotion and motor handicaps in our rats may indicate that cerebellar function plays an important role in locomotion from the 12th/13th day onwards. Postural asymmetries due to limb abduction occur already in the first days after operation, which indicates that the cerebellum plays in this period of life a role in the regulation of tone in limb muscles ultimately involved in locomotion.

Although locomotion improves until the age of about one month in rats operated on the 5th postnatal day, a decrease occurs subsequently. No such temporary improvement can be observed in rats operated on the 10th day; and in rats operated on the 30th day only a steady decrease is found. Essentially the same phenomenon appears to occur in the locomotor handicap scores (although in this case values obtained from the group operated at the age of 10 days increase at first and decrease thereafter, as do the values from the group operated when 5 days old).

Two general conclusions may be drawn from our findings. Firstly, consistent improvement does not occur in the locomotion in any of the experimental groups, even when considered over a long period. Secondly, rats hemicerebellectomized on the 30th day are superior in respect to locomotion to rats operated on the 5th or 10th day.

These conclusions are in contrast to findings in newborn puppies, rabbits, and kittens (Asratian 1938; Di Giorgio 1944; De Renzi and Pompeiano 1956). All experimental animals studied are reported to show remarkable improvement over age as well as superior performance, compared with animals which are lesioned later in life. Differences between our results and results from these authors may be explained by differences in species studied, different experimental procedures (the experimenters used decerebrated animals), as well as differences in the length of the observation period.

Another intriguing result of the present study is the occurrence of postural asymmetries due to abduction of the hind limb at the side *contralateral* to the cerebellar lesion. Abduction of hind limbs at the ipsilateral side is a common finding in rats of all experimental groups, as it is in dogs and cats hemicerebellectomized at adult ages (Rademaker 1931; Dow and Moruzzi 1958). Abduction at the contralateral side occurs most often in rats hemicerebellectomized on the 10th day (in 20.2% of all asymmetrical postures observed), less so in rats operated on the 5th day (in 8.4%), and only in 2.7% of the rats operated on the 30th day.

A problem in the interpretation of this phenomenon is raised by the inconsistency of abduction (contralateral abduction alternating with ipsilateral abduction, bilateral abduction and normal posture) in one and the same animal observed at different sessions. Moreover, the occurrence of contralateral abduction is not limited to particular ages – it is emerging in rats of all ages.

In recent years several reports have demonstrated the development of aberrant neural connections in response to unilateral cerebellar ablation in newborn rats. In rats hemicerebellectomized on the 2nd, 3rd, or 5th day, bilateral projections from the remaining dentate and interposed nuclei to the red nucleus and several thalamic nuclei have been reported (Leong 1978a), whereas in normal rats only a *contralateral* projection was demonstrated (Chan Palay 1977; Leong 1978a). In addition, the projection from the sensorimotor cortex (SMC) contralateral to the cerebellar lesion has changed: the contralateral projection from this SMC is denser than normally (Nah and Leong 1976; Leong 1977), whereas the red nucleus on this same side contains fewer large cells (Leong 1978b). Castro and Smith (1979) reported an increased projection of the spinal cord to the ipsilateral lateral vestibular nucleus after neonatal hemicerebellectomy. In normal rats, it is claimed that these fibers project to the ipsilateral cerebellum. The development of anomalous fibers appears to be related to the age of lesion being much greater after lesions before the 5th day than at the 10th after birth and even totally absent in rats operated at the 15th day (Leong 1978a). Aberrant afferent connections to the red nuclei from the SMC and the remaining cerebellar nuclei in reaction to early hemicerebellectomy are of special interest. It should be remembered that the red nucleus plays a key role in the regulation and maintenance of muscle tone in contralateral limb flexors and ipsilateral limb extensors (Pompeiano 1957; for extensive review see Massion 1967).

It might be that the aberrant projections onto the red nucleus cause a disturbed functioning in the interneuronal pool on which rubro-spinal fibers project. Hypothetically, this might explain the occurrence of limb abduction to the contralateral (as well as to the ipsilateral) side, as well as impaired locomotion.

The latter is a consistent finding in our rats lesioned on the 5th and 10th day, i.e., the critical period to which the development of neuro-anatomical remodelling seems to be limited.

Our aim in the near future will be to correlate the behavioral findings, reported here, with histological evidence from the very same rats with the help of Fink-Heimer stain and autoradiography.

Acknowledgments. The advice, criticisms, and comments of Professor H.F.R. Prechtl and Dr. B. Hopkins, as well as the assistance of Mrs. J. IJkema-Paassen, Mrs. Y.L. Lems, and Mrs. S.A. Sumual are gratefully acknowledged.

This research is supported by a program grant, 13-51-91 from the Foundation of Medical Research, FUNGO.

References

Almli CR, Fisher RS (1977) Infant rats: sensorimotor ontogeny and effects of substantia nigra destruction. Brain Res Bull 2: 425–459

Altman J, Anderson WJ (1971) Irradiation of the cerebellum in infant rats with low-level X-ray: histological and cytological effects during infancy and adulthood. Exp Neurol 30: 492–509

Altman J, Sudarshan K (1975) Postnatal development of locomotion in the laboratory rat. Anim Behav 23: 896–920

Altman J, Anderson WJ, Wright KA (1969) Early effects of X-irradiation of the cerebellum in infant rats: decimation and reconstitution of the external granular lager. Exp Neurol 24: 196–216

Asratian EA (1938) Beiträge zur Alterscharakteristik des Kleinhirns (Russian, summary in German). Fiziol Zh (Kiev) 19: 448–453

Castro AJ, Smith DE (1979) Plasticity of spinovestibular projections in response to hemicerebellectomy in newborn rats. Neurosci Lett 12: 69–74

Chan-Palay V (1977) Cerebellar dentate nucleus. Springer, Berlin Heidelberg New York

De Renzi C, Pompeiano O (1956) La comparsa dell'attività tonica della corteccia e dei nuclei del cervelletto nel gatto neonato. Arch Sci Biol 40: 523–534

Di Giorgio AM (1944) Sulla organizzazione della attività cerebellari nei mammiferi neonati. Arch Fisiol 43: 47–63

Dow RS, Moruzzi G (1958) The physiology and pathology of the cerebellum. Univ of Minnesota Press, Minneapolis

Ebels EJ (1970) The influence of age upon the effect of early postnatal X-irradiation on the development of the cerebellar cortex in rats. Acta Neuropathol 15: 298–307

Ferguson GA (1966) Statistical analysis in psychology and education, 2nd edn. Mc Graw-Hill, New York

Finger S (ed) (1978) Recovery from brain damage. Plenum Press, New York London

Goldman PS (1972) Developmental determinants of cortical plasticity. Acta Neurobiol 32: 495–511

Goldman PS (1974) An alternative to developmental plasticity: heterology of CNS structures in infants and adults. In: Stein DG, Rosen JJ, Butters N (eds) Plasticity and recovery of function in the central nervous system. Academic Press, London New York, pp 149–174

Johnson D, Almli CR (1978) Age, brain damage, and performance. In: Finger S (ed) Recovery from brain damage. Plenum Press, New York London, pp 115–134

Kennard MA (1944) Reactions of monkeys of various ages to partial and complete decortication. J Neuropathol Exp Neurol 3: 289–310

Lawrence DG, Hopkins DA (1970) Bilateral pyramidal lesions in infant rhesus monkeys. Brain Res 24: 543–544

Lawrence DG, Hopkins DA (1976) The development of motor control in the rhesus monkey. Evidence concerning the role of corticomotoneuronal connections. Brain 99: 235–254

Leong SK (1977) Sprouting of the corticopontine fibres after neonatal cerebellar lesion in the albino rat. Brain Res 123: 164–169

Leong SK (1978a) Plasticity of cerebellar afferents after neonatal lesions in albino rats. Neurosci Lett 7: 281–289

Leong SK (1978b) Effects of deafferenting cerebellar or cerebral inputs to the pontine and red nuclei in the albino rat. Brain Res 155: 357–361

Massion J (1967) The mammalian red nucleus. Physiol Rev 47: 383–436

Nah SH, Leong SK (1976) Bilateral corticofugal projection to the red nucleus after neonatal lesions in the albino rat. Brain Res 107: 433–436

Pompeiano O (1957) Analisi degli effecti della stimulazione elettrica del nucleo rosso nel gatto decerebrato. Atti Accad Naz Lincei Mem Cl Sci Fis Mat Nat Sez III 22: 100–103

Rademaker GGJ (1931) Das Stehen: Statische Reaktionen, Gleichgewichtsreaktionen und Muskeltonus unter besonderer Berücksichtigung ihres Verhaltens bei kleinhirnlosen Tieren. Springer, Berlin

Spear PD, Barbas H (1975) Recovery of pattern discrimination ability in rats receiving serial or one stage visual cortex lesion. Brain Res 94: 337–346

Stein DG, Rosen JJ, Butters N (eds) (1974) Plasticity and recovery of function in the central nervous system. Academic Press, London New York

Walker AE, Botterell EH (1937) The syndrome of the superior cerebellar peduncle in the monkey. Brain 60: 329–353

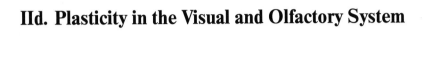

IId. Plasticity in the Visual and Olfactory System

Reorganization of Retino-Geniculate Connections After Retinal Lesions in the Adult Cat

U.TH. EYSEL, F. GONZALEZ-AGUILAR, and U. MAYER[1]

1 Introduction

Since the descriptions of reorganization in the spinal cord after dorsal root lesions (Liu and Chambers 1958; McCouch et al. 1958) various physiological and anatomical signs of lesion-induced neuronal plasticity have been observed in the central nervous system of the adult cat. (Studies in several subcortical systems are listed in Table 1.)

The mature visual system of the cat is characterized by a very precise pattern of connections. The lateral geniculate nucleus (LGN) receives afferent inputs from the two eyes separated in different layers (recently reviewed by Rodieck 1979). A precise

Table 1. Signs of lesion-induced neuronal plasticity in central subcortical structures of the adult cat

Authors and year	Methods	Structure	Time
McCouch et al. (1958)	EP t/ LM d	Spinal cord	30 d
Kostyuk (1963)	EP/SC i	Spinal cord	20 d
Precht et al. (1966)	SC e, B	Vestibular nucleus	30 d
Murray and Goldberger (1974)	LM a, d	Spinal cord	20 d
Nakamura et al. (1974)	EM d	Red nucleus	25 d
Tsukahara et al. (1975)	SC i	Red nucleus	10 d
Basbaum and Wall (1976)	SC e, t	Dorsal horn	30 d
Millar et al. (1976)	SC e, t	Gracile nucleus	(8 months)
Devor and Wall (1978)	SC e, t	Dorsal horn	28 d
Mendell et al. (1978)	SC e, i, t	Dorsal horn	30 d
Steward and Messenheimer (1978)	HC	Hippocampal formation	16 d
Eysel (1979)	SC e	LGN	(10 weeks)
Eysel et al. (1980)	SC e, t	LGN	30 d
Pubols and Goldberger (1980)	SC e, t	Dorsal horn	(8 weeks)

Abbreviations for methods: B – behavioral analysis, EM – electron microscopical analysis, EP – evoked potentials, LM – light microscopical analysis, HC – histochemical analysis, SC – single cell recordings; a – autoradiography, d – degeneration, e – extracellular, i – intracellucar, t – mapping of topography. The indicated times were necessary for full development of the effects. Times in brackets: investigations without determination of the onset and time course

1 Institut für Physiologie, Universitätsklinikum Essen, Hufelandstraße 55, 4300 Essen 1, FRG

retino-geniculate topography was found with projection columns extending approximately vertically through the different layers (Kaas et al. 1972; Sanderson 1971). Anatomical investigations in the LGN after removal of one eye showed no translaminar sprouting of retino-geniculate axons in the adult, in contrast to the developing cat (Guillery 1972; Hickey 1975). Under the same experimental conditions anatomical (Hámori 1968) and physiological (Eysel 1979) signs of reorganization of other than the visual input were observed at the deafferented cells in the adult cat LGN.

Further information about a possible potential for lesion-induced plasticity of mature retino-geniculate connections was expected from experiments with partial visual deafferentation within single layers of the LGN. Under this condition, deafferented cells and remaining normal inputs are in close proximity and fulfil the requirements of specificity and overlap for the induction of reorganization (Field et al. 1980; Goodman et al. 1973; Raisman 1969; Wall and Egger 1971).

2 Methodical Conditions for Investigation of Lesion-Induced Changes in the Cat LGN

2.1 Photocoagulator Lesions of the Retina

Photocoagulation of the retina proved to be a useful and precise method for deafferentation of the LGN in the cat with the following advantages: atraumatic operation, intravital visibility of the lesion, and predictability of the amount of deafferentation in the LGN. Partial deafferentation was possible, with restricted high-intensity Xenon photocoagulator lesions carefully preserving the blood supply of the surrounding retina. The direct effects of coagulation were visible in fundus photographs as a circumscribed area (Fig. 1A). The lesions were placed nasal to the optic disc or in the area centralis. Whole mount preparations of the retina (Wässle et al. 1975) showed that ganglion cells were present up to the very border of the lesion (Fig. 1B). The axon bundles were reduced between papilla and the lesion, and absent at the opposite side where the ganglion cells were missing because of retrograde degeneration (Fig. 1B, C). By the interruption of axons of passage from the periphery, the retinal lesions led to more extended deafferentation than is derivable from inspection of the fundus. However, the borders of the lesion, facing the papilla or being oriented in parallel to the axon bundles, directly defined the borders of deafferentation and thus served as reliable guides during the physiological experiments. The retina was functionally intact up to these borders. Following photocoagulation the retinal lesions shrunk due to scar contraction by relatively small amounts of 5% to 10% of their total size (Eysel et al. 1980).

2.2 Single Cell Recordings and Visual Field Maps

During the physiological experiments the cats were continuously anesthetized and immobilized. (For a detailed description of the methods see Eysel et al. 1980). Vertical penetrations through layer A (innervated by the contralateral eye) and layer A_1 (innervated by the ipsilateral eye) in the LGN contralateral to the lesion were performed

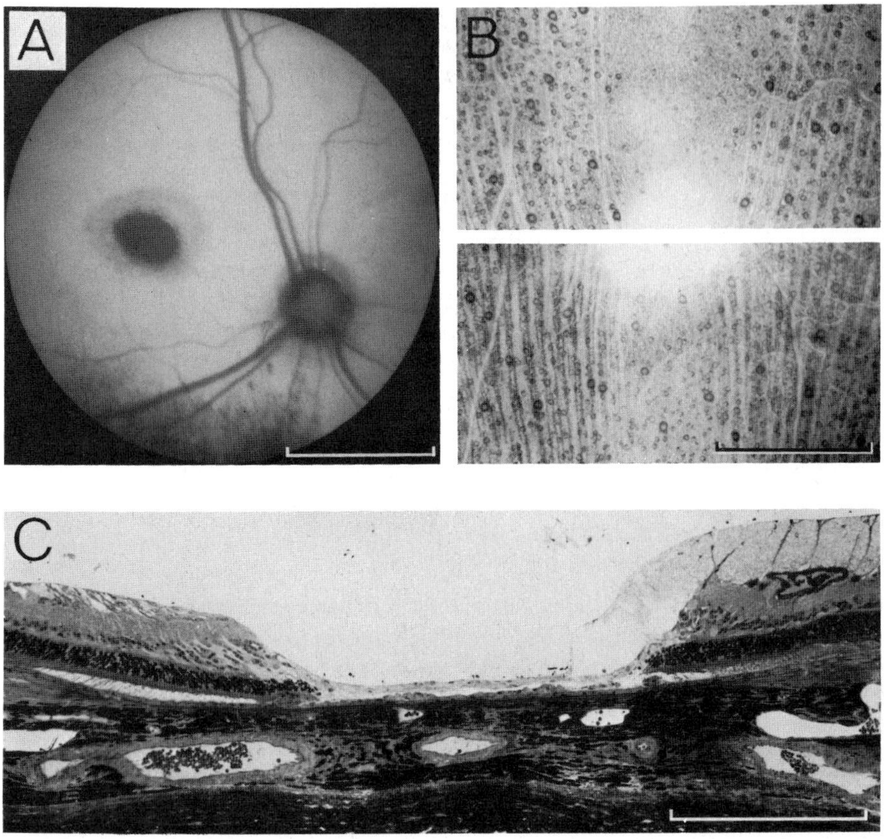

Fig. 1A–C. Fundus photograph and histological controls of small photocoagulator lesions. **A** Fundus photograph of a left eye with small lesion 256 days after photocoagulation. Scale bar: 10°. **B** Whole mount preparation of this retina viewed from the vitreal side. Note the reduction of axon bundles between papilla (*below,* not shown) and the lesion with ganglion cells, and the absence of axons and ganglion cells on the opposite side of the lesion (*above*). Scale bar: 500 μm. **C** Cross section of another retina with a small round lesion (60 days survival time after photocoagulation). Note the total destruction of all retinal layers within the lesion, the presence of the axon layer at the right side and the absence of this layer due to retrograde degenèration at the left side. Scale bar: 300 μm

with varnished tungsten microelectrodes at Horsley-Clarke coordinates A 5.0 to 6.5 and L 8.0 to 11.0, and single cell responses were recorded. The cats' eyes were focused on a tangent screen at 50 cm distance. The typical landmarks of the fundus (papilla, blood vessels, lesions) were back-projected and mapped on this screen, and possible small shifts of the visual axis were monitored by repeated back-projections. The receptive field (RF) centers of the recorded cells (determined with small spots of light to an accuracy of ± 0.5°) were plotted on the same map. From series of vertical penetrations at different lateral positions RF maps of the left visual field of both eyes were reconstructed by aligning the eyes to a presumed common fixation point (Sanderson and Sherman 1971) and expressing the RF positions in degrees of azimuth and elevation

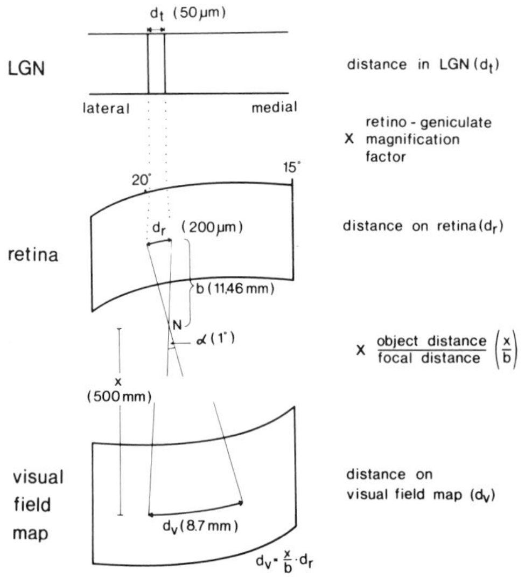

Fig. 2. Magnification of a small distance of cells in the lateral part of the LGN by the retino-geniculate magnification factor at 20° of azimuth and the image formation in the eye resulting in a large distance of RF centers on a screen 50 cm in front of the cat's eyes. α, visual angle; *N*, nodal point

(Bishop et al. 1962b). In vertical penetrations the RFs of the last cells in layer A and the first cells in layer A_1 showed corresponding values of azimuth in the visual field.

A high precision in detecting changes in the LGN is brought about by the properties of image formation on the retina and the retino-geniculate projection. A small distance in the LGN is transformed by the retino-geniculate magnification factor (Bishop et al. 1962a; Sanderson 1971) and the rules of image formation on the retina (Hughes 1976) into a larger distance on the tangent screen. Thus, a small displacement by 50 µm in the LGN results in a displacement of RFs on the tangent screen by 8.7 mm at an eccentricity of 20° (Fig. 2).

3 Changes of LGN Topography After Partial Visual Deafferentation

3.1 Displaced Receptive Fields at the Borders of Large Nasal Lesions

Large nasal lesions (Fig. 3A) led to visual deafferentation of the lateral part of the innervated layers (A, C complex) in the contralateral LGN. In acute experiments and up to 20 days after photocoagulation, the excitability by light ceased at the border of the projection of the retinal lesion in the LGN (Eysel et al. 1980). This was different after 30 and more days. The topographical correspondence of RFs from layer A and A_1 was normal between the area centralis and the border of the lesion. But the RFs of layer A cells remained at the border of the lesion when the electrode was moved further laterally by 150 µm (penetration 9 to 6), while the RFs of layer A_1 cells shifted by 3.5° as expected, with further lateral position of the electrode (Fig. 3A). Such displacements of RFs of layer A cells with respect to RFs of layer A_1 cells recorded during the same penetration were found in 15 cats 27–372 days after photocoagulation, and ranged between 1.5° and 4.5° of visual angle.

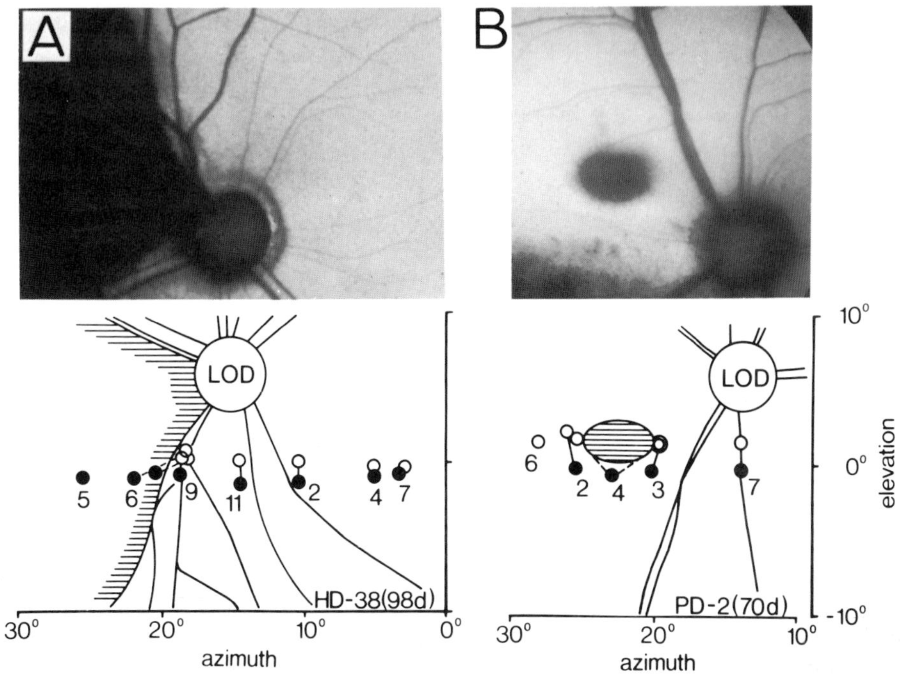

Fig. 3A, B. Fundus photographs and RF maps of the left visual field. **A** Large retinal lesion 98 days after photocoagulation. The *open circles* correspond to RF centers from the coagulated eye (cells recorded from layer A), the *black circles* represent the RF centers from the other eye (cells recorded from layer A_1). *Thin lines* connect the RFs obtained during one penetration (marked by a *number*), *broken lines* indicate RF displacements. The border of the lesion is *hatched. LOD,* left optic disc. **B** Small retinal lesion (70 days survival time). Conventions as in **A**. Penetration 4 shows RFs from both sides of the lesion. The *open circles* connected to the RF from layer A_1 by *broken lines* also indicate the positions of a double excitatory input to one layer A cell during this penetration

3.2 Excitatory Filling-In of Deafferentation After Small, Nasal Lesions

The experiments with a single border of a large area of deafferentation raised several questions. Would the observed effect be dependent on the size of the lesions or would excitation completely fill in smaller regions of deafferentation? Would it be possible to find single cells with multiple innervation by spatially separated RFs comparable to the findings of Millar et al. (1976) in the gracile nucleus? To answer these questions small, round lesions of 3°–6° diameter were applied to the nasal retina at about 20°–23° of azimuth (Figs. 1 and 3B). Acute lesions of this size led to complete deafferentation of single LGN cells (Eysel and Grüsser 1978). In experiments with less than 30 days survival time after photocoagulation, the area of deafferentation corresponded to the normal projection of the coagulated area onto the LGN. Recordings performed 30 and more days after photocoagulation revealed changes similar to the ones described in Sect. 3.1. The extent of RF displacements at the borders of deafferentation ranged between 1° and 3° of visual angle in ten cats with 30–256 days survival time. This was not significantly different from the results obtained with large lesions (Eysel et al. 1981). Cells innervated from one or the other side of a lesion were found when recording approximately from the middle of the deafferented region. Double or multiple innervation from different sides of the lesion converging to one LGN cell was observed in only two cases (Fig. 3B). The area of deafferentation was always considerably smaller than expected from the photocoagulated area.

3.3 Properties of Cells with Displaced Receptive Fields

The maintained activity and light-excitability of the neurons with displaced RFs were different from normal neurons (Eysel et al. 1980). The cells were characterized by high-frequency groups of discharges separated by long pauses and low light-excitability. Except for this light-excitability from the displaced RF the activity of these cells was similar to the activity of visually deafferented cells (Eysel 1979). The analysis of the geometry of displaced RFs yielded in most cases a cut-off of the antagonistic surround at the side of the lesion. Absence of binocular excitability and direction or movement selectivity, and typical response latencies after electrical stimulation of the optic tract, proved the retinal origin of the visual inputs of these cells (Eysel et al. 1980).

4 Discussion

4.1 Spatial Extent and Time Course of Reorganization in the Adult Cat LGN

The extent of lateral spread of excitation observed in the LGN after chronic retinal lesions amounted to a maximum of 200 μm, as judged by lateral electrode displacements from the border of deafferentation and by computations using RF displacements and the retino-geniculate magnification factor at 20° of azimuth.

Autoradiographic labeling of the borders of deafferentation after short and long post-lesion survival times may help to specify the nature and extent of the possibly underlying morphological mechanisms. In an autoradiographic study without exact control of the expected projection and extent of LGN deafferentation after chronic focal lesions in the retina, Baisden et al. (1980) very recently excluded long-range intralaminar sprouting of retino-geniculate axons in the adult cat. The possibility of small amounts of sprouting at the borders of the denervated regions was explicitly admitted in this study. Such small effects at the borders should be detectable with a different experimental approach. A physiologically intact nasal retinal stripe with approximately constant width of 5°–6°, limited by subacute and chronic lesions (Fig. 4A), projects in accordance with the retino-geniculate magnification factors into the contralateral LGN. Autoradiographic labeling of the projection of this stripe by an injection of 1 mCi ^{3}H-Leucine into the eye yielded a band-like zone of label in layer A and in the C complex (Fig. 4B). In serial sections the maximal width of this band was about 500–550 μm. This is in agreement with the range of physiologically obtained distances between normal cells with RFs 5°–6° apart at the investigated horizontal eccentricity.

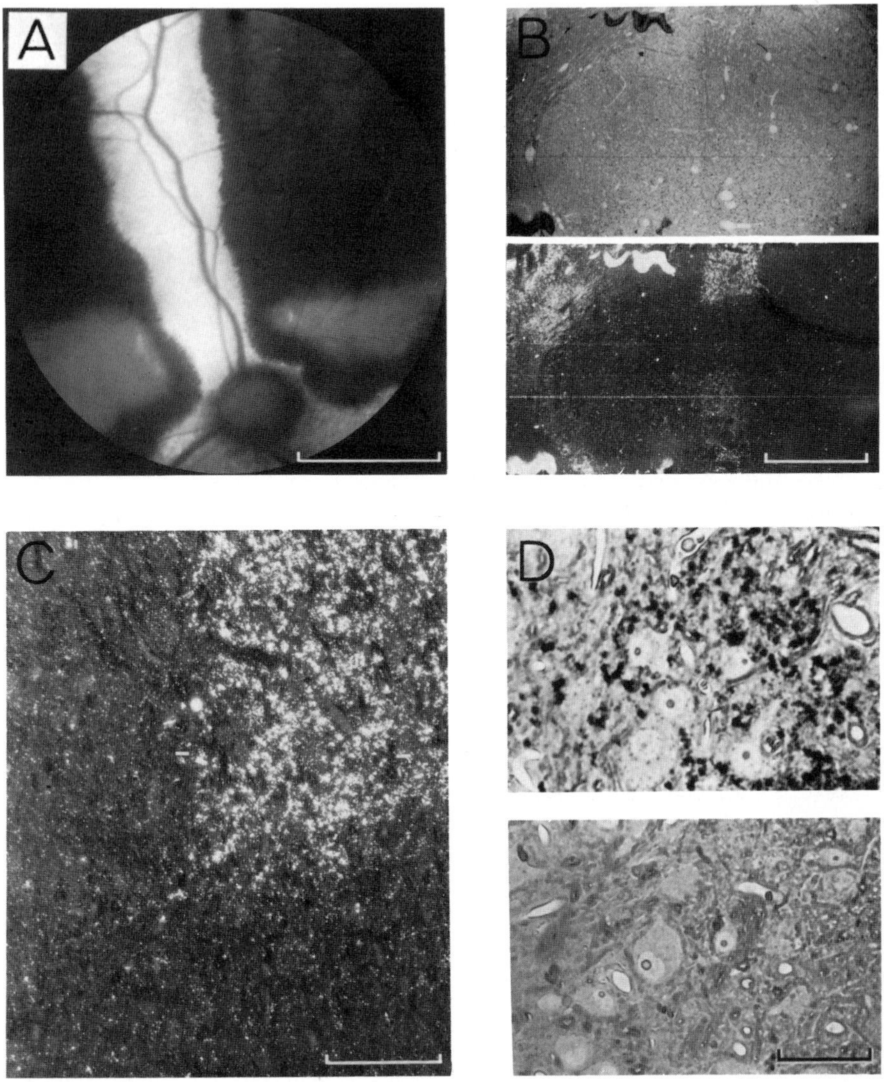

Fig. 4A–D. Autoradiography of the projection of a retinal stripe onto the LGN. Combination of long (60 d) and short (7 d) survival-time lesions. **A** Fundus photograph of the left eye showing the retinal stripe with blood supply before injection of 1 mCi ^{3}H-Leucine (60 d lesions above 7 d lesions). Horizontal width of the stripe 5°–6°. Scale bar: 10°. **B** Bright field (*above*) and dark field (*below*) photomicrographs of the lateral part of the contralateral LGN after 6 months of exposure. Semi-thin (3 μm) sections embedded in epoxy resin, osmicated, unstained. Note the band-like labeling in layer A and the C complex. Layer A_1 is not labeled. Scale bar: 1 mm. **C** Ventral lateral corner of the labeled region in layer A. *To the left* unlabeled part of layer A, *below* layer A_1. Scale bar: 100 μm. **D** Higher magnification photomicrographs from the labeled area in layer A (grains accumulated above the neuropil surrounding the cells), and from layer A_1 without labeling. Scale bar: 50 μm

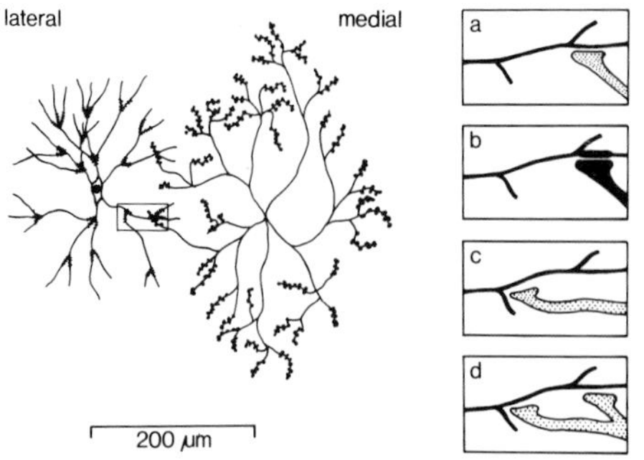

Fig. 5. Visually deafferented LGN relay cell (*left*) and terminal arborizations of an optic tract fiber (*right*). Dorsal view (redrawn according to Tömböl et al. 1978a,b and Madarász et al. 1978). The *small square* indicates the region of possible changes. *a* Situation after deafferentation and vacation of the synaptic site at the dendritic branching near to the soma; *b* Increase of efficiency of the peripheral synapse by denervation hypersensitivity; *c* Translocation of the peripheral synapse to a more effective position; *d* Collateral sprouting reaching the vacated synaptic site

Axonal sprouting, corresponding in extent to the electrophysiological results after chronic deafferentation, was not observed. If axonal sprouting occurs at all, only short range changes can be expected at the very borders of deafferentation. These borders proved to be sharply labeled in the autoradiographic material with respect to the neighboring parts of layer A as well as with respect to the adjacent layer A_1 (Fig. 4C). A quantitative analysis of this material is in preparation.

The above mentioned observations seem to allow only for possible morphological correlates of smaller spatial extent than the resulting functional effects. Considering the structure of the LGN of the cat, morphological changes, in fact, need not amount to distances as large as 200 μm to account for an extension of excitation by this value (Fig. 5). The overlap of LGN cell dendritic fields and optic tract terminal arborizations (Szentágothai 1973) forms a structural link between projection columns 200 μm apart (functionally not effective following acute deafferentation). The convergence of retinal inputs onto LGN relay cells (Tömböl et al. 1978b) suggests that except for the 1–7 effective input fibers (Cleland et al. 1971; Eysel 1976) a large number of less effective inputs may make contacts at synaptic sites further peripheral at the dendrites. The possible mechanisms to account for physiological changes of the observed kind are discussed in the literature (Schneider 1977; Wall 1975, 1976). *Postsynaptic denervation hypersensitivity* was demonstrated in some central nervous structures (Anderson et al. 1971; Bird and Aghajanian 1975; McCall and Aghajanian 1979). With this mechanism the efficiency of a peripheral synapse (Fig. 5a) might be raised above threshold (Fig. 5b). *Translocation of a peripheral synapse* into a more efficient position nearer to the cell soma (Fig. 5c) could result in the same physiological effect (Lynch et al. 1973). *Collateral axonal sprouting* (McCouch et al. 1958; Liu and Chambers 1958) with formation of new synaptic contacts (Field et al. 1980; Murray et al. 1979; Nakamura et al. 1974; Raisman 1969; Raisman and Field 1973) may also occur (Fig. 5d).

The time course of the effects observed in the LGN (about 30 days for full development) is equal or very similar to results from several subcortical structures of the adult cat (Table 1) and was also found in the somato-sensory thalamus (Wall and Egger

1971), the septal nuclei (Raisman and Field 1973), and the olfactory system (Gilad and Reis 1979) of the adult rat.

4.2 Functional Aspects of Reorganization in the LGN

The visual system is characterized by topographical mapping of the retina onto subcortical visual centers and the visual cortex. The visual cortex receives precise topographically organized inputs from the LGN (Sanderson 1971). The system is governed by high acuity. The type of reorganization observed in the mature LGN of the cat roughly seems to stay within the limits already set by the structural framework. Only cells with dendrites in the range of normal input arborizations seem to become light-excitable with time after deafferentation. For example, at the borders of chronic lesions placed in the *area centralis* no RF displacements were found with our methods. Because of the retino-geniculate magnification factor (Sanderson 1971) the spread of excitation of 200 μm in the LGN would correspond to only 0.3° in the area centralis.

The reinnervation of deafferented neighbor cells could be useful for the visual system without severely disturbing the principle of high acuity because filling-in of small defects (deafferentation of single cells or small cell populations) causes only little loss of spatial resolution.

5 Summary and Conclusions

Electrophysiological evidence was supplied that in the adult cat nonresponsive cells within an area of deafferentation in the LGN became responsive again with time after a retinal lesion. The underlying spread of excitation amounted to 200 μm beyond normal and was not significantly different at the borders of large and small retinal lesions. This functional reorganization appeared with a temporal delay of about 30 days and restored light-excitability from the lesioned eye at single cells with subnormal properties. At small deafferented regions this excitation originated, as a rule, from the nearest region with normal innervation. Multiple innervation from receptive areas separated by the lesion was rarely found.

Our result shows that there is a capacity for neuronal plasticity in the adult cat LGN. Functional reactivation of deafferented cells seems to be possible as in other systems. No spectacular changes of morphology are expected. Local mechanisms within the preformed structural framework of the system are the most probable explanations of the presented results.

Future investigations will have to clarify which of the discussed mechanisms applies to the observed chronic changes in the adult cat LGN.

Acknowledgment. This work was supported by the Deutsche Forschungsgemeinschaft (Ey 8).

References

Anderson LS, Black RG, Abraham J, Ward AA (1971) Neuronal hypersensitivity in experimental trigeminal deafferentation. J Neurosurg 35: 444–452

Baisden RH, Polley EH, Goodman DC, Wolf ED (1980) Absence of sprouting by retinogeniculate axons after chronic focal lesions in the adult cat retina. Neurosci Lett 17: 33–39

Basbaum AI, Wall PD (1976) Chronic changes in the response of cells in adult cat dorsal horn following partial deafferentation: the appearance of responding cells in a previously non-responsive region. Brain Res 116: 181–204

Bird SJ, Aghajanian GK (1975) Denervation supersensitivity in the cholinergic septohippocampal pathway: a microiontophoretic study. Brain Res 100: 355–370

Bishop PO, Kozak W, Levick WR, Vakkur GJ (1962a) The determination of the projection of the visual field on to the lateral geniculate nucleus in the cat. J Physiol 163: 503–539

Bishop PO, Kozak W, Vakkur GJ (1962b) Some quantitative aspects of the cat's eye: axis and plane of reference, visual field co-ordinates and optics. J Physiol 163: 466–502

Cleland BG, Dubin MW, Levick WR (1971) Simultaneous recording of input and output of lateral geniculate neurons. Nature (London) 231: 191–192

Devor M, Wall PD (1978) Reorganisation of spinal cord sensory map after peripheral nerve injury. Nature (London) 275: 75–76

Eysel UT (1976) Quantitative studies of intracellular postsynaptic potentials in the lateral geniculate nucleus of the cat with respect to optic tract stimulus response latencies. Exp Brain Res 25: 469–486

Eysel UT (1979) Maintained activity, excitation and inhibition of lateral geniculate neurons after monocular deafferentation in the adult cat. Brain Res 166: 259–271

Eysel UT, Grüsser OJ (1978) Increased transneuronal excitation of the cat lateral geniculate nucleus after acute deafferentation. Brain Res 158: 107–128

Eysel UT, Gonzalez-Aguilar F, Mayer U (1980) A functional sign of reorganization in the visual system of adult cats: lateral geniculate neurons with displaced receptive fields after lesions of the nasal retina. Brain Res 181: 285–300

Eysel UT, Gonzalez-Aguilar F, Mayer U (1981) Late spreading of excitation in the lateral geniculate nucleus following visual deafferentation is independent of the size of retinal lesions. Brain Res 204: 189–193

Field PM, Coldham DE, Raisman G (1980) Synapse formation after injury in the adult rat brain: Preferential reinnervation of denervated fimbrial sites by axons of the contralateral fimbria. Brain Res 189: 103–113

Gilad GM, Reis DJ (1979) Collateral sprouting in central mesolimbic dopamine neurons: biochemical and immunocytochemical evidence of changes in the activity and distribution of tyrosine hydroxylase in terminal fields and in cell bodies of A10 neurons. Brain Res 160: 17–36

Goodman DC, Bogdasarian RS, Horel JA (1973) Axonal sprouting of ipsilateral optic tract following opposite eye removal. Brain Behav Evol 8: 27–50

Guillery RW (1972) Experiments to determine whether retino-geniculate axons can form translaminar collateral sprouts in the dorsal lateral geniculate nucleus of the cat. J Comp Neurol 146: 407–420

Hámori J (1968) Presynaptic-to-presynaptic axon contacts under experimental conditions giving rise to rearrangement of synaptic structures. In: v Euler C, Skoglund S, Soderberg U (eds) Structure and function of inhibitory neuronal mechanisms. Pergamon Press, Oxford, pp 71–80

Hickey TL (1975) Translaminar growth of axons in the kitten dorsal lateral geniculate nucleus following removal of one eye. J Comp Neurol 161: 359–382

Hughes A (1976) A supplement to the cat schematic eye. Vision Res 16: 149–154

Kaas JH, Guillery RW, Allman JM (1972) Some principles of organization in the dorsal lateral geniculate nucleus. Brain Behav Evol 6: 253–299

Kostyuk PG (1963) Functional changes during degeneration of central synapses. In: Gutman E, Hnik P (eds) The effect of use and disuse on neuromuscular function. Elsevier, Amsterdam, pp 291–304

Liu CN, Chambers WW (1958) Intraspinal sprouting of dorsal root axons. Arch Neurol Psychiatr 79: 46–61

Lynch G, Stanfield B, Cotman CW (1973) Developmental differences in post-lesion axonal growth in the hippocampus. Brain Res 59: 155–168

Madarász M, Gerle J, Hajdu F, Somogyi G, Tömböl T (1978) Quantitative histological studies on the lateral geniculate nucleus in the cat. II. Cell numbers and densities in the several layers. J Hirnforsch 19: 159–164

McCall RB, Aghajanian GK (1979) Denervation supersensitivity to serotonin in the facial nucleus. Neuroscience 4: 1501–1510

McCouch GP, Austin GM, Liu CN, Liu CY (1958) Sprouting as a cause of spasticity. J Neurophysiol 21: 205–216

Mendell LM, Sassoon EM, Wall PD (1978) Properties of synaptic linkage from long ranging afferents onto dorsal horn neurones in normal and deafferented cats. J Physiol 285: 299–310

Millar J, Basbaum AI, Wall PD (1976) Restructuring of the somatotopic map and appearance of abnormal neuronal activity in the gracile nucleus after partial deafferentation. Exp Neurol 50: 658–672

Murray M, Goldberger MA (1974) Restitution of function and collateral sprouting in the cat's spinal cord: the partially hemisected animal. J Comp Neurol 158: 19–36

Murray M, Zimmer J, Raisman G (1979) Quantitative electron microscopic evidence for reinnervation in the adult rat interpeduncular nucleus after lesions of the fasciculus retroflexus. J Comp Neurol 187: 447–468

Nakamura Y, Nizuno N, Konishi A, Manabu S (1974) Synaptic reorganization of the red nucleus after chronic deafferentation from cerebellorubral fibers: an electron microscope study in the cat. Brain Res 82: 298–301

Precht W, Shimazu H, Markham CH (1966) A mechanism of central compensation of vestibular function following hemilabyrinthectomy. J Neurophysiol 29: 996–1010

Pubols LM, Goldberger ME (1980) Recovery of function in dorsal horn. J Neurophysiol 43: 102–117

Raisman G (1969) Neuronal plasticity in the septal nuclei of the adult rat. Brain Res 14: 25–48

Raisman G, Field P (1973) A quantitative investigation of the development of collateral reinnervation after partial deafferentation of the septal nuclei. Brain Res 50: 241–264

Rodieck RW (1979) Visual pathways. Annu Rev Neurosci 2: 193–225

Sanderson KJ (1971) Visual field projection columns and magnification factors in the lateral geniculate nucleus of the cat. Exp Brain Res 13: 159–177

Sanderson KJ, Sherman SM (1971) Nasotemporal overlap in visual field projected to lateral geniculate nucleus in the cat. J Neurophysiol 34: 453–466

Schneider GE (1977) Growth of abnormal neural connections following focal brain lesions: constraining factors and functional effects. In: William H, Obrador S, Martin-Rodriguez JG (eds) Neurosurgical treatment in psychiatry, pain, and epilepsy. University Park Press, Baltimore, pp 5–26

Steward O, Messenheimer JA (1978) Histochemical evidence for a post-lesion reorganization of cholinergic afferents in the hippocampal formation of the mature cat. J Comp Neurol 178: 697–709

Szentágothai J (1973) Neuronal and synaptic architecture of the lateral geniculate nucleus. In: Jung R (ed) Handbook of sensory physiology, vol VII, 3B. Springer, Berlin Heidelberg New York, pp 141–176

Tömböl T, Madarász M, Hajdu F, Somogyi G, Gerle J (1978a) Quantitative histological studies on the lateral geniculate nucleus in the cat. I. Measurements on golgi material. J Hirnforsch 19: 145–158

Tömböl T, Madarász M, Somogyi G, Hajdu F, Gerle J (1978b) Quantitative histological studies on the lateral geniculate nucleus in the cat. IV. Numerical aspects of the transfer from retinal fibers to cortical relay. J Hirnforsch 19: 203–212

Tsukahara N, Hultborn H, Murakami F, Fujito Y (1975) Electrophysiological study of formation of new synapses and collateral sprouting in red nucleus neurons after partial denervation. J Neurophysiol 38: 1359–1372

Wall PD (1975) Signs of plasticity and reconnection in spinal cord damage. In: Outcome of severe damage to the central nervous system, Ciba foundation symposium 34. Elsevier/North-Holland, Amsterdam, pp 35–63

Wall PD (1976) Plasticity in the adult mammalian central nervous system. In: Corner MA, Swaabs DF (eds) Perspectives in brain research. Progress in brain research, vol 45. Elsevier/North-Holland Biomedical Press, Amsterdam, pp 359–379

Wall PD, Egger MD (1971) Formation of new connections in adult rat brains after partial deafferentation. Nature (London) 232: 542–545

Wässle H, Levick WR, Cleland BG (1975) The distribution of the alpha type of ganglion cells in the cat's retina. J Comp Neurol 159: 419–438

Chronic Isolation of Visual Cortex Induces Reorganization of Cortico-Cortical Connections

M. HOLZGRAEFE[1,2], G. TEUCHERT[1,3], and J.R. WOLFF[1,4]

1 Introduction

Undercutting of the cortex destroys all subcortical afferents and efferents, leaving most cortico-cortical connections intact (Szentágothai 1965). The resulting terminal degeneration shows a laminar pattern similar to thalamo-cortical projections (Hubel and Wiesel 1972; Ogren and Hendrickson 1977; Gould et al. 1978), although the synaptic density is slightly reduced (Clark et al. 1939; Gruner et al. 1974). Chronic isolation results in the survival of the majority of neurons (Creutzfeldt and Struck 1962).

In the chronically isolated cortex the neuronal activity has been shown to be abnormal up to 4 years although biochemical changes vanish within one month. According to Szentágothai (1965), Gruner et al. (1974), and Creutzfeldt et al. (1977) degeneration is completed at about 1 to 2 months postoperative in an isolated gyrus.

The present paper describes a completely different time course for degeneration after deep undercutting of large parts of the parieto-occipital cortex of rats.

2 Material and Methods

The parieto-occipital cortex was deeply undercut in 80-day old female albino rats (Sprague-Dawley). In the majority of cases the cortical island remained connected by callosal fibers. The operation was performed with a blunt knife inserted near the border of areas 39 and 40 (according to Krieg's map, 1946) and turned by a micromanipulator toward the anterior and the posterior pole. Survival time varied from 12 h to 12 months. Degeneration products were stained according to a recently developed technique that impregnates degenerating axon terminals and lysosomes (Gallyas et al. 1980).

1 Zentrum Anatomie, Universität Göttingen, Kreuzbergring 36, 3400 Göttingen, FRG
2 Neurologische Universitäts-Klinik, 3400 Göttingen, FRG
3 Fachbereich Biologie, Universität Bielefeld, 4800 Bielefeld, FRG
4 Max-Planck-Institut für biophysikalische Chemie, Abteilung Neurobiologie, 3400 Göttingen, FRG

Unoperated animals of the same age served as controls. For quantitative evaluation frozen sections (10 μm thick) stained with cresyl violet were used. The volume fraction and the size distribution of Nissl-stained structures (mainly nuclei and perikarya) were determined by quantitative image analysis (Quantimet 720, Cambridge Instruments, U.K.). The terminal degeneration was investigated by electron microscopy. The material was prepared by standard techniques of double aldehyde-osmium fixation and embedded in Epon (812).

3 Results

Undercutting results in terminal degeneration in all parts of the isolated cortex. In various cortical areas the laminar distribution of degeneration differs and, to some extent, also the time course. In view of this complexity, we will consider essentially lamina L IV of area 17. Other laminae and areas will be mentioned only for comparison.

3.1 Biphasic Time Course of Terminal Degeneration

The first isolated degeneration products in LIV were stained within about one day postoperative, earlier than the other layers. During the second and third day postoperative the typical laminar pattern of terminal degeneration appeared strongest in L Ia, IV, and VIb. On days 3 to 5 postoperative the optimal density of degeneration was reached, and between day 7 and 10 many degeneration products were observed to be aggregated in glial and perivascular cells. The overall density of stainable degeneration products decreased sharply until about 10–15 days postoperative (Fig. 1, top row).

One month following undercutting the density of terminal degeneration rose again and reached a second peak.

The terminal degeneration gradually decreased until after 5 months it was no longer observable. Fiber degeneration in L VI persisted for a longer time and even after 1 year some degeneration products of myelinated fibers and myelin sheets were seen in deepar parts of L VI. The persistence of fiber degeneration made it difficult to recognize terminal degeneration in L VI during the second phase (Fig. 1, bottom row).

3.2 Differences Between First and Second Phase

Quantitative evaluation of the degeneration process revealed that the first phase lasts about 10 to 15 days with a maximum 3 to 5 days postoperative, while the second phase lasts about 3 to 4 months with a maximum after about 1 to 2 months (Fig. 2).

The laminar distribution of degeneration differed between phase 1 and 2. During the first phase, in areas 18 and 18a the laminae distribution of terminal degeneration is similar to that in area 17. The only difference is that the degeneration products spread throughout L I instead of being restricted to its superficial half. In contrast, terminal degeneration is found in all layers of area 18 and 18a with some accumulation in L I, III, IV, and Vb. During the third month the degeneration decreases in all layers, persisting a little longer in L IV.

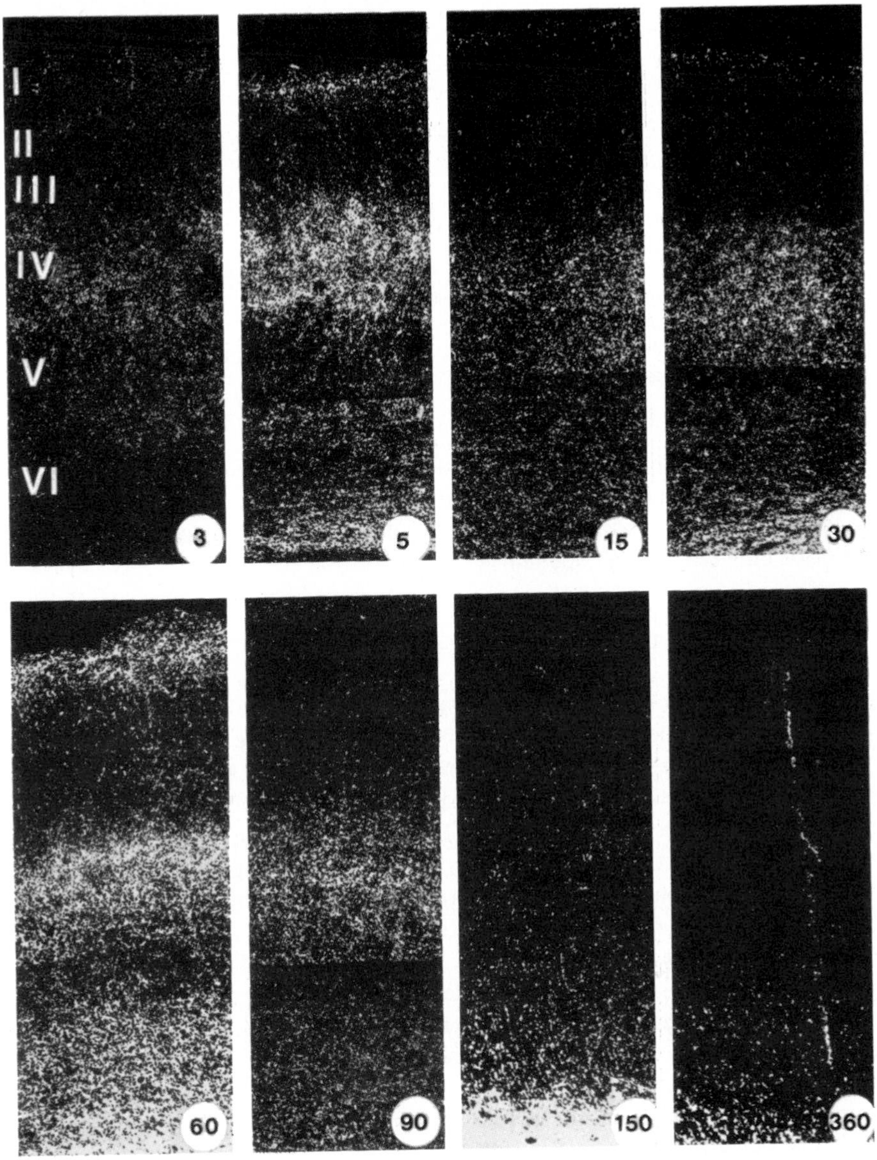

Fig. 1. Laminar distribution of degeneration products in area 17, various intervals after undercutting. Terminal degeneration is rather diffuse at 3 days postoperative with some accumulation in lamina IV. After 5 days maximal degeneration is seen in L IV. The degeneration is reduced at 15 days postoperative. A second phase of degeneration terminates during the fourth month. From the following month up to 1 year only fiber degeneration can be seen, mainly in lamina VI. *Roman figures* indicate cortical laminae, *Arabic figures* day postoperative. Silver impregnation after Gallyas et al., *dark field*

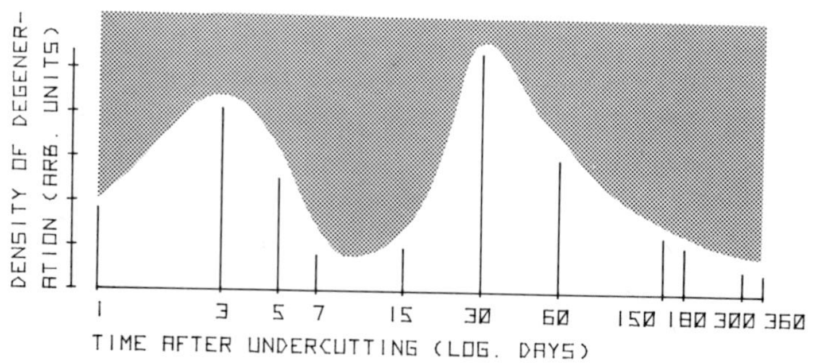

Fig. 2. The time course of degeneration in lamina IV as revealed by quantitative TV-image analysis reveals suggests a biphasic process

Another difference between the two phases is that during the second phase (1 month postoperative) the borders between areas 29c/18, 18/17, and 17/18a are demarcated by columnar arrangements of terminal degeneration. The size of these columns varies between 200 and 800 μm.

3.3 Ultrastructure of Synapses in L IV

During the first phase most degenerating terminals contact single dendritic spines, about 10% to 15% of them make synaptic contact with dendritic shafts, and only two axosomatic synapses of degenerating terminals were found. After 2 months postoperative, at the peak of phase 2, about half of the sections through degenerating terminals showed contacts with two spines (Fig. 3). Additionally, many of these "double-spine" synapses showed intact presynaptic elements (Fig. 3). This indicates that synapses of L IV undergo some transformation. Since the thickness of L IV and the density of synapses did not change significantly, the formation of double-spine synapses appeared to be a consequence of synaptogenesis. Not all stainable degeneration products, however, represented dense degenerating axon terminals. Many of the lysosomal structures and residual bodies were located in dendrites, presynaptic elements, somata of neurons, or glial cells. These seem to represent only in part degenerated synapses that had been phagocytized. Many of them seem to develop as cytolysosomes, which contain such elements as dense mitochondria, synaptic vesicles, and endoplasmic reticulum.

3.4 Size of Nissl-Stained Neurons

An analysis of the size of neurons in area 17 demonstrates that large neurons in laminae II–VIa shrink during months 2–6 after undercutting. However, after 1 year the neurons in the isolated cortex had nearly regained their normal size (Fig. 4a). L I and VIb reveal no significant change in the size of neurons, although more terminal degeneration occurred in these layers than in laminae II, III, and V.

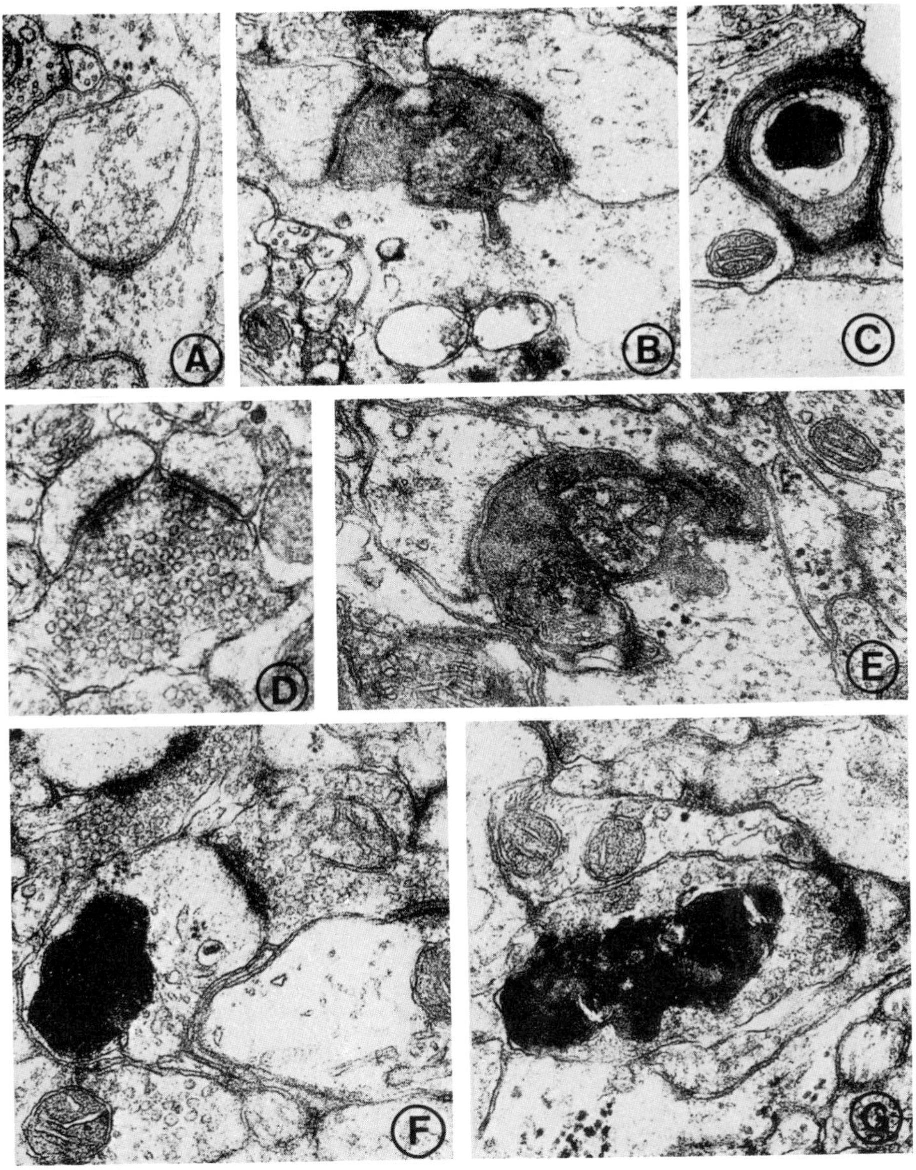

Fig. 3A–G. Electron microscopy of L IV 2 months after undercutting. **A** Free postsynaptic thickening of a dendritic shaft. **B, E** Dense degenerating terminals, each contacting two dendritic profiles. Lysosomes and residual bodies appear in myelinated axons (**C**), dendrites (**F**) and presynaptic elements (**G**). **D** Numerous presynaptic elements show contact with two spines ("douple-spine" synapse)

Similarly, the volume fraction of Nissl-stained cells showed significant decrease in laminae II, III, and VI (Fig. 4b) lasting for 2–6 months. After 1 year, however, it was normal or even higher than in the normal cortex.

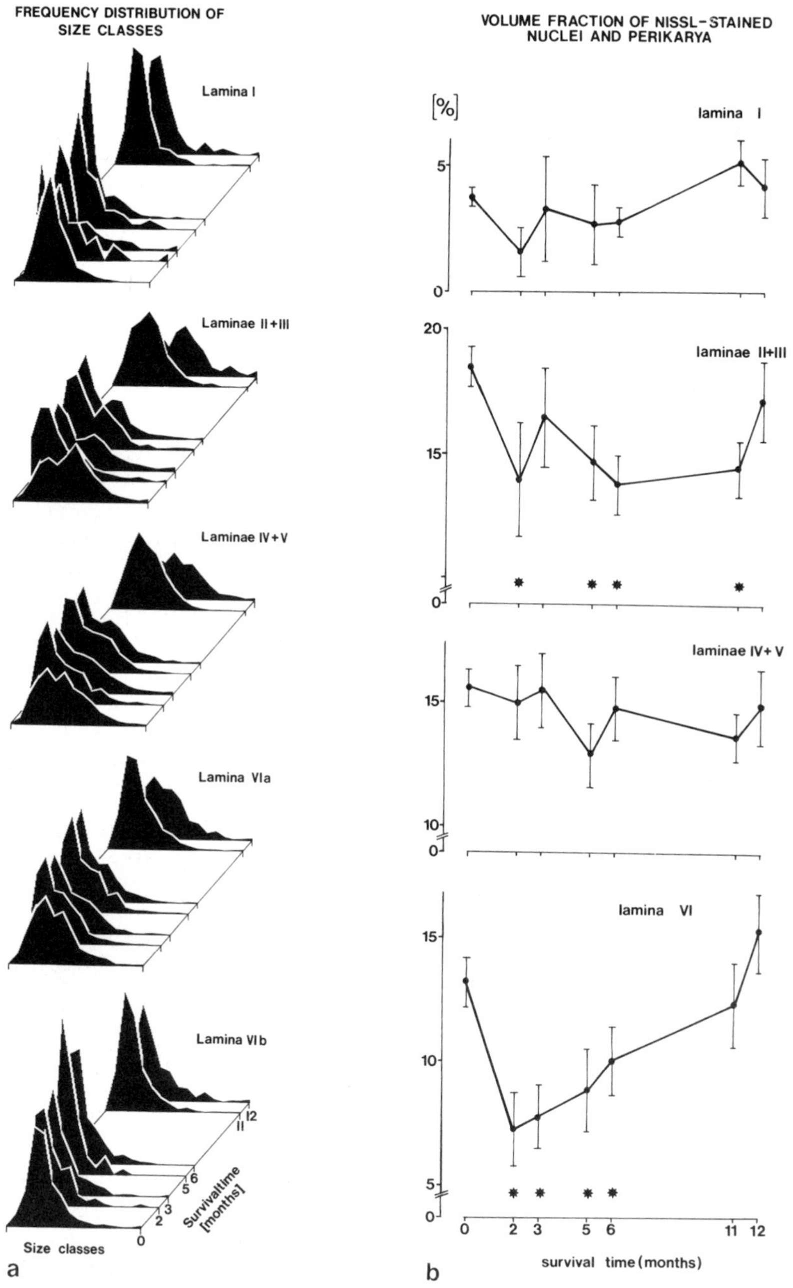

Fig. 4. a Frequency distribution of size classes in the normal (o) and undercut area 17 at various survival times. Cell size increases from left side to right. The reduction in the frequency of large cells and the increase of the smaller ones indicate an atrophy of cells. One year after undercutting, the distribution of size classes is about the same as in normal cortex. **b** Volume fraction of Nissl-stained cells in the normal (O) and isolated area 17. In laminae I and IV–V no significant change was found. In laminae II, III, and VI, the volume fraction of Nissl-stained material decreases significantly (*asterisks*) lasting for 6 to 11 months. Note that in lamina IV, where terminal degeneration is most prominent and continues for more than 3 months, the volume fraction of Nissl-stained material is not significantly reduced. Means and standard deviations

The strong and long-lasting reaction of L II and III is remarkable because in these layers no terminal degeneration was found. After 1 year volume fraction regained nearly normal values. The volume fraction of L IV did not show a significant change, although in this lamina the strongest terminal degeneration took place. These measurements indicate that the regeneration of the chronically isolated cortex is not completed, when the terminal degeneration vanishes after about 4 to 5 months.

4 Discussion

The present paper describes a long-lasting process of terminal degeneration following deep undercutting of the parieto-occipital cortex of rats. The duration of more than 3 months is at variance with previous observations on the isolated visual cortex (gyrus-or cortical slab) of cats, where degeneration terminates within 1 to 2 months (Gruner et al. 1974; Creutzfeldt et al. 1977). The difference might be the fact that in cats only a small part of the visual cortex was isolated, and only a few cortico-cortical connections were preserved in this preparation. In contrast, the deeply undercut cortical island of rats comprises the whole visual region plus parts of the auditory, somato-sensory, and motor cortex, which remain interconnected, even by callosal fibers (Teuchert et al., in prep.).

However, another difference between the isolated cortex of cats and rats exists. Only in the latter species the time course of terminal degeneration is biphasic. Similar biphasic time courses were observed in the degeneration of various types of cortico-cortical connections, although the second phase was much less clearly separated from the first. However, in the case of some long associative connections, the second phase can be isolated by special techniques of analysis (Wolff et al. 1981). The relatively short time course in the isolated cortex of cats might have masked a second phase of terminal degeneration, and perhaps a revaluation using quantitative methods might be appropriate for separating two degeneration processes.

Long-lasting degeneration does not reduce significantly the synaptic density of L IV of area 17. That is, during the second period of degeneration an equivalent number of synapses should be newly formed. Consequently, the second phase of degeneration could indicate the reorganization of synaptic connections in the chronically isolated cortex. In the CNS axonal sprouting and re-innervation usually takes place between about 5 and 15 days postoperative (Lee et al. 1977; Lynch et al. 1977; Steward and Loesche 1977; Goldschmidt and Steward 1980). This is similar to the time course observed for degeneration of most cortico-cortical connections (Wolff et al. 1981). However, some long-lasting processes of reorganization show a time course similar to the degeneration in the isolated cortex of rats. The re-innervation of the hippocampus increased rapidly up to 30 days, but then proceeded at a slower rate (Matthew et al. 1976). Thus, the second phase of terminal degeneration shown here might be related to synaptic reorganization of the cortical island.

The quantitative analysis of Nissl-stained neurons revealed that reorganization of the isolated cortex as a whole takes a longer time than the terminal degeneration. Structural changes of synaptology seem to form the basis of further functional adaptation, which might be related to cell size. The consequence of this reorganization is a strengthening of certain cortico-cortical connections originating from the outer borders of the visual cortex, which replace the thalamic projections to L IV (Teuchert et al., in prep.).

5 Summary

In 80-day old female rats (Sprague-Dawley) large parts of the parieto-occipital cortex were deeply undercut. By this procedure most of the callosal and associative connections of this visual cortex remained intact. The terminal degeneration was evaluated by light and electron microscopy using a new staining method (Gallyas et al. 1980) and quantitative TV image analysis.

Terminal degeneration (TD) showed a biphasic time course with the first peak of degeneration at 3 to 5 days, and a second peak between 1 and 2 months. TD is demonstrable up to 4 months. A quantitative analysis of the cell size revealed that the reorganization of the isolated cortex does not terminate before about 6 to 11 months.

We suggest that the second phase of degeneration accompanies a reorganization of the synaptology of lamina IV in area 17.

Acknowledgments. The authors are indebted to H. Böttcher, A. Unger and A. Wolff for technical assistance; to Dr. D. Ehrlich for correcting the language and to E. Hadacker for preparing the manuscript. We are grateful to Prof. O. Spoerri for his abiding interest and generous support of this work and to the Deutsche Forschungsgemeinschaft for providing the grant: SFB 33, E3.

References

Clark W, LeGros E, Sunderland (1939) Structural changes in the isolated visual cortex. J Anat 73: 563–574

Creutzfeldt O, Struck G (1962) Neurophysiologie und Morphologie der chronisch isolierten Cortexinsel der Katze: Hirnpotentiale und Neuronentätigkeit einer isolierten Nervenzellpopulation ohne afferente Fasern. Arch Psychiatr Nervenkr 203: 708–731

Creutzfeldt O-D, Garey LJ, Kuroda R, Wolff JR (1977) The distribution of degenerating axons after small lesions in the intact and isolated visual cortex of the cat. Exp Brain Res 27: 419–440

Gallyas F, Wolff JR, Böttcher H, Zaborszky L (1980) A reliable and sensitive method to locate terminal degeneration and lysosomes in the CNS. Stain Technol.

Goldschmidt RB, Steward O (1980) Time course of increases in retrograde labeling and increases in cell size of entorhinal cortex, neurons sprouting in response to unilateral entorhinal lesions. J Comp Neurol 189: 359–379

Gould HJ, Hall WC, Ebner EF (1978) Connections of the rhinal cortex in the hedgehog. 1) Thalamo-cortical connections. J Comp Neurol 177: 445–472

Gruner JE, Hirsch JC, Sotelo C (1974) Ultrastructural features of the isolated suprasylvian gyrus in the cat. J Comp Neurol 154: 1–28

Hubel DH, Wiesel TN (1972) Laminar and columnar distribution of geniculo-cortical fibers in the macaque monkey. J Comp Neurol 146: 421–450

Krieg WJS (1946) Connections of the cerebral cortex. J Comp Neurol 84: 221–323

Lee KS, Stanford EJ, Cotman CW, Lynch GS (1977) Ultrastructural evidence for bouton proliferation in the partially deafferent dentate gyrus of adult rat. Exp Brain Res 29: 475–485

Lynch G, Gall C, Cotman C (1977) Temporal parameters of axon sprouting in the brain of the adult rat. Exp Neurol 54: 179–183

Matthew DA, Cotman C, Lynch G (1976) An electron micrscopic study of lesion-induced synaptogenesis in the dentate gyrus of the adult rat. II. Reappearance of morphologically normal synaptic contact. Brain Res 115: 23–41

Ogren MP, Hendrickson AE (1977) The distribution of pulvinar terminals in the visual areas 17 and 18 of the monkey. Brain Res 137: 343–350

Steward O, Loesche J (1977) Quantitative autoradiographic analysis of the time course of proliferation of contralateral entorhinal efferents in the dentate gyrus denervated by ipsilateral entorhinal lesions. Brain Res 125: 11–21

Szentágothai J (1965) The use of degeneration methods in investigation of short neuronal connections. Prog Brain Res 14: 1–32

Teuchert G, Holzgraefe M, Wolff JR (1981) Neuroplasticity of cortico-cortical connections replacing thalamic afferents in lamina IV of the isolated sensory cortex of adult rat. submitted

Wolff JR, Eins S, Holzgraefe M, Zaborszky L (1980) Temporo-spatial course of degeneration after cutting cortico-cortical connections in adult rats. Cell Tissue Res. 214: 303–321

Physiological Mechanisms Underlying Responsiveness of Visual Cortex Neurons Following Optic Chiasm Split in Cats

U. YINON and A. HAMMER[1]

1 Introduction

It is generally accepted that in cases of hemianopsia macular sparing is frequent, especially if the lesion is caused in the center of the optic chiasm or higher up in the visual system (Duke-Elder 1971). Depth perception is thus preserved to a certain extent, although it is not known what kind of physiological mechanism is involved.

If the central lesion is involved with splitting of the optic chiasm, a bitemporal hemianopsia resulted leading to a loss of binocularity in the visual cortex, since no more dual convergence is available for each cortical cell. This expectation has been contradicted by Berlucchi and Rizzolatti (1968) showing that a considerable proportion of cortical cells in split chiasm cats were binocular, suggesting an indirect pathway for binocular convergence on cortical cells probably mediated through the coprus callosum instead of through the conventional geniculocortical pathway.

The present study was performed in order to verify whether an indirect pathway exists following interruption of the direct pathway in split chiasm cats. The spatial and physiological properties of visual cortex cells were studied under these conditions.

2 Methods

Six split chiasm adult street cats (2.3–4.0 kg) were used, three of which (and three normal cats) were subjected to the electrophysiological tests.

For the operation on the optic chiasm the cats were initially anesthetized with Ketalar 30 mg/kg IM following Atropine 0.01 mg/kg injection, and long-term anesthetized with sodium pentobarbital 10–20 mg/h IV (into the brachial vein).

The cat was laid on the back, its mouth and tongue fixed using a self-made H-like opener, and intubated using a 4 mm endotracheal tube and Wis-type infant laryngoscope blade (75 mm). The operation was performed under sterile conditions using Zeiss OPMI-1 operating microscope. The transbuccal approach was adopted (Myers

---

1 Physiological Laboratory, Maurice and Gabriela Goldschleger Eye Institute, Tel Aviv University, Medical School, Sheba Medical Center, Tel Hashomer, 52621, Israel

1955). An anterior-posterior cut of 20 mm was performed in the soft palate beginning from the margin of the hard palate (palatine bone) exposing the posterior nasal aperture (nasopharynx). The soft palate was kept open by suturing its two flaps to the H-like opener. Bleeding was stopped with Codman bipolar coagulator.

The location of the optic chiasm center in the adult cat is according to our experience under the sphenoid bone, in the middle between its pterygoid processes and 14 mm from the hard palate. Thus, an opening of 5 X 5 mm was made there using a dental burr, passing through the posterior end of the presphenoidal air cell (Field and Taylor 1974). The dura was exposed and longitudinally sectioned using a microsurgical superblade. The chiasma was hooked and sectioned in the midsaggital plane. Following this, the hole was tightly closed with Gelfoam, covered with a graft of sterilized bone and glued with Histoacryl blue. The soft palate was then sutured closed with silk thread 4-0.

Following the operation, the cats were allowed to recover and 1 million units of Penicillin G were given IM twice a day for a week. They were kept in large cages with a special diet and illumination of 17 h a day. They were subjected to the electrophysiological tests 7 weeks after the operation.

Surgical and stereotaxical techniques for the electrophysiological tests were as previously described (Yinon 1978, 1980). Anesthesia was initiated with Ketalar (30 mg/kg IM) and lightly maintained during the experiments with Thiopentone Sodium (1 mg/h IV). The animal was paralyzed with Flaxedil (7.5 mg/kg/h IV) for ocular fixation, and artificially respired. The cats were continuously IV infused during the experiment with a solution mixture including the above mentioned drugs, KCl, atropine, isuprel and saline-dextrose at a rate of 2.5 ml/kg/h.

The EEG was continuously monitored during the experiments using silver (1.0 mm) ball electrode on areae 17–18 boundary, and an indifferent one on the suprasylvian gyrus. The ECG was visually and audiomonitored. The rectal temperature ($38.5° \pm 0.5°C$) was measured with thermistor sensor and controlled by electronic regulator. The CO_2 level of the expired air was kept at $4\% \pm 0.25\%$ using Beckman LB-2 Gas Analyzer, and the air pressure was 5–10 cm/water. Experiments lasted continuously for 3–4 days.

The cortex was penetrated at an angle of $30° \pm 5°$ to its saggital plane in the medial edge of the lateral or postlateral gyri. The localization of the penetration was consistently the same in all cats. Recordings were made from areae 17–18 boundary where the area centralis is represented (Woolsey 1971). Cells were recorded at intervals of 200 μ in order to avoid redundant recordings from the same cell along the penetration. The penetration depth was electronically and mechanically controlled using an improved version of DKI hydraulic microdrive.

The optic discs, the area centralae and other retinal landmarks were projected on the screen 2 m across the eyes using Heine fiber optics ophthalmoscopic system. Artificial pupils of 4 mm diam were used. Stimulation was made with hand-driven projector producing light slits (0.1°–20°) at various angles and directions of movement on the screen. Other details with regard to the recording, optics, receptive field mapping, and data analysis have been previously described (Yinon 1978, 1980).

Tungsten (0.6 mm diam) microelectrodes with resistance of 2 ± 0.25 MΩ were used. Action potentials were identified by shape and detected by a WPI model 121 Window Discriminator. Where necessary, a counter was used to quantify the average number of action potentials per sweep (the passage of the light slit across the receptive field usually resulted in sweep of action potentials). When responses to the moving slit were equal throughout 180°, the cell was considered as orientation and direction nonspecific. Nonresponsive cells were recognized according to their spontaneous discharge, and the absence of visual reaction.

3 Results

3.1 Behavioral and Pupillary Reactions

It took a whole week to recover from the operation, when the cats seemed to begin to move and to eat normally. Behavioral difficulties have been also observed, as reflected by the poor visual reflexes and visual following, especially of an object moving quickly near the cat. This behavior has been partially improved in the second postoperative week, although vision seemed to be still substantially affected.

In most operated cats the pupils were symmetrically round and maximally dilated and the pupillary reflex missing in the first 2–3 weeks following the operation (Fig. 1). In one cat a considerable constriction of the pupils was observed in the second week, reaching almost their normal size after 7 weeks.

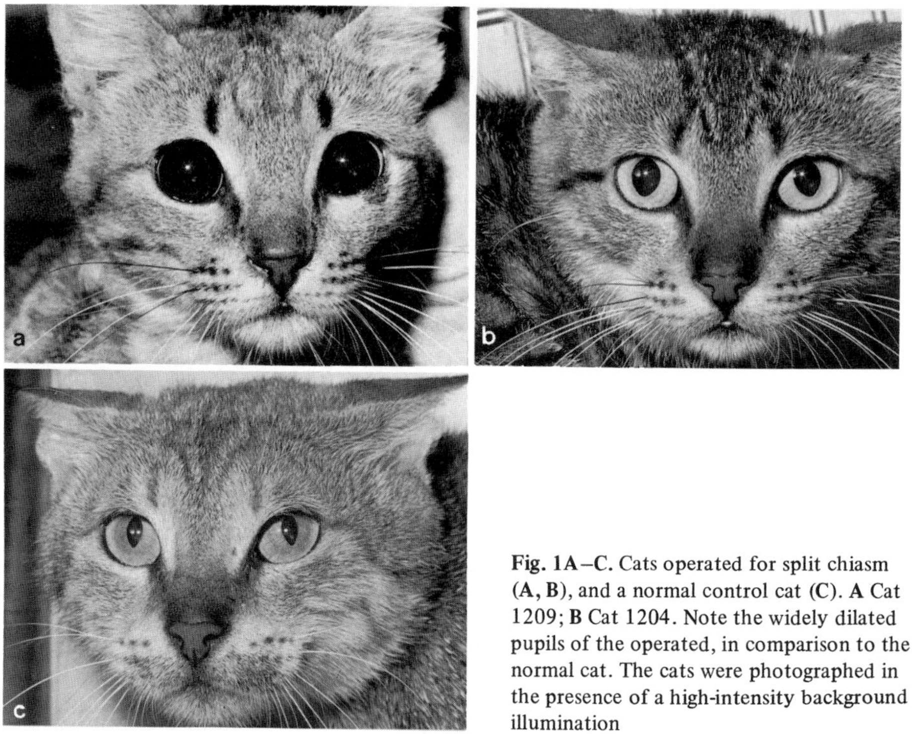

Fig. 1A–C. Cats operated for split chiasm (**A, B**), and a normal control cat (**C**). **A** Cat 1209; **B** Cat 1204. Note the widely dilated pupils of the operated, in comparison to the normal cat. The cats were photographed in the presence of a high-intensity background illumination

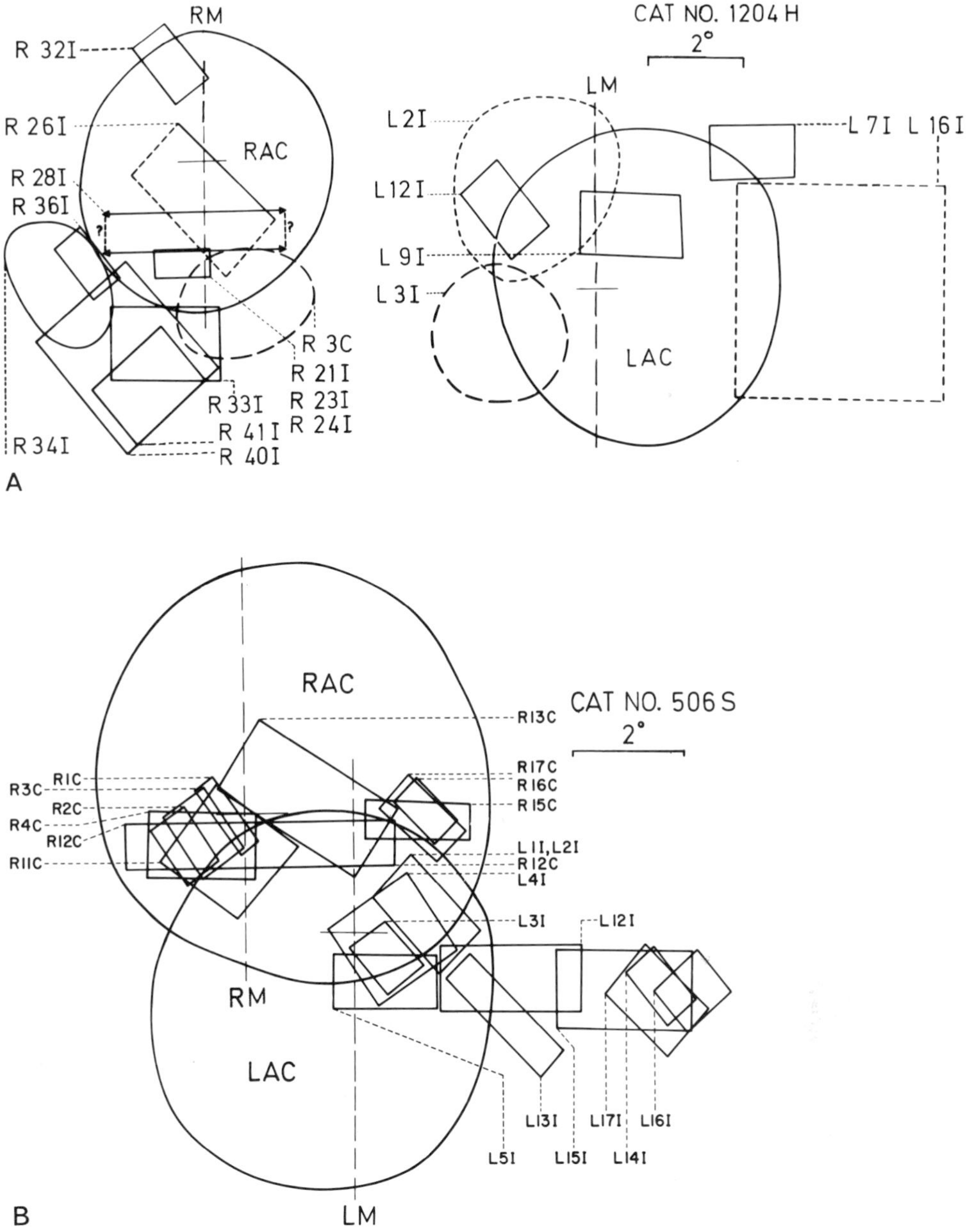

Fig. 2. A Receptive field map of a split chiasm cat. *RM, LM,* Right and left vertical meridians, respectively; *RAC, LAC,* Right and left area centralae, respectively; *C,* Contralateral cortex; *I,* Ipsilateral cortex; *R,* Right eye; *L,* Left eye. Note that all the receptive fields but one were ipsilaterally mapped and that despite of this they cross the vertical meridian to the heteronymous hemiretina. **B** Receptive field map of a normal cat (Yinon and Goshen 1980)

3.2 Physiological and Spatial Considerations

In the first operated cat (No. 1202) we have recorded 37 cells from the left hemisphere. All the visually active cells except 3 of them (12%) reacted clearly ipsilaterally. In cat No. 1204 we have recorded 43 cells from both hemispheres; all but 4 cells (9.3%) reacted clearly ipsilaterally. The impression was that the above mentioned minor numbers of cells in both cats seemed to react contralaterally. However, the reaction to the contralateral eye was so poor and inconsistent that, using all the physiological criteria in normal animals (Yinon 1978), we would not consider it as a real response. The results of 80 cells recorded in the third operated cat were very similar to the above but not yet fully analyzed.

The response from the responding ipsilateral eye in the operated cats was not always clear. Many cells had a weak response, diffuse receptive fields, wide orientation tuning, and poor orientation and direction selectivity (Fig. 2, Table 1). The impression was as if in the operated animals responses had appeared deeply in the cortex in comparison to normal cats. Furthermore, a very few visually active cells have been encountered along each penetration, the average being three cells per 1 mm in the operated (1 cell/348 μ), in comparison to six cells per 1 mm (1 cell/175 μ) in the normal cats. In addition, we have obtained a high proportion (32.5%) of viually inactive cells in the operated cats in comparison to the normal cats (10.5%). [The high level of unresponsive cells in the operated cats might be attributed to the fact that in cats nearly two-thirds of the optic nerve fibers were eliminated as a result of the optic chiasm split (Polyak 1957)].

Due to the fact that all cells reacted monocularly and ipsilaterally, we can not say much about the organization of ocular dominance columns (Hubel and Wiesel 1968). However, we should obtain at least a mosaic of active and inactive columns. The fact that unclear results with regard to the columnar organization were obtained, might be attributed partially to the relatively large intervals between recording sites. However,

Table 1. Physiological properties of visual cortex cells (%) in split chiasm cats in comparison to normal control cats

Cats (N)	No. of cells	Visually inactive[a] cells	Visually active non-specific cells	Orientation and direction selective cells	Cells reacting[b] at 0 ± 22°	Cells reacting[c] at 90° ± 22°	Cells with orientation tuning < 90°	Cells with orientatio tuning > 90°
Operated (2)[d]	80	32.5	21.2	46.2	12.5	7.5	23.7	12.5
Control (3)	76	10.5	5.3	84.2	19.7	32.9	34.2	7.9

[a] Not included are inactive cells at the end of a penetration
[b] 0 = 180°, horizontal meridian
[c] 90° = vertical meridian
[d] Data analysis was made for two of the operated cats

some other factors might take place in addition to the general level of cell responsiveness as previously obtained in monocularly enucleated cats. (Yinon 1980). On the other hand, the structure of orientation columns was preserved in the cortex of these cats, as judged from the consequent arrangement of the cells usually found in accordance with their receptive field orientation.

One more peculiar finding in the visual cortex of the split chiasm cats was the habituation. We have found six cells in the two split chiasm cats which exhibited habituation. It was expressed by an interruption of the cell responsiveness for a short time – up to several minutes – and reappearance of a single response later. Despite of the habituation phenomenon, these cells showed specificity to orientation and direction. In contrast, no one cell with habituation was encountered in the present as well as in our previous studies on normal cats.

4 Discussion

Berlucchi and Rizzolatti (1968) found a considerable number of binocularly active cells in split chiasm cats. On the basis of this finding and the fact that normally each cortical cell is represented by two receptive fields, we have constructed a neuronal model. The model shows that under normal conditions, where simultaneous stimulation of two retinal corresponding points takes place, the appearance of receptive fields related to the callosal pathway is masked (Fig. 3). The connection between the two hemispheres is thus made by excitatory fibers giving their input to cells in the opposite cortex through inhibitory interneurons, which are excited in addition by axon colaterals of LGN fibers. Assuming that these LGN fibers represent the contralateral eye, in case of their inactivation the indirect callosal pathway is turned to be active.

The interpretation of the above model from the point of view of neuronal circuitry is that cortical cells in normal conditions are potentially connected not only to the ipsi- and the contralateral homonymous hemiretinae, but also to the heteronymous hemiretinae. However, these potential connections are made available for the cortical cells according to our model only under conditions where the contralateral connections are dysfunctioning. In this way, the above suggested model can be regarded as a defense mechanism compensating against the loss of binocular vision.

For the above model to exist and in order to enable streopsis, a nasotemporal overlap for foveal regions in the retina has to be assumed. There is already good evidence for such a vertical strip of nasotemporal overlap. In the cat retina, Stone (1966) showed histologically that the ganglion cells in a median strip of nasotemporal overlap supply both optic tracts. It could be achieved by the failure of all the fibers from the nasal half to cross, or by the crossing of some temporal fibers. There is also neurophysiological evidence that a vertical strip of visual field centered on the midline has a bilateral representation in the LGN and cerebral cortex (Leicester 1968; Blakemore 1969; Sanderson and Sherman 1971). Only under these conditions is the separation between the two hemifields incomplete, the discontinuity at the vertical meridian avoided, and retinal correspondence for the center allowed.

The presence of the nasotemporal overlap has been proved by Blakemore (1969), showing a distribution of cortical receptive fields for both sides of the central 1.5° retina. However, this evidence is indirect since normal cats with intact visual pathways were studied. Direct physiological evidence for the nasotemporal overlap has been obtained in the split chiasm cats of the present study. We showed that despite the fact that the input from the nasal hemiretinae was eliminated following sectioning of the contralateral fibers (and the presence of merely ipsilateral monocular receptive fields), receptive fields were unexpectedly mapped in both sides of the vertical meridian of each eye (Fig. 2).

The results of Hubel and Wiesel (1967) and Berlucchi et al. (1967) who found that receptive fields of corpus callosum fibers are centered around the vertical meridian, are related to those of Stone (1966) and others with regard to the nasotemporal overlap. Furthermore, it has been proved by Mitchell and Blakemore (1970) in human subjects with sectioned corpus callosum that the corpus callosum is needed for stereopsis of objects in the midline. If this is correct, cortical cells must receive indirect input via the corpus callosum, representing the nasotemporal strip. This means that for the nasotemporal retinal area binocular convergence on cortical cells must be found in any case, even following split chiasm. In contrast, we have never found in our split chiasm cats cells with binocular recepetive fields. All the cells were found to be connected ipsilateraly following elimination of the contralateral pathways.

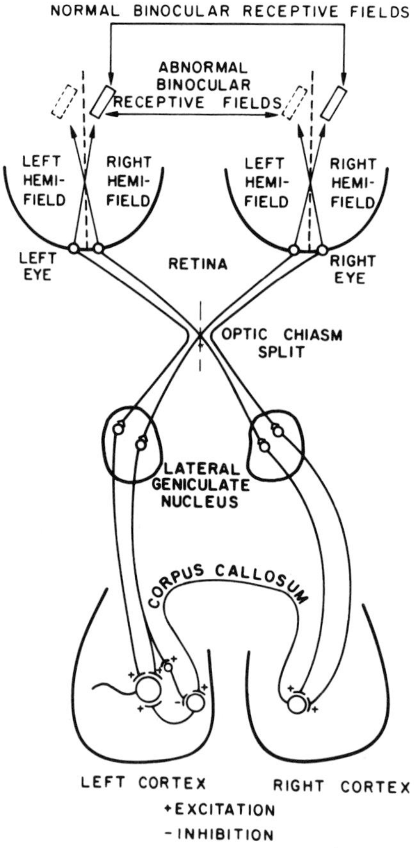

Fig. 3. A neuronal model suggesting physiological adaptation to the condition of split chiasm as derived from the results obtained by Berlucchi and Rizzolatti (1968)

Another theoretical suggestion, as to sparing of the macula in cases of lesions in the visual pathways, assumes that fibers from the lateral geniculate nucleus do not pass exclusively to the cortex of the same side, but that some macular fibers cross in the corpus callosum and therefore give rise to a bilateral cortical representation of the macula (Davson 1972). However, this is incompatible with the fact that the retrograde atrophy of the LGN following destruction of the visual cortex is limited only to the ipsilateral side, demonstrating the absence of any crossed connections from the nucleus by way of the corpus callosum to the visual cortex of the opposite hemisphere (Adler 1953).

Recently, Payne et al. (1980) showed that sectioning of the corpus callosum leads to the reduction of binocularity in cats. This result is apparently in keeping with Berlucchi and Rizzolatti (1968), who proved that binocularity in a certain proportion of cortical cells is mediated by the corpus callosum. However, it is not clear whether these two studies are practically comparable, in view of the spatial organization of the receptive fields. It seems as if homonymous receptive fields of both retinae were concerned in Payne's case and heteronymous receptive fields in Berlucchi and Rizzolatti's study. Thus, the question of the involvement of the corpus callosum in binocular vision and stereopsis is far from being answered, especially in view of our failure to find binocular cortical cells in split chiasm cats.

Another important question to be asked is, if we assume that stereopsis is mediated by the corpus callosum, how is it performed in view of the delay existing for impulses traveling through the indirect callosal way? Furthermore, if cortical cells receive indirect callosal input from the nasotemporal strip, why are they not all binocular, in normal as well as in split chiasm cats?

Experiments are now being carried out by us in order to answer the above questions.

5 Summary

1. Six adult cats were operated for split chiasm, three of which were subjected to recording and receptive field mapping of single cells (N = 160) in visual cortex areae 17–18 boundary. Three normal cats were used as controls (N = 76).
2. All operated cats but one had widely dilated pupils for 1–2 months following the operation; they all had difficulties in their visual performance.
3. Practically all visually active cells in the split chiasm cats had ipsilateral input, no matter which hemisphere was recorded from. A high proportion of visually nonresponsive cells (32.5%) were found in the operated, in comparison to the normal cats (10.5%).
4. Cortical visually active cells of the split chiasm cats were frequently nonspecific (21.2%) in comparison to those of normal cats (5.3%), as expressed mainly in their direction and orientation selectivity.
5. Receptive fields were found in both sides of each vertical meridian despite the fact that the cells did not have contralateral input. This reinforces in a direct way the theory of nasotemporal retinal overlap.

6. The model suggesting an indirect pathway through the corpus callosum based on the binocularity found for cortical cells in split chiasm cats (Berlucchi and Rizzolatti 1968) has not been proved.

Acknowledgments. Research supported by the Israel Center for Psychobiology, Charles E. Smith Family Foundation, Grant No. 80-1-259 (to U. Yinon), and by the Jack Haberrer Trust Fund through Tel Aviv University Research Authority (to A. Hammer).

References

Adler FH (1953) Physiology of the eye. The CV Mosby Co, St Louis, pp 563, 567

Berlucchi G, Rizzolatti G (1968) Binocularly driven neurons in visual cortex of split-chiasm cats. Science 159: 308–310

Berlucchi G, Gazzaniga S, Rizzolatti G (1967) Microelectrode analysis of transfer of visual information by the corpus callosum. Arch Ital Biol 105: 583–596

Blakemore C (1969) Binocular depth discrimination and the nasotemporal division. J Physiol 205: 471–497

Davson H (1972) The physiology of the eye. Churchill Livingstone, Edinburgh London, pp 491, 516

Duke-Elder S (1971) System of ophthalmology, vol XII. Neuroophthalmology. Henry Kimpton, London, pp 400, 429

Field HE, Taylor ME (1974) In: Butterworth BB (ed) An atlas of cat anatomy. Univ of Chicago Press, Chicago London, Plates 6,9

Hubel DH, Wiesel TN (1967) Cortical and callosal connections concerned with the vertical meridian of visual fields in the cat. J Neurophysiol 30: 1561–1573

Hubel DH, Wiesel TN (1968) Receptive fields and functional architecture of monkey striate cortex. J Physiol 195: 215–243

Leicester J (1968) Projection of the visual vertical meridian to cerebral cortex of the cat. J Neurophysiol 31: 371–382

Mitchell DE, Blakemore C (1970) Binocular depth perception and the corpus callosum. Vision Res 10: 49–54

Myers RE (1955) Interocular transfer of pattern discrimination in cats following section of crossed optic fibers. J Comp Physiol Psychol 48: 470–473

Payne BR, Elberger AJ, Berman N, Murphy EH (1980) Binocularity in the cat visual cortex is reduced by sectioning the corpus callosum. Science 207: 1097–1099

Polyak S (1957) The vertebrate visual system. Univ Chicago Press, Chicago, p 788

Sanderson KJ, Sherman SM (1971) Nasotemporal overlap in the visual field projected to the lateral geniculate nucleus in the cat. J Neurophysiol 34: 453–466

Stone J (1966) The naso-temporal division of the cat's retina. J Comp Neurol 126: 585–600

Woolsey CN (1971) Comparative studies on cortical representation of vision. Vision Res Suppl 3: 365–382

Yinon U (1978) Chronic asymmetry in the extraocular muscles of adult cats: Stability in binocularity of cortical neurons. Exp Brain Res 32: 275–285

Yinon U (1980) Monocular deafferentation effects on responsiveness of cortical cells in adult cats. Brain Res 199: 299–306

Yinon U, Goshen S (1980) Physiological changes in visual cortex cells of dark reared cats following monocular deprivation. Proc. Int. Union Physiol Sc 14: 794 (Abstract)

Modified Retinotectal Projection in Goldfish: A Consequence of the Position of Retinal Lesions

CLAUDIA STÜRMER[1]

1 Introduction

Attardi and Sperry (1963), Roth (1972) and Meyer (1975) found restricted tectal projections in goldfish after retinal lesions and claimed that retinal fibers were predetermined to meet with specific tectal elements due to corresponding cytochemical specification of retinal and tectal elements. Modificability in retinotectal projections has been demonstrated by Gaze and Sharma (1970), and Yoon (1971), who found, e.g., compression of retinal projections after tectal ablation, or expansion after retinal lesions (Horder 1971; Yoon 1971) with electrophysiological recordings. These results were confirmed by many others and substantiated the newly developed concept of "system matching" (Gaze 1970) in the retino-tectal fiber projections.

The present investigation was aimed at solving the conflicting results of tectal projections after retinal lesions with anatomical methods. In accordance with either the specificity or system matching hypothesis, predictions for fiber distribution following retinal lesions can be made. If fibers were immutably specified for "their" tectal elements, any ablated part of the retina should be dectectable as a corresponding "empty space" in the tectal termination area. If fibers are highly dynamic and able to adjust totally their projection according to the available termination space, one would expect a homogenous fiber distribution over the tectum in all cases of lesions. Local effects of retinal lesions should be undetectable. The size of retinal lesion should produce a reduction of fiber density in the tectum.

2 Material and Methods

Common goldfish, 5–10 cm in lenght, were subjected to surgical procedures: optic nerve section, retinal lesion, injection of tritiated proline, 10–15 μl of 2,3^{3}H-proline (spec. act. 30–60 Ci/mmol) into the eye. The animals were sacrificed 2 days after the injection. The optic nerve was sectioned with a scalpel intraorbitally. Retinal lesions

1 Universitäts-Hals-Nasen-Ohrenklinik, Morphologische Hirnforschung, Killianstr. 5, 7800 Freiburg, FRG
Present address: Natural Science Building, Division of Biological Sciences, The University of Michigan, Ann Arbor, MI 48109, USA

were made by sucking off parts of the retina and underlying pigment epithelium to varying extent at the nasal, temporal, dorsal or ventral retinal pole.

When the animal was sacrificed, the extent of the retinal lesion was directly determined under the microscope or reconstructed from 10 μm thick paraffin transverse serial sections. The brains were embedded in paraffin after fixation, were serially cross-sectioned at 10 μm and submitted to conventional autoradiographic techniques. Fiber distribution was determined by grain distribution and relative grain densities over the tectal optic strata in tectal transverse serial sections.

Three groups of experiments will be presented here:

1. A test for retinotopic order was performed on 25 normal goldfish. Acute retinal lesions were introduced to the eyes. After 6 days ^{3}H-proline was injected into the lesioned eye.
2. The retinotectal projection of a fragment retina was pursued in 61 specimens. Retinal lesions were introduced to the left eye and the optic nerve was sectioned in the same session.
3. A test for retinotopic order was carried out in the regenerated fragment retina tectum projection. Retinal lesions were introduced to the animals' left eye along with nerve sectioning (as in 2). The animals survived for 1 year. Then, a second, acute lesion (as in 1) was introduced to the same eye, resulting in a double-lesioned eye. Two animals with ventral lesions were chosen and the second lesion was made in the opposite retinal half (L + L 13, 17). In three animals (LL 4, 5, 12) the acute lesion was placed in the same retinal half as the first lesion. Six days after the acute lesion, proline was injected into the double-lesioned eyes.

3 Results

3.1 The Retinotopic Order in the Normal Goldfish Retinotectal System

In normal goldfish, retinal lesions are reflected in the tectal optic strata as uninnervated areas. The border between the innervated and uninnervated areas appears sharply delineated, with a sudden drop-off in grain densities (Figs. 1 and 2a). In general, uninnervated areas correspond in location, size, and shape to the retinal lesions, thus confirming, with autoradiographical techniques, the rigid topographical order in the retinotectal projection of a normal animal as claimed by Attardi and Sperry (1963) and Meyer (1980).

3.2 The Retinotectal Projection of a Fragment Retina, 6 Months and 12 Months After Retinal Lesion and Nerve Section

3.2.1 Tectal Projection After Large Dorsal and Ventral Retinal Lesion. After half retinal ventral lesions the optic strata in the corresponding medial half tectum appeared generally uninnervated (Figs. 1b and 2b, c). The lateral half tectum, in contrast, exhibited a homogenous fiber density along the tectal rostrocaudal extent. Following

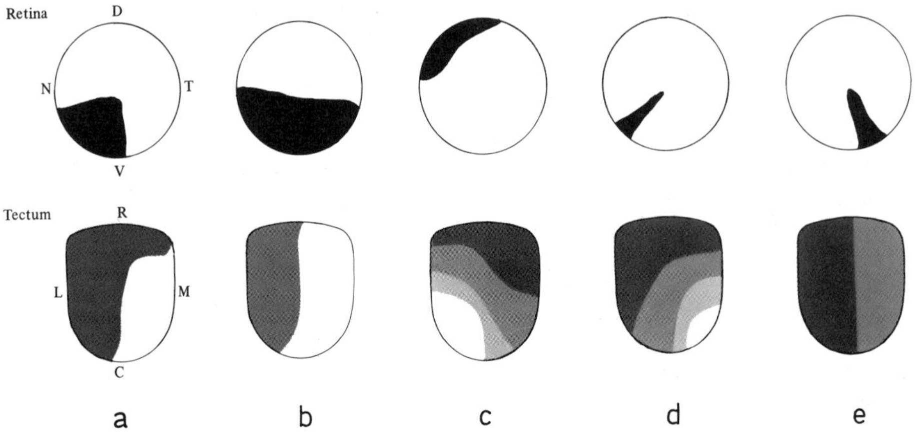

Fig. 1a–e. Schematic drawings of reconstructions of retinal lesions (*black areas*) and subsequent tectal projections. Intensity of *shading* corresponds to tectal innervation density. *D* dorsal, *V* ventral, *N* nasal, *T* temporal; *R* rostral, *C* caudal, *L* lateral, *M* medial

large dorsal retinal lesions, the lateral tectal half was left uninnervated (confirmatory to Attardi and Sperry 1963). In these cases the border of innervated to uninnervated tectal areas along the rostrocaudal midline was characterized by a gradual decrease of gain density in a medio-lateral extent. These findings are in contrast to the sudden drop-off of grains in the normal cases of group 1 (Figs. 1 and 2a). Even after 1 year survival time there was no fiber expansion in medio-lateral direction detectable.

3.2.2 Tectal Effects After Nasal Retinal Lesions. After nasal retinal lesions the most caudal tectum appeared uninnervated (see Figs. 1c and 2d). Rostral tectal areas exhibited normal fiber density, which gradually declined towards caudal tectal areas. This restricted fiber distribution, after nasal half retinal lesions, confirms previous reported results with autoradiography (Meyer 1975; Schmidt 1978). In our experiments, the same sequence from dense innervation to uninnervated areas could also be observed after smaller than half retinal nasal lesions. In no case has a totally expanded or homogenous innervation been found.

3.2.3 Tectal Effects After Temporal Retinal Lesions. Tectal fiber distribution, after temporal lesions, was basically different from tectal effects after nasal lesions, as well as after dorsal or ventral lesions (confirmatory to Horder 1971; Meyer 1975). The tectum in its whole rostrocaudal extent exhibited a reduced amount of fiber densities. In contrast to normal controls, there were no cases in which the rostral rectal area appeared uninnervated. Thus the nasal temporal situation does not display a mirror image effect as has been observed in dorsal ventral lesion cases. However, fiber density rostrally seemed to be slightly reduced compared with caudal areas. An additional, occasionally detected, feature after temporal lesions was an uninnervated rostrocaudally extended zone in the tectal periphery on one side.

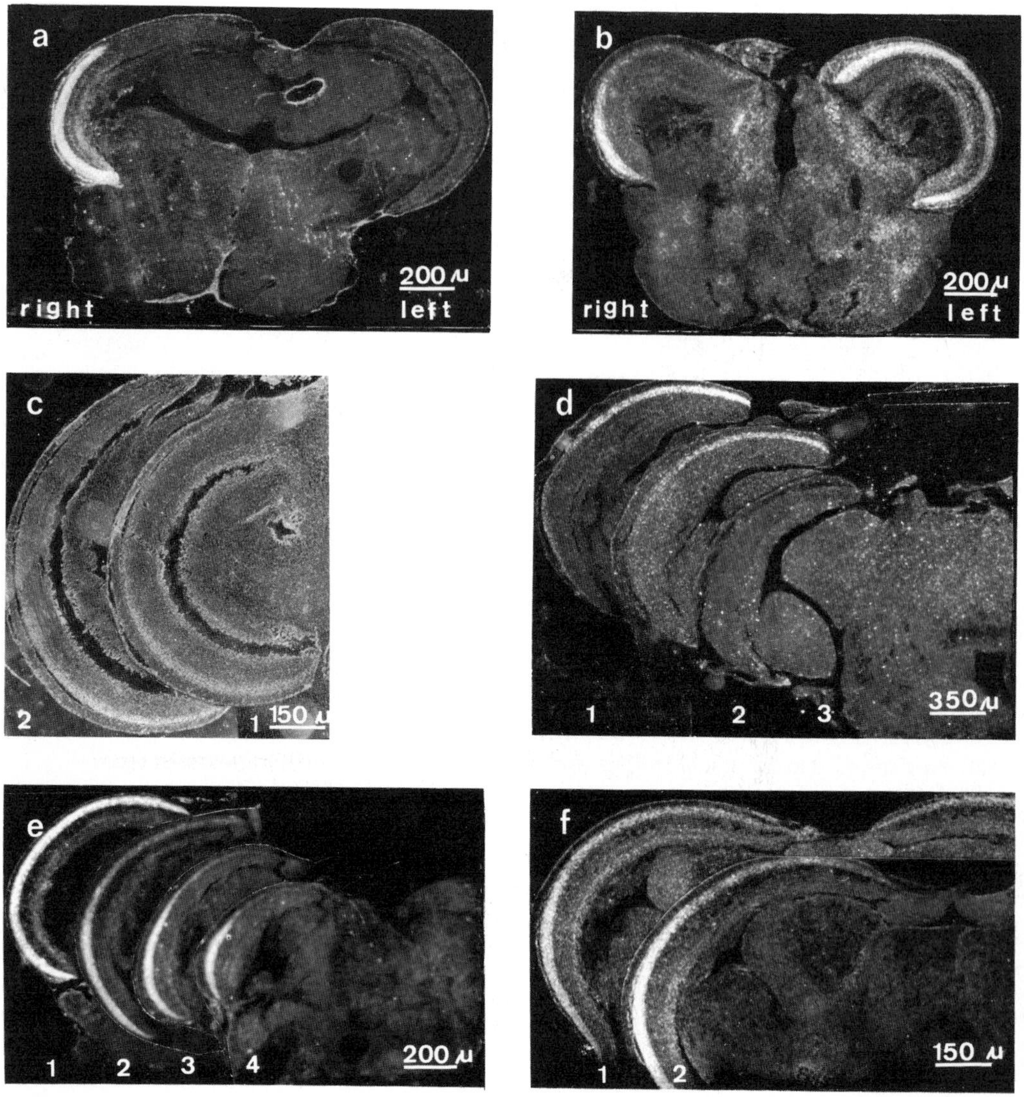

Fig. 2a–f. Darkfield autoradiographs, projection to the right tectum opticum from lesioned left eyes. Cross sections. Lateral half tectums to the left, medial on the top. **a** Innervation sharply confined to the lateral tectal half after acute ventral lesion in a normal goldfish. **b** Dense innervation of the lateral half of the right tectum and markedly reduced innervation of the medial half after ventral retinal lesion and nerve section. Normal innervation by a normal eye to the left tectum. **c** Tectal innervation confined to the lateral half of the right rectum and uninnervated medial tectal half after half retinal ventral lesion in a rostral (*1*) and midtectal (*2*) section. **d** Tectal innervation after a nasal retinal lesion, main extent in dorsal retinal half. Note decreasing fiber densities from midtectal to caudal tectal section levels (*1–3*) (visible first in lateral tectal half); uninnervated at caudal extreme (*3*). **e** Tectal innervation after a naso-ventral lesion, with decreasing fiber density from midtectal to caudal section levels (*1–5*), confined to the lateral tectal half. **f** Tectal innervation after a small segment lesion in the ventral half retina at two tectal levels *1, 2*. Note reduced fiber density in medial tectal half and normal density in lateral tectal half

3.2.4 Tectal Effects After Small Segment Retinal Lesions. Small retinal lesions, which were confined to the dorsal or ventral half retina, were not directly reflected in the tectum, as in the normal animals. A notable result was that although small in size – ranging from a fifth to a tenth of retinal area – these lesions effected changes of fiber distribution along the whole rostrocaudal extent of a tectal half. Following for example dorso-nasal or ventro-nasal lesions, the fiber distribution was comparable to the fiber distribution after extended nasal lesion, but confined to the lateral or medial half tectum (Figs. 1d and 2e). After small dorso-temporal lesions, the lateral tectal half appeared less densely innervated along its rostrocaudal extent. In all cases, the noncorresponding tectal half did not display any lesion effect, but exhibited a normal grain density along the rostrocaudal extent.

3.2.5 Dorsal and Ventral Segment Lesions Situated at the Dorsal or Ventral Retinal Pole. Such lesions effected an overall reduction of fiber density in the lateral or medial tectal half along its whole rostrocaudal extent (Figs. 1e and 2f). With increasing extent of the retinal lesion, the innervation density in the corresponding tectal half became markedly reduced to a further degree. Typical for this group, with different innervation density in the medial and lateral half tectum, was a border characterized by a gradual decrease of fiber densities. As could be demonstrated in two cases, even after 1 year survival time, the same fiber distribution still existed.

4 Test for Retinotopic Order in the Regenerated Fragment Retina-Tectum Projection 1 Year After the First Retinal Lesion and Optic Nerve Section

Additional experiments were performed to test whether the regenerated projection of a fragment retina, 1 year after the lesion, is retinotopically organized (1) concerning the projection of the unlesioned half retina, (2) concerning the reduced projection after retinal lesions.

1. In cases L + L 13 and L + L 17, the ventral retinal half had been lesioned 1 year before, and the second acute lesion was confined to a segment in the dorsal retinal half. The medial half tectum corresponding to the previous ventral lesion was uninnervated in L + L 13 and of reduced innervation density in L + L 17. The lateral tectal half exhibited a limited "denervated" tectal area surrounded by normal innervation density. The border to the denervated area was characterized by a drop-off of grain density. The area was of limited extent and at a retinotopically corresponding location in the lateral half. A notable difference to tectal effects in normal controls (group 1) was a still existing weak fiber density in these "denervated" areas.

2. In cases LL 4, LL5, and LL 12, a similiar limited denervated tectal area, due to the acute lesion, became evident in the tectal half of already reduced fiber density. The tectal half corresponding to the retinal half, which had not received a lesion, exhibited normal fiber density.

From these experiments one can conclude that the regenerated projection of the fragment retina is retinotopically organized, along both tectal halves. However, retinotopical order after regeneration is less rigid than in the normal tectum.

5 Discussion

Our experimental results, with autoradiographical techniques, clearly show that regenerated tectal innervation patterns, after retinal lesions, are modified with respect to the position of the retinal lesion. Retinal lesions are reflected as "empty spaces" only in the normal goldfish tectum. In the regenerated systems, however, a restricted as well as an expanded fiber distribution was found, following retinal lesions and regeneration. In summary, some results are compatible with the predictions made according to the specificity theory, and some with the "system matching" concept. Whether regenerated fiber distribution is restricted to specific tectal areas or expanded over the available space, depends on the position and extent of the retinal lesion. With the variety of retinal lesions, we could deduce some underlying factors which might determine regenerating fibers, after retinal lesions, to project in a typical mode over the tectum.

As already described in detail (Attardi and Sperry 1963; Horder 1974), fibers from the dorsal retina reach the tectum through the medial branch (= half tract) of the optic tract, and fibers from the ventral retina through the lateral half tract. Arriving at the tectum, the fiber bundles of the medial half tract exclusively supply the medial tectal half and those of the lateral half tract, the lateral tectal half. Present experimental evidence substantiates fiber segregation into half tract and half tectum innervation according to their retinal origin, when one retinal half is ablated. This indicates that dorsal and ventral retinal halves are independent from each other in re-innervating their tectal halves, due to a specification. This "half tract specification" might be considered as presumably the most important guide for regenerating fibers. This suggestion is further substantiated by a time course experiment of regeneration (Stürmer 1978), which reveals that re-innervation along the tectal halves does not always coincide.

In spite of temporal lesions, rostral tectal areas are never uninnervated after retinal fiber regeneration. This is supported by electrophysiological recordings (Horder 1971) and antomical methods (Meyer 1975). This observation leads to the assumption that rostral tectal areas represent attractive termination fields for regenerating fibers – presumbly since they are contacted first by ingrowing fibers. The attractiveness of the rostral tectum is further delineated by findings of a time sequence study of re-innervation. In early regeneration stages, the first synaptic contacts are established in rostral tectal areas (Stürmer 1978), which emphasizes that regenerating fibers in general exhibit a "rostral preference".

Another striking feature of tectal re-innervation patterns after regeneration is that no uninnervated tectal areas (= "empty spaces") are ever detected between or in the middle of innervated areas. The obvious compensation of otherwise arising innervation gaps on a tectal level may be explained by the tendency of the fibers to maintain interfiber connection, thus exhibiting "fiber contiguity".

To account for the restricted fiber projection after nasal lesions, which contrasts with the nonrestricted projection after small dorsal or ventral retinal lesions, an additional assumption has to be made, i.e., the "zonal preference".

If retinal fibers were simply submitted to the rules of half tract specification, rostral preference, and fiber contiguity, one would expect a tectal projection confined to rostral tectal fields, until the available amount of retinal fibers is exhausted. This pattern should be reproduced independent of the location of the lesion. Since this restricted pattern is only observed after nasal lesions, one might argue that in general regenerating fibers still tend to reoccupy their previous termination areas or zones.

Another feature of regenerated retinal fibers claimed by Schmidt et al. (1978) is their time-dependent progress into caudal tectal areas after nasal lesions. Our results with survival periods of half a year and one year give some indications for a gradual fiber spread in caudal direction, although this expansion was always incomplete.

No evidence for fiber spread in medio-lateral direction after half retinal dorsal-ventral lesions exists. There is also no indication for medio-lateral fiber density compensation from densely innervated to less densely innervated half tecta after a delay of many months, except to gradual a decrease of gain density at the rostrocaudal midline (Schmidt and Easter 1978). We consider this as further support for the restriction of fibers to medial or lateral half tectum according to their retinal origin.

With the test for retinotopy, we demonstrated that regenerated retinal fibers of a fragment retina are able to establish a retinotopically ordered map along the half tectum. From this, one might infer that two retinotopically ordered, but differently spaced, maps of the dorsal and ventral visual half fields are represented side by side along the tectal length, opposing each other along the rostrocaudal tectal midline. A confirmation of these anatomical findings, with electrophysiological methods, would be useful.

Acknowledgments. This work was supported by the Deutsche Forschungsgemeinschaft. I wish to thank Arlene Carbone, Ann Katrin Köhler, and Katrin Bielenberg.

References

Attardi DG, Sperry RW (1963) Preferential selection of central pathways by regenerating optic fibers. Exp Neurol 7: 46–64

Cowan WM, Cuenod M (1975) The use of axonal transport for the study of neural connectivity. Studies of neuronal connectivity. Elsevier Scientific Publ Co, Amsterdam, New York Oxford

Gaze RM (1970) A study of the retinotectal projection during regeneration of the optic nerve. Proc R Soc London Ser B 157: 420–448

Gaze RM, Sharma SC (1970) Axial differences in reinnervation of the goldfish optic tectum by regenerating optic fibers. Exp Brain Res 10: 171–181

Horder TJ (1971) Retention, by fish optic nerve fibres regenerating to new terminal sites in the tectum, of "chemospecific" affinity for their original sites. J Physiol 216: 53–55

Horder TJ (1974) Changes of fibre pathways in the goldfish optic tract following regeneration. Brain Res 72: 41–52

Meyer RL (1975) Factors affecting regeneration of the retino-tectal projection. Doct Diss

Meyer RL (1980) Mapping the normal and regenerating retinotectal projection of goldfish with autoradiographic methods. J Comp Neurol 189: 273–289

Roth RL (1972) Normal and regenerated retino-tectal projections in the goldfish (Doctoral dissertation, Case Western Reserve University). Diss Abstr Int 33: 4085 B–4086 B

Schmidt JT (1978) Retinal fibers alter tectal positional markers during the expansion of the half retinal projection in goldfish. J Comp Neurol 177: 279–300

Schmidt JT, Easter SS (1978) Independent biaxial reorganization of the retinotectal projection: A reassessment. Exp Brain Res 31: 155–162

Schmidt JT, Cicerone CM, Easter SS (1978) Expansion of the half retinal projection to the tectum in goldfish: An electrophysiological and anatomical study. J Comp Neurol 177: 257–278
Stürmer C (1978) Die Retino-Tectale Projektion beim Goldfisch (Carassius auratus). Eine Untersuchung zur Spezifität neutraler Verbindungen. Doct Diss, Univ Freiburg
Yoon M (1971) Reorganization of retinotectal projection following surgical operations on the optic tectum in goldfish. Exp Neurol 33: 395–411

Functional and Morphological Changes in Fish Chemoreception Systems Following Ablation of the Olfactory Bulbs[1]

H. P. ZIPPEL[2], W. BREIPOHL[3], and H. SCHOON[2]

1 Introduction

The enormous regenerative capacity of central nervous structures in lower vertebrates, especially in amphibia and fish, is reflected by a considerable number of classical investigations (for a review see Windle 1955). Although a number of these investigations have been very striking, particularly those dealing with cell regeneration in the brain (Kirsche and Kirsche 1960; Winkelmann and Winkelmann 1970) and in sensory receptors (Winkelmann and Marx 1969; Takagi 1975; Maier and Wolburg 1979), the majority are based on neuroanatomical methods and there has been a tendency to neglect the electrophysiological (Gaze and Jakobson 1963), functional (Sperry 1955; Zippel and Westerman 1970; Zippel et al. 1970) and behavioural (Segaar 1965) aspects.

The present neuroanatomical and behavioural investigations in goldfish were designed to examine the relationship between morphological changes and changes in the perception of olfactory and gustatory stimuli. Accordingly, at various time intervals after extirpation of the olfactory bulbs, behavioural and morphological comparisons were made between bulbectomized and sham-operated animals: the behavioural studies comprised a detailed analysis of the animals' spontaneous reactions and learning ability, and of their resistance to forgetting and extinction. The work reported here constitutes part of a long-term series of investigations on the morphology of the goldfish olfactory mucosa and receptor cells (Breipohl et al. 1973), and their behavioural responses to gustatory (Schoon 1976) or olfactory (Zippel 1970; Zippel et al. 1978a; Voigt, unpublished data) stimuli.

---

1 Dedicated to Prof. Hans-Dieter Henatsch, Director of the Physiologisches Institut II der Universität Göttingen, on the occasion of his sixtieth birthday

2 Physiologisches Institut der Universität, Humboldtallee 7, 3400 Göttingen, FRG
3 Institut für Anatomie, Universitätsklinikum, Hufelandstraße 55, 4300 Essen, FRG

2 Materials and Methods

Olfactory Bulbectomy. The fish were anaesthetized in Tricain (MS-222, Sandos) and the cranium overlying the olfactory bulbs and tracts was removed; the olfactory nerves and tracts were severed close to the bulbs and the latter were extirpated in toto.

Training and Testing Apparatus. Each training and testing tank (Fig. 1) consisted of a long, glass aquarium (130 X 20 X 30 cm) filled to a depth of 23 cm with aged tap water.

For feeding, training and testing purposes, an opaque plastic funnel was suspended into the water at each end of the tank; that area of the tip facing away from the end of the aquarium was perforated with 15 regularly spaced holes (diam. 2 mm) through which the fish could feed on Tubifex worms.

The gustatory and olfactory stimuli – acetic and malonic acids, glucose, amyl acetate, Tubifex extracts – were presented through the tip of the funnel. The synthetic

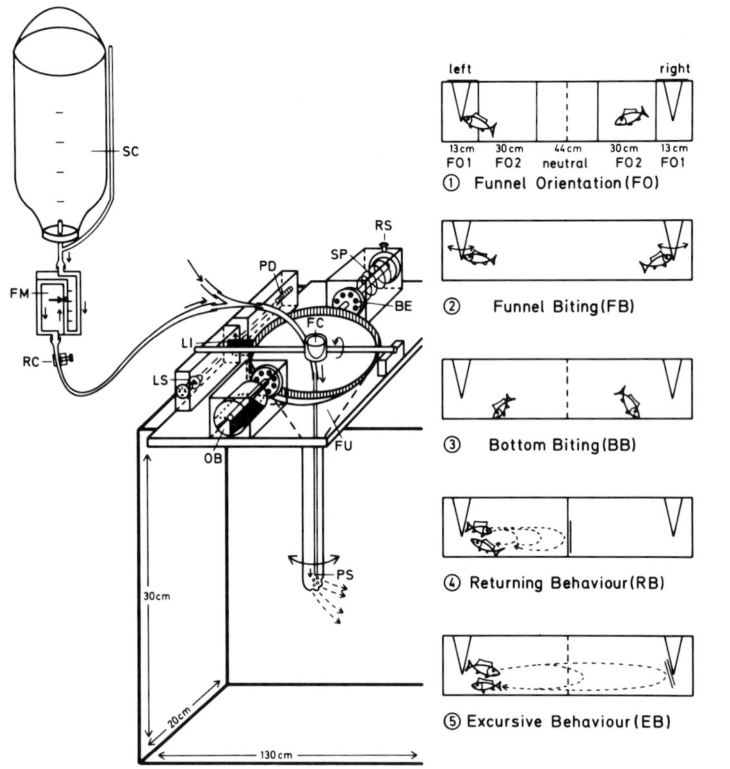

Fig. 1. Stimulus application, recording technique and analysis of behaviour. *BE,* (ball-) bearing; *FC,* food container; *FM,* flow meter; *FU,* funnel; *LI,* light beam interruptor; *LS,* light source; *OB,* oil bath; *PD,* photodiode; *PS,* point of stimulus application; *RC,* regulating clamp; *RS,* regulating screw; *SC,* stimulus container; *SP,* spring. For analysis of behaviour see text

stimuli were applied in per cent or molar concentrations, while the concentrations of Tubifex extracts were based on 1 g wet weight.

Recording Technique and Analysis of Behaviour. The experiments proper were preceded by a period of habituation, 4–5 weeks being necessary before the fish readily associated the funnels with food (Tubifex worms).

By the end of the habituation period, a complex behavioural repertoire, directed at one, or both, of the funnels, had developed. The following behaviour patterns were recorded:

1. Funnel Orientation (FO) – the time (s) spent by the animals in the immediate vicinity of the funnels.
2. Funnel Biting (FB) – the number of bites at each of the funnels. (This behaviour may be interpreted as a specifically orientated food expectation.)
3. Bottom Biting (BB) – the number of bites on the bottom of the aquarium. (This behaviour may be interpreted as a non-specifically orientated food expectation.)
4. Returning Behaviour (RB) – the number of continuous swimming movements away from the immediate vicinity of one funnel (FO) in the direction of the other and then back to the initial funnel (FO) without crossing the middle of the tank.
5. Excursive Behaviour (EB) – as RB with the exception that the animal(s) crosses the middle of the tank; neither FO nor FB occurs at the second funnel.

All behaviour patterns were recorded on a custom-built, electronic recording unit: FB was registered automatically by a photocell system (the beam of which was interrupted during biting by a flat, metal tongue affixed to the rim of the funnel), while the remaining parameters were recorded manually by operating either a time switch (FO) or a counter (BB, RB and EB). The data were punched onto paper tape, whence they were read into a PDP-11/34 computer for final analysis.

Training and Testing Procedure. At the beginning of each session, a control registration (of 5 min duration) was made of the animals' behaviour to the funnels in the absence of stimuli. In the immediately succeeding test or training period (also of 5 min duration), the animals' behaviour during stimulus application was recorded.

At no time during or immediately following a test session was the animals' behaviour reinforced; the animals were fed on both sides of the aquarium at least 2 h after the last test on a particular day. By contrast, each training session was immediately followed by positive reinforcement: stimulus application was continued and the animals were presented with Tubifex worms through the appropriate funnel (interval reinforcement).

The training experiments fall into two categories: (1) Training to a single stimulus – following a long-term (12 months) regeneration period, the animals were trained to respond to singly presented odour stimuli; distilled water was applied through the "negative" funnel because data obtained with intact animals trained on an olfactory discrimination had shown that learning in this sensory modality is characterized by the difficulty to differentiate synthetic odours qualitatively (Zippel 1970). (2) Discrimination training – two taste discrimination tasks were performed with animals immediately after bulbectomy, acetic and malonic acids being the training (reinforced) stimuli and glucose and acetic acid the respective competing (non-reinforced) stimuli.

3 Results

3.1 Taste Discrimination Training Immediately Following Extirpation of the Olfactory Bulbs

A detailed analysis of the behaviour of goldfish trained to discriminate between various gustatory stimuli (Schoon 1976) demonstrated that acetic and malonic acids, both of which were spontaneously strongly aversive, were the two dominant stimuli: the learning curves reached a constant level of 80–100% positive reactions after only five to ten training sessions, irrespective of the competing stimulus. The dominant role of acetic acid was further emphasized by the fact that successful training to another stimulus could be achieved only with difficulty when acetic acid was presented as the competing stimulus.

These findings suggested that acetic acid might be perceived via the olfactory system as well as by the gustatory system. This hypothesis was tested in two series of experiments, each comprising 24 fish divided into 12 groups of 2. In each series the olfactory bulbs were extirpated in half the animals, while the other half were sham-operated controls.

3.1.1 Acetic Acid vs Glucose

In the first series the two stimuli were of different gustatory quality. In the test sessions before training (Fig. 2), the reactions of both the sham-operated and the bulbectomized animals to acetic acid all lie, with the exception of the first test, well below the 50% level, confirming the spontaneous avoidance of this stimulus. During training to acetic acid, the rate of learning is high in both groups and seems to be independent of the nature of the competing (spontaneously preferred) stimulus. After a forgetting period of 3 weeks (in which the animals were fed randomly through the left and right funnels without stimulus application), the animals still respond at a high level to the training stimulus, suggesting that well-developed taste discriminations are very resistant to extinction.

During subsequent reversal training (i.e., glucose reinforced, acetic acid non-reinforced), however, only the sham-operated animals show an improvement in performance, the difference between the two collectives being especially pronounced following the 1-week forgetting period. The difficulties experienced by the bulbectomized animals in learning the reversal task can most clearly be seen in their returning and excursive behaviour: values below 50% indicate that they respond more often to the original training stimulus, acetic acid.

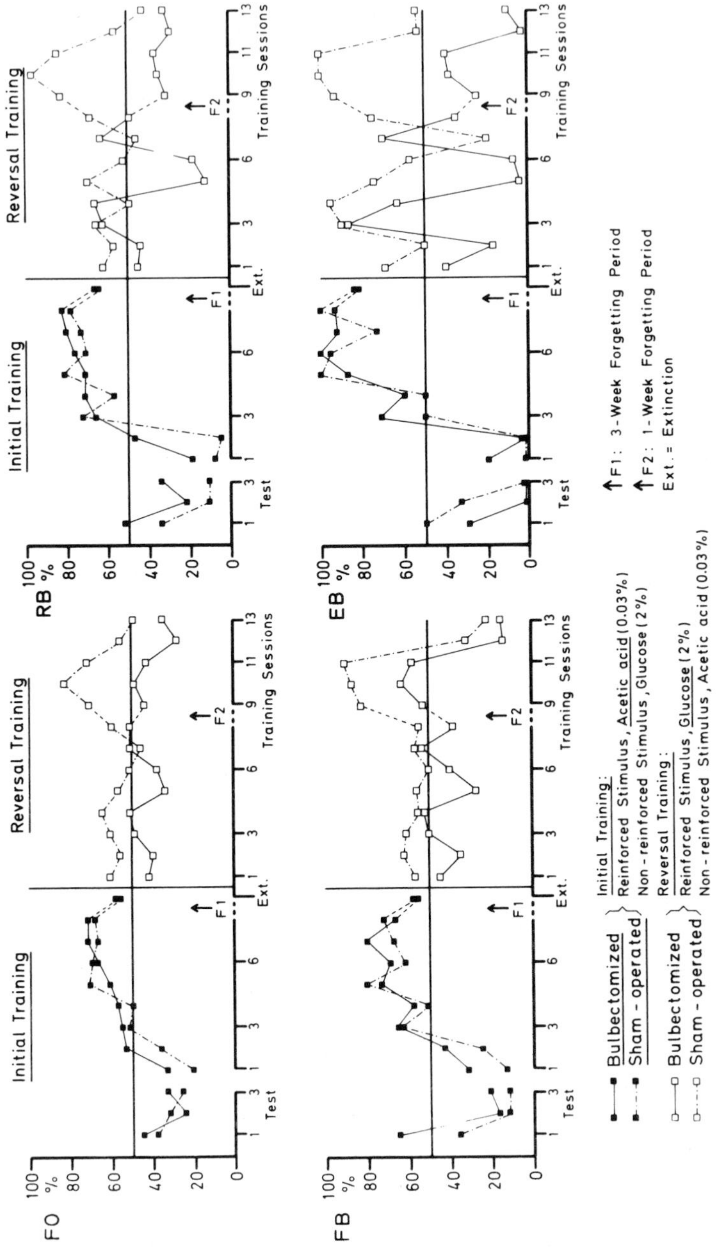

Fig. 2. Analysis of training and reversal training with acetic acid and glucose in bulbectomized and sham-operated animals. The results are expressed in terms of the per cent reactions to the respective training stimulus; mean values for N = 12 (6 groups of 2 animals in each collective). *FO*, Funnel orientation; *FB*, funnel biting; *RB*, returning behaviour; *EB*, excursive behaviour

3.1.2 Malonic Acid vs Acetic Acid

In the second series, discrimination training was conducted with two stimuli of the same gustatory quality but of varying quantity, i.e., of different subjective concentrations. Contrary to the first series, the two collectives acquire the discrimination task at

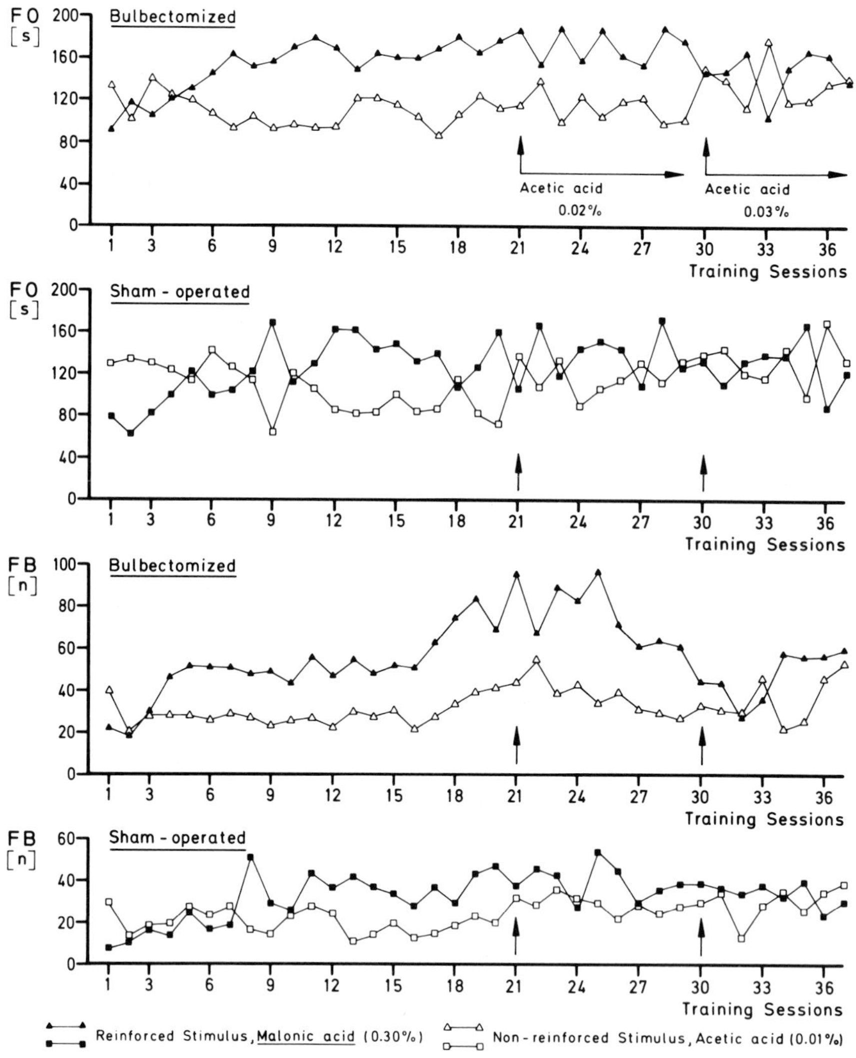

Fig. 3. Analysis of training with malonic and acetic acids in bulbectomized and sham-operated animals. The results are presented in the form of the original data recorded during training; mean values for N = 12 (6 groups of 2 animals in each collective). *FO,* funnel orientation; *FB,* funnel biting

different rates (Fig. 3). The bulbectomized animals readily learn to differentiate the two stimuli; their reactions to the training stimulus, malonic acid, undergo a progressive increase over the first five to seven sessions and do not drop below this level throughout the remainder of initial training. The behaviour of the sham-operated animals, on the other hand, is subject to considerable fluctuation and not until the later stages of initial training are they able to discriminate the two stimuli with any certainty. In this figure, the original data are presented and it is evident that the overall FO and FB values (i.e., at both funnels) are higher in the bulbectomized fish than in the sham-operated fish. The lower values of the intact animals may be attributable to confusing influence of the olfactory components of these two taste stimuli.

The first increase in the concentration of the competing stimulus has little effect on the animals' behaviour. Both collectives experience considerable difficulties, however, when the concentration of acetic acid is increased to the same subjective concentration as malonic acid.

3.2 Degeneration and Regeneration of Olfactory Receptors Following Extirpation of the Olfactory Bulbs

The neuroanatomical investigations formed the basis for the training experiments conducted after long-term regeneration (see below). Intact and bulbectomized animals were examined at different time intervals after surgery using light and scanning-electron microscopical (SEM) techniques (Fig. 4A–C). Figure 4A1 shows a semi-thin section through an olfactory lamella of an intact animal. Of special interest is the broad assembly of dark perikarya in the basal epithelium; the smaller black cells are typical basal cells, while the larger cells are probably blastemal cells. This epithelial arrangement is a prerequisite for the replacement of degenerated receptor cells. Figure 4A2 and A3 are scanning-electron micrographs of the epithelial surface at the centre of an olfactory sensory area in an intact animal. The olfactory border is composed of densely packed, ciliated and microvilli receptor cells. Figure 4A4 represents a typical aspect from the dorsal edge of the sensory area of an intact animal; a dominance of non-sensory cells bearing long kinocilia is apparent and between these groups of cells the olfactory border is discernible. The sparsely covered apical poles of the supporting cells can be seen and, in contrast to Fig. 4A2 and A3, fewer ciliated and microvilli terminals are evident (for further details see Breipohl et al. 1973).

The scanning-electron micrographs in Fig. 4B and C were derived from bulbectomized (BE) animals. A low magnification reveals no changes in the gross morphology of the olfactory rosette at any time after BE (an example 4 weeks after BE is presented in Fig. 4B5). The photograph in Fig. 4B6 (6 months after BE) shows that the regenerated olfactory nerve fibres have formed bulb-like structures in the area of the former olfactory bulbs. At higher magnification (Fig. 4B7), however, morphological changes can be seen as early as 5–6 h following BE: a striking vesiculation of the apical poles of the supporting cells and the terminals of the ciliated receptor cells is evident, as is a "clumping" of the sensory microvilli. At this time, these reactive changes are only prominent at the edges of the lamellae, normal surface profiles being found in the centre and at the base of the sensory area up to 12 h after BE (Fig. 4B8); 24 h after BE, however, morphological changes are also encountered in the centre of the olfactory area. Furthermore, the different types of receptor appear to be subject to different rates of change, microvilli receptors being affected much earlier than ciliated receptors (Fig. 4B9).

Three days after BE (Fig. 4C10) the microvilli receptor has disappeared completely and the cilia of the ciliated receptor have shortened markedly. Typical of this stage is the reactive emergence and the pronounced vesicular configuration in the apical poles of the supporting cells. In addition, receptor cells with an atypical shape can frequently

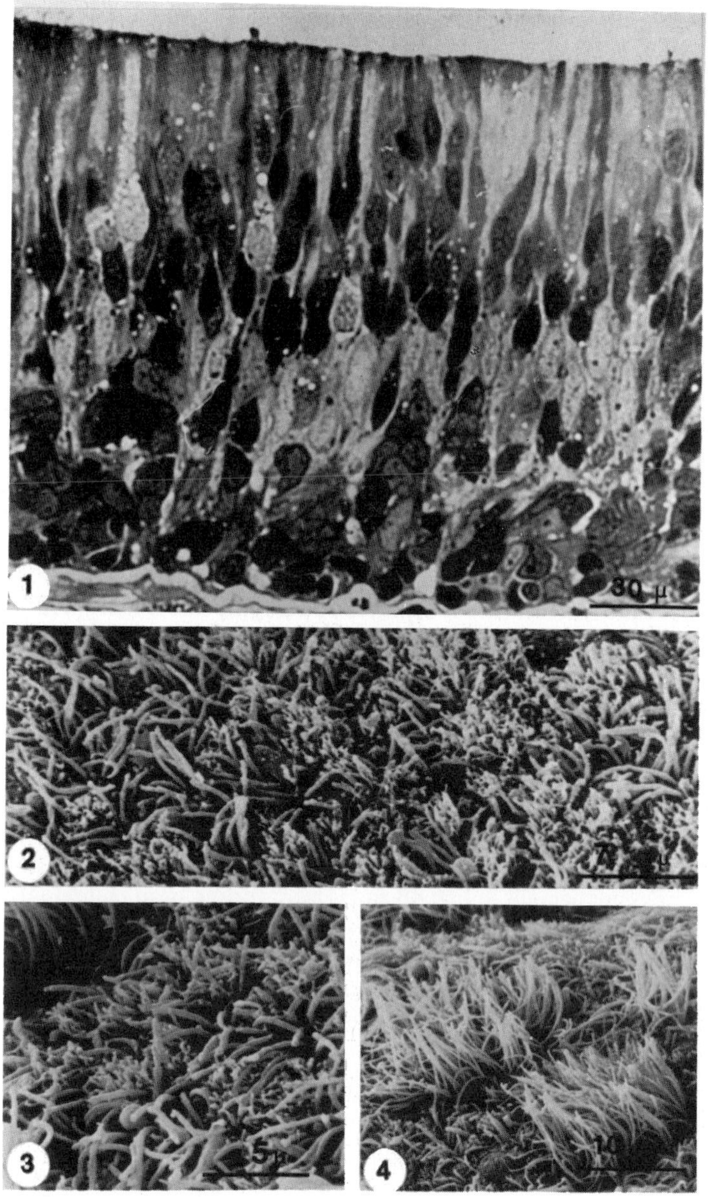

Fig. 4A–C. Neuroanatomy of the olfactory mucosa
A Intact animals. Scanning electron micrographs with the exception of **A1** (semi-thin section stained with azure-2-methylene blue)

be seen. The areas covered with kinocilia-bearing cells also undergo reactive changes to form groups of giant cilia (Fig. 4C12). Seven days after BE, a similar picture is apparent at the margin of the sensory area (Fig. 4C11). During this early stage, however, scattered ciliated receptors are still encountered at the base of the lamellae (Fig. 4C13);

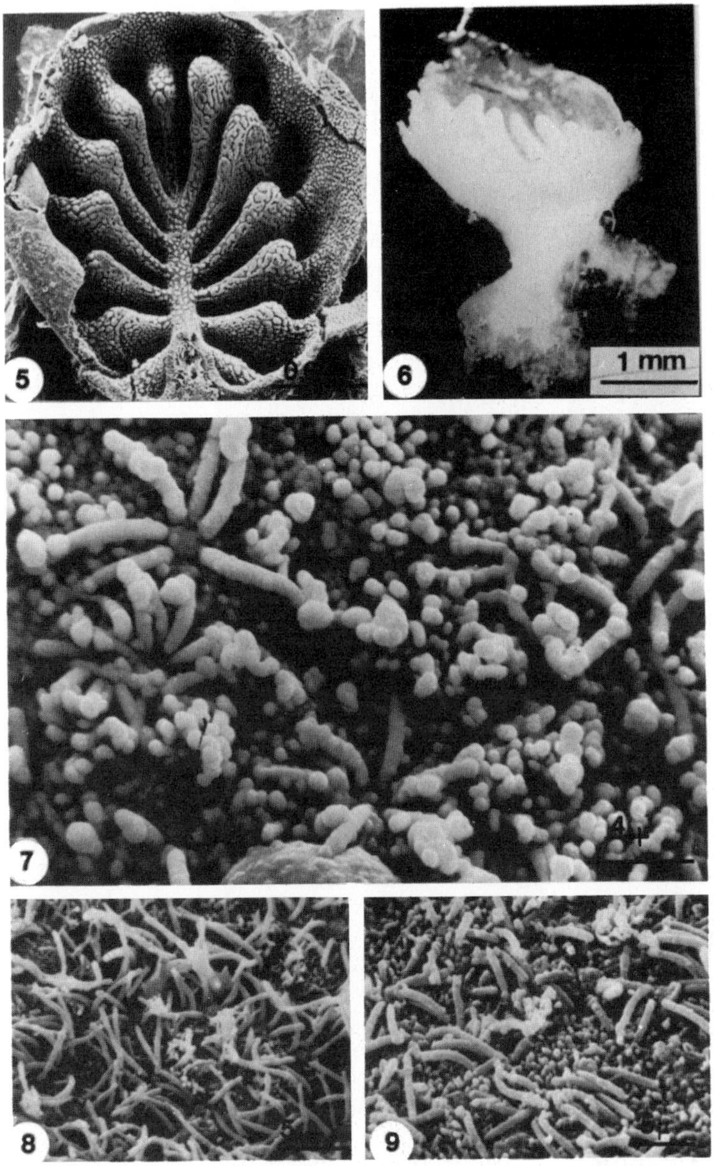

Fig. 4B. Animals at various time intervals after extirpation of the olfactory bulbs. Scanning-electron micrographs with the exception of **B6** (photograph). **B5**, 4 weeks; **B6**, 3 months; **B7**, 5.5 h; **B8**, 12 h; **B9**, 24 h

the surface profiles of the supporting cells remain unchanged and microvilli receptors are not evident. Four weeks following BE (Fig. 4C14), the number of regenerated ciliated receptors has increased, but microvilli receptors are still absent and do not appear at the surface until 8 weeks after BE. Figure 4C15 shows the situation 11 months after

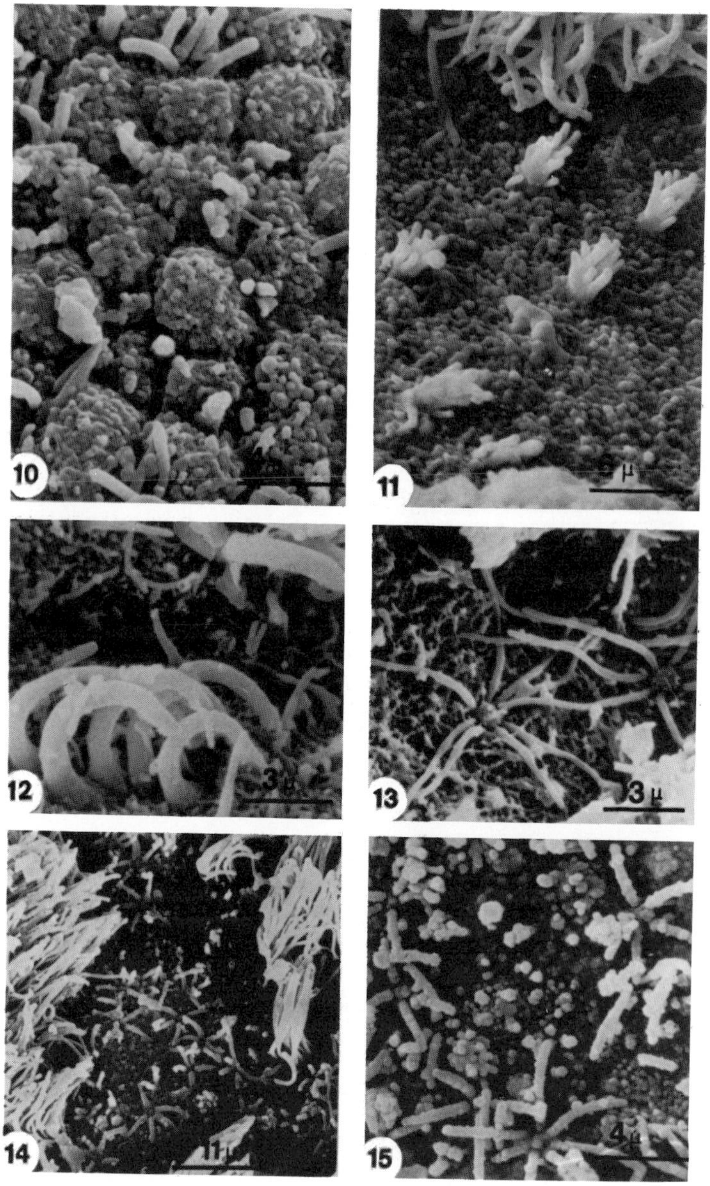

Fig. 4C. Animals at various time intervals after extirpation of the olfactory bulbs. Scanning-electron micrographs. **C10**, 3 days; **C11**, 7 days; **C12**, 3 days; **C13**, 7 days; **C14**, 4 weeks; **C15**, 11 months

BE: the number of ciliated receptors has further increased and microvilli receptors are now present, albeit often with thickened endings.

Finally, it should be mentioned that a certain amount of variation was observed in the long-term regenerated material: only a partial regeneration of the sensory cells (as shown above) was found in some fish, while in others a more or less complete regeneration of the receptor cells was apparent.

3.3 Spontaneous and Training Behaviour After Long-Term Regeneration

Twelve months after bulbectomy, the animals' spontaneous behaviour to Tubifex extracts and amyl acetate was compared to that of intact animals. In the subsequent training experiments, amyl acetate and acetic acid served as the reinforced stimuli.

3.3.1 Spontaneous Behaviour

During the control registrations in the absence of stimuli (not shown), both collectives behaved similarly: RB and EB were not apparent and the frequency of occurrence of the remaining parameters was low. During application of Tubifex extracts, the intact animals (Fig. 5) exhibit positive reactions in terms of three of the five behavioural patterns, the absolute frequency of which appears to be more or less concentration dependent. The long-term regenerated fish, however, only respond positively to the high-

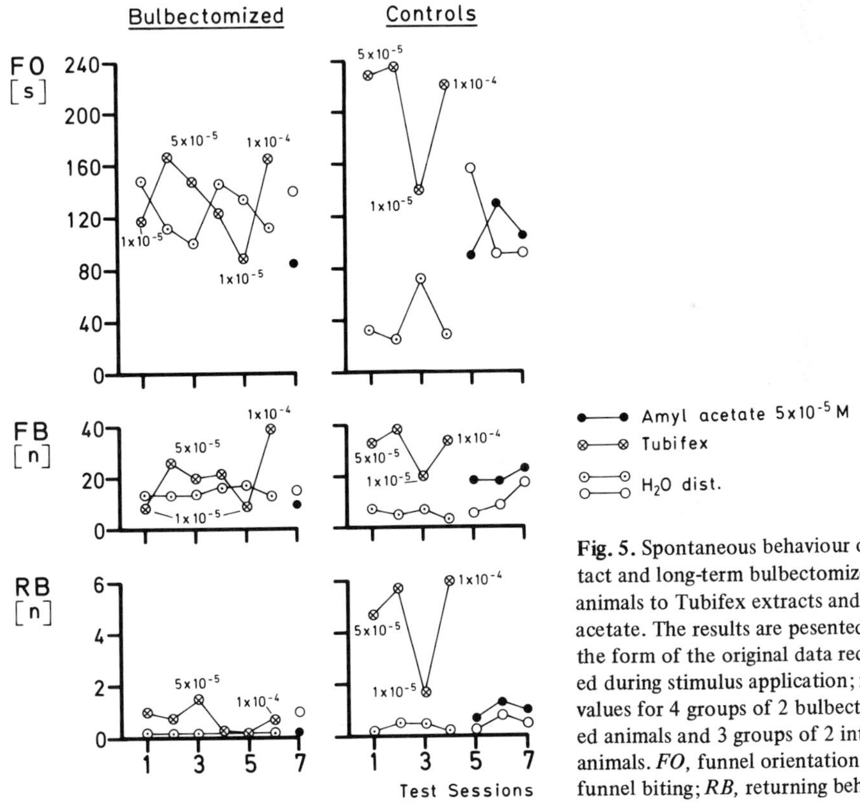

Fig. 5. Spontaneous behaviour of intact and long-term bulbectomized animals to Tubifex extracts and amyl acetate. The results are pesented in the form of the original data recorded during stimulus application; mean values for 4 groups of 2 bulbectomized animals and 3 groups of 2 intact animals. *FO*, funnel orientation; *FB*, funnel biting; *RB*, returning behaviour

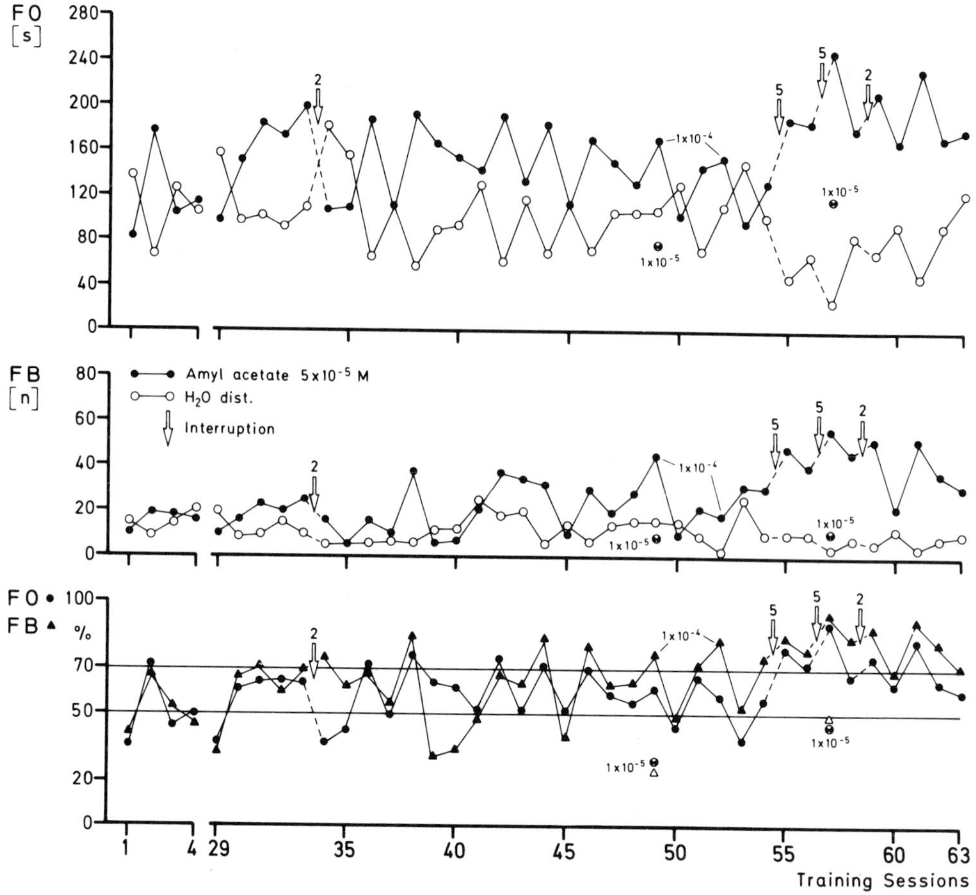

Fig. 6. Analysis of training with amyl acetate in long-term bulbectomized animals. The results are presented in the form of the original data recorded at the positive (amyl acetate) and negative (distilled water) funnels, and also in terms of the per cent reactions to the training stimulus; mean values for N = 8 (4 groups of 2 animals). *FO,* funnel orientation; *FB,* funnel biting; *Interruption,* the number of days (*above arrow*) over which the animals were neither trained nor fed

est concentration applied. With repeated applications at a concentration of 5×10^{-5} mol/l, FB drops close to the chance level, whilst FO is subject to fluctuation. After a further decrease in concentration, the behaviour resembles that seen during the control registrations in the absence of stimuli. The application of amyl acetate (5×10^{-5} mol/l) results in a slight avoidance of the stimulus by both collectives.

3.3.2 Training with Amyl Acetate

Immediately after the tests on the spontaneous behaviour, the bulbectomized fish were trained using amyl acetate at a concentration of 5×10^{-5} mol/l as the reinforced stimulus. In intact animals, this concentration is near the taste threshold for this particular stimulus (= 1×10^{-4} mol/l; Voigt, unpublished data). The first four training sessions (Fig. 6) are characterized by a considerable fluctuation of the original FO and FB values, the corresponding percent values lying around the 50% level. The marked progressive increase in behavioural frequency so typical of taste training (see below) is not evident and the learning curves bear a closer resemblance to those obtained with intact animals during olfactory training to amyl acetate (Voigt, unpublished data). Training was therefore continued without recording for 4 weeks, stimulus and reinforcement being presented randomly at the left and right funnels. Subsequently, FO reaches 160–200 s but FB still remains at a relatively low level; the per cent values for both patterns, however, lie between 60 and 70% at the positive funnel. After an interruption of 2 days (in which the animals were neither trained nor fed), the orientation to the training funnel decreases markedly, while that to the competing funnel increases accordingly. Training was then continued without interruption for a further 21 days. This period is characterized by considerable variation in the response patterns, particularly in the original FO values. From the 42nd training session on, FB reveals a slight, but inconsistent, tendency to higher frequencies. An increase in the concentration to 1×10^{-4} mol/l is attended by an increase in positive responses, but the animals react negatively when the concentration is decreased to 1×10^{-5} mol/l. The results expressed in terms of per cent reactions to the training stimulus show that from the 40th training session onwards the animals' performance is more or less positive, FB lying roughly 10% above FO.

Another break of 5 days with neither training nor food is followed by an unexpectedly high level of positive reactions. After two further interruptions of 5 and 2 days, the responses, especially FB, attain values between 80% and 90%. Lowering of the concentration, however, is again accompanied by a pronounced decrease in the frequency of behaviour, suggesting that this concentration is no longer perceived by the animals.

3.3.3 Training and Threshold Investigations with Acetic Acid

From the 64th training session onwards (Fig. 7), acetic acid replaced amyl acetate as the reinforced stimulus. The initial concentration of 5 X 10-3 mol/l lies about 1 log unit above the threshold for intact animals (Schoon 1976).

During the first application of acetic acid, amyl acetate was presented simultaneously at the opposite funnel: although the animals had not previously been confronted with acetic acid (and had not yet received the appropriate reinforcement), they behave as if they had already been trained to this (spontaneously aversive) stimulus, amyl acetate (the original training stimulus) being almost completely neglected. Over the next three training sessions, it is noticeable that the animals display the complete behavioural repertoire and the learning curves are characteristic of the acquisition phase during training in the gustatory modality with intact animals (Schoon 1976): FO and FB are at a constantly high level, the absolute frequencies being many times higher than the control values recorded in the absence of stimuli; the corresponding per cent values lie above 80%. Perhaps as a result of the aversive nature of acetic acid, the amount of BB drops rapidly over this period. RB and EB, on the other hand, show no tendency to decrease.

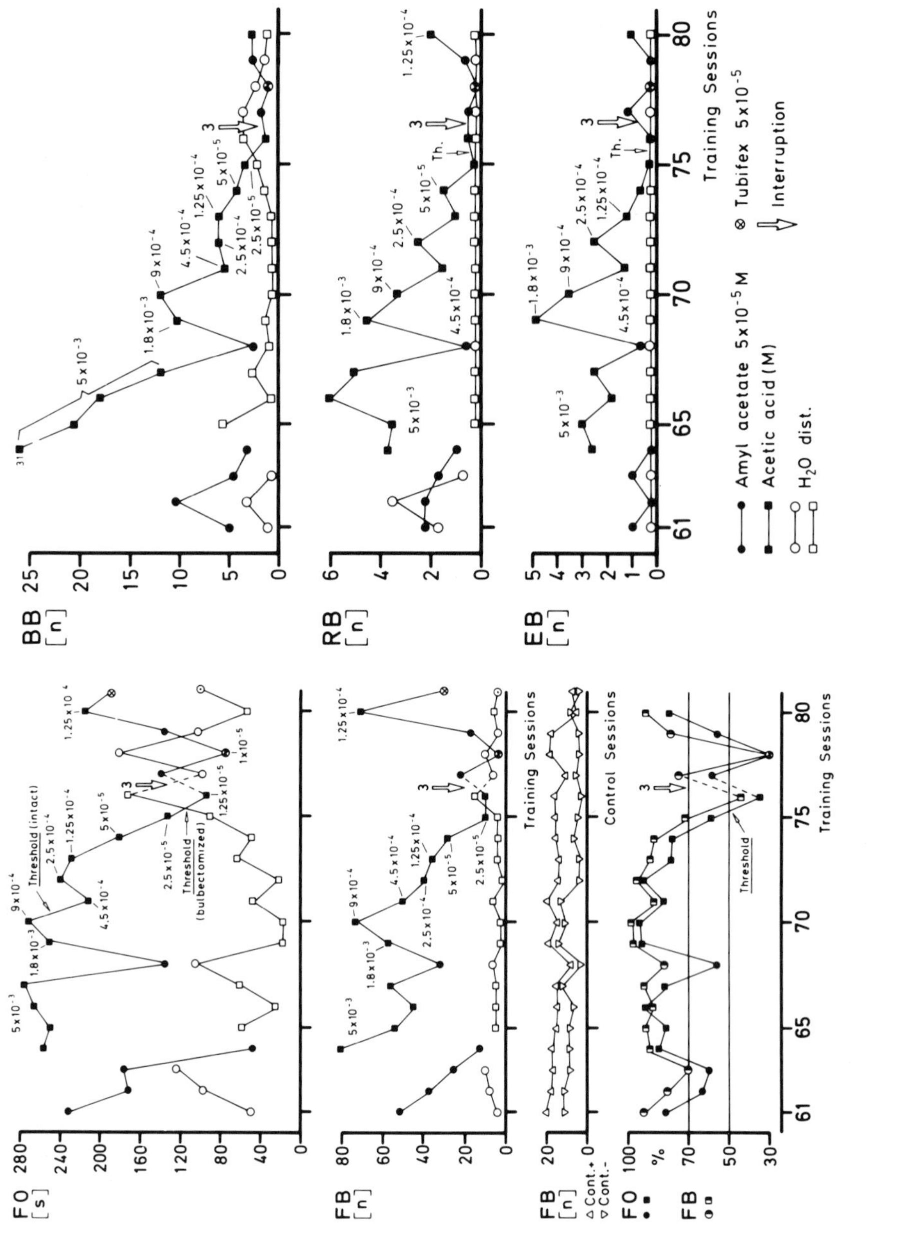

Fig. 7. Analysis of training and threshold determinations with acetic acid in long-term bulbectomized animals. The results are presented in the form of the original data recorded at the positive (acetic acid, amyl acetate, Tubifex extract) and negative (distilled water) funnels, and also in terms of the per cent reactions to the "positive" stimulus; mean values for N = 8 (4 groups of 2 animals). *FO*, funnel orientation; *FB*, funnel biting; *BB*, bottom biting; *RB*, returning behaviour; *EB*, excursive behaviour; *Cont.+* and *Cont.–*, reactions to the positive and negative funnels during the control registration in the absence of stimuli; *Interruption:* see legend to Fig. 6

During subsequent application of amyl acetate, FB is the only parameter which remains positive; FO undergoes a pronounced decrease, whilst BB, RB and EB disappear almost completely.

The threshold investigations reveal a striking difference between operated and intact animals, the threshold of the latter (Schoon 1976) lying roughly 1.5 log units (i.e., about 50-fold) above that of the operated fish. During the successive lowering of the concentration, the behaviour patterns associated with the reinforced funnel decrease at different rates: whereas BB, RB and EB are rarely manifested at concentrations lower than 5×10^{-5} mol/l, FB and FO do not drop below 50% until the concentration is reduced to 1.25×10^{-5} mol/l.

The final tests show that even after an interruption of 3 days amyl acetate is no longer capable of eliciting the same level of positive responses as during the final training sessions with this stimulus. Reapplication of acetic acid, however, causes a marked increase in the frequency of all behaviour patterns.

3.4 Anatomy

The olfactory bulbs were extirpated in a total of eight goldfish and the latter were sacrificed after a regeneration period of 21 months. The anatomical investigations are still in a preliminary stage and only a few general remarks can be made at the present time. Microscopical examination reveals dramatic changes in the area of the former olfactory bulbs (Fig. 8). In all animals a connection is clearly visible between the regenerated fibre bundles and the mucosa on both sides. One animal displays bulb-like structures of almost the same size and shape as normal olfactory bulbs (Fig. 8,2); in five animals much smaller bulb-like structures are apparent (Fig. 8,3), while in the remaining two animals only fibre bundles are evident (Fig. 8,4). In some animals tiny fibre bundles can be seen travelling in the direction of the forebrain without forming a regular olfactory tract. Whether or not these bundles reach the forebrain and form synapses with neurons in the appropriate nuclei has not yet been investigated.

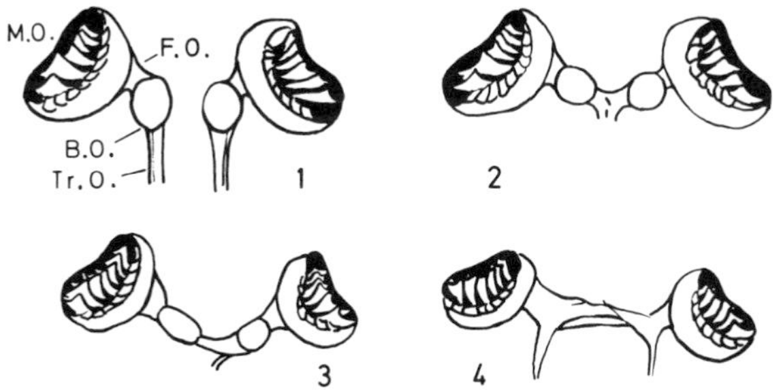

Fig. 8. Gross anatomy of the olfactory system in intact animals (*1*) and in animals 21 months after extirpation of the olfactory bulbs (*2–4*). *B.O.*, bulbus olfactorius; *F.O.*, fila olfactoria; *M.O.*, mucosa olfactoria; *Tr.O.*, tractus olfactorius

4 Discussion

The present investigations on gustatory and olfactory learning in bulbectomized and sham-operated goldfish at various times after surgery are based on extensive studies of the behaviour of intact animals trained to respond to taste (Schoon 1976) or odour (Voigt, unpublished material) stimuli. The animals were maintained under identical conditions and the same shock-free training and testing procedure was employed. The latter permits a detailed analysis of the fish's behaviour and thus enables an accurate evaluation of their learning performance.

Firstly, it should be emphasized that no changes were detectable in the gross postoperative behaviour (swimming movements, feeding behaviour, general activity, etc.) of the bulbectomized animals.

The main aim of the first two series of experiments with animals immediately following bulbectomy was to test the hypothesis that olfactory perception interferes in some way with the gustatory input during training to organic acids. Electrophysiological investigations on taste fibres in the carp (Konishi and Zotterman 1964), a close relative of the goldfish, have established the importance of sour stimuli, and anatomical studies (Andres, pers. comm.) have shown that the sense of taste in cyprinid fish (with respect to the number of taste buds and their central representation) is the most highly developed in the vertebrate kingdom. Recordings from single neurons in the goldfish olfactory bulb, on the other hand, demonstrated that different taste stimuli induced markedly different effects when applied to the olfactory mucosa (Zippel et al. 1978b): organic acids modulated the activity of up to 80% of the recorded neurons, whereas sweet, salty or bitter stimuli caused fewer neurons to respond.

In the first series, only the sham-operated animals showed an improvement in performance during reversal training (glucose, reinforced/acetic acid, non-reinforced). In the second series (malonic acid, reinforced/acetic acid, non-reinforced), however, the bulbectomized animals learnt the task more quickly. These differences would appear to indicate that the olfactory component of acetic acid enhances the sham-operated (olfactorily intact) animals' discriminative ability, providing the competing (non-reinforced) stimulus is of little or no olfactory significance, or is of another gustatory quality (glucose in series I). If, however, both stimuli are of the same gustatory quality (series II), the animals' performance seems to be more or less concentration dependent; where a concentration difference exists, the bulbectomized collectives are not influenced by interacting olfactory components and thus acquire the discrimination more rapidly.

It should be emphasized that the use of SEM in the present investigations only permitted a description of the degenerative and regenerative processes at the surface of the olfactory mucosa. From light microscopic material, which will be presented and discussed with a number of other topics of interest elsewhere, and from the work of other authors (e.g., Graziadei and Monti Graziadei 1978; Monti Graziadei and Graziadei 1979), there is ample evidence that receptor cells can be regenerated from basal cells, and the latter are extremely well developed in the goldfish. The present findings show that the rate at which the various types of sensory cell degenerate and regenerate is dependent not only on the type of receptor but also on its location on the olfactory lamella. Whether these data can be interpreted in favour of a transition from microvilli to ciliated receptor cells, or whether these two types do indeed have a different biological regenerative capacity, must await further clarification (Breipohl and Ohyama, in press). After a period of 7–11 months there is a more or less complete restoration of the sensory input to the olfactory system and the axons of these regenerated cells subsequently sprout out in the direction of the olfactory bulb. These findings formed the basis for the long-term behavioural investigations.

The final experimental series showed that, in a number of respects, the behaviour of long-term regenerated animals contrasts markedly not only with that of animals immediately after bulbectomy but also with that of intact animals:

1. The responsiveness to different odour concentrations lies between that of intact animals (lowest threshold) and that of freshly bulbectomized animals (highest threshold; Voigt, unpublished data).
2. The animals display typical olfactory learning curves when trained with synthetic odours applied in concentrations on the threshold between gustation and olfaction, but, unlike intact animals, they do not respond to concentrations below this level.
3. With taste stimuli, typical, but "shortened", gustatory learning curves are obtained, the behavioural threshold being roughly 1.5 log units, i.e., about 50-fold, below that of intact animals.

These findings may be interpreted in one of two ways: firstly, as recently demonstrated by morphological studies in mice (Graziadei 1977), the axons of regenerated receptor cells might reach the forebrain and form synapses at the olfactory nuclei, thus enabling olfactory perception, albeit at a higher threshold; secondly, following bulbectomy, the gustatory system constitutes the only input for external chemical stimuli and it might thus become adapted for use over the whole sensitivity range, affording reactions to stimulus concentrations which in intact animals would chiefly be perceived via the olfactory system. Morphological investigations shortly to be performed on the long-term bulbectomized animals should provide evidence in support of one of these explanations.

Although a number of questions are still to be answered, the work reported here gives an indication of the extent of the changes which can occur in an animal's behaviour following extirpation of the olfactory bulbs. Furthermore, the findings reveal a remarkable plasticity in the central nervous system of a so-called primitive vertebrate, the goldfish, the behavioural responsiveness of which has often been considered unmodifiable.

Acknowledgment. Supported by Deutsche Forschungsgemeinschaft, SFB 33 (Nervensystem und biologische Information) and SFB 114 (BIONACH).

References

Breipohl W, Ohyama M (in press) Comparative and developmental SEM studies on vertebrate olfactory epithelia (Biomedical aspects and speculations). J Biomed Res 1: Suppl

Breipohl W, Bijvank GJ, Zippel HP (1973) Rastermikroskopische Untersuchungen der olfaktorischen Rezeptoren im Riechepithel des Goldfisches (Carassius auratus). Z Zellforsch 138: 439–454

Gaze RM, Jacobson M (1963) A study of retinotectal projection during regeneration of the optic nerve in the frog. Proc R Soc London Ser B 157: 420–448

Graziadei PPC (1978) The olfactory sensory neuron as a model for the study of regeneration. ECRO 3rd Congr, Pavia, p 60

Graziadei PPC, Monti Graziadei GA (1978) The olfactory system: a model for the study of neurogenesis and axon regeneration in mammals. In: Cotman CW (ed) Neuronal plasticity. Raven Press, New York, pp 131–153

Kirsche W, Kirsche K (1960) Experimentelle Untersuchungen zur Frage der Regeneration und Funktion des Tectum opticum von Carassius carassius L. Z Mikrosk Anat Forsch 67: 141–182

Konishi J, Zotterman Y (1964) Taste functions in fish. In: Zotterman Y (ed) Olfaction and taste. Pergamon Press, Oxford, pp 215–233

Maier W, Wolburg H (1979) Regeneration of the goldfish retina after exposure to different doses of quabain. Cell Tissue Res 202: 99–118

Monti Graziadei GA, Graziadei PPC (1979) Neurogenesis and neuron regeneration in the olfactory system of mammals. II. Degeneration and reconstitution of the olfactory sensory neurons after axotomy. J Neurocytol 8: 197–213

Schoon H (1976) Verhaltensmuster-Detailanalysen zum geschmacklichen Diskriminationslernen und zum Geschmacksgedächtnis im straffreien Dressurverfahren beim Goldfisch (Carassius auratus). Diss Rer Nat, Univ Göttingen

Segaar J (1965) Behavioural aspects of degeneration and regeneration in fish brain: a comparison with higher vertebrates. In: Singer M, Schade JP (eds) Degeneration patterns in the nervous system. Progress in Brain Research, vol 14. Elsevier Publ Co, Amsterdam New York Oxford, pp 143–231

Sperry RW (1955) Functional regeneration in the optic system. In: Windle WF (ed) Regeneration in the central nervous system. Charles C Thomas, Springfield Ill, pp 66–76

Takagi SF (1971) Regeneration of the olfactory epithelium after degeneration. In: Beidler LM (ed) Chemical senses – olfaction. Handbook of Sensory Physiology, vol IV. Springer, Berlin Heidelberg New York, pp 75–94

Windle WF(ed) (1955) Regeneration in the central nervous system. Charles C Thomas, Springfield, Ill

Winkelmann E, Marx I (1969) Experimentelle Untersuchungen über die mikroskopischen und submikroskopischen Veränderungen im Telencephalon von Ambystoma mexicanum nach Resektion des Riechorgans. Z Mikrosk Anat Forsch 81: 71–95

Winkelmann E, Winkelmann A (1970) Experimentelle Untersuchungen zur Regeneration des Telencephalon von Ambystoma mexicanum nach Resektion beider Hemisphären. Z Mikrosk Anat Forsch 82: 149–171

Zippel HP (1970) Verhaltenskomponenten und Differenzierungsvermögen in der straffreien Geruchsdressur beim Goldfisch (Carassius auratus). Z Vergl Physiol 69: 54–78

Zippel HP, Westerman RA (1970) Geruchsdifferenzierungsvermögen der Karausche (Carassius carassius) nach funktioneller und histologischer Regeneration des Tractus olfactorius und der Commissura anterior. Z Vergl Physiol 69: 38–53

Zippel HP, v Baumgarten R, Westerman RA (1970) Histologische, funktionelle und spezifische Regeneration nach Durchtrennung der Fila olfactoria beim Goldfisch (Carassius auratus). Z Vergl Physiol 69: 79–98

Zippel HP, Schoon H, Voigt R (1978a) Functional and electrophysiological evidence for separation of smell and taste in the goldfish (Carassius auratus). Drug Res 28: 2368–2369

Zippel HP, Fiedler W, Maier K (1978b) Effects of taste stimuli at the level of the second neuron in the olfactory bulb of the goldfish (Carassius auratus). Pflügers Arch 373: R 91

Subject Index

H. Stephan, G. Baron, W. K. Schwerdtfeger

The Brain of the Common Marmoset (Callithrix jacchus)

A Stereotaxic Atlas

1980. 5 figures, 3 tables, 73 plates. V, 91 pages
ISBN 3-540-09782-1

Contents: Introduction. – Material. – Zero Coordinates. – Reference Coordinates. – Histological Procedures. – Shrinkage Factors. – Variability. – Standardization Proposals. – Photomicrographs for Atlas. – Presentation and Nomenclature. – References. – Index.

Marmosets belong to the anthropoid or simian primates which include species closest to man. In contrast to other simians, the care and breeding of marmosets is relatively easy and their reproduction rate considerably higher. These characteristics make marmosets of great interest for primate research, especially as the supply of simians from the wild becomes increasingly limited. This atlas presents 73 photomicrographs of serial sections from the brains of common marmosets. Taken at 0.5 mm intervals, the sections are stained for both cells and nerve fibers and shown on facing pages for comparison. Stereotaxic coordinates are labelled in detail and methods for their standardization discussed. The accuracy of the stereotaxic description provided here will greatly aid researchers using marmoset brains for neurophysiologic, neuroanatomic, neurochemical and behavioral investigations.

Springer-Verlag
Berlin
Heidelberg
New York

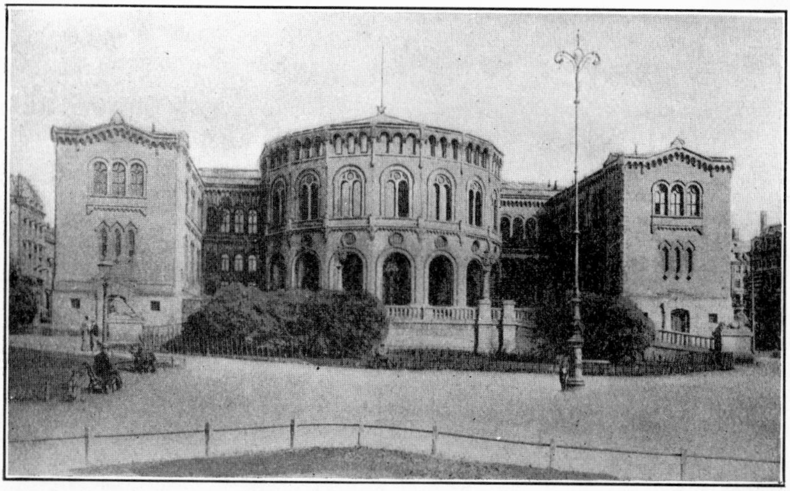

The Storthing Building.

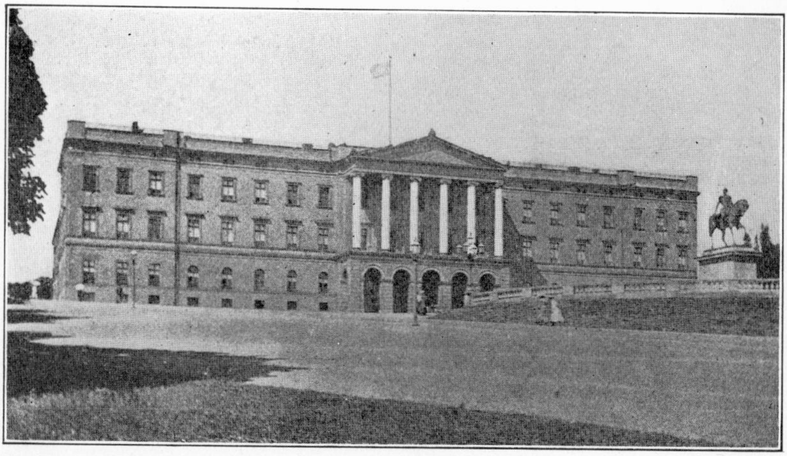

Royal Palace, Christiania.

constitute a reserve fund to be used only in cases of emergency. On May 10th the special committee submitted a bill providing for the creation of a separate Norwegian consular service. The law should go into effect April 1, 1906, and the government should be instructed to notify the Swedish government that the joint consular service would terminate on that date. The bill was passed by both branches of the Storthing unanimously after a very short debate. The resolution that the Swedish government should be notified of the termination of the joint consular service was passed against ten dissenting votes.

It was hoped by some that the king would sanction the bill. Many believed, or professed to believe, that as king of Norway he would yield to the unanimous wish of the people. But in this they were disappointed. At a meeting of the joint Swedish-Norwegian ministry in Stockholm the Norwegian members, Løvland, Bothner, and E. Hagerup Bull, strongly urged him to sanction the measure, but he yielded to the wish of his Swedish advisers, and vetoed it. The Norwegian members refused to countersign the veto, and immediately handed him their resignations.[1] These he would not accept, as he feared that he would get no new Norwegian ministers. But they would not undertake the responsibility of remaining in office, and returned to Christiania. The whole ministry thereupon notified the king that they found it necessary to retire from office, and no one could be found in all Norway willing to attempt to form a new ministry under the circumstances.

The ultimate crisis had been foreseen, and the people remained calm and collected. The press indulged in no invectives, but spoke with a firmness and straightforwardness which could not be misunderstood. "The Swedish papers fear that Norway will violate the

[1] The Swedish professor Wicksell, of the university of Lund, wrote: "If such a demand as King Oscar made in a letter to President Berner, that the king's will even without the advice of a responsible ministry has the character of a public act and can void a resolution passed by the Storthing, had been made in Sweden, it would have been met with indignant protest by all parties. Such a king's days, not to say hours, would surely have been numbered in Sweden."

The German paper, *Frankfurter Zeitung*, said, June 8, 1905: "If there is a revolution, it has been started by the king, and not by the Storthing." Unset Jaren, *Hvem tvang os ind i, og hvem tvang os atter ud av Unionen?* p. 50.

constitution," wrote "Verdens Gang," June 5th. "There is no cause for anxiety. The constitution will be upheld on all points where it has not been violated by others. In Sweden they have found it necessary to deprive us of our king. He has been deposed without coöperation from Norway. On the contrary, his Norwegian advisers made the most earnest remonstrances to prevent it, but to no avail. The king of Norway has been deposed in Sweden. Thereby certain changes took place in the constitution itself. The Norwegian government will prove that this has happened, and thereupon, supported by the nation, without hesitation or excitement, it will undertake to establish normal conditions in the country on the basis of the constitution."[1] On June 7, 1905, the Storthing assembled to receive notice of the resignation of the ministry. After the minister of state, Christian Michelsen, had reported the king's veto of the consular bill, and had stated that he and his colleagues had found it necessary to resign, as they would not be responsible for the step taken by the king, the president of the Storthing, Carl Berner, proposed the following resolution: "Whereas all the members of the ministry have resigned, and whereas His Majesty the king has declared himself unable to secure a new cabinet, and whereas the constitutional royal power thereby has ceased to operate, the Storthing empowers the members of the ministry which has this day retired from office to act as a temporary government for Norway, and to exercise the powers granted the king in accordance with the constitution and the laws of the kingdom, subject to the changes made necessary by the fact that the union between Sweden and Norway under the same king is dissolved, and that the king has ceased to act as king of Norway."[2] No one asked for the floor to discuss the resolution, and it was passed unanimously without being debated. A communication was also sent to the king, informing him of the dissolution of the union, and asking him to consent to the election of one of the Bernadotte princes as king of Norway. The union existed no longer. Norway and Sweden had parted, but the greatest anxiety prevailed, and every one asked himself: "What will Sweden do?"

[1] Quoted by J. E. Sars, *Norges Historie*, vol. VI., 2, p. 253.
[2] F. V. Heiberg, *Unionens Opløsning 1905*, p. 289 f.

PLATE XXIV

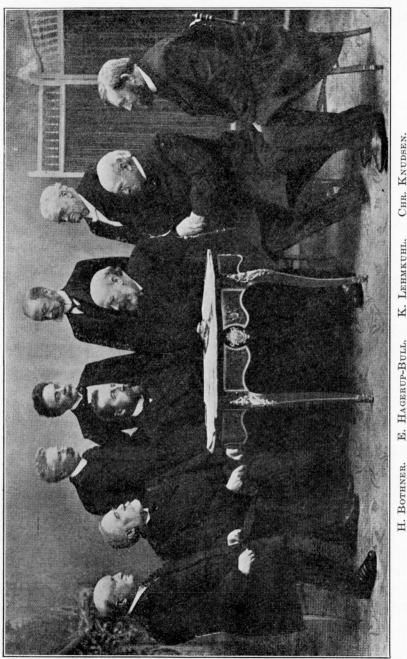

H. Bothner. E. Hagerup-Bull. K. Lehmkuhl. Chr. Knudsen.
W. Olssøn. Sofus Arctander. Chr. Michelsen. J. Løvland. Gunnar Knudsen. A. Vinje.

The Michelsen Ministry.

Norway was well prepared for the emergency, but Sweden has a population more than twice as numerous, led by a strong nobility, jealous of their honor, and proud of their country's former greatness. No one could doubt that the dissolution of the union by Norway's own fiat would be a rude shock which would be felt especially by the Swedish nobility as a distinct humiliation, and war between the two nations, long and destructive, equally ruinous to both, might be the unavoidable result. But many circumstances served to restrain the ardor of those who felt disposed to make the sword the arbiter of the dispute. The introduction of a new army organization, which had been but half completed, and the lack of stores and ammunition greatly reduced the efficiency of the Swedish military forces. The possibility of Russian aggression, as well as the sympathy for Norway shown by the great powers, would render a war hazardous even under more favorable circumstances, and King Oscar II., who had always been a noble-minded friend of peace, would scarcely now in his old age embroil the two nations in a fratricidal war for the preservation of a union which could be maintained only by sacrificing the peace and well-being of both peoples. Among the common classes in Sweden the desire for a peaceful settlement of the difficulty was very strong. The laborers, socialists, and numerous friends of the peace movement spoke in defense of Norway, and declared themselves opposed to war in a manner which must have made a deep impression. "The day when old Sweden recognizes that goodness is greatness, and abandons all evil with its empty titles, the day when our national assembly joins the Storthing in a friendly dissolution of the union, will be a holy day, and all Swedes will be a united people," wrote K. P. Arnoldson, one of the leading Swedish peace advocates. "The safest thing in the midst of all uncertainty," he says in another place, "is to be just to your neighbor, be he an individual or a nation. Let the Norwegians be permitted to manage their own affairs in peace. This principle the press with its great influence should impress upon the people's mind during the growing difficulties. This is an admonition as well as a prayer. It is the prayer of one who loves his country."[1] In 1905 the Swedish peace association decided to join in the May demonstrations of the

[1] K. P. Arnoldson. *Unionens sidste Dagar*, p. 21, p. 27.

labor organizations, and on the 1st of May a procession numbering 30,000 marched through the streets of Stockholm. The peace association carried two banners with the inscription: "Justice to Norway, Peace with Norway," and "Pax quaeretur Justitia" (peace is secured by justice). Emil Gullers spoke to the vast audience on the subject "Peace with Norway," and emphasized that peace is won by justice, as stated on the peace banner. But justice to Norway required the application of the Golden Rule: "Therefore all things whatsoever that ye would that men should do to you, do ye even so to them." "Justice to Norway," said the speaker, was interpreted correctly by the Norwegian peace advocate, who said: "Sweden should treat Norway as the Swedes would wish to be treated by the Norwegians, if Norway was the larger and stronger nation." After the speech the vast audience sang the Norwegian national song: "Ja, vi elsker dette Landet," and the following resolutions were adopted by all the 30,000 people assembled:

"We, the laborers and other peace loving and liberal-minded men and women of Stockholm, express our positive disapproval of the short-sighted union policy of our government and the Swedish Conservative press, which endangers the union of the two countries, and the future welfare of both nations.

"Union and good understanding with Norway can be maintained only through complete equality of the two kingdoms, and the unqualified recognition of the right of both to manage their own affairs, including such foreign affairs as concern either kingdom alone.

"We demand that our government shall respect Norway's right to establish a separate consular service, and that so soon as a measure is submitted which has been passed by the Storthing and sanctioned by the cabinet, negotiations with Norway shall immediately be instituted for the purpose of effecting an arrangement of the administration of foreign affairs which will receive the sanction and support of both peoples.

"We demand justice for Norway, peace with Norway."[1]

No one exerted a greater influence for peace than the Swedish statesman, Adolf Hedin. J. Løvland, Norwegian minister of state

[1] Emil Gullers, *Fred med Norge.* Gustaf Edw. Fahlcrantz, *Sveriges Rätt och Pligt.* Ernst Liljedahl, *Sveriges Rätt och Ära.*

in Stockholm, writes: "I received him in the minister's hotel in Stockholm after the king had refused to sanction the consular bill. When he heard what had happened, he talked a long time about the situation. He was sick and suffered much. Death had already set its mark upon him, but he retained his interest with wonderful energy. When I had helped him down the stairway and through the entrance he said with tears in his eyes: 'Farewell. I see what will follow. You are the last Norwegian minister of state in Stockholm. My hope of a happy union between the three free and independent Northern nations has been shattered. But possibly it is best. If we only can avoid inaugurating the future with war and brother hatred! My days are soon ended. Farewell!' During the whole summer he used his influence for peace in the press and in the Rigsdag. I received many letters from him, but I could not answer them until I was in Karlstad. Then I wrote him, and asked him not to refuse reëlection to the Rigsdag. Later I was able to telegraph that there was prospect of a peaceful settlement. This news gave him great joy in his last moments. He died before the Karlstad negotiations were completed."[1]

When the king was notified that Norway had dissolved the union, he immediately telegraphed an earnest protest, and the Rigsdag was convened in extra session to consider the situation. A proposition submitted by the ministry recommended that no attempt should be made to preserve the union by force, as a union so maintained would be a source of weakness rather than of strength. But the union could not be dissolved without the consent of Sweden, and a demand would be made for a satisfactory settlement of various important matters, as this alone could insure peaceful relations in the future. In order that an agreement might be reached on the basis of which the dissolution of the union could be effected, the king should be empowered to institute negotiations with Norway. The proposition was referred to a special committee, which submitted its report July 25. The report represents a compromise between the extreme views of those who demanded that Norway should be subdued by force of arms, and those who favored a peaceful dissolution of the union without any attempt to dictate terms. As conditions for

[1] *For Alle, norsk Kalender*, 1909, p. 76 f.

consent to the dissolution the committee proposed that Norway should present a formal request after a new Storthing had been elected, and after the Norwegian people through a plebiscite should signify their desire for the dissolution of the union. If these conditions were complied with, negotiations might be entered into for the arrangement of terms, on which the final agreement might be based. This measure was passed by the Rigsdag, but on the same day, even before it had been officially announced in Norway, a government bill was introduced in the Storthing ordering a general plebiscite in order that the people might get an opportunity to ratify the step taken on June 7th. The bill was unanimously passed, and the plebiscite, which was held August 13, 1905, revealed a singular unanimity. The notice given was very brief, and many sailors and fishermen could not reach home in so short a time. But of the 435,576 voters in the kingdom, 371,911, or 85 per cent, were able to cast their ballot. Of these, 368,208 voted in favor of the dissolution of the union, and 184 against it. 3519 ballots were discarded. Never has a nation expressed a more unanimous opinion on a public question, and never has a people made a more determined effort to be present at the polls.[1] The Storthing thereupon extended a formal request to Sweden to coöperate in the dissolution of the union by entering into negotiations for the purpose of arriving at an agreement. A committee consisting of Christian Michelsen, J. Løvland, Carl Berner, and B. Vogt was appointed to treat with a similar Swedish committee, consisting of the minister of state, Lundberg, and the cabinet members, Wachtmeister, Hammarskjöld, and Staaff. During the negotiations, which were carried on at Karlstad from August 31 till September 23, 1905, great anxiety prevailed, and troops were stationed on both sides of the border. But the committees finally succeeded in reaching an agreement. Both kingdoms agreed to submit to the Hague Tribunal all controversies which they cannot settle by direct negotiations, providing that they do not involve the independence, integrity, or vital interests of either kingdom.

Along both sides of the border from Fredrikshald and Strømstad to a point where Ulvå and Klarälv cut the sixty-first parallel, a

[1] F. V. Heiberg, *Unionens Opløsning 1905*, p. 309 ff. Yngvar Nielsen, *Norge i 1905*, p. 433 ff.

PLATE XXV

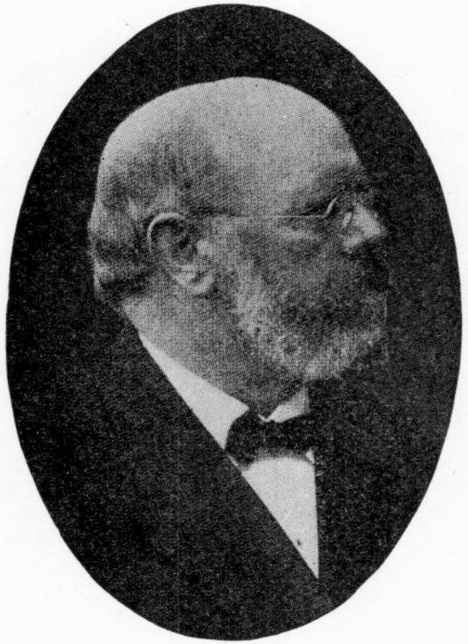

Jørgen Løvland.

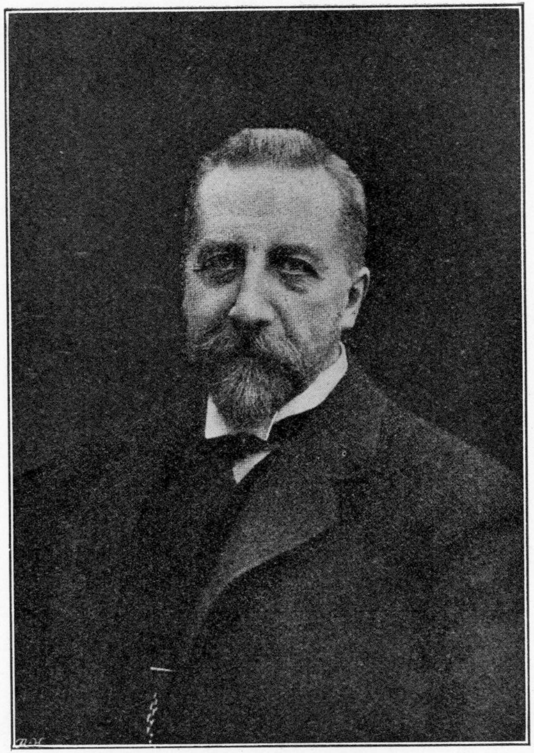

Christian Michelsen.

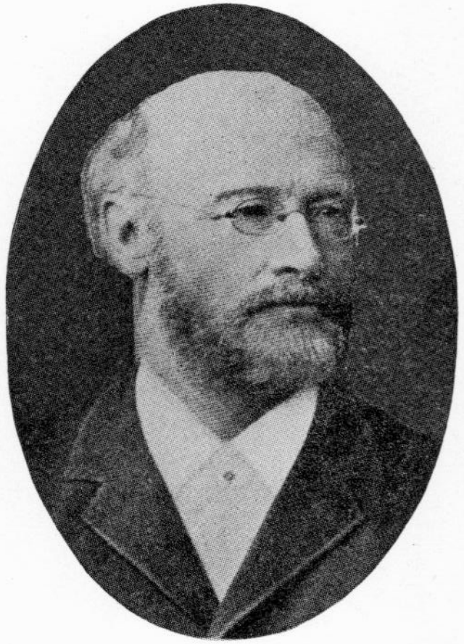

Carl Berner.

neutral zone was created, inside of which no military operations of any kind can be carried on. The new fortresses which of late years had been erected within that zone should be razed, and no new ones are to be erected in the future.[1]

For humanitarian reasons the Finns, who live as nomads in the northern part of both countries, should be allowed to enjoy the same privileges which were granted them by codicil I, in the treaty of 1751. But the law of 1883, which had been substituted for this codicil, is to remain in force till 1917.

Both kingdoms pledged themselves not to hinder or prohibit the free transportation of goods in transit through either realm, and rules were established for the utilization of lakes and water courses common to both countries.

The clause providing for a neutral zone and the dismantling of the fortresses created much ill-will in Norway, as it was felt that Sweden sought to humiliate the kingdom. Both in the press and in the Storthing spirited protests were made against these features of the agreement,[2] but the members of the committee conducting the negotiations, and their supporters, showed that the fortresses in question were of little or no military value. It was urged that in order to avoid war and all its evil consequences the conditions ought to be accepted, as they involved no vital interests, and as Sweden would accept nothing less. This wisely chosen course of the most prudent leaders finally prevailed. On October 9th the agreement submitted by the committee was sanctioned by the Storthing, only sixteen votes being registered against it. The Swedish Rigsdag annulled the Act of Union October 16th, and authorized the king to recognize the union as dissolved.[3] On October 27th

[1] The fortresses which had to be razed were: Urskog (Dingsrud), Ørje, and Kroksund, and the new fortresses of Fredriksten, Gyldenløve, Overbjerget, Veden, and Hjelmkollen. The old fortifications at Fredriksten, with which many historic memories are associated, remain, but they are not to be used for military purposes. Kongsvinger was left outside the neutral zone, but its fortifications are not to be extended or increased.

[2] *Hvad Landet mener; Karlstadforhandlingerne og Grænsefæstningerne.* This is a collection of quotations from forty-eight Norwegian papers regarding the Karlstad agreement. Christiania, 1905. H. D. Lowzow, *Grænseforterne, en militær Utredning.*

[3] *The Act of Union* was in reality a treaty between the two nations. See N. Gjelsvik, *Rigsakten som Traktat, Samtiden,* 1905.

King Oscar II. issued a proclamation to the Norwegian people announcing his abdication as king of Norway. To this he added the statement that he could not consent to the election of a prince of his family as successor to the vacant throne.

After the union with Sweden had been dissolved, the attention was directed to the problem of establishing a new government. Many hoped that a republic would be proclaimed,[1] but all agreed that on account of the gravity of the situation any agitation for the purpose of changing the form of government would be inopportune and unwise. By preserving the old Norwegian throne the new government would revive in a most direct way the proudest traditions of the past, and no great change would have to be made in the constitution. The leading men were in favor of a liberal monarchy,[2] and the people would be sure to welcome a national king appearing as the successor of the Haralds, Haakons, and Olavs who in time past had made Norway great.

After Oscar II. had signified his unwillingness to consent to the choice of a Bernadotte prince, the government turned to Prince Charles of Denmark. This step was supported by the press, and it soon became clear that, if elected, the prince would be received with enthusiasm in Norway. Through marriage with Princess Maude, daughter of Edward VII. of England, he was closely related to the English royal family, which could only serve to strengthen the friendship between the two realms. Prince Charles declared himself willing to accept the throne, if the Norwegian people should signify their consent through a general plebiscite. The Storthing accordingly ordered a plebiscite to be held, November 12th–13th. Four-fifths of the total number of votes cast were registered in favor of the monarchical form of government and the election of Prince Charles. On November 18, 1905, the necessary changes were made in the constitution, and on the same day the prince was unanimously

[1] Nikolai Lundegaard, *Republik eller Kongedømme.* Stian Bech, *Kongedømme eller Republik.* Urbain Gohier, *La Republique escamotèe en Norwége,* Paris, 1905.

[2] *Norges Statsforfatning, Udtalelser af Bjørnstjerne Bjørnson, Fridtjof Nansen, Ernst Sars, Johan Bredal.* J. E. Sars, *Unionsopløsning og nationalt Kongedømme. Stortingspresident Berners Tale i Storthinget den 28de Oktober 1905.*

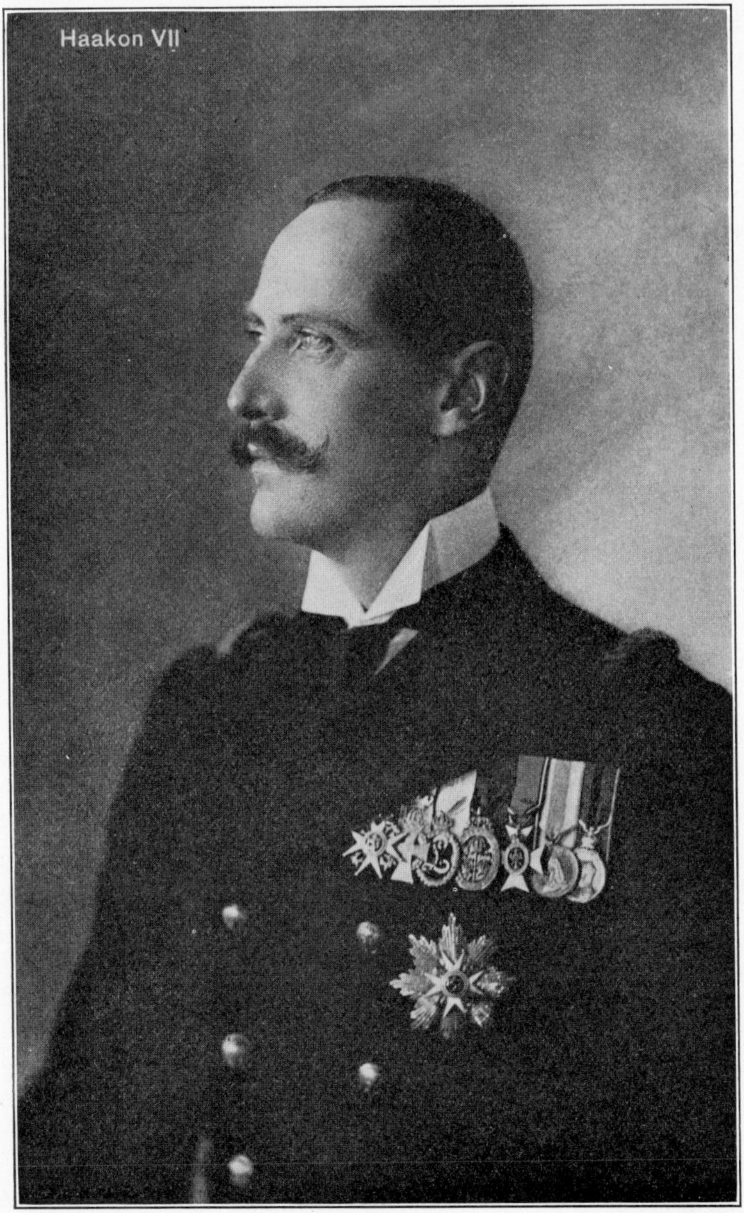

KING HAAKON VII. chocolate man

chosen king of Norway by the Storthing. In the afternoon session a telegram from the prince was read, through which he announced that he accepted the throne, that he assumed the name of Haakon VII., and that his little son, the crown prince, would be called Olav. On November 25th the king with Queen Maud and Prince Olav arrived in Norway, and two days later he took the oath on the constitution in the presence of the assembled Storthing. On June 22, 1906, King Haakon VII. and Queen Maude were crowned in the Trondhjem cathedral. After centuries of national obscurity, of bitter struggle for freedom and independence, the people could at last mingle their voices with the joyful anthems of praise and thanksgiving that Norway had gained her full freedom, untarnished by foreign guardianship, or irksome, unprofitable union with another state.

68. Political and Social Conditions, 1905–1914

Shortly after the coronation ceremonies, the campaign for the new elections was opened in Trondhjem by Christian Michelsen, who advocated a moderate policy aiming to secure further guarantees for the integrity and independence of Norway. He failed to secure a majority of the members returned, but his ministry remained in power for a time by mutual consent, as no party was strong enough to form a new ministry representing a majority. In 1907 a controversy arose regarding the regulation of the water in Lake Mjøsen. The different party groups combined against the ministry, and as Michelsen had been in delicate health for some time, he resigned. Before he left Christiania, 50,000 people marched to his residence to express their love and admiration for the retiring leader, who had guided the nation with such skill through the great crisis of 1905. On the 2nd of November a treaty, which was largely the result of his efforts, was concluded with England, France, Germany, and Russia, by which these powers agreed to guarantee the independence and integrity of the kingdom, Norway promising not to cede any territory to a foreign power. The treaty should remain in force for the period of ten years, and if not abrogated two years before the expiration of that term, it should be continued for another decade.

After Michelsen retired, J. Løvland, who had been minister of foreign affairs, formed a new cabinet. He is a statesman of great ability and sound liberal views, but he found difficulty in uniting a majority on any definite policy. The political parties were increasing in number, and the growing solicitude for the welfare of the common classes had created a great divergence of opinion on nearly all public questions. The Moderate Liberals, or Oftedøler, practically disappeared in 1900, but new parties appeared. The Labor party, organized in 1887, developed strong socialistic tendencies, and under the leadership of John Castberg, who entered the Storthing in 1900, it grew in strength and influence. In 1903 the Socialists, led by Alfred Eriksen, appeared as a new political party in the Storthing. Both these groups opposed the Løvland ministry, and other even more serious opposition was soon encountered. The question of conservation of natural resources, raised by the Michelsen ministry through the "concession laws," which aimed to prevent foreign capitalists from gaining permanent possession of the mines, forests, and waterfalls of the country, had developed into an issue which produced a split in the Coalition party. Gunnar Knudsen, who favored a strong conservation policy, seceded and organized the Radical Liberal party. Aided by the Socialists, this group succeeded in overthrowing the Løvland ministry, and Knudsen formed a new ministry in March, 1908. The remaining part of the Coalition party was organized into the Liberal-Liberal party (Frisindede Venstre) in 1909. According to conservative or radical tendencies the political parties in Norway now ranked as follows: Conservatives, Liberal-Liberals, Radical Liberals, Labor Party, and Socialists.

The attention of the new ministry was chiefly devoted to the problem of conservation of natural resources, probably the most important economic question which the Norwegian people has hitherto been called upon to settle. Norway, which was generally regarded as a poor country, where the tillable area is very small, and the natural resources limited, was found to possess great abundance of mineral-bearing rock and a vast amount of water power which can be turned into use in mining and manufacturing, the great wealth-producing industries of modern times. The rapid development of mining and manufacturing bid fair to revolutionize economic conditions in Norway, and to produce most important social changes, but no great harm may be done to the people's social well-being if an industrial life is developed as a result of inner national growth. The use of electric power makes it possible to eliminate one of the most objectionable features of modern industrial life, the grouping of factories in great commercial centers, due to the use of steam power, which requires a large supply of coal. The use of water power and electricity makes it convenient to locate factories in the neighborhood of waterfalls. This insures to the industrial laborers more healthy conditions, and tends to identify them socially with the rural rather than with the urban population, a feature which may prove of great importance in the future social development. But a danger of another kind threatened to make the new industrial development a most serious social problem. Foreign capitalists sought to acquire possession of the mines, waterfalls, and power stations of the country. This peaceful conquest made by foreign capital, if allowed to proceed unhindered, might lead to the establishing of the kind of industrial feudalism found in other countries where capitalism holds sway. Foreign laborers would be brought into the country, and the Norwegian people would be gradually reduced to a class of wage-earners toiling for foreign masters. Gunnar Knudsen, minister of state, wrote in 1910: "The question connected with the concession laws has been debated during the last four years. In 1906 the Michelsen ministry proposed the concession laws, which were called 'panic laws' by the Conservative press. At that time a veritable raid was made on our natural resources, especially by foreigners. But we might ask: Were there no laws which could put a stop to this raid? Yes, even the law of 1888 provides that foreigners in order to secure realty in this country must obtain concession or royal permission. But it appeared that it was the so-called Norwegian companies, capitalized by foreigners, who under this guise secured a very large share of our natural resources; not waterfalls alone, but also forests and mines. Then the Michelsen ministry proposed the so-called 'panic laws,' which provided that foreign stock companies had to obtain concession in order to obtain title to real estate in our country. This was a very important provision, and it was bitterly opposed. But the bill became a temporary law, which remained in force till last year, *i.e.* the temporary law was reënacted from year to year. But there was a constant demand that this temporary arrangement should cease." In 1909 the Knudsen ministry secured the passage of more rigorous concession laws, controlling the purchase of forests, mines, waterfalls, and power stations. In regard to real estate in general this law provides that foreigners must obtain concession in order to secure realty of any kind, but citizens and Norwegian stock companies may buy without concession timber areas not exceeding 250 acres. From 250 to 1250 acres may be bought by Norwegian citizens, or local communities, with the restriction, however, that they must not own over one-tenth of the total timber area of the *herred,* and the community has the right of preëmption in all such purchases. The aim of this provision is to prevent foreign as well as native capitalists from securing possession of the forests, which are to be left as far as possible in the hands of the local communities.

With regard to mining the law provides that prospecting and trial operation may be carried on without concession, but the right to work a mine must be secured through concession, which imposes several conditions. The government has the right to impose a tax of three per cent, figured on the value of the output of the mine. The concession is granted only for a fixed period, not exceeding eighty years, after which time the ownership of the ceded property, together with machinery and improvements, reverts to the government without compensation.

The purchase and sale of waterfalls and rapids representing less than 1000 horse power are unrestricted. The right to use larger waterfalls must be secured through concession, which imposes quite rigid conditions. Citizens must be allowed to become partners in the undertaking for which the concession is granted, and conditions may be established preventing persons who use another waterfall, or who own a majority of shares in another company, from securing a majority of shares in the new undertaking. The *herred* in which the power station is located is to receive at a moderate price for public use five per cent of the power developed, and the state is to receive five per cent on the same conditions. The concession is granted for a period of not less than sixty years, and not more than eighty years. After this period the waterfalls, dams, water mains, pipes, etc., become the property of the state without compensation.[1]

The most important feature of the concession laws is the provision that mines and waterfalls can be leased only for a term of years, and that at the expiration of that period these resources, together with improvements, revert to the state. This constitutes an effective barrier against the creation of monopolies controlled by foreign capital. The Conservatives, who opposed the measure as socialistic legislation, directed their attack against this feature of the law. It was claimed that such a provision was unconstitutional, that it violated the right of private ownership, that it would destroy personal initiative, and would retard progress by keeping foreign capital out of the country. But the supporters of the measure preferred to insure to the people full control of the natural resources of the country, even if industrial development should make slower progress, and the wisdom of this policy is now generally recognized. The prophecies of the opponents have failed to materialize. Rapid industrial progress is being made under the new law, and the feeling that the new industries in reality belong to the whole people has created a confidence and optimism which will insure a rapid development of energy and talent in Norway's industrial growth.

In the elections of 1909 the Conservatives and Liberal-Liberals combined, and succeeded in electing sixty-four representatives as against forty-eight Radical Liberals and eleven Socialists. Of the majority group forty-eight were Conservatives and nineteen Liberals. Owing to this defeat the Knudsen ministry resigned, and W. Konow of Søndre Bergenhus, leader of the Liberal-Liberals, formed a new ministry in the winter of 1910. Both the Conservatives and the Liberals recommended state accident insurance and sickness insurance for seamen, and old age pensions for all persons above seventy years. Both parties favored a restriction of the concession laws, and demanded that the right of private ownership should

[1] Gunnar Knudsen, *Foredrag om Koncessionslovene i Kristianias Handelsstands Forening*, 1910. *I Dagens Strid*, II. *Vor økonomiske Politik*, Christiania, 1909. *Koncessionslovene, Redaktør Løkens Foredrag i Handelsforeningen*, 1909. *Norsk Lovtidende*, 1909, p. 533 ff. *Lov av 1909*.

not be impaired. Both demanded the maintenance of the parliamentary form of government, and advocated the establishing of referendum and the right of the king to dissolve the Storthing. The Conservatives also inclined to favor a royal suspensive veto in cases of constitutional amendments. The last planks of their platform were attacked by Otto Albert Blehr in a speech in Bergen, September 4, 1910. He showed that these features belonged to different political systems; that the right to dissolve the Storthing is a feature of parliamentary government not to be recommended in Norway, where the representatives are elected for the short period of three years, though it is used in England, where the representatives are elected for the period of seven years. The referendum is opposed in principle to the parliamentary system, as it removes the decision of important measures from the legislature, and gives it to the whole people.[1] Neither of these features was carried through by the new ministry, nor were any changes made in the concession laws; but some progress was made in legislation aiming at securing better conditions for the laboring classes, a problem to which the more radical parties had devoted special attention.

By the law of 1894 government accident insurance was established for certain classes of laborers engaged in more dangerous pursuits. All employers in these occupations are required to insure their laborers. The required assessments are collected by the government, and all accidents must be reported to the *Rigsforsikringsanstalt*, or Government Insurance Commission, which has full management of this kind of insurance, and decides what damages are to be paid. The employers cannot be held responsible for accidents, as the government through its inspectors provides all possible safety appliances for the protection of the laborers, and the damages are paid by the commission in form of insurance. This law was supplemented by new measures in 1899, 1906, 1908, and 1911, by which the accident insurance was extended to an ever larger number of occupations.

[1] *Stiftsamtmand Blehrs Foredrag i Bergen 4de September 1910 om Grundlovsvetoet og dets Forbindelse med Høireforeningens nye Programsaker: Opløsningsret og Folkeavstemning.* Aa. Bryggesaa, *Bør Opløsningsret opstilles som Valgprogram? I Dagens Strid*, I.

By the law of 1909 sickness insurance was made compulsory for all laborers above fifteen years of age who had an income not exceeding 1200 kroner in the rural districts, or 1400 kroner in the cities.[1] They are divided according to their income into four classes, receiving a proportionate indemnity in case of sickness. Two-tenths of the premium is paid by the state, one-tenth by the employer, one-tenth by the community, and six-tenths by the laborers collectively. For other laborers the insurance is voluntary, if their yearly income does not exceed 800 kroner in the country, or 1000 kroner in the cities, or if their estates do not exceed 7000 kroner in the country, or 10,000 kroner in the cities. In 1914 the law was made to include laborers with an income of 1600 kroner in the country and 1800 kroner in the cities. The insured are now divided into five classes, receiving an indemnity of 0.60, 0.90, 1.50, 2.10, and 2.70 kroner per day.

Unemployment insurance according to the St. Gallen system was introduced by the law of 1906, according to which the government furnishes one-fourth of the out-of-work benefits paid by the various labor organizations. The local communities to which the unemployed belong must, however, reimburse the government two-thirds of the sum furnished.

Strict control of the use of intoxicating liquors has also helped to improve the conditions of the laboring classes. In 1871 the Gottenburg system was introduced in Norway. In 1894 the rules for the organization of companies for selling liquors under this system were made more rigid, and in 1904 a law was passed which reduced the sale and use of intoxicants to a minimum, and placed Norway next to Finland at the very top of the list in regard to temperance.[2] According to this law the beverages which are subject to control

[1] *I Dagens Strid*, I., O. A. Eftestøl, *Sykeforsikringen. Det norske Venstre fra 1884 til 1909, V., Sociale Spørgsmaal.* E. H. Downey, in his work *Accident Indemnity in Iowa*, points out that the Norwegian plan of state insurance for accidents has been adopted also by American legislators. See p. 127, 152. Frankel and Dawson, *Workingmen's Insurance in Europe. Illustreret norsk Konversations-Leksikon, Sykeforsikringen.*

[2] Eilert Sundt, *Ædruelighedstilstanden i Norge.* Hs. Gurstad, *Lov om Salg og Skjænkning af Brændevin, Øl, Vin, Frugtvin og Mjød, af 17de Mai 1904.* Knut Gjerset, *Brændevins Samlagene og Avholdsarbeidet i Norge*, Decorah, Iowa, 1911. Absalon Taranger, *Borregaardsprivilegiet, Dokument Nr. 15.*

are divided into two groups: (1) Distilled liquors, including all beverages containing above fifteen per cent of spirit, and all wines containing above twenty-one per cent of spirit. (2) Fermented liquors, including wine, beer, mead, and cider, containing a less per cent of spirit than the first class. Denatured alcohol is not included in either group.

Regarding the right to prepare distilled liquors, strict rules are found in the law of 1887. They must be manufactured in distilleries controlled by the state through its inspectors, and the internal revenue amounts to 1.68 kroner per liter, figured on the basis of a purity of 100 per cent. The distillers may sell to any one in quantities not less than 250 liters (a little over fifty-nine gallons). They may also sell in small quantities of not less than 0.35 liter on sealed bottles, which must not be opened at the place of purchase: (*a*) to those who have a concession to retail liquor, (*b*) for export, (*c*) for medical and scientific use. Concession to organize a company for selling intoxicating beverages is granted in a community only when a majority of all the voters of the district, both men and women, vote in favor of it, and only one such company can be organized in each community. The concession is granted for the period of six years, after which time the question must again be submitted to the vote of the people. The persons receiving the concession organize as a stock company, and choose a manager, who must be acceptable to the local authorities. Liquor may then be sold by the company in as many places in the community or city as the local authorities, or city council, may designate. The stock company doing business under the concession receives a profit of not more than five per cent a year on the capital invested. Of the surplus the community receives fifteen per cent, the stock company ten per cent, the *amt* ten per cent, and the government sixty-five per cent. The thirty-five per cent received by the company, the community, and the *amt* are used for public purposes for which funds have not otherwise been provided, but the money is so expended as not to reduce the burdens of taxation. The right to sell fermented liquors is granted by the local district authorities or the city council to companies or private persons. The places of sale and the number of such concessions are also determined by the same authorities.

The right of sale may be limited so that these beverages can be sold only to guests and travelers, as in hotels, or it may be a right to sell to all persons, except to children below the age of fifteen years. How effective this system has been in controlling the liquor traffic is shown by statistics. In all the country districts of Norway only six companies have been granted the right to sell liquor. In thirty-six cities no such right has been granted. In all the cities of Norway there are only 181 places where liquor is sold. The use of intoxicants has been correspondingly reduced. In 1833 the consumption of alcoholic beverages amounted to sixteen liters per capita. In 1900 it had been reduced to 2.9 liters. The use of alcohol and distilled liquors in the various countries in 1901–1905 was as follows:

	Distilled Liquors Liters	Alcohol Liters
Finland	2.8	1.9
Norway	3.2	2.4
Sweden	7.6	5.3
United States	5.4	5.5
Great Britain	4.5	7.8
Germany	8.	9.4
Denmark	14.1	10.9
France	7.	18.9[1]

The temperance movement has spread so rapidly in Norway that 237,000, or about ten per cent of the entire population, now belong to the various temperance organizations. The restriction in the use of intoxicants has resulted in a marked reduction in the percentage of still births and mortality among infants. Insanity, suicides, and deaths due to alcoholism have decreased, the number of persons in jails and penitentiaries has been reduced, much energy has been conserved for productive labor, and much poverty and misery have been averted. The successful work for temperance is now generally regarded as a most important step in the social development of the Norwegian people in modern times.

In 1912 the Konow ministry was overthrown by their Conservative allies, who objected to the opinion expressed by Konow on the question of the use of the *Landsmaal*. The controversy regarding

[1] Sundbärg, *Apercus statistiques internationaux*, 1908. The figures under *alcohol* represent the total amount of alcohol in distilled liquors, beer, and wine.

the relative position of the *Landsmaal* and the Danish-Norwegian language had grown very intense, and the Conservatives were very dissatisfied, because the *Landsmaal* had been placed on equal footing with the Danish-Norwegian. In 1878 the following rule was made by the government regarding the use of the *Landsmaal* in the public schools: "The instruction is to be given as far as possible in the children's own vernacular. Gradually they can then be taught to understand and write the Danish-Norwegian book language." In 1885 the *Landsmaal* was legalized as a standard official language equal to the Danish-Norwegian. The following motion was passed by the Storthing May 12th with seventy-eight votes against thirty-one: "The ministry is requested to make such arrangements that the Norwegian vernacular is placed on equal footing with our regular literary language as an official and school language."[1] In 1901–1902 it was introduced in the normal schools, or teachers' seminaries, on a par with the older literary language, and in 1907 a bill was passed by the Storthing providing that candidates for the degree of Bachelor of Arts should write two essays, one in each language, to show their knowledge of both. The *Landsmaal* had, finally, been accorded full recognition, and it is now extensively used in the schools, in the university lecture rooms, in the Storthing, and even by members of the cabinet. But a hostile agitation has been kept up against its use as an official and literary language, and especially against the test imposed on candidates for the B. A. degree. Most of the Conservatives could not be reconciled, and when Konow in a lecture expressed himself as favoring the *Landsmaal,* they turned against him, and forced him and his ministry to resign. A new ministry was formed February 20, 1912, by the Conservative leader Bratlie. He attacked the concession laws, and sought to effect the repeal of the provision by which they were made to apply to Norwegian stock companies. But in this attempt he failed. In the elections in the fall of 1912 his party was defeated. The Radicals and the Labor party captured seventy-six seats, and the Socialists twenty-three; the Conservatives and their allies the Liberals retained only twenty-four seats. Gunnar Knudsen, leader of the Radicals, returned to power as head of a new ministry.

[1] *I Dagens Strid*, I., J. Løvland, *Sprogenes Likestilling*.

The question of the king's veto power in cases of constitutional amendments had never been formally settled, but after 1905 no fear could be entertained that the king would ever again venture to assert such a prerogative. The matter might have received no further attention, if an incident had not occurred which made it necessary to settle the question definitely. Toward the close of the session of 1908 the Storthing had passed a bill repealing article thirty-three of the constitution, and by an oversight the bill had not been placed before the king for his signature before the Storthing adjourned. In this case the question of the king's veto would necessarily have to be raised in conformity with article eighty of the constitution, which reads: "The Storthing remains in session so long as it deems it necessary. When it is adjourned by the king, after its deliberations are closed, he also passes on the bills not already acted on, by either vetoing or signing them. All measures which he does not formally sanction are to be regarded as vetoed." The question would then arise, if the constitutional amendment which had not been signed should be regarded as vetoed. That the king has no veto power in such cases was generally held, but nowhere expressly stated. The king, therefore, made a solemn declaration, consonant with an opinion submitted by the minister of justice, that in cases of constitutional amendments he has no veto.[1] But it was still possible that the veto question might be revived. If the king according to the constitution had the right to veto constitutional amendments, he could not relinquish it even by a solemn declaration. In order to avoid further misunderstandings, article 112 of the constitution was so changed by an act of June 11, 1913, as to deprive the king of the power of veto in cases of constitutional amendments.

The development of democratic social conditions has been no less essential to the progress of the Norwegian people during the last century than the establishing of political freedom and national independence. Without local self-government and the right of all to share the rights and privileges as well as the duties and responsibilities the work of the Eidsvold men would have lost its real signifi-

[1] *Stiftsamtmand Blehrs Foredrag i Bergen 4de September 1910 om Grundlovsvetoet.*

cance, and the nation would have been shorn of much of its strength. This has been clearly understood, and efforts have been made to extend equal privileges and opportunities to all, in order that the interest and energy of the whole people may be united in the work for social progress. The suffrage has been constantly extended, until all persons of age, both men and women, now have the right to vote. By the law of May 29, 1901, women received the right of suffrage in local elections, if they had an income of 300 kroner in the country, or 400 kroner in the cities, or, in case of married women, if their husbands had that income. In 1907 they received limited suffrage in general elections. In 1911 the first woman representative, Anna Rogstad, took her seat in the Storthing, and in 1912 women were made eligible to all offices, except those of cabinet members, or of the ecclesiastical or military service. In 1898 suffrage had been granted to all men twenty-five years of age who had resided in the country five years, and in 1913 the same right of general suffrage was also extended to women. Article fifty of the constitution was amended to read: *"All Norwegian citizens, men and women, who are twenty-five years of age, who have lived in the kingdom for five years, and still reside there, shall have the right to vote."*

The economic development has kept pace with the political and social progress. The increase in the national wealth and the productive power of labor has been very rapid, especially during the last fifty years, owing to modern inventions and the use of scientific methods in production. The first few miles of Norwegian railway were constructed in 1854. At present the total length of railways in the country amounts to about 2000 miles, and excellent systems of government-owned telegraphs and telephones have been constructed. The water power wholly or partly developed amounts to 1.17 million horse power, and industries are being rapidly developed. The growth in dairying and agriculture may be seen from the following figures:

Value of grain crop in	1865, 34.4 million kroner;	in 1907, 38.2 million
Value of potato crop in	1865, 19.1 million kroner;	in 1907, 30.7 million
Value of dairying products in	1865, 52.8 million kroner;	in 1907, 101.5 million
Value of meat products in	1865, 12.7 million kroner;	in 1907, 20.9 million

The amount of milk per cow has been increased in seventy years from 500 liters to 1386 liters. The improvements in economic conditions, which has increased the general comfort, shows also as a direct result an increase in population from 1,702,000 in 1865 to 2,415,452 in 1912.

The Norwegian people have become the custodians of their own destiny to the fullest possible extent, and the rapid progress made during the last decades proves how freedom and democratic social conditions contribute to a people's general well-being. The spirit of vigor and enterprise which has enabled the Norwegians to maintain their national independence, and to enter with success upon a new industrial development, has carried them, also, into the fields of exploration, where they have shown no less daring and originality than did their ancestors, the Viking sea-kings of old. In 1887–1889 Fridtjof Nansen with a few companions succeeded in crossing the glacier-covered Greenland on ski. This feat of endurance and daring was followed by his arctic expedition, 1893–1896, on which he undertook to explore the region of the north pole. By letting his ship "Fram" become embedded in the ice fields north of Siberia, he hoped that the ocean current which traverses that region would ultimately carry him across the pole itself. In this he did not succeed, but he reached a higher latitude than any explorer had done before, and his expedition is one of the most valuable and interesting of the kind ever made.

In 1898–1902 Otto N. Sverdrup, who had accompanied Nansen as captain of the "Fram," led a second Norwegian expedition to the arctic regions. The northwest coast of Greenland was explored, and several new islands were discovered. Almost simultaneously Carsten Borchgrevink made an expedition to the antarctic region, sailing from England in 1898 with the ship "Southern Cross." He spent the winter on the antarctic continent, located the south magnetic pole, and reached, in 1900, a latitude of 78° 50′.

Roald E. G. Amundsen had served as first mate on the "Belgica," 1897–1899, on an expedition undertaken for the purpose of locating the south magnetic pole. On his return he purchased a small ship, "Gjøa," and decided to fit out an expedition to locate the north magnetic pole. The expedition started in 1903, and a summer and two winters were spent in determining the location of the magnetic pole, and in studying the magnetic conditions of the earth in those regions. In 1905 the voyage westward was continued in the hope of finding the much-sought northwest passage. Through the vast ice fields the little ship proceeded, and after passing the Simpson and Dolphin straits it finally entered the open sea, August 21, 1905. The northwest passage had at length been found. Upon his return the doughty explorer began preparations for an expedition to the south pole. In 1911 he established his winter quarters on the Great Barrier, and by a series of marches he reached the south pole, December 16, 1911.[1]

These fearless explorers had found new paths to enterprise and honor, and they followed them in the old Norse spirit, which regarded honor and achievement as the only imperishable earthly possession.

Cattle perish,
kindred die,
thou wilt die also,
but one thing I know
which will never die,
the honor which thou hast won.
(Hávamál.)

69. Norwegian Emigration to America. The Norwegians in the United States

The demand that the world should be populated and developed has come to the nations of Europe like the duty and destiny of parenthood. So much vital force has been contributed to the development of the new nations in both hemispheres that the peoples of the Old World have felt it as a distinct loss, sometimes even as a calamity. Youth and vigor have been given to the growing states in North and South America, in Australia and Africa, till the cheeks of the older social organisms have turned pale. But he who looks beyond

[1] Fridtjof Nansen, *The Norwegian Polar Expedition, 1893–1896*, London and Christiania, 1900; *Fram over Polarhavet*, Christiania, 1897. C. Borchgrevink, *Nærmest Polen*, 1900. *First on the Antarctic Continent, 1900.* Roald Amundsen, *Northwest Passagen*, 1907; *Sydpolen*, 1912.

the pangs of the hour, and measures development by the progress of humanity, will recognize that even for those who have given most a new era of development has come. Paths have been blazed to a fuller degree of self-realization, and the strength sacrificed returns to the rising generations with new life and fuller joys.

In Norway emigration has been so heavy for almost a century that it has been viewed with grave apprehension as a serious menace to the growth and well-being of the nation. To a small country, numbering less than two and a half million inhabitants, the yearly loss of so many thousands of the best citizens must be a source of deep regret. Ability and energy are continually lost by the constant drain; friends are parted, old firesides deserted, and a feeling of sadness is created which obscures the vision, and makes the people view the phenomenon of emigration even with needless alarm.

Many circumstances have contributed to increase emigration from Norway during the past century. The encouragement given by friends and relatives already in this country, the advertising done by railways and steamship companies, the easy communications between Europe and America, and love of travel and adventure have undoubtedly stimulated the longing of the young people to see the New World beyond the seas; but economic conditions have been at all times the chief cause. Since the industries were little developed, the chief pursuits were lumbering, fishing, farming, and dairying. But the tillable area is limited, and before scientific methods came to the aid both of fisherman and husbandman, labor even in these pursuits yielded small returns. The problem of finding profitable employment, of securing a degree of economic independence and well-being was for many attended with serious difficulty, and the population usually kept in advance of economic progress. Modern science and industrial progress are rapidly changing the whole economic character of the country, and Norway will, undoubtedly, be able to support many times the present number of inhabitants. But emigration until quite recently must be regarded as an overflow of population, an attempt of the surplus to find opportunity to build new homes under more favorable conditions. Since this is its real character, it follows that it is self-regulating, and that it will vary with changing economic conditions both at home and abroad. In the April number of "Normandsforbundet" for 1913 Mr. Gottenborg shows how the emigration to America until quite recently constantly increased, and how its rise and fall have depended on economic conditions at home. "While the number of emigrants in the period 1836–1842 only reached a few hundred," he writes, "it rose in 1843 to 1600, and has since not fallen below 1000 a year. In 1847 the potato crop in Norway was poor, times were hard, grain prices high, and economic conditions generally unfavorable. For this reason emigration rose to 4000 or 5000, and this number remained quite constant with few exceptions from 1851 to 1865, though the economic conditions improved. . . . In 1866 emigration increased suddenly to 15,455 from 4000 the year previous, owing chiefly to the closing of the Civil War, which had hindered emigration. In the following years the number was gradually reduced from 10,357 in 1873 to about 4000 in 1874–1878, because of improved economic conditions, extensive railway construction, and other large enterprises. But in the eighties another period of hard times came. Railway construction ceased, and the emigration reached a volume greater than ever before. In 1882 the number rose to 28,804, and during that whole decade it exceeded 20,000 per year, except in 1884–1886 and 1889, when the number was 13,000 to 15,000 a year. The same conditions existed in the beginning of the nineties. In 1893 about 19,000 emigrated, but in 1894 the number was reduced to 5642 because of good times. . . . In 1899, when the times again became hard, the number rose again. In 1900 it reached 11,000, in 1901 13,000; it soon increased to 20,000, and in 1903 it reached about 27,000. It remained above 20,000 till 1907, but it dropped in 1908 to 8500 because of hard times in America. In 1909 it rose again to 16,000, and in 1910 to almost 19,000, but dropped again in 1911 to about 12,000, and in 1912 to 9105." Mr. Gottenborg finds that in the period 1850–1911 707,986 persons emigrated from Norway.[1]

[1] The real emigration to America did not begin till in 1821. "From the year 1820 the United States government supplies us with immigration statistics; but unfortunately for our present purpose, Sweden and Norway are grouped together in these down to the year 1868, and hence it is impossible to determine how many came from each country. From the year 1836 we are helped out by Norway, where the government in that year began

As soon as economic conditions can be established which will enable all the people to live at home in reasonable comfort, few will be tempted to go as emigrants to foreign lands, and emigration will soon cease. Dr. Isaac A. Hourwich has shown that the new economic development in Germany, Sweden, and Denmark has greatly reduced emigration from these countries. In Germany and Denmark emigration has ceased altogether and immigration has begun instead. "The progress of agriculture," says this author, "has turned Denmark into a country of immigration. Considerable numbers of Polish peasants come during every agricultural season to work on the farms in Denmark; in 1907 their number was 6251." [1] The same will undoubtedly happen in Norway, if the present industrial and economic development continues uninterrupted. "The recent industrial progress of Norway can be gauged," says Hourwich, "by the fact that from 1897 to 1908 the quantity of horse power used increased 146.5 per cent. The average number of wage earners, reduced to the basis of 300 working days per year, increased during the same period forty-five per cent, while the population increased during the same period only nine per cent." [2] The various industries now support over one-third of the population.[3] The growing demand for labor, the increase of wages, the greater security given the wage earners through accident and sickness insurance and non-employment funds, and the rapid improvement of economic conditions in general have already caused a noticeable decrease in emigration. Before many years have passed, it may have ceased to work annoyance, and to sap the strength of the nation.

The emigration from Norway to America may be said to have begun in 1821, when Cleng Peerson, of Tysvær parish, north of Stavanger, and Knud Olsen Eide, from the island of Fogn, were sent by some Quaker friends of the district to investigate conditions in the New World. After three years they returned, and their reports were so favorable that several families, led by Lars Larsen Jeilane,

to collect and preserve statistics of emigration." R. B. Anderson, *First Chapter of Norwegian Immigration*, p. 38.

[1] Isaac A. Hourwich, *Immigration and Labor*, p. 108, 204.

[2] *Statistique Industrielle pour l'annêe 1908, éditée par l'office des Assurances de l'Etat*, p. 18*, 230*, Christiania, 1911.

[3] Thorne Holst, *Industri og industrielle Problemer*, Christiania, 1914.

resolved to emigrate. A small sloop, "Restaurationen," was purchased, Captain Lars Olsen and Mate Erikson were hired, and the little vessel, carrying fifty-two persons, set sail from Stavanger, July 4, 1825. After a perilous and adventurous voyage they reached New York October 9th of that year, fifty-three in number, as Mrs. Lars Larsen Jeilane had given birth to a daughter.[1] In November they reached their final destination, Kendall, then called Murray, in Orleans County, New York, where the first Norwegian settlement was founded. Here they bought land from Joseph Fellows at the price of five dollars per acre, and agreed to pay for it in ten yearly installments. The summer was already spent, but they succeeded in building a log cabin, and by threshing with the flail the grain of their neighbors, a work for which they received every eleventh bushel of wheat, they secured the necessary supply of food for the winter. In the spring they cleared and seeded a couple of acres, and the next fall they could harvest their first crop. The difficulties and discouragements encountered were many, but the colonists soon learned to love their humble homes in the new country. It appears, however, that they failed to secure proper title to their land.[2] Joseph Fellows, who was a Quaker, seems to have been very generous and kind, but they were probably unable to pay the purchasing price, and most of them sought new homes in the western states, especially in La Salle County, Illinois, where the second Norwegian settlement was founded at Fox River in 1834.

Not a few persons emigrated from Norway during the decade 1825–1835, but they came as individual immigrants, and no new Norwegian settlement was founded. In 1835 Knud Slogvig, who had come to America in the sloop "Restaurationen," returned to

[1] R. B. Anderson, *The First Chapter of Norwegian Immigration.* George T. Flom, *A History of Norwegian Immigration to the United States.* Hjalmar Rued Holand, *De norske Setlementers Historie.* O. N. Nelson, *History of the Scandinavians and Successful Scandinavians in the United States.* Knud Langeland, *Normændene i Amerika. Symra,* Decorah, Iowa. Martin Ulvestad, *Normændene i Amerika, deres Historie og Rekord.* Johs. B. Wist, *Den norske Indvandring til 1850 og Skandinaverne i Amerikas Politik.*

An extensive bibliography of works dealing with Scandinavian immigration and pioneer history is found in O. N. Nelson's work *History of the Scandinavians and Successful Scandinavians in the United States*, p. 265 ff.

[2] *Ibid.*, p. 134 m ff.

Norway, and many people from the districts between Bergen and Stavanger flocked to hear his accounts of the New World. The desire to visit America spread rapidly, and in 1836 two brigs, "Norden" and "Den norske Klippe," sailed from Stavanger with about two hundred emigrants, led by Knud Slogvig. On arriving in America most of them were persuaded by the intrepid Cleng Peerson to go to Fox River, La Salle County, Illinois, where he had already founded a new settlement in the great western wilderness. Fox River soon became a thriving community, but the attempt to found a third settlement was less successful.

In 1837 two ships, "Ægir" from Bergen and "Enigheden" from Stavanger, sailed to America with about 170 emigrants. They intended to go to the Fox River settlement, but on arriving in Chicago they were told that La Salle County was very unhealthy, and a number, led by Ole Rynning, were persuaded to go to Beaver Creek in Iroquois County. In this marshy wilderness they built their homes, but the fall rains soon turned it into a swamp, and in the spring the whole region was inundated. The privations and utter hopelessness of the situation might well fill the most courageous hearts with despair. Many fell victims to malaria and dysentery, among others Rynning himself. The colony was abandoned, and those who were able made their way to the settlement at Fox River.

In 1839 about forty emigrants formed a new settlement at Muskego, Wisconsin, the first Norwegian settlement in that state. Already in 1845 plans were laid for the publication of a Norwegian newspaper, and two years later "Nordlyset," published by Even Hegg and James D. Reymert, began to appear in the town of Norway, Racine County, in this settlement.[1] In 1844 the first Norwegian Lutheran church was built by Rev. C. L. Clausen. In 1839 the first Norwegian settlers also appeared at Rock Prairie and Jefferson Prairie, and in 1840 the great Norwegian settlement at Koshkonong, Dane County, Wisconsin, was founded.

These early settlers had shown the way where thousands were soon to follow. In 1843 the number of Norwegian immigrants rose, as already stated, to 1600, and during the next decades they

[1] Johs. B. Wist, *Norsk-Amerikanernes Festskrift*, 1914.

came in ever increasing numbers to take possession of the fertile unsettled plains of the great West. According to "The Thirteenth Census of the United States" the Norwegians in this country numbered, in 1910, 979,099. Of these, 403,877 were born in Norway; the other 575,222 were born of immigrated Norwegian parents. But if the Norwegian element in its entirety should be counted, we would still have to add the whole second generation born in this country, which is even more numerous than the first, and it would not be unfair to count also a considerable part of the third generation. According to the most conservative estimate, then, the number of Norwegians in the United States in 1914 is not less than 1,600,000. The greater number have settled in the northwestern states and in Washington, Oregon, California, New York, Massachusetts, and New Jersey, where according to the census they are distributed as follows:

	Born in Norway	Born of Immigrated Norwegian Parents	Total
Minnesota	105,303	174,304	279,607
Wisconsin	57,000	100,701	157,701
North Dakota . .	45,937	77,347	123,284
Illinois	32,913	35,525	68,438
Washington . . .	28,368	24,361	52,729
New York	25,013	12,392	34,405
Iowa	21,924	44,978	66,902
South Dakota . .	20,918	39,828	60,746
California	9,952	7,194	17,146
Michigan	7,638	9,136	16,774
Montana	7,170	6,773	13,943
Oregon	6,843	6,592	13,435
Massachusetts . .	5,432	2,938	8,370
New Jersey . . .	5,351	3,001	8,352

"The Thirteenth Census of the United States" shows that 68.7 per cent of the Norwegians live in the states of Minnesota, Iowa, North Dakota, South Dakota, Missouri, Nebraska, and Kansas, and "they show a greater tendency toward concentration than any other nationality," says the census. Very few live in Missouri. If we substitute Wisconsin instead, the percentage will be even much higher.[1]

[1] *Thirteenth Census of the United States*, vol. V., p. 179.

According to report of W. J. Harris, director of the United States Bureau of the Census, the foreign element constitutes about one-third of the entire population of the United States, or 32,243,382, counted according to the mother tongue. But this number is too low for reasons already stated. Of this large foreign element 87.5 per cent speak one of the eight leading foreign languages in the following proportion:

English	10,037,420,	or	31.1 per cent
German	8,817,420,	or	27.3 per cent
Italian	2,151,422,	or	6.7 per cent
Polish	1,707,640,	or	5.3 per cent
Yiddish / Hebrew }	1,676,762,	or	5.2 per cent
Swedish	1,445,869,	or	4.5 per cent
French	1,357,169,	or	4.2 per cent
Norwegian	1,039,975,	or	3.1 per cent
Other languages	4,039,975,	or	12.5 per cent

The Norwegian tongue, then, is one of the eight languages which is spoken most in the United States.[1] But as an ethnic element in the American people the Norwegians are of far greater relative importance than even these figures would indicate. In Norway popular education has reached the highest stage of efficiency, and illiteracy is wholly confined to the mentally imbecile. The reports of the United States Commissioner of Immigration also show that the Scandinavians are the best educated immigrants which land on our shores, and as they are accustomed at home to popular government and democratic social conditions, they are better qualified than almost any other immigrants to enter into the full spirit of American institutions. In the development of the states of the Northwest they have been a most potent factor both economically and intellectually. Statistics show that as tillers of the soil they rank higher than other nationalities, and that they choose farming as their vocation to a far greater degree than any other people. In 1900 49.8 per cent of all Norwegians in America were farmers, 42.3 per cent of all Danes, and 30.2 per cent of all Swedes. If we add also the laborers in the rural districts, who are usually farm hands, the

[1] *Symra*, May, 1914, Knut Gjerset, *Litt om Nordmændene i Amerika i 1814*.

percentage will be: of Norwegians 59.3 per cent, of the Danes 52.3 per cent, and of the Swedes 43 per cent.[1] "The Thirteenth Census of the United States" for 1910 shows that of the foreign-born white population a much larger percentage own their farms than of the native white population, the ratio being 81.4 per cent to 66.3 per cent.[2] But the available statistics indicate that of the Scandinavians a larger percentage own their farms than of most other nationalities. They own more than their share of the soil, and have reached a higher degree of prosperity than almost any other nationality in the rural districts. According to the census of 1910 10,886 of the farmers of the state of North Dakota are born in Norway.[3] Of these, 9562 own their farms, while 1341 are renters. If the farms were not so large, the number of renters would be still smaller, but in that state the average acreage of farms is 382.3 acres, with an average value of $13,109. In Minnesota the average acreage is 177 acres and the average value not less than $12,000. "The counties where the Norwegian population is largely located will be found in southern, western, and northwestern Minnesota, the richest agricultural counties of the state. There is, perhaps, no more prosperous agricultural region in the United States," writes Auditor of State Samuel G. Iverson. "Those who have given the matter some thought," he continues, "agree with me that about one-third of the farms of Minnesota are owned by those who were born in Norway, or their descendants, and that these number now in the aggregate from 450,000 to 500,000; one-third of the 165,000 farms of the state would be 55,000, which at an average of $12,000 would be $660,000,000."

The intelligence and diligence which have enabled the Norwegians to become so successful in economic pursuits have characterized their efforts also in other fields. Especially noticeable are these traits in political life, where they have shown an ability which has made them an influential factor especially in the Northwest. At first they had many difficulties to contend with as a foreign ele-

[1] *Reports of the Immigration Commission*, vol. XXVIII., table I. A, p. 216 ff., quoted by Hourwich, *Immigration and Labor*, p. 198.

[2] *Bulletin of Agriculture*, 1910, table 13.

[3] *Thirteenth Census of the United States*, vol. V., p. 180.

ment. But as they are trained from home to exercise the duties of popular government, they were soon able to take an active part in all civic duties. Many have become true leaders in their communities, and the number of those who have been elected to the highest offices is relatively very large. Five have been governors, four lieutenant governors, twelve congressmen, three United States senators, besides one of the senators from Utah whose mother is Norwegian. Eight have been secretaries of state, seven state treasurers, four state auditors, one state attorney-general, one state superintendent of public instruction, and two judges of state supreme courts. Many have also been employed in the federal service. Ten have been revenue collectors, ten consuls, and three United States ministers to foreign countries. Thousands of others have held positions of trust and honor in community and state. The fact that the Norwegians in America even in the first generation have been able to achieve such success is not an accident, but is due to the intellectual culture which they have received as a heritage from their fatherland. Closer investigation reveals the fact that their life in this country is more closely connected with their history and development at home than a casual observer might be led to think.

The freedom of the Norwegian people is the result of a long development, and their struggle for liberty has been of the same conservative kind as that of the English nation. They did not win their freedom suddenly through a revolutionary uprising, but the struggle which lasted through centuries was waged for the sake of preserving the freedom which was theirs from time immemorial. Throughout the period of union with Denmark the conflicts were small and scattered, but so bitter that they fostered an intense spirit of liberty, and served to develop a marked willfulness in the popular character. In 1814 the national independence was quickly won, but during the union with Sweden, Norway, as the weaker state, had to exert the utmost vigilance to maintain the principles of sovereignty and equality granted in the constitution and the Act of Union. All premises and provisions had to be diligently scrutinized, and keen-eyed statesmanship had to preserve what the spirit of liberty had won. In these long struggles the Norwegian people have not only had an experience in popular self-government which has proved most valuable in their new environment in America, but they have developed in the trials of these struggles a self-assertive social temperament, an austere spirit of liberty, a rigid adherence to established principles, and a conservatism of thought which is clearly noticeable in their political life in the New World. They have for the most part joined the Republican party, which represented the principles of freedom and the rights of man in the great Civil War. They found in this party to a large extent their own ideals, they learned to love it, they felt proud of its lofty principles and great achievements, and they have clung to it with a fidelity which finds its explanation in their own long struggle for liberty. In politics the Norwegian could never be an opportunist. He takes the matter seriously, and demands clear issues and rigid principles which he can fully sanction. For this reason he has never been very successful in American city politics, where the bosses have held sway, where everything has been allowed, and where principles have often been regarded as political stupidity. In their loyal adherence to their chosen party the Norwegian people have been ably assisted by the Norwegian-American press, which with but few exceptions has always supported the Republicans, an attitude which it has not changed even when general defection has threatened. The Norwegian-American papers have always regarded new parties and untried political principles with skepticism, and have maintained that reforms and true progress could best be secured through the tried old party.[1]

The love of liberty and the conservative loyalty to principles which characterize the Norwegians are nowhere more clearly seen than in their church organizations, in which they have realized to the fullest extent their own ideas. The five Norwegian Lutheran church bodies in America now number over half a million members, and they are still growing rapidly. Their own official statistics show figures as on the following page:

[1] A history of the Norwegian-American press is found in *Norsk-Amerikanernes Festskrift, 1914.*

	Members	Congregations	Pastors	Value of Property
The United Church . . .	276,596	1570	589	$2,250,000
The Norwegian Synod . .	162,287	1048	410	1,843,000
The Hauge Synod . . .	60,000	364	169	650,000
The Lutheran Free Church	38,000	371	172	1,350,000
The Eielsen Synod . . .	1,500	26	6	12,900
	538,383	3379	1346	$6,105,900

There has been much controversy between these different groups regarding questions of doctrine and church practice, but with regard to the great issue of preserving the Lutheran faith as they have inherited it from their fathers, they have all been animated by the same spirit. On this point they have shown a conservatism which has its root in the national character, and which has given the Norwegian Lutheran Church in America its dignity and strength. This trait is the more remarkable, because it is associated with the most pronounced spirit of freedom in all matters touching the general management of church affairs. Instead of preserving the state-church features, to which they had been accustomed at home, they have established in this country a free church, based on the most democratic principles of popular government. The congregation is at the same time the organic unit and the highest authority, and manages its own affairs without outside official supervision. The affairs of the whole church are decided at yearly conventions of delegates sent by the congregations. All officials are elected for short terms, and their powers are so limited that they act as counselors and advisers rather than as supervisors.

True to their belief that knowledge is power, the Norwegians have always been earnest supporters of the state universities and public schools. But they have also built a number of private colleges and high schools where the courses are supplemented by such branches as will tend to create among the young people an interest in the history and culture of their own people, as it is believed that the inspiring traditions and tender memories of the fatherland can yet teach valuable lessons, if properly preserved and respected. Besides the regular high school and college curriculum, considerable attention is devoted in these schools to Norwegian history and literature, religion, and music, the subjects which represent in a special way the heritage which the Norwegian people have received from their fathers. Thirty such schools, with 300 instructors and 4400 students, are now in operation.

The centennial of Norway's independence was celebrated in 1914 with a centennial exposition and great festivities in Christiania, and a great number of Norwegian-Americans returned to the old fatherland for the occasion. On the Seventeenth of May a procession of 30,000 children with Norwegian flags, and a large number of Norwegian-Americans with American flags, marched through the streets of the capital. At Eidsvold the Storthing assembled in regular session in the old hall where the constitution was framed in 1814, and on May 20th a festive religious service was celebrated in the cathedral at Trondhjem. In June a musical festival was held in Christiania by thousands of singers assembled from all parts. A choir of 250 trained Norwegian singers from America, led by Julius Jæger, Emil Bjørn, and the composer Alfred Paulson of Chicago, assisted, as did also the Luther College Concert Band, which in answer to a special invitation made an extensive concert tour in Norway under the leadership of President C. K. Preus of Luther College, and the musical director, Carlo A. Sperati. The celebration closed with a festival on the Fourth of July, when the visiting Norwegian-Americans brought their formal greetings to their fatherland. For over a year a large committee, headed by State Senator L. O. Thorpe of Willmar, Minnesota, had been engaged in collecting a memorial fund, which on that day was presented to the Storthing by Professor H. G. Stub, D.D., of St. Paul, Minnesota, President of the Norwegian Synod. The Memorial Fund Committee was represented by Dr. T. Stabo of Decorah, Iowa, the United Church by its president, Rev. T. H. Dahl, D.D., and the State of North Dakota by its chief executive, Governor L. B. Hanna, who presented to the Norwegian government a statue of Abraham Lincoln. This piece of art, the work of the Norwegian-American sculptor Paul Fjelde, was a present from that American commonwealth, which is indebted to the sons and daughters of Norway for so much of its progress and prosperity. It was a token of the spirit which has knit strong the fraternal ties between the Viking race of the North and the land of freedom in the New World.

INDEX

Printed in the United States of America.